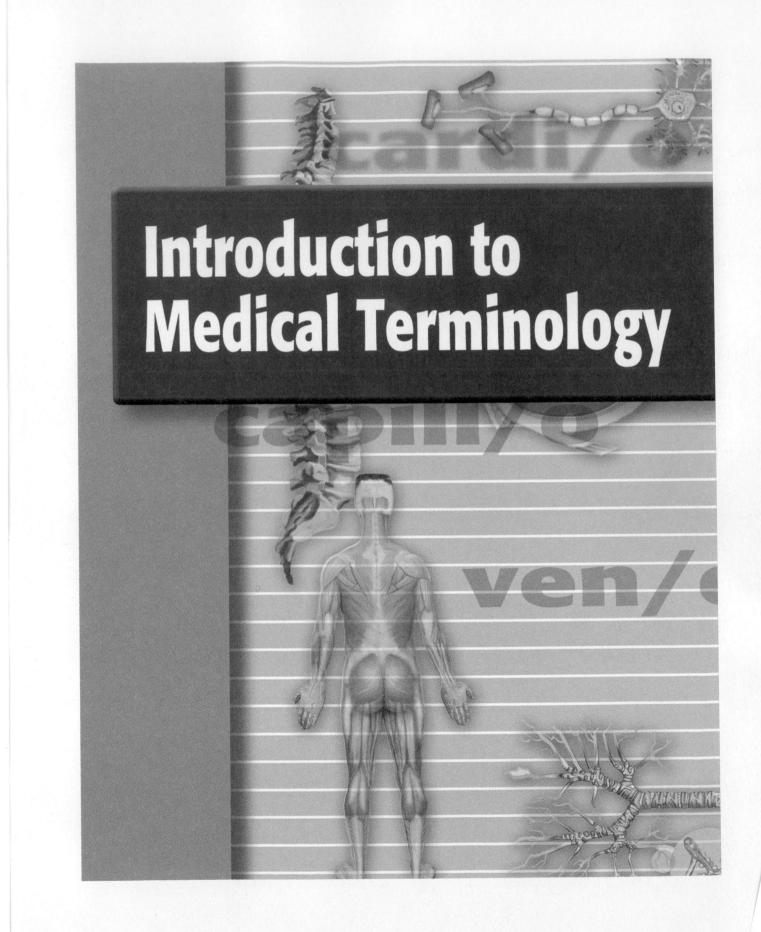

Introduction to Medical Terminology

Introduction to Medical Terminology

Ann Ehrlich
Carol L. Schroeder

THOMSON

DELMAR LEARNING

Australia Canada Mexico Singapore Spain United Kingdom United States

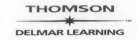

Introduction to Medical Terminology

by Ann Ehrlich and Carol L. Schroeder

Executive Director, Healthcare Business Unit:
William Brottmiller

Executive Editor:
Cathy L. Esperti

Acquisitions Editor:
Sherry Gomoll

Developmental Editor:
Deb Flis

Executive Marketing Manager:
Dawn F. Gerrain

Channel Manager:
Jennifer McAvey

Marketing Coordinator:
Mona Caron

Editorial Assistant:
Jennifer Conklin

Executive Production Manager:
Karen Leet

Art/Design Coordinator:
Robert Plante

Production Coordinator:
Catherine Ciardullo

Project Editor:
David Buddle

Library of Congress Cataloging-in-Publication Data
Introduction to medical technology / Ann Ehrlich, Carol L. Schroeder.
    p. ; cm.
Includes index.
  ISBN 1-4018-1137-X
1. Medicine—Terminology.
  [DNLM: 1. Medicine—Terminology—English. WB 15 R698I 2004] I. Schroeder, Carol L.
  R123 .R64 2004
  610' .1'4—dc21   2002073641

Contents

CHAPTER 14

The Reproductive Systems

CHAPTER 15

Diagnostic Procedures and Pharmacology

APPENDIX A

Prefixes, Word Roots (Combining Forms), and Suffixes

APPENDIX B

Abbreviations and Meanings

APPENDIX C

Glossary of Pathology and Procedures

Preface

TO THE STUDENT

This is an exciting time to be entering a healthcare profession! On every level, there are almost limitless opportunities to be part of a caring profession, helping people and fully expressing your own special talents and abilities. However, entering a healthcare field is somewhat like going to a foreign country. You cannot really understand what is happening until you learn the language.

Here's the good news: Learning medical terms is much easier than learning a whole new language. In fact, you already know quite a few of the words, such as *appendicitis* and *tonsillectomy*. Even new terms become a lot easier with the discovery that many of them are made up of interchangeable word parts, used over and over again in different combinations. Once you understand this principle, you will be well on your way to "translating" even the toughest medical terms—including terms you have never seen before. You will be amazed to see how quickly your vocabulary grows!

This textbook, the Student Activity CD-ROM, and the accompanying Student Workbook make the process of learning medical terminology as simple as possible. Review the introductory sections including How to Use This Book and How to Use the Student Activity CD-ROM so that you can find your way around easily. Once you get comfortable with the materials, you will find yourself learning faster than you ever imagined possible!

CHAPTER ORGANIZATION

INTRODUCTORY CHAPTERS

Start your studies with Chapters 1 and 2. These chapters provide the foundation that enables you to master the rest of the book. Chapter 1 introduces key word parts—the building blocks of most medical terms. Chapter 2 introduces more word parts and provides an overview of the basic terms used throughout the health field.

If you are using the Student Workbook, after reading these chapters you will want to complete the Word Part Review section that follows Chapter 2 in the workbook. These exercises will tell you whether you have mastered the concept of these all-important building blocks.

BODY SYSTEM CHAPTERS

Chapters 3 through 14 are organized according to body systems—one chapter per system. Each chapter begins with the structures and functions of that system so that you can relate them to the pathology and diagnostic and treatment procedures that follow. Chapter 15, Diagnostic Procedures and Pharmacology, introduces basic diagnostic procedures, imaging procedures and positioning, and pharmacology.

APPENDICES

Appendix A, Prefixes, Word Roots (Combining Forms), and Suffixes, is a handy reference for most medical word parts. When you do not recognize a word part, look it up here. Appendix B, Abbreviations and Meanings, is an extensive list of abbreviations and their commonly accepted meanings. Abbreviations are important in medicine, and using them *accurately* is even more important! Appendix C, Glossary of Pathology and Procedures, is a ready reference to quickly find any of the more than 1,500 pathology and procedure terms introduced in the text.

STUDENT ACTIVITY CD-ROM

This computer component is an exciting way to gain additional practice in working with medical terms. The exercises and games provided will help you remember even the most difficult terms. See How to Use the Student Activity CD-ROM for details.

EXTENSIVE TEACHING AND LEARNING PACKAGE

WORKBOOK TO ACCOMPANY INTRODUCTION TO MEDICAL TERMINOLOGY

Order No. 1-4018-1140-X

The Student Workbook contains many features to make learning medical terminology easier. There is a chapter in the workbook to accompany each textbook chapter. The workbook includes the following features:

- **Learning Exercises.** A wide variety of questions and challenges have been provided to help you master the concepts and terms that have been introduced in the chapter. Space has been included in this section for you to write your answers. Writing the correct medical terminology, instead of just selecting a letter in a multiple-choice question, will reinforce your learning.

- **Word Part Review Section.** This section, which is included after Chapter 2, helps you evaluate how well you are mastering the word parts.

- **Comprehensive Medical Terminology Review.** This section, which is included after Chapter 15, helps you prepare for the final examination. It includes study tips, practice exercises, and a simulated final test.

- **Flashcards.** The flashcards are printed on heavy stock and are located at the back of the workbook. Remove these pages from the workbook and separate them into the flash cards for a great study aid. Tips for using the flashcards also are included in the workbook.

INSTRUCTOR'S MANUAL TO ACCOMPANY INTRODUCTION TO MEDICAL TERMINOLOGY

Order No. 1-4018-1138-8

The Instructor's Manual features the very latest in classroom activities and tests:

- **Course Planning Tips.** This section contains suggestions and samples for developing a 16-week syllabus and course plan.

- **Tips for New Teachers.** Information and creative suggestions are included to help new teachers and their students excel in the classroom. Even experienced teachers will want to read this section to look for fresh, new ideas.

- **Chapter Resources.** Many resources and activities for each chapter are grouped together. When planning your classes, simply turn to that chapter's resource guide to see what is available.

- **Answer Keys for Exercises.** Every chapter in the text includes a set of five Review Time questions, and the Student Workbook features 100 exercises per chapter. The answer keys for both are provided in this manual.

- **Classroom Quizzes.** Each chapter in this manual provides you with two 25 question quizzes and the correct answers.

- **Review Session Activities.** These are special activities to help students review Chapters 1 through 8 for the mid-term and Chapters 9 through 15 for the final exam. The Student Activity CD-ROM includes a Comprehensive Medical Terminology Review section. The Student Workbook has a similar section that is located after Chapter 15. Answer keys for the Comprehensive Medical Terminology Review practice activities are included in the Instructor's Manual.

- **Mid-Term and Final Exams plus Answer Keys.** This manual includes a 100-question mid-term test and a 150-question final exam. These tests are designed for either machine or manual grading, and the answer keys are provided.

COMPUTERIZED TESTBANK TO ACCOMPANY INTRODUCTION TO MEDICAL TERMINOLOGY

Order No. 1-4018-1139-6

By offering 1,500 questions, 100 for each chapter, this CD-ROM testbank assists you in creating personalized chapter, mid-term, and final examinations.

Features include

- An interview mode or "wizard" to guide you through the steps to create a test in less than five minutes
- The capability to edit questions or to add an unlimited number of questions
- Online (Internet-based) testing capability
- Online (computer-based) testing capability
- A sophisticated word processor
- Numerous test layout and printing options
- Groups of questions linked to common narratives

DELMAR'S MEDICAL TERMINOLOGY FLASH!: COMPUTERIZED FLASHCARDS

Order No. 0-7668-4320-3

Learn and review over 1,500 medical terms using this unique electronic flashcard program. Flash! is a computerized flashcard-type question and answer association program designed to help users learn correct spellings, definitions, and pronunciations. Graphics and audio clips make it a fun and easy way for users to learn and test their knowledge of medical terminology.

DELMAR'S MEDICAL TERMINOLOGY IMAGE LIBRARY CD-ROM, 2ND EDITION

Order No. 1-4018-1009-8

This CD-ROM is an ideal resource to enhance your classroom presentation of medical terminology. This CD-ROM contains 600 graphic files that can be incorporated into a software program presentation, used directly from the CD-ROM or used to make color transparencies.

Acknowledgments

Thanks to Dorothy Winger, HOSA adviser and CNA instructor, who allowed us to visit her class and answered many questions. Special thanks also go to Don Jacobsen for his help in "pronouncing" the terms used in this text. Thanks also go to the editorial and production staff of Delmar Learning for their professional, yet personalized, assistance throughout the planning and production processes.

We are particularly grateful to the individuals who shared their life stories for the Career Profiles in this text and to the reviewers. Their insights, comments, suggestions, and attention to detail were very important in making certain that this book is "on target" for health career students.

Ann Ehrlich

Carol L. Schroeder

REVIEWERS

Janet Gower, RN
California Teacher of the Year 2002
Ygnacio Valley Health Careers Partnership Academy
Ygnacio Valley High School
Concord, California

Marie Moran, RN
Instructor
Institute of Business and Medical Centers, Inc.
Fort Collins, Colorado

Kathleen Park, MEd, MT (ASCP), EMSC
EMS/MLT Director
Alternative Certification of Educators (ACE) Teacher Educator
Lamar State College-Orange
Orange, Texas

Martha Young-Jones, RN, BSN, MA, MS
Assistant Principal Adult Counseling Services
Jordan-Locke Community Adult School
Los Angeles Unified School District
Division of Adult and Career Education
Los Angeles, California

How to Use This Book

Introduction to Medical Terminology helps you learn and remember medical terms with surprising ease. The key lies in the following features:

1 Body System Overview

The first page of each body system chapter is a chart giving an overview of the major structures, related word roots, and functions most important to that system.

2 Vocabulary List

The second page of each chapter is a 90-term vocabulary list. These are the key terms for that chapter. Next to each term is a box so you can check off each term as you have learned it. This list also is used with the Audio Activity on the Student Activity CD-ROM.

3 Learning Objectives

The beginning of each chapter lists learning objectives to help you understand what is expected of you as you read the text and complete the exercises.

4 Illustrations

Full-color illustrations, complete with detailed labeling, help clarify the text and contain important information of their own. Review each illustration carefully for easy and effective learning.

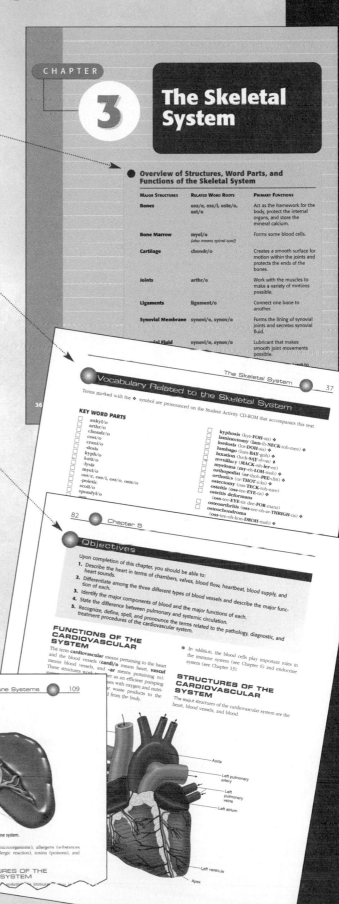

CHAPTER

3

The Skeletal System

Overview of Structures, Word Parts, and Functions of the Skeletal System

MAJOR STRUCTURES	RELATED WORD ROOTS	PRIMARY FUNCTIONS
Bones	oss/e, oss/i, oste/o, ost/o	Act as the framework for the body, protect the internal organs, and store the mineral calcium.
Bone Marrow	myel/o (also means spinal cord)	Forms some blood cells.
Cartilage	chondr/o	Creates a smooth surface for motion within the joints and protects the ends of the bones.
Joints	arthr/o	Work with the muscles to make a variety of motions possible.
Ligaments	ligament/o	Connect one bone to another.
Synovial Membrane	synovi/o, synov/o	Forms the lining of synovial joints and secretes synovial fluid.
Synovial Fluid	synovi/o, synov/o	Lubricant that makes smooth joint movements possible.

The Skeletal System   37

Vocabulary Related to the Skeletal System

Terms marked with the ❖ symbol are pronounced on the Student Activity CD-ROM that accompanies this text.

KEY WORD PARTS

- ankyl/o
- arthr/o
- chondr/o
- cost/o
- crani/o
- -desis
- kyph/o
- kratt/o
- -lysis
- myel/o
- oss/e, oss/i, ost/o, oste/o
- -poietic
- scoli/o
- spondyl/o

- kyphosis (kye-**FOH**-sis) ❖
- laminectomy (lam-ih-**NECK**-toh-mee)
- lordosis (lor-**DOH**-sis) ❖
- lumbago (lum-**BAY**-goh) ❖
- luxation (luck-**SAY**-shun) ❖
- myalita (**MACK**-sih-ler-ee) ❖
- myeloma (**my**-eh-**LOH**-mah) ❖
- orthopedist (or-thoh-**PEE**-dist) ❖
- orthotics (or-**THOT**-icks) ❖
- osteitis (oss-tee-**EYE**-tis) ❖
- osteitis deformans (oss-tee-**EYE**-tis dee-**FOR**-manz) ❖
- osteoarthritis (oss-tee-oh-ar-**THRIGH**-tis) ❖
- osteochondroma (oss-tee-oh-kon-**DROH**-mah) ❖

82   Chapter 5

Objectives

Upon completion of this chapter, you should be able to:

1. Describe the heart in terms of chambers, valves, blood flow, heartbeat, blood supply, and heart sounds.
2. Differentiate among the three different types of blood vessels and describe the major function of each.
3. Identify the major components of blood and the major functions of each.
4. State the difference between pulmonary and systemic circulation.
5. Recognize, define, spell, and pronounce the terms related to the pathology, diagnostic, and treatment procedures of the cardiovascular system.

FUNCTIONS OF THE CARDIOVASCULAR SYSTEM

The term **cardiovascular** means pertaining to the heart and the blood vessels (**cardi/o** means heart, **vascul/o** means blood vessels, and **-ar** means pertaining to). These structures work together as an efficient pumping system that supplies the cells with oxygen and nutrients and carries away waste products to the organs that remove them from the body.

• In addition, the blood cells play important roles in the immune system (see Chapter 6) and endocrine system (see Chapter 13).

STRUCTURES OF THE CARDIOVASCULAR SYSTEM

The major structures of the cardiovascular system are the heart, blood vessels, and blood.

The Lymphatic and Immune Systems   109

Spleen
Splenic artery
Splenic vein
Liver
Small intestine
Stomach
Large intestine

FIGURE 6.5 The spleen performs many important functions related to the immune system.

• A **lymphangioma** (lim-**fan**-jee-**OH**-mah) is a benign abnormal collection of lymphatic vessels forming a mass (**lymphangi** means lymph vessel and **-oma** means tumor).

• **Lymphedema** (lim-feh-**DEE**-mah) is an abnormal accumulation of lymphatic fluid that causes swelling usually in the arms or legs (**lymph** means lymph and

ease-producing microorganisms), allergens (substances producing an allergic reaction), toxins (poisons), and malignant cells.

STRUCTURES OF THE IMMUNE SYSTEM

Unlike other body systems, the immune system

Aorta
Left pulmonary artery
Left pulmonary veins
Left atrium
Left ventricle
Apex

- A **lymphangioma** (lim-**fan**-jee-**OH**-mah) is a benign abnormal collection of lymphatic vessels forming a mass (**lymphangi** means lymph vessel and **-oma** means tumor).
- **Lymphedema** (lim-feh-**DEE**-mah) is an abnormal accumulation of lymphatic fluid that causes swelling usually in the arms or legs (**lymph** means lymph and **-edema** means swelling). Compare with lipedema in Chapter 12.
- **Primary lymphedema,** which is a hereditary disorder, may occur at any time in life. It can affect any of the limbs.
- **Secondary lymphedema** is caused by identifiable factors such as the surgical removal or radiation of the lymph nodes in the treatment of cancer. This affects the limb nearest the treatment.
- **Splenomegaly** (**splee**-noh-**MEG**-ah-lee) is an enlargement of the spleen (**splen/o** means spleen and **-megaly** means abnormal enlargement). Notice that the word root for spleen is spelled with only one *e*).
- **Splenorrhagia** (**splee**-noh-**RAY**-jee-ah) is bleeding from the spleen (**spleen/o** means spleen and **-rrhagia** means bleeding).

ease-producing microorg
producing an allergic re
malignant cells.

STRUCTURES
IMMUNE SYS

Unlike other body syste
contained within a sin
Instead, it depends on
body systems (Figure 6.6

Tonsils and adenoids

Lymphatic vessels

Bone marrow

The im
systems.

5 ## Sounds Like Pronunciation System

The sounds like pronunciation makes pronunciation easy by respelling the word with syllables that you can understand and say at a glance. Simply pronounce the term just as it appears in parentheses, accenting the syllables as follows:

- **Primary (strongest) accent:** capital letters and bold type
- **Secondary accent:** lowercase letters and bold type

6 ## Word Parts

Because word parts are such an important part of learning medical terminology, whenever a term made up of word parts is introduced, the definition is followed (in parentheses) by the word parts highlighted in color and defined.

7 ## Career Opportunities

As you learn medical terminology, you will want to give some thought as to what career you want to pursue after graduation. This section, near the end of each chapter, will give you some ideas to consider.

8 ## Health Occupation Profile

Read the real-life experiences of healthcare workers to find out how they selected their career, what they do, and how they like it. Their words may inspire your own career choice!

TREATMENT PROCEDURES RELATED TO PREGNANCY AND CHILDBIRTH

- An **Apgar score** is an evaluation of a newborn infant's physical status by assigning numerical values (0 to 2) to each of five criteria: (1) heart rate, (2) respiratory effort, (3) muscle tone, (4) response stimulation, and (5) skin color. The newborn is evaluated at one and five minutes after birth, and a total score of 8 to 10 indicates the best possible condition.
- A **cesarean delivery,** also known as a **cesarean section** (seh-**ZEHR**-ee-un **SECK**-shun) or **C-section,** is the delivery of the child through an incision in the maternal abdominal and uterine walls.
- The vaginal delivery of a subsequent child after a cesarean birth is referred to as a **VBAC** (vaginal birth after cesarean).
- An **episiotomy** (eh-**piz**-ee-**OT**-oh-mee) is a surgical incision of the perineum and vagina to facilitate delivery and prevent laceration of the tissues (**episi** means vulva and **-otomy** means a surgical incision). A **laceration** (**lass**-er-**AY**-shun) is a jagged tear of the tissue.
- An **episiorrhaphy** (eh-**piz**-ee-**OR**-ah-fee) is a sutured repair of an episiotomy (**episi/o** means vulva and **-rrhaphy** means to suture).

Career Opportunities

In addition to the medical specialties already discussed, some of the health occupations involving the treatment of the reproductive systems include

- **Midwife:** assists in labor and delivery. A certified nurse midwife (CNM) is an RN with specialized training in obstetrics and gynecology who provides primary care in normal pregnancies and deliveries.
- **Doula:** provides emotional, physical, and informational support to the mother before and during labor and delivery
- **Sonographer** or **ultrasound technologist:** conducts ultrasound tests to show the development and condition of the fetus
- **Registered nurse Mother/Baby Unit (RN-MBU):** an RN who specializes in maternity and newborn care
- **Childbirth educator:** teaches expectant parents about prenatal care, childbirth, and infant care
- **Mammographer:** a radiographer who specializes in performing mammograms
- **Genetics counselor:** works with members of a healthcare team to provide information and support to families regarding the risks of birth defects or genetic disorders

FUNCT

TREATMENT PROCEDURES RELATED TO PREGNANCY AND CHILDBIRTH

- An **Apgar score** is an evaluation of a newborn infant's physical status by assigning numerical values (0 to 2) to each of five criteria: (1) heart rate, (2) respiratory effort, (3) muscle tone, (4) response stimulation, and (5) skin color. The newborn is evaluated at one and five minutes after birth, and a total score of 8 to 10 indicates the best possible condition.
- A **cesarean delivery,** also known as a **cesarean section** (seh-**ZEHR**-ee-un **SECK**-shun) or **C-section,** is the delivery of the child through an incision in the maternal abdominal and uterine walls.
- The vaginal delivery of a subsequent child after a cesarean birth is referred to as a **VBAC** (vaginal birth after cesarean).
- An **episiotomy** (eh-**piz**-ee-**OT**-oh-mee) is a surgical incision of the perineum and vagina to facilitate delivery and prevent laceration of the tissues (**episi** means vulva and **-otomy** means a surgical incision). A **laceration** (**lass**-er-**AY**-shun) is a jagged tear of the tissue.
- An **episiorrhaphy** (eh-**piz**-ee-**OR**-ah-fee) is a sutured repair of an episiotomy (**episi/o** means vulva and **-rrhaphy** means to suture).

Career Opportunities

In addition to the medical specialties already discussed, some of the health occupations involving the treatment of the reproductive systems include

- **Midwife:** assists in labor and delivery. A certified nurse midwife (CNM) is an RN with specialized training in obstetrics and gynecology who provides primary care in normal pregnancies and deliveries.
- **Doula:** provides emotional, physical, and informational support to the mother before and during labor and delivery
- **Sonographer** or **ultrasound technologist:** conducts ultrasound tests to show the development and condition of the fetus
- **Registered nurse Mother/Baby Unit (RN-MBU):** an RN who specializes in maternity and newborn care
- **Childbirth educator:** teaches expectant parents about prenatal care, childbirth, and infant care
- **Mammographer:** a radiographer who specializes in performing mammograms
- **Genetics counselor:** works with members of a healthcare team to provide information and support to families regarding the risks of birth defects or genetic disorders

Health Occupation Profile: CERTIFIED NURSE MIDWIFE

Maureen Darcey is a certified nurse midwife. "I started out as a nurse in orthopedics at a small hospital. When I became the night supervisor, I was often needed in labor and even catch their times couldn't get to the hospital in time, so I would help women in labor and being present with them at such babies. I loved supporting these women through their labor and delivery. I decided to enroll in the SUNY Downstate Medical Center midwifery program and became a certified nurse midwife.

"Midwives are able to function independently and to offer complete well-woman healthcare throughout a woman's life—from a young girl's first menses through and postpartum. The primary focus is on obstetrical care: prenatal, labor and delivery, and beyond menopause. Midwives do not approach birth as a natural process and invite a woman to trust her own body. Midwives do not independently handle high-risk birth situations requiring medical intervention, but for a birth without complications, we help create a homelike environment where birth is honored as a special family event."

9 Study Break

Put down your pencil—there is no quiz on this one. The Study Break is a brief and amusing pause in your studies before you go on to review the important information in the chapter.

10 Review Exercises

At the end of each chapter, there is a review exercise section with five questions. Each requires a written response (on a separate piece of paper) and a discussion response. These review exercises give you opportunities to practice communicating with patients (using lay terms) and communicating with other healthcare professionals (using correct medical terminology). As you progress through the text, these exercises become increasingly challenging.

11 Optional Internet Exercises

Two Internet exercises are included at the end of each chapter. One requires you to go to a specific web site. The other requires you to search a particular topic relating to the chapter. These exercises give you practice using the Internet.

12 The Human Touch: Critical Thinking Exercise

Located at the end of each chapter is a "real-life" mini-story that involves patients and pathology to help you practice critical thinking skills and encourage you to view each patient as a person. These stories are a fun classroom activity for discussion of the hot issues in medical care today. There are no right or wrong answers, just questions to get you started using the new terms you have learned.

Chapter 14

STUDY BREAK

The period of *gestation* for the development of a human fetus in the uterus is usually around nine months (253–300 days). The fact that women are limited to about one pregnancy a year is an important factor in determining human population growth.

Imagine how many people there might be on the planet if the human gestation period were that of a

- Wolf (60–63 days)
- Rabbit (30–35 days)
- Mouse (19–30 days)

Another factor limiting human population is the relatively low number of children born to most mothers. Our population would truly explode if every mother matched the record set by Mrs. Feodor Vassilyev of Russia in the eighteenth century: 69 children, including 16 pairs of twins, 7 sets of triplets and 4 sets of quadruplets!

Review Time

Write the answers to the following questions on a separate piece of paper or in your notebook. In addition, be prepared to take part in the classroom discussion.

1. **Written assignment:** Describe why sexually transmitted diseases are sometimes referred to as venereal diseases.
   Discussion assignment: What are the most common STDs?

2. **Written assignment:** Using terms a physician would understand, describe the male and female sterilization procedures.
   Discussion assignment: How would you explain each of these procedures to a patient?

3. **Written assignment:** Describe the phase of the menstrual cycle during which the female is most likely to become pregnant.
   Discussion assignment: How would you explain this concept to a couple who want this information to help with birth control planning?

4. **Written assignment:** Using terms a patient would understand, describe the difference between preeclampsia and eclampsia.
   Discussion assignment: Why is prenatal care so important in detecting and controlling these conditions?

5. **Written assignment:** Report on your research about the person for whom Apgar scores were named. Include in your report his or her full name and dates.
   Discussion assignment: How are these scores used to evaluate the physical status of a newborn?

Optional Internet Activity

The goal of this activity is to help you learn more about medical terminology while improving your Internet skills. Select one of these two options and follow the instructions.

1. **Internet Search:** Search for information about PMS. Write a brief (one- or two-paragraph) report on something new you learned here and include the address of the web site where you found this information.

2. **Web Site:** To learn more about sexually transmitted diseases, go to this web address: http://www.4woman.gov/. Search on Frequently Asked Questions and find Sexually Transmitted Diseases. Write a brief (one- or two-paragraph) report on something new you learned here.

The Reproductive Systems   273

The Human Touch: Critical Thinking Exercise

The following story and questions are designed to stimulate critical thinking through class discussion or as a brief essay response. There are no right or wrong answers to these questions.

"But Sam, you promised!" Jamie Chu began.

"Please don't get so upset," her husband interrupted. "I know I agreed to a vasectomy, but Grandmother may have a point. I do not have a son. Our family name has to be considered. I just feel that we should think about this."

"But Sam, we already discussed it. You're scheduled for the procedure." It seemed to Jamie that they had already spent plenty of time considering the number of children they wanted and talking about various contraceptive methods. Jamie had problems taking the pill, and Sam didn't like using a condom. A tubal ligation could have been the answer, but Jamie had a fear of not waking up from the anesthesia. Besides, she had been the one to go through two pregnancies and childbirths. Sam had reluctantly agreed that it was his turn to take responsibility for family planning.

Their two daughters, two-year-old Nanya and her big sister Nadya, made the perfect size family, Jamie thought. She had grown up in a large family. A lot of her childhood was spent taking care of her brothers and sisters, and she rarely had her mother's undivided attention. She didn't want that for her children.

Sam's story was different. Before his parents immigrated to America they had had four daughters. His father was so proud when he was born, a son to carry on the family tradition.

It had taken quite a long time to convince Sam that a family of only daughters could be considered complete. And now Grandmother was questioning that decision.

Suggested Discussion Topics

Which partner is responsible for birth control and why?

XV

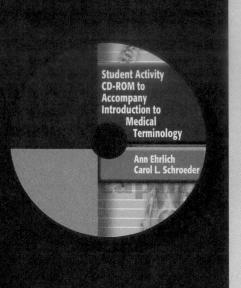

How to Use The Student Activity CD-ROM

The Student Activity CD-ROM was designed as an exciting enhancement to *Medical Terminology for Health Professions, 4th edition* to help you learn difficult medical terms. As you study each chapter in the text, be sure to explore the corresponding unit on the CD-ROM.

Each chapter is divided into two major sections: exercises and fun and games. Exercises can be used for additional practice, review, or self-testing. Fun and games provide an opportunity to play and practice through a variety of activities.

Getting started is easy. Follow the simple directions on the CD label to install the program on your computer. Then take advantage of the following features:

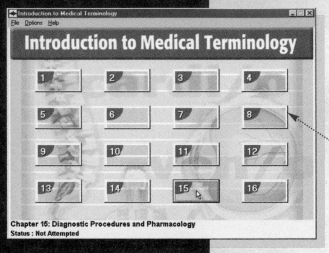

1 Main Menu

The main menu follows the chapter organization of the text exactly—which makes it easy for you to find your way around. Just click on the button for the chapter you want, and you'll come to the chapter opening screen.

Toolbar

The Back button at the top left of every screen allows you to retrace your steps, while the Exit button gets you out of the program quickly and easily. As you navigate through the software, check the toolbar for other features that help you use individual exercises or games.

Online Help

If you get stuck, just press F1 to get help. The online help includes instructions for all parts of the Student Activity CD-ROM.

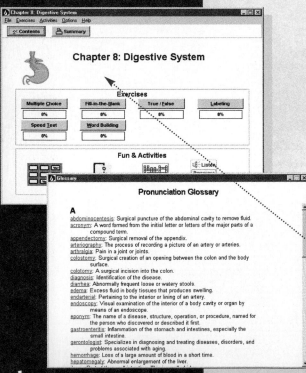

2 The Chapter Screen

Here you have the opportunity to choose how you want to learn. Select one of the exercises for additional practice, review, or self-testing. Or click on a game to practice the terms for that chapter in a fun format.

3 Exercises

The Student Activity CD-ROM acts as your own private tutor. For each exercise, it chooses from a bank of over 800 questions covering all 15 chapters and the Medical Term inology Review. Putting these exercises to work for you is simple:

- Choose a multiple choice, fill-in-the-blank, or labeling exercise, whichever one appeals to you.

- You'll encounter a series of 10 questions for each exercise format; each question gives you two chances to answer correctly.

- Instant feedback tells you whether you're right or wrong —and helps you learn more quickly by explaining why an answer was correct or incorrect.

- The Student Activity CD-ROM displays the percentage of correct answers on the chapter screen. An on-screen score sheet (which you can print) lets you track correct and incorrect answers.

- Review your previous questions and answers in an exercise for more in-depth understanding. Or start an exercise over with a new, random set of questions that gives you a realistic study environment.

- When you're ready for an additional challenge, try the timed Speed Test. Once you've finished, it displays your score and the time you took to complete the test, so you can see how much you've learned.

4 Fun & Games

To have fun while reinforcing your knowledge, enjoy each of the six simple games on this disk. You can play alone, with a partner, or on teams.

- Concentration: match terms to their corresponding definitions under the cards as the seconds tick by.

- Hangman: review your spelling and vocabulary by choosing the correct letters to spell medical terms before you're "hanged."

- Crossword Puzzles: using the definition clues provided, fill in the medical terms to complete each puzzle. A click of the Check button highlights incorrect answers in blue.

- Medical Terminology Championship Game: challenge your classmates and increase your knowledge by playing this Jeopardy style question-and-answer game.

- Listening Activity: Select medical terms and listen to them to master the pronunciation.

- Drag & Drop: Both word building and art labeling exercises are included to help you learn in an interactive environment.

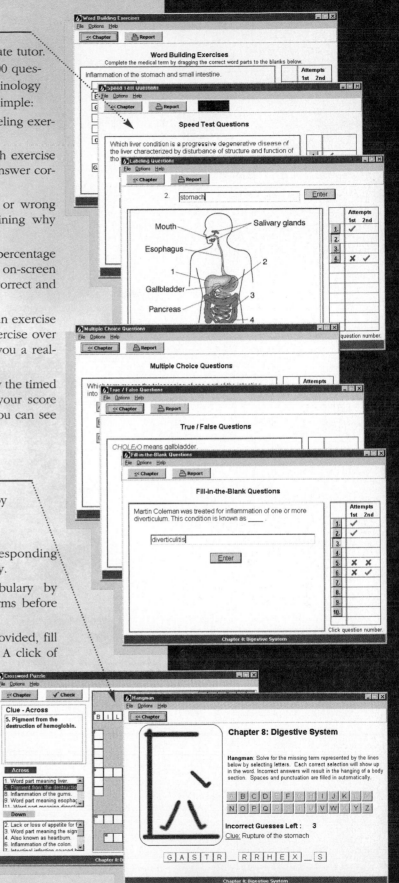

CHAPTER

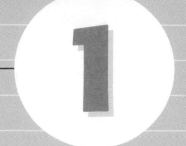

Introduction to Medical Terminology

● Overview of Introduction to Medical Terminology

Word Parts Are the Key!
Introduction to word parts and how they create complex medical terms.

Word Roots
The word parts that usually indicate the part of the body involved.

Suffixes
The word parts that usually indicate the procedure, condition, disorder, or disease.

Prefixes
The word parts that usually indicate location, time, number, or status.

Determining Meanings on the Basis of Word Parts
Use knowledge of word parts to decipher medical terms.

Medical Dictionary Use
Guidelines to make the use of a medical dictionary easier.

Pronunciation
Learn the easy-to-use Sounds-Like pronunciation system.

Spelling Is Always Important
Discover how one wrong letter can change the entire meaning of a term!

Using Abbreviations
Caution is important when using abbreviations.

Singular and Plural Endings
Unusual singular and plural endings used in medical terms.

Basic Medical Terms
Terms used to describe disease conditions.

Look-Alike Sound-Alike Terms and Word Parts
Clarify confusing terms that look or sound alike.

Vocabulary Related to Medical Terminology

Terms marked with the ❖ symbol are pronounced on the Student Activity CD-ROM that accompanies this text.

KEY WORD PARTS

- [ ] **-algia**
- [ ] **dys-**
- [ ] **-ectomy**
- [ ] **hyper-**
- [ ] **hypo-**
- [ ] **-itis**
- [ ] **-osis**
- [ ] **-ostomy**
- [ ] **-otomy**
- [ ] **-plasty**
- [ ] **-rrhage**
- [ ] **-rrhaphy**
- [ ] **-rrhea**
- [ ] **-rrhexis**
- [ ] **-sclerosis**

KEY MEDICAL TERMS

- [ ] **abdominocentesis** (ab-**dom**-ih-noh-sen-**TEE**-sis) ❖
- [ ] **acronym** (**ACK**-roh-nim) ❖
- [ ] **appendectomy** (**ap**-en-**DECK**-toh-mee) ❖
- [ ] **appendicitis** (ah-**pen**-dih-**SIGH**-tis)
- [ ] **arteriogram** (ar-**TEER**-ee-oh-gram)
- [ ] **arteriography** (**ar**-tee-ree-**OG**-rah-fee) ❖
- [ ] **arterionecrosis** (ar-**tee**-ree-oh-neh-**KROH**-sis)
- [ ] **arteriosclerosis** (ar-**tee**-ree-oh-skleh-**ROH**-sis)
- [ ] **arthralgia** (ar-**THRAL**-jee-ah) ❖
- [ ] **atheroma** (**ath**-er-**OH**-mah)
- [ ] **cardiac** (**KAR**-dee-ack)
- [ ] **colostomy** (koh-**LAHS**-toh-mee) ❖
- [ ] **colotomy** (koh-**LOT**-oh-mee) ❖
- [ ] **diagnosis** (**dye**-ag-**NOH**-sis) ❖
- [ ] **diarrhea** (**dye**-ah-**REE**-ah) ❖
- [ ] **edema** (eh-**DEE**-mah) ❖
- [ ] **endarterial** (**end**-ar-**TEE**-ree-al) ❖
- [ ] **endoscopy** (en-**DOS**-koh-pee) ❖
- [ ] **eponym** (**EP**-oh-nim) ❖
- [ ] **erythrocytes** (eh-**RITH**-roh-sights)
- [ ] **gastralgia** (gas-**TRAL**-jee-ah)
- [ ] **gastroenteritis** (**gas**-troh-en-ter-**EYE**-tis) ❖
- [ ] **gastrosis** (gas-**TROH**-sis)
- [ ] **gerontologist** (**jer**-on-**TOL**-oh-jist) ❖
- [ ] **hemorrhage** (**HEM**-or-idj) ❖
- [ ] **hepatomegaly** (**hep**-ah-toh-**MEG**-ah-lee) ❖
- [ ] **hypertension** (**high**-per-**TEN**-shun)
- [ ] **hypotension** (**high**-poh-**TEN**-shun)

- [ ] **ileum** (**ILL**-ee-um) ❖
- [ ] **ilium** (**ILL**-ee-um) ❖
- [ ] **infection** (in-**FECK**-shun) ❖
- [ ] **inflammation** (**in**-flah-**MAY**-shun) ❖
- [ ] **interstitial** (**in**-ter-**STISH**-al) ❖
- [ ] **intramuscular** (**in**-trah-**MUS**-kyou-lar) ❖
- [ ] **laceration** (**lass**-er-**AY**-shun) ❖
- [ ] **lesion** (**LEE**-zhun) ❖
- [ ] **leukocytes** (**LOO**-koh-sights)
- [ ] **ligation** (lye-**GAY**-shun) ❖
- [ ] **lithotomy** (lih-**THOT**-oh-mee) ❖
- [ ] **melanosis** (**mel**-ah-**NOH**-sis) ❖
- [ ] **mycosis** (my-**KOH**-sis) ❖
- [ ] **myelopathy** (my-eh-**LOP**-ah-thee) ❖
- [ ] **myopathy** (my-**OP**-ah-thee) ❖
- [ ] **myorrhaphy** (my-**OR**-ah-fee)
- [ ] **myorrhexis** (**my**-oh-**RECK**-sis)
- [ ] **neonatology** (**nee**-oh-nay-**TOL**-oh-jee) ❖
- [ ] **neuritis** (new-**RYE**-tis) ❖
- [ ] **neuroplasty** (**NEW**-roh-**plas**-tee) ❖
- [ ] **otolaryngology** (**oh**-toh-**lar**-in-**GOL**-oh-jee) ❖
- [ ] **otorhinolaryngology** (**oh**-toh-**rye**-noh-**lar**-in-**GOL**-oh-jee) ❖
- [ ] **palpation** (pal-**PAY**-shun) ❖
- [ ] **palpitation** (**pal**-pih-**TAY**-shun) ❖
- [ ] **perinatal** (**pehr**-ih-**NAY**-tal) ❖
- [ ] **poliomyelitis** (**poh**-lee-oh-**my**-eh-**LYE**-tis) ❖
- [ ] **postnatal** (pohst-**NAY**-tal) ❖
- [ ] **prenatal** (pre-**NAY**-tal) ❖
- [ ] **prognosis** (prog-**NOH**-sis) ❖
- [ ] **prostate** (**PROS**-tayt) ❖
- [ ] **prostrate** (**PROS**-trayt) ❖
- [ ] **pyelitis** (**pye**-eh-**LYE**-tis) ❖
- [ ] **pyoderma** (**pye**-oh-**DER**-mah) ❖
- [ ] **pyrosis** (pye-**ROH**-sis) ❖
- [ ] **subcostal** (sub-**KOS**-tal) ❖
- [ ] **supination** (**soo**-pih-**NAY**-shun) ❖
- [ ] **suppuration** (**sup**-you-**RAY**-shun) ❖
- [ ] **supracostal** (**sue**-prah-**KOS**-tal) ❖
- [ ] **suturing** (**SOO**-chur-ing) ❖
- [ ] **symptom** (**SIMP**-tum) ❖
- [ ] **syndrome** (**SIN**-drohm) ❖
- [ ] **tonsillectomy** (**ton**-sih-**LECK**-toh-mee) ❖
- [ ] **tonsillitis** (**ton**-sih-**LYE**-tis)
- [ ] **trauma** (**TRAW**-mah) ❖
- [ ] **triage** (tree-**AHZH**) ❖
- [ ] **viral** (**VYE**-ral) ❖
- [ ] **virile** (**VIR**-ill) ❖

Objectives

Upon completion of this chapter, you should be able to:

1. Identify the roles of the three types of word parts in forming medical terms.
2. Analyze unfamiliar medical terms using your knowledge of word parts.
3. Describe the steps in locating a term in a medical dictionary.
4. Define the commonly used prefixes, word roots, and suffixes introduced in this chapter.
5. Pronounce medical terms correctly using the Sounds-Like system.
6. Recognize the importance of always spelling medical terms correctly.
7. State why caution is important when using abbreviations.
8. Recognize, define, spell, and pronounce the medical terms in this chapter.

WORD PARTS ARE THE KEY!

Learning medical terminology is much easier once you understand how word parts work together to form medical terms. This book includes many aids to help you to continue reinforcing your word-building skills.

● The types of word parts and the rules for their use are explained in this chapter. Learn these rules and follow them!

● Each time a term is introduced, the definition is followed, in parentheses, by the word parts in **blue** with their meanings.

● In your Student Workbook, the Learning Exercises for each chapter include a Challenge Word Building section. These sections will help you develop your skills in working with word parts.

● In your workbook, after the Chapter 2 Learning Exercises, there is a Word Part Review section. This section provides additional word part practice and enables you to evaluate your progress toward mastering the meanings of these word parts.

THE THREE TYPES OF WORD PARTS

Three types of word parts may be used to create medical terms. Guidelines for their use are shown in Table 1.1.

● **Word roots** contain the basic meaning of the term. They usually, *but not always*, indicate the involved body part.

● **Suffixes** usually, *but not always*, indicate the procedure, condition, disorder, or disease. A suffix always comes at the end of a word.

● **Prefixes** usually, *but not always*, indicate location, time, number, or status. A prefix always comes at the beginning of a word.

WORD ROOTS

Word roots act as the foundation of most medical terms. They usually, *but not always*, describe the part of the body that is involved (Figure 1.1). Some of the word roots that indicate color are shown, with their combining vowels, in Table 1.2.

Table 1.1

WORD PART GUIDELINES

1. A word root cannot stand alone. A suffix must be added to complete the term.

2. The rules for the use of combining vowels apply when a suffix is added to a word root. These rules are explained in Table 1.3.

3. When a prefix is necessary, it is always placed at the beginning of the word.

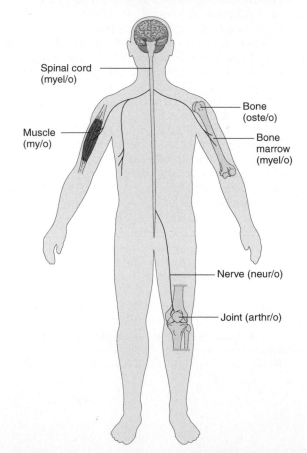

FIGURE 1.1 A word root usually indicates the involved body part.

COMBINING VOWELS

A combining vowel may be needed between the word root and suffix to make the medical term easier to pronounce. The rules for using combining vowels are explained in Table 1.3

- The letter **O** is the most commonly used combining vowel.
- When a word root is shown with a back slash and a combining vowel, such as **cardi/o**; this format is referred to as a **combining form** (**cardi/o** means heart).

Table 1.2

WORD ROOTS INDICATING COLOR	
cyan/o means blue	**Cyanosis** (**sigh**-ah-**NOH**-sis) is a blue discoloration of the skin caused by a lack of adequate oxygen (**cyan** means blue and **-osis** means condition).
erythr/o means red	**Erythrocytes** (eh-**RITH**-roh-sights) are mature red blood cells (**erythr/o** means red and **cytes** means cells).
leuk/o means white	**Leukocytes** (**LOO**-koh-sights) are white blood cells (**leuk/o** means white and **-cytes** means cells).
melan/o means black	**Melanosis** (**mel**-ah-**NOH**-sis) is any condition of unusual deposits of black pigment in different parts of the body (**melan** means black and **-osis** means condition).
poli/o means gray	**Poliomyelitis** (**poh**-lee-oh-**my**-eh-**LYE**-tis) is a viral infection of the gray matter of the spinal cord that may result in paralysis (**poli/o** means gray, **myel** means spinal cord, and **-itis** means inflammation).

Table 1.3

RULES FOR USING COMBINING VOWELS
1. A combining vowel *is used* when the suffix begins with a consonant.
For example, when **neur/o** (nerve) is joined with the suffix **-plasty** (surgical repair), the combining vowel O *is used* because **-plasty** begins with a consonant.
Neuroplasty (**NEW**-roh-**plas**-tee) is the surgical repair of a nerve (**neur/o** means nerve and **-plasty** means surgical repair).
2. A combining vowel *is not used* when the suffix begins with a vowel (a, e, i, o, u).
For example, when **neur/o** (nerve) is joined with the suffix **-itis** (inflammation), the combining vowel *is not used* because -**itis** begins with a vowel.
Neuritis (new-**RYE**-tis) is an inflammation of a nerve or nerves (**neur** means nerve and **-itis** means inflammation).
3. A combining vowel *is always used* when two or more root words are joined.
For example, when **gastr/o** (stomach) is joined with **enter/o** (small intestine), the combining vowel *is used* with **gastr/o**. However, when the suffix **-itis** (inflammation) is added, the combining vowel *is not used* with **enter/o** because **-itis** begins with a vowel.
Gastroenteritis (**gas**-troh-en-ter-**EYE**-tis) is an inflammation of the stomach and small intestine (**gastr/o** means stomach, **enter** means small intestine, and **-itis** means inflammation).
4. A prefix does not require a combining vowel. Do not place a combining vowel between a prefix and the word root.

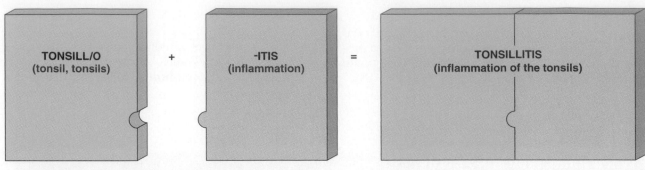

FIGURE 1.2 A word plus a suffix creates a new term.

COMMONLY USED WORD ROOTS

Because word roots describe body parts, most of them are specific to body systems.

- Many of these word roots are introduced in this chapter and in Chapter 2.
- Learning these word roots *now* will make your study of the other chapters much easier!

SUFFIXES

A suffix is added to the end of a word root to complete the term. Suffixes usually, but not always, indicate the procedure, condition, disorder, or disease (Figure 1.2):

- For example, **tonsill/o** means tonsils. A suffix is added to complete the term and to tell what is happening to the tonsils.
- **Tonsillitis** (**ton**-sih-**LYE**-tis) is an inflammation of the tonsils (**tonsill** means tonsils and **-itis** means inflammation).
- A **tonsillectomy** (**ton**-sih-**LECK**-toh-mee) is the surgical removal of the tonsils (**tonsill** means tonsils and **-ectomy** means surgical removal).

SUFFIXES MEANING "PERTAINING TO"

- Some suffixes complete the term by changing the word root into an **adjective** (a word that describes a noun). Many of these suffixes are defined as "pertaining to."
- For example, **cardiac** (**KAR**-dee-ack) is an adjective that means pertaining to the heart (**cardi** means heart and **-ac** means pertaining to).
- The "Pertaining to" table, at the beginning of Appendix A, makes such suffixes easy to find.

SUFFIXES AS NOUN ENDINGS

- Some suffixes complete the term by changing the word root into a **noun** (a word that is the name of a person, place, or thing).
- For example, the **cranium** (**KRAY**-nee-um) is the portion of the skull that encloses the brain (**crani** means skull and **-um** is a noun ending).

- Other suffixes in this group are defined as *noun endings*. These suffixes also are listed in a table at the beginning of Appendix A.

SUFFIXES MEANING ABNORMAL CONDITION

- Some suffixes have a general meaning of "abnormal condition or disease."
- For example, **-osis** means an abnormal condition or disease. **Gastrosis** (gas-**TROH**-sis) means any disease of the stomach (**gastr** means stomach and **-osis** means abnormal condition).
- These suffixes are also listed in a table at the beginning of Appendix A.

SUFFIXES RELATED TO PATHOLOGY

Pathology (pah-**THOL**-oh-jee) means the study of disease, and the suffixes related to pathology describe specific disease conditions:

- **-algia** means pain and suffering. **Gastralgia** (gas-**TRAL**-jee-ah) means pain in the stomach (**gastr** means stomach and **-algia** means pain).
- **-dynia** also means pain. **Gastrodynia** (gas-troh-**DIN**-ee-ah) also means pain in the stomach (**gastr/o** means stomach and **-dynia** means pain).
- **-itis** means inflammation. **Gastritis** (gas-**TRY**-tis) is an inflammation of the stomach (**gastr** means stomach and **-itis** means inflammation).
- **-malacia** means abnormal softening. **Arteriomalacia** (ar-**tee**-ree-oh-mah-**LAY**-shee-ah) is the abnormal softening of the walls of an artery or arteries (**arteri/o** means artery, and **-malacia** means abnormal softening). (Notice that **-malacia** is the opposite of **-sclerosis.**)
- **-megaly** means enlargement. **Hepatomegaly** (hep-ah-toh-**MEG**-ah-lee) is the abnormal enlargement of the liver (**hepat/o** means liver and **-megaly** means enlargement).
- **-necrosis** means tissue death. **Arterionecrosis** (ar-**tee**-ree-oh-neh-**KROH**-sis) means the tissue death of an artery or arteries (**arteri/o** means artery and **-necrosis** means tissue death).

- **-sclerosis** means abnormal hardening. **Arteriosclerosis** (ar-**tee**-ree-oh-skleh-**ROH**-sis) is the abnormal hardening of the walls of an artery or arteries (**arteri/o** means artery and **-sclerosis** means abnormal hardening). (Notice that **-sclerosis** is the opposite of **-malacia.**)

- **-stenosis** means abnormal narrowing. **Arteriostenosis** (ar-**tee**-ree-oh-steh-**NOH**-sis) is the abnormal narrowing of an artery or arteries (**arteri/o** means artery and **-stenosis** means abnormal narrowing).

SUFFIXES RELATED TO PROCEDURES

Suffixes related to procedures identify a procedure that is performed on the body part identified by the word root:

- **-centesis** is a surgical puncture to remove fluid for diagnostic purposes or to remove excess fluid. **Abdominocentesis** (ab-**dom**-ih-noh-sen-**TEE**-sis) is the surgical puncture of the abdominal cavity to remove fluid (**abdomin/o** means abdomen and **-centesis** means a surgical puncture to removal fluid).

- **-ectomy** means surgical removal. An **appendectomy** (**ap**-en-**DECK**-toh-mee) is the surgical removal of the appendix (**append** means appendix and **-ectomy** means surgical removal).

- **-graphy** means the process of recording a picture or record. **Arteriography** (ar-tee-ree-**OG**-rah-fee) is the process of recording a picture of an artery or arteries (**arteri/o** means artery and **-graphy** means to record).

- **-gram** means record or picture. An **arteriogram** (ar-**TEER**-ee-oh-gram) is the record produced by arteriography (**arteri/o** means artery and **-gram** means record).

- **-plasty** means surgical repair. **Myoplasty** (**MY**-oh-plas-tee) is the surgical repair of a muscle (**myo** means muscle and **-plasty** means surgical repair).

- **-scopy** means visual examination. **Endoscopy** (en-**DOS**-koh-pee) is the visual examination of the interior of a body cavity or organ by means of an endoscope (**endo-** means within and **-scopy** means visual examination).

THE DOUBLE RR'S

Suffixes beginning with two Rs, which are often referred to as the **double RRs,** are particularly confusing. They are grouped together here to help you understand the word parts and to remember the differences:

- **-rrhage** and **-rrhagia** mean bursting forth, as in an abnormal excessive fluid discharge or bleeding. **Hemorrhage** (**HEM**-or-idj) means the loss of a large amount of blood in a short time (**hem/o** means blood and **-rrhage** means bursting forth). *Note:* **-rrhage** and **-rrhagia** both refer to the flow of blood. To remember this suffix, think of how rage may lead to a bloody fight.

- **-rrhaphy** means to suture or stitch. **Myorrhaphy** (my-**OR**-ah-fee) means to suture a muscle wound (**my/o** means muscle, and **-rrhaphy** means to suture). To remember this suffix, think of r-r-wrap as if you were going to wrap the injury in sutures.

- **-rrhea** means an abnormal flow or discharge and refers to the abnormal flow of most body fluids. **Diarrhea** (**dye**-ah-**REE**-ah) is abnormally frequent loose or watery stools (**dia-** means through and **-rrhea** means abnormal flow). *Note:* Although **-rrhea** and **-rrhage** both describe an abnormal flow, they are *not* used interchangeably because **-rrhea** does *not* refer to the flow of blood.

- **-rrhexis** means rupture. **Myorrhexis** (my-oh-**RECK**-sis) means the rupture of a muscle (**my/o** means muscle and **-rrhexis** means rupture). To remember this suffix, think of the *X* as being ready to rupture and fly apart.

PREFIXES

A prefix is added to the beginning of a word to change the meaning of that term (Figure 1.3). Prefixes usually, but not always, indicate location, time, or number. The term **natal** (**NAY**-tal) means pertaining to birth (**nat** means birth, and **-al** means pertaining to). The following examples show how a prefix changes the meaning of this term:

- **Prenatal** (pre-**NAY**-tal) means the time and events before birth (**pre-** means before, **nat** means birth, and **-al** means pertaining to) (Figure 1.4).

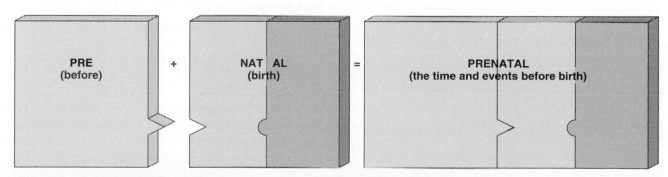

FIGURE 1.3 A prefix added to a word root plus a suffix changes the meaning of the term.

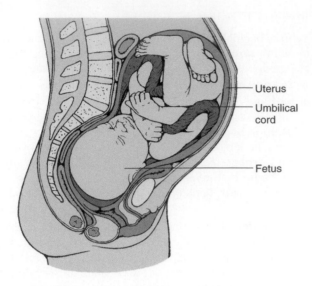

FIGURE 1.4 The term *prenatal* refers to the events that occur before birth. Shown here is a diagram of a developing child in the uterus before birth.

- Uterus
- Umbilical cord
- Fetus

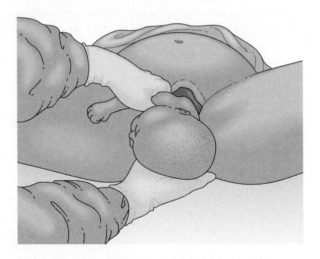

FIGURE 1.5 The term *perinatal* refers to the time and events around birth. As shown here, in a normal delivery the baby's head emerges first.

- **Perinatal** (**pehr**-ih-**NAY**-tal) refers to the time and events surrounding birth (**peri-** means surrounding, **nat** means birth, and **-al** means pertaining to). This is the time just before, during, and just after birth (Figure 1.5).
- **Postnatal** (pohst-**NAY**-tal) means the time and events after birth (**post-** means after, **nat** means birth, and **-al** means pertaining to) (Figure 1.6).

CONTRASTING AND CONFUSING PREFIXES

Some prefixes are confusing because they are similar in spelling but opposite in meaning. The more common prefixes of this type are summarized in Table 1.4.

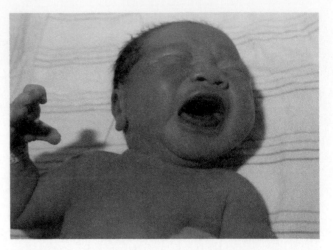

FIGURE 1.6 The term *postnatal* refers to the time and events after birth. As shown here, a healthy newborn has a lusty cry.

DETERMINING MEANINGS ON THE BASIS OF WORD PARTS

Knowing the meaning of the word parts often makes it possible to figure out the definition of an unfamiliar medical term.

TAKING TERMS APART

To determine a word's meaning by looking at the component pieces, you must first separate it into word parts.

- Always start at the end of the word, with the suffix, and work toward the beginning.
- As you separate the word parts, identify the meaning of each. Identifying the meaning of each part should give you a definition of the term.
- Because some word parts have more than one meaning, it also is necessary to determine the context in which the term is being used. As used here, *context* means to determine which body system this term is referring to.
- If you have any doubt, use your medical dictionary to double-check your definition.

An Example

Look at the term **otorhinolaryngology** as shown in Figure 1.7. It is made up of three combining forms plus a suffix. Here are the words parts as the term is taken apart, beginning at the end.

- The suffix **-ology** means the study of.
- The word root **laryng** means larynx and throat. The combining vowel *is not used* here because the word root is joining a suffix that begins with a vowel.
- The combining form **rhin/o** means nose. The combining vowel *is used* here because **rhin/o** is joining another word root.

Table 1.4

CONTRASTING AND CONFUSING PREFIXES	
ab- means away from.	**ad-** means toward or in the direction of.
Abnormal means not normal or away from normal.	**Addiction** means drawn toward or a strong dependence on a drug or substance.
dys- means bad, difficult, painful.	**eu-** means good, normal, well, or easy.
Dysfunctional means an organ or body part that is not working properly.	**Euthyroid** (you-**THIGH**-roid) means a normally functioning thyroid gland.
hyper- means excessive or increased.	**hypo-** means deficient or decreased.
Hypertension (**high**-per-**TEN**-shun) is higher than normal blood pressure.	**Hypotension** (**high**-poh-**TEN**-shun) is lower than normal blood pressure.
inter- means between or among.	**intra-** means within or inside.
Interstitial (**in**-ter-**STISH**-al) means between, but not within, the parts of a tissue.	**Intramuscular** (**in**-trah-**MUS**-kyou-lar) means within the muscle.
sub- means under, less, or below.	**supra-** means above or excessive.
Subcostal (sub-**KOS**-tal) means below a rib or ribs.	**Supracostal** (**sue**-prah-**KOS**-tal) means above or outside the ribs.

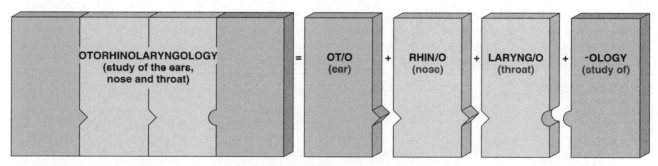

FIGURE 1.7 A medical term may be taken apart to determine its meaning.

- The combining form **ot/o** means ear. The combining vowel *is used* here because **ot/o** is joining another word root.

- Together they form **otorhinolaryngology** (oh-toh-**rye**-noh-**lar**-in-**GOL**-oh-jee), which is the study of the ears, nose, and throat (**ot/o** means ear, **rhin/o** means nose, **laryng** means throat, and **-ology** means study of).

- Because this is such a long name, this specialty is frequently referred to as **ENT** (ears, nose, and throat) or is shortened to **otolaryngology** (**oh**-toh-**lar**-in-**GOL**-oh-jee).

MEDICAL DICTIONARY USE

Learning to use a medical dictionary is an important part of mastering the correct use of medical terms. The following tips for dictionary use apply whether you are working with a traditional book form dictionary or an electronic dictionary on your computer.

GUESSING AT MEANINGS

When you are able to guess at the meaning of a term on the basis of the word parts that make it up, you must always double check for accuracy because some terms have more than one meaning. For example, look at the term **lithotomy** (lih-**THOT**-oh-mee):

- On the basis of word parts, **lithotomy** means a surgical incision for the removal of a stone (**lith** means stone, and **-otomy** means a surgical incision). This meaning is discussed further in Chapter 9.

- However, **lithotomy** is also the name of an examination position in which the patient is lying on the back with the feet and legs raised and supported in stirrups. This term is discussed further in Chapter 15.

This possible confusion is only one of the many reasons why a medical dictionary is an important medical terminology tool.

IF YOU KNOW HOW TO SPELL THE WORD

When starting to work with an unfamiliar dictionary, spend a few minutes reviewing its use guide, table of contents, and appendices. The time you spend reviewing now will be saved later when you are looking up unfamiliar terms.

- On the basis of the first letter of the word, start in the appropriate section of the dictionary. Look at the top of the page for clues. The top left word is the first term on the page. The top right word is the last term on the page.

- Next, alphabetically look for words that start with the first and second letters of the word you are researching. Continue looking through each letter until you find the term you are looking for.

- When you think you have found it, check the spelling very carefully letter by letter, working from left to right. Terms with similar spellings have very different meanings.

- When you find the term, carefully check *all* of the definitions.

IF YOU DO NOT KNOW HOW TO SPELL THE WORD

- Listen carefully to the term and write it down. If you cannot find the word on the basis of your spelling, start looking for alternative spellings based on the beginning sound as shown in Table 1.5. *Note:* All of these examples are in this text. However, you could practice looking them up in the dictionary!

LOOK UNDER CATEGORIES

Most dictionaries use categories such as *Diseases* and *Syndromes* to group disorders with these terms in their title. For example

- *Venereal disease* would be found under *Disease, venereal.* These sexually transmitted diseases are discussed further in Chapter 14.

- *Fetal alcohol syndrome* would be found under *Syndrome, fetal alcohol.* This condition is discussed further in Chapter 2.

- When you come across such a term and cannot find it listed by the first word, the next step is to look under the appropriate category.

Table 1.5

GUIDELINES TO LOOKING UP UNFAMILIAR TERMS

If It Sounds Like	It May Begin With	Example
F	F	**flatus** (**FLAY**-tus)
	PH	**phlegm** (**FLEM**)
J	G	**gingivitis** (**jin**-jih-**VYE**-tis)
	J	**jaundice** (**JAWN**-dis)
K	C	**crepitus** (**KREP**-ih-tus)
	CH	**cholera** (**KOL**-er-ah)
	K	**kyphosis** (kye-**FOH**-sis)
	QU	**quadriplegia** (**kwad**-rih-**PLEE**-jee-ah)
S	C	**cytology** (sigh-**TOL**-oh-jee)
	PS	**psychologist** (sigh-**KOL**-oh-jist)
	S	**serology** (seh-**ROL**-oh-jee)
Z	X	**xeroderma** (zee-roh-**DER**-mah)
	Z	**zygote** (**ZYE**-goht)

PRONUNCIATION

A medical term is easier to understand and remember when you know how to pronounce it properly. To help you to pronounce terms, we have identified each new term in the text in **bold**. The term is followed (in parentheses) by a commonly accepted pronunciation and then the definition.

- In this Sounds-Like pronunciation system, the word is respelled using normal English letters to create sounds that are familiar. To pronounce a new word, just say it as it is spelled in the parentheses.

- The part of the word that receives the primary (most) emphasis when you say it is shown in capital letters and bold. For example, **edema** (eh-**DEE**-mah) means excess fluid in body tissues, causing swelling.

- A part of the word that receives secondary emphasis when you say it is shown in lowercase letters and bold. For example, **appendicitis** (ah-**pen**-dih-**SIGH**-tis) means an inflammation of the appendix (**appendic** means appendix and **-itis** means inflammation).

A WORD OF CAUTION

Frequently, there is more than one correct way to pronounce a medical term!

- The pronunciation of many medical terms is based on their Greek, Latin, or other foreign origin. However, there is a trend toward pronouncing terms as they would sound in English.

- The result is having more than one "correct" pronunciation for a term. In the text, sometimes an alternative pronunciation is included to reflect these changes.

- Both are correct, and the difference is a matter of preference. However, your instructor will tell you which pronunciation to use in your course.

SPELLING IS ALWAYS IMPORTANT

Accuracy in spelling medical terms is extremely important!

- Changing just one or two letters can completely change the meaning of a word—and this difference literally could be a matter of life or death for the patient.

- The section Look-Alike Sound-Alike Terms and Word Parts later in this chapter will help you become aware of some terms and word parts that are frequently confused.

USING ABBREVIATIONS

Abbreviations are frequently used as a shorthand way to record long and complex medical terms, and Appendix B contains an alphabetized list of many of the more commonly used medical abbreviations.

- Abbreviations can also lead to confusion and errors! Therefore, it is important that you be very careful when using or translating an abbreviation.

- For example, the abbreviation *BE* means both *below elbow* and *barium enema*. Just imagine what a difference a mix-up here would make for the patient!

- Because the same abbreviation may have more than one meaning, it is important that you be very careful when using or translating an abbreviation. To be safe, always follow this rule: *When in doubt, spell it out.*

SINGULAR AND PLURAL ENDINGS

Many medical terms have Greek or Latin origins. As a result of these different origins, there are unusual rules for changing a singular word into a plural form. In addition, English endings have been adopted for some commonly used terms.

- Table 1.6 on page 12 provides guidelines to help you better understand how these plurals are formed.

- Also, throughout the text when a term with an unusual singular or plural form is introduced, both forms are included. For example, a **phalanx** (**FAY**-lanks) is one bone of the fingers or toes (Figure 1.8) (plural, **phalanges**).

BASIC MEDICAL TERMS

Some of the basic medical terms used to describe diseases and disease conditions are shown in Table 1.7 on page 13.

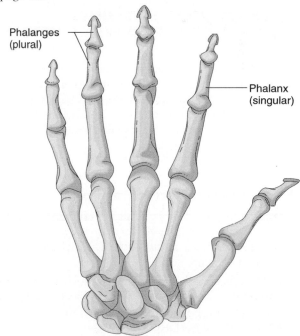

Phalanges (plural)

Phalanx (singular)

FIGURE 1.8 **A phalanx is one finger or toe bone. Two or more of these bones are called phalanges.**

Table 1.6

GUIDELINES TO UNUSUAL PLURAL FORMS

Guideline	Singular	Plural
1. If the term ends in **a**, the plural is usually formed by adding an **e**.	bursa vertebra	bursae vertebrae
2. If the term ends in **ex** or **ix**, the plural is usually formed by changing the **ex** or **ix** to **ices**.	appendix index	appendices indices
3. If the term ends in **is**, the plural is usually formed by changing the **is** to **es**.	diagnosis metastasis	diagnoses metastases
4. If the term ends in **itis**, the plural is usually formed by changing the **is** to **ides**.	arthritis meningitis	arthritides meningitides
5. If the term ends in **nx**, the plural is usually formed by changing the **x** to **ges**.	phalanx meninx	phalanges meninges
6. If the term ends in **on**, the plural is usually formed by changing the **on** to **a**.	criterion ganglion	criteria ganglia
7. If the term ends in **um**, the plural usually is formed by changing the **um** to **a**.	diverticulum ovum	diverticula ova
8. If the term ends in **us**, the plural is usually formed by changing the **us** to **i**.	alveolus malleolus	alveoli malleoli

*If you are in doubt as to how a plural is formed, **look it up** in a medical dictionary!*

LOOK-ALIKE SOUND-ALIKE TERMS AND WORD PARTS

One confusing part of learning medical terminology is dealing with words and word parts that look and sound much alike. This section highlights some frequently used terms and word parts that you may find confusing. Pay particular attention to these terms and word parts as you encounter them in the text.

arteri/o, ather/o, AND arthr/o

- **arteri/o** means artery. **Endarterial** (**end**-ar-**TEE**-ree-al) means pertaining to the interior or lining of an artery (**end-** means within, **arteri** means artery, and **-al** means pertaining to).
- **ather/o** means plaque or fatty substance. An **atheroma** (**ath**-er-**OH**-mah) is a fatty deposit within the wall of an artery (**ather** means fatty substance and **-oma** means tumor).
- **arthr/o** means joint. **Arthralgia** (ar-**THRAL**-jee-ah) means pain in a joint or joints (**arthr** means joint and **-algia** means pain).

ILEUM AND ILIUM

- The **ileum** (**ILL**-ee-um) is part of the small intestine. (Remember, il**e**um with an **e** as in int**e**stine.)
- The **ilium** (**ILL**-ee-um) is part of the hip bone. (Remember, il**i**um with an **i** as in h**i**p.)

INFECTION AND INFLAMMATION

- An **infection** (in-**FECK**-shun) is the invasion of the body by a pathogenic (disease-producing) organism. The infection may remain localized or may be systemic (affecting the entire body).
- **Inflammation** (**in**-flah-**MAY**-shun) is a localized response to an injury or destruction of tissues. The cardinal signs (indications) of inflammation are (1) *redness* (erythema), (2) *heat*, (3) *swelling* (edema), and (4) *pain*. These are caused by extra blood flowing into the area as part of the healing process.
- The suffix **-itis** means inflammation. However, it also is often used to indicate infection.

LACERATION AND LESION

- A **laceration** (**lass**-er-**AY**-shun) is a torn, ragged wound.

Table 1.7

BASIC MEDICAL TERMS

A **sign** is evidence of disease, such as fever, that can be observed by the patient and by others.

A **symptom** (**SIMP**-tum), such as pain or a headache, can be observed only by the patient.

A **syndrome** (**SIN**-drohm) is a set of the signs and symptoms that occur together as part of a specific disease process.

A sign is **objective** because it can be evaluated or measured by others.

A symptom is **subjective** because it can be evaluated or measured only by the patient.

Diagnosis (**dye**-ag-**NOH**-sis) is the identification of the disease (plural, **diagnoses**).
To **diagnose** is the process of reaching a diagnosis.

A **differential diagnosis** attempts to determine which one of several diseases may be producing the symptoms.

Prognosis (prog-**NOH**-sis) is a forecast or prediction of the probable course and outcome of a disorder (plural, **prognoses**).

An **acute** disease or symptom has a rapid onset, a severe course, and a relatively short duration.

A **chronic** disease or symptom of long duration. Although such diseases may be controlled, they are rarely cured.

A **remission** is the partial or complete disappearance of the symptoms of a disease without having achieved a cure. A remission is usually temporary.

Some diseases are named for the **condition described.** For example, **chronic fatigue syndrome (CFS)** is a persistent overwhelming fatigue that does not resolve with bed rest.

An **eponym** (**EP**-oh-nim) is a disease, structure, operation, or procedure named for the person who discovered or described it first. For example, **Alzheimer's disease** is named for Alois Alzheimer, a German neurologist who lived from 1864 to 1915. (See Chapter 10.)

An **acronym** (**ACK**-roh-nim) is a word formed from the initial letter or letters of the major parts of a compound term. For example, the acronym **laser** stands for **l**ight **a**mplification by **s**timulated **e**mission of **r**adiation. (See Chapter 12.)

- A **lesion** (**LEE**-zhun) is a pathologic change of the tissues due to disease or injury.

MUCOUS AND MUCUS

- **Mucous** (**MYOU**-kus) is an adjective that describes the specialized mucous membranes that line the body cavities.
- **Mucus** (**MYOU**-kus) is a noun and is the name of the fluid secreted by the mucous membranes.

myc/o, myel/o, AND my/o

- **myc/o** means fungus. **Mycosis** (my-**KOH**-sis) means any disease caused by a fungus (**myc** means fungus and **-osis** means abnormal condition).
- **myel/o** means bone marrow *or* spinal cord. **Myelopathy** (my-eh-**LOP**-ah-thee) is any pathologic change or disease in the spinal cord (**myel/o** means spinal cord and **-pathy** means disease).

- **my/o** means muscle. **Myopathy** (my-**OP**-ah-thee) is any pathologic change or disease of muscle tissue (**my/o** means muscle and **-pathy** means disease).

-ologist AND -ology

- **-ologist** means specialist. A **gerontologist** (jer-on-**TOL**-oh-jist) is a specialist in diagnosing and treating diseases, disorders, and problems associated with aging (**geront** means old age and **-ologist** means specialist).
- **-ology** means the study of. **Neonatology** (nee-oh-nay-**TOL**-oh-jee) is the study of disorders of the newborn (**neo-** means new, **nat** means birth, and **-ology** means study of).

-ostomy AND -otomy

- **-ostomy** means to surgically create an artificial opening. A **colostomy** (koh-**LAHS**-toh-mee) is the surgical creation of an opening between the colon and the body surface (**col** means colon and **-ostomy** means an artificial opening).

- **-otomy** means cutting into or a surgical incision. A **colotomy** (koh-**LOT**-oh-mee) is a surgical incision into the colon (**col** means colon and **-otomy** means a surgical incision).

PALPATION AND PALPITATION

- **Palpation** (pal-**PAY**-shun) is an examination technique in which the examiner's hands are used to feel the texture, size, consistency, and location of certain body parts. This is discussed further in Chapter 15.
- **Palpitation** (**pal**-pih-**TAY**-shun) is a pounding or racing heart. This is discussed further in Chapter 5.

PROSTATE AND PROSTRATE

- **Prostate** (**PROS**-tayt) refers to a male gland that lies under the urinary bladder and surrounds the urethra.
- **Prostrate** (**PROS**-trayt) means to collapse and be lying flat or to be overcome with exhaustion.

pyel/o, py/o, AND pyr/o

- **pyel/o** means renal pelvis (which is part of the kidney). **Pyelitis** (**pye**-eh-**LYE**-tis) is an inflammation of the renal pelvis (**pyel** means renal pelvis and **-itis** means inflammation).
- **py/o** means pus. **Pyoderma** (**pye**-oh-**DER**-mah) is any pus-producing disease of the skin (**py/o** means pus and **-derma** means skin).
- **pyr/o** means fever or fire. **Pyrosis** (pye-**ROH**-sis), also known as **heartburn,** is discomfort due to the regurgitation of stomach acid upward into the esophagus (**pyr** means fever or fire and **-osis** means abnormal condition).

SUPINATION AND SUPPURATION

- **Supination** (**soo**-pih-**NAY**-shun) is the act of rotating the arm so that the palm of the hand is forward or upward. It also means the act of assuming the supine (lying down) position.
- **Suppuration** (**sup**-you-**RAY**-shun) is the formation or discharge of pus.

SUTURING AND LIGATION

- **Suturing** (**SOO**-chur-ing) is the act of closing a wound or incision by stitching or a similar means.
- **Ligation** (lye-**GAY**-shun) is the act of binding or tying off blood vessels or ducts.

TRIAGE AND TRAUMA

- **Triage** (tree-**AHZH**) is the medical screening of patients to determine their relative priority of need and the proper place of treatment. For example, emergency personnel arriving on an accident scene must identify which of the injured require care first

and must determine where they can be treated most effectively.

- **Trauma** (**TRAW**-mah) means wound or injury. These are the types of injuries that might occur in an accident, shooting, natural disaster, or fire.

VIRAL AND VIRILE

- **Viral** (**VYE**-ral) means pertaining to a virus (**vir** means virus or poison and **-al** means pertaining to).
- **Virile** (**VIR**-ill) means possessing masculine traits.

Career Opportunities: Setting Your Goals

Learning about medical terminology is essential to a wide range of health occupations, from transplant surgeon to dance therapist. As you learn about the different body systems and fields of medical care, think about which jobs sound most appealing to you. Look in the library and on the Internet for detailed information about careers you might want to pursue.

Some health occupations require only a high school diploma and a willingness to learn on the job, whereas others require a college degree and many years of postgraduate study. Table 1.8 can help you plan your future in the health occupation you choose.

In the chapters to come, there will be many career ideas for you to consider. Most involve direct contact with patients; others deal with vital behind-the-scenes work, such as keeping accurate medical records and maintaining complex life-saving equipment. A few examples are:

- **Medical records administrator (RA):** plans the systems for storing and obtaining medical records
- **Medical records** or **health information technician:** organizes and codes patient records, gathers statistical or research data, and records information
- **Medical records clerk:** files and retrieves patient records
- **Medical billing clerk:** sends invoices to patients and insurance companies, listing the procedures and tests that have been performed
- **Medical transcriptionist:** works with doctors and other health professionals to record data and prepare reports
- **Medical illustrator, photographer,** or **writer:** helps create books, newspaper and magazine articles, informational brochures for patients, and other print materials in the medical field
- **Health unit clerk:** performs administrative and secretarial tasks in a healthcare facility such as a hospital, clinic, or nursing home

(continues)

- **Administrative medical assistant:** works in a physician's office or clinic as a receptionist or office manager

- **Insurance underwriter** or **assistant:** processes claims for medical, disability, and other health-related claims

- **Biomedical equipment technician (BET):** installs, tests, services, and maintains the various types of equipment essential for medical diagnosis and treatment, such as x-ray machines, incu-bators, dialysis machines, heart-lung machines, and respirators

- **Biomedical researcher:** works in a laboratory setting to explore and test new drug therapies

- **Pharmaceutical sales representative:** provides drug information and samples to medical personnel on behalf of the manufacturer

- **Mortuary worker:** prepares bodies for burial or cremation, plans funeral services, and helps console the bereaved

Table 1.8

EDUCATION AND LEVELS OF TRAINING

Career Level	Educational Requirement	Examples
Aide or Assistant	One or more years of combined classroom and/or on-the-job training	Dental assistant Medical assistant Nurse assistant
Nurse (LPN, LVN) or Technician	Two-year associate's degree, special health occupations education, or three to four years of on-the-job training	Dental hygienist Medical laboratory technician Surgical technician
Registered Nurse (RN), Technologist, or Therapist	Three to four years of college plus work experience, usually a bachelor's degree; however, a master's degree may be required	Medical laboratory technologist Physical therapist Speech therapist
Professional	Postgraduate education in medical specialty (master's or doctorate degree)	Dentist Medical doctor Psychologist

STUDY BREAK

Learning word parts can help you understand more than just medical words. It might come in handy to know that intramural sports are those played within the walls, or confines, of the school (*intra-* = within, and *mural* = pertaining to walls). You could point out that substandard work is not acceptable (*sub* = below, standard).

Try making up a few silly words to play around with word parts and amuse your friends. Start by figuring out the meaning of these made-up words:

- Hyperhungry
- Rhinobop
- Leukomelano TV

You could even string together a lot of word parts to make an impressive nonsense word like "super-califragilisticexpialidocious!"

Health Occupation Profile: ADMINISTRATIVE MEDICAL ASSISTANT

Brad Hamilton, 33, is a certified medical assistant (CMA). "My introduction to medical assisting began when I took a health occupations course in high school. I knew I wanted a career in health care, but I didn't know whether I wanted to work with patients or would like an administrative role better. Since medical assistants are trained in both areas, after graduation I enrolled in a medical assisting program. For me, this was a great career choice. (Being one of the few guys in the class wasn't bad either!)"

"My first job was working as a clinical assistant in a private practice. I enjoyed working with patients, but I liked the administrative side of the job best, so I started taking business courses in the evenings. This educational background, plus my work experience, helped me move into a supervisory position at a large private clinic. I love what I'm doing and feel that my job gives me the best of both worlds in health care."

Review Time

Write the answers to the following questions on a separate piece of paper or in your notebook. In addition, be prepared to take part in the classroom discussion.

1. **Written assignment:** Describe the differences between a **sign** and a **symptom.**

   Discussion assignment: Why are both types of observations important diagnostic indicators?

2. **Written assignment:** Use your own words to define the term **triage.**

   Discussion assignment: What are the kinds of situations in which triage would be important?

3. **Written assignment:** Use your word part skills to determine the meaning of the term **cardiopulmonary** (**pulmon/o** means lungs) and then state the definition and identify the word parts that make up this term.

   Discussion assignment: What rules relating to the use of combining vowels are used in this term?

4. **Written assignment:** Use your medical dictionary to research the eponym **Graves' disease** and report on the name, and dates, of the physician for whom this disease is named.

   Discussion assignment: What is the meaning of the term **eponym?**

5. **Written assignment:** Compare the terms **diagnosis** and **prognosis.**

   Discussion assignment: How is information about both the diagnosis and prognosis important to the patient and to his family?

Optional Internet Activity

The goal of this activity is to help you learn more about medical terminology while improving your Internet skills. Select one of these two options and follow the instructions.

1. **Internet Search:** Search for information about the Health Occupations Students of America (HOSA). Write a brief (one- or two-paragraph) report on something new you learned here and include the address of the web site where you found this information.

2. **Web Site:** To learn more about a health occupation of interest to you, go to this web address: **http://stats.bls.gov/oco/.** Click on the letter of the occupation of greatest interest to you and find it in the alphabetical list. Write a brief (one- or two-paragraph) report on something new you learned here. Be certain to include in your report the name of the occupation you researched.

The Human Touch: Critical Thinking Exercise

The following story and questions are designed to stimulate critical thinking through class discussion or as a brief essay response. There are no right or wrong answers to these questions.

Baylie Hutchins sits at her kitchen table with her medical terminology book opened to the first chapter, highlighter in hand. Her two-year-old son, Mathias, plays with a box of Animal Crackers in his highchair, some even finding his mouth. "Arteri/o, ather/o, and arthr/o," she mutters, lips moving to shape unfamiliar sounds. "They're too much alike, and they mean totally different things." Mathias sneezes loudly, and spots of Animal Cracker rain on the page, punctuating her frustration.

"Great job 'Thias," she says wiping the text with her finger. "I planned on using the highlighter to mark with, not your lunch." Mathias giggles and peeks through the tunnel made by one small hand.

"Mucous and mucus," she reads aloud, each sounding the same. Then she remembers her teacher's tip for remembering the difference: "The long word's the membrane, and the short one's the secretion."

Mathias picks up an Animal Cracker and excitedly shouts, "Tiger, Mommy! Tiger!" "That's right, 'Thias. Good job!"

Turning back to the page she stares at the blue words -rrhagia, -rrhaphy, -rrhea, and -rrhexis. Stumbling over the pronunciation, Baylie closes her eyes and tries to silence the voices in her head. "You can't do anything right," her ex-husband says. "Couldn't finish if your life depended on it," her mother's voice snaps.

Baylie keeps at it. "Rhin/o means nose," highlighting those three words, "and a rhinoceros has a big horn on his nose."

"Rhino!" Mathias shouts, holding up an Animal Cracker. Baylie laughs. We both have new things to learn, she realizes. And we can do it!

Suggested Discussion Topics

1. Baylie needs to learn medical terminology if she wants a career in the medical field. What study habits would help Baylie accomplish this task?

2. A support group could help empower Baylie to accomplish her goals. What people would you suggest for this group and why?

3. How can this textbook and other resource materials help her (and you) learn medical terminology?

4. Discuss strategies the instructor could use, and has already used, to help Baylie improve her terminology skills.

5. Discuss how previous educational or learning experiences influence a student's approach to learning a new skill or subject.

Student Workbook and Student Activity CD-ROM

1. Go to your **Student Workbook** and complete the Learning Exercises for this chapter.

2. Go to the **Student Activity CD-ROM** and have fun with the exercises and games for this chapter.

2 The Human Body in Health and Disease

● Overview of the Human Body in Health and Disease

Anatomic Reference Systems	Descriptive terms used to describe the location of body planes, directions, and cavities.
Cytology	The structures of cells, chromosomes, DNA, and genetics.
Histology	The study of the tissues, which are composed of cells that join together to perform specific functions.
Glands	Specialized cells that secrete material used elsewhere in the body.
Organs and Body Systems	Body parts organized into systems according to function.
Pathology	Study of structural and functional changes caused by disease.

Vocabulary Related to the Human Body in Health and Disease

Terms marked with the ❖ symbol are pronounced on the Student Activity CD-ROM that accompanies this text.

KEY WORD PARTS

- ☐ aden/o
- ☐ adip/o
- ☐ caud/o
- ☐ cephal/o
- ☐ col/o
- ☐ coron/o
- ☐ cyt/o
- ☐ hepat/o
- ☐ hist/o
- ☐ hyster/o
- ☐ lapar/o
- ☐ nephr/o
- ☐ oste/o
- ☐ path/o
- ☐ retr/o

KEY MEDICAL TERMS

- ☐ abdomen (ab-DOH-men or AB-doh-men) ❖
- ☐ abdominal (ab-DOM-ih-nal)
- ☐ abdominopelvic (ab-dom-ih-noh-PEL-vick) ❖
- ☐ adenectomy (ad-eh-NECK-toh-mee) ❖
- ☐ adenitis (ad-eh-NIGH-tis) ❖
- ☐ adenoma (ad-eh-NOH-mah) ❖
- ☐ adenomalacia (ad-eh-noh-mah-LAY-shee ah) ❖
- ☐ adenosclerosis (ad-eh-noh-skleh-ROH-sis) ❖
- ☐ adenosis (ad-eh-NOH-sis) ❖
- ☐ adipose (AD-ih-pohs) ❖
- ☐ anaplasia (an-ah-PLAY-zee-ah) ❖
- ☐ anatomy (ah-NAT-oh-mee) ❖
- ☐ anomaly (ah-NOM-ah-lee) ❖
- ☐ anterior (an-TEER-ee-or) ❖
- ☐ aplasia (ah-PLAY-zee-ah) ❖
- ☐ ascites (ah-SIGH-teez) ❖
- ☐ caudal (KAW-dal) ❖
- ☐ cephalic (seh-FAL-ick) ❖
- ☐ chromosomes (KROH-moh-sohmes) ❖
- ☐ communicable (kuh-MEW-nih-kuh-bul) ❖
- ☐ congenital (kon-JEN-ih-tahl) ❖
- ☐ coronal (koh-ROH-nal)
- ☐ cytology (sigh-TOL-oh-jee) ❖
- ☐ cytoplasm (SIGH-toh-plazm)
- ☐ deoxyribonucleic (dee-ock-see-rye-boh-new-KLEE-ick) ❖
- ☐ distal (DIS-tal)
- ☐ dorsal (DOR-sal)
- ☐ dysplasia (dis-PLAY-see-ah) ❖

- ☐ endemic (en-DEM-ick) ❖
- ☐ endocrine (EN-doh-krin) ❖
- ☐ epidemic (ep-ih-DEM-ick) ❖
- ☐ epidemiologist (ep-ih-dee-mee-OL-oh-jist) ❖
- ☐ epigastric (ep-ih-GAS-trick)
- ☐ epithelial (ep-ih-THEE-lee-al) ❖
- ☐ etiology (ee-tee-OL-oh-jee) ❖
- ☐ exocrine (ECK-soh-krin) ❖
- ☐ geneticist (jeh-NET-ih-sist) ❖
- ☐ hemophilia (hee-moh-FILL-ee-ah) ❖
- ☐ histologist (hiss-TOL-oh-jist)
- ☐ histology (hiss-TOL-oh-jee) ❖
- ☐ homeostasis (hoh-mee-oh-STAY-sis) ❖
- ☐ hyperplasia (high-per-PLAY-zee-ah) ❖
- ☐ hypochondriac (high-poh-KON-dree-ack)
- ☐ hypogastric (high-poh-GAS-trick)
- ☐ hypoplasia (high-poh-PLAY zee-ah) ❖
- ☐ iatrogenic (eye-at-roh-JEN-ick) ❖
- ☐ idiopathic (id-ee-oh-PATH-ick) ❖
- ☐ iliac (ILL-ee-ack)
- ☐ infectious (in-FECK-shus) ❖
- ☐ inguinal (ING-gwih-nal) ❖
- ☐ laparoscopy (lap-ah-ROS-koh-pee) ❖
- ☐ lumbar (LUM-bar)
- ☐ membrane (MEM-brain)
- ☐ mesentery (MESS-en-terr-ee) ❖
- ☐ midsagittal (mid-SADJ-ih-tal) ❖
- ☐ nosocomial (nos-oh-KOH-mee-al) ❖
- ☐ nucleus (NEW-klee-us)
- ☐ pandemic (pan-DEM-ick) ❖
- ☐ parietal peritoneum (pah-RYE-ch-tal pehr-ih-toh-NEE-um) ❖
- ☐ pathologist (pah-THOL-oh-jist)
- ☐ pathology (pah-THOL-oh-jee) ❖
- ☐ pelvic (PEL-vick) ❖
- ☐ peritoneum (pehr-ih-toh-NEE-um) ❖
- ☐ peritonitis (pehr-ih-toh-NIGH-tis) ❖
- ☐ phenylketonuria (fen-il-kee-toh-NEW-ree-ah) ❖
- ☐ physiology (fiz-ee-OL-oh-jee) ❖
- ☐ posterior (pos-TEER-ee-or) ❖
- ☐ proximal (PROCK-sih-mal) ❖
- ☐ retroperitoneal (ret-roh-pehr-ih-toh-NEE-al) ❖
- ☐ sagittal (SADJ-ih-tal)
- ☐ thoracic (thoh-RAS-ick) ❖
- ☐ transverse (trans-VERSE) ❖
- ☐ umbilical (um-BILL-ih-kal) ❖
- ☐ ventral (VEN-tral) ❖
- ☐ visceral (VIS-er-al) ❖

Upon completion of this chapter, you should be able to:

1. Define anatomy and physiology and use anatomic reference systems to identify the anatomic position, body planes, directions, and cavities.
2. Recognize, define, spell, and pronounce the terms related to the abdominal cavity and peritoneum.
3. Recognize, define, spell, and pronounce the terms related to the structure, function, pathology, and procedures of cells, tissues, and glands.
4. Define the terms associated with genetics including mutation, genetic engineering, and genetic counseling.
5. Differentiate between genetic and congenital disorders and identify examples of each.
6. Identify the body systems in terms of their major structures, functions, and related word parts.
7. Recognize, define, spell, and pronounce the terms related to types of diseases and the modes of disease of transmission.

ANATOMIC REFERENCE SYSTEMS

Anatomic reference systems are used to describe the location and functions of body parts. These reference systems include body planes, body directions, body cavities, and structural units.

ANATOMY AND PHYSIOLOGY DEFINED

- **Anatomy** (ah-**NAT**-oh-mee) is the study of the structures of the body.
- **Physiology** (**fiz**-ee-**OL**-oh-jee) is the study of the functions of these structures.

THE ANATOMIC POSITION

Descriptions of the body are based on the **anatomic position.** In this position, the individual is

- Standing up so that the body is erect.
- Facing forward.
- Holding the arms at the sides.
- Turning the hands with the palms toward the front.

BODY PLANES

Body planes are imaginary vertical and horizontal lines that are used to divide the body into sections for descriptive purposes.

Vertical Planes

- A **vertical plane** is an up-and-down line that is at a right angle to the horizon.
- The **midsagittal plane** (mid-**SADJ**-ih-tal), also known as the **midline,** is the vertical plane that divides the body, from top to bottom, into *equal* left and right halves (Figure 2.1).

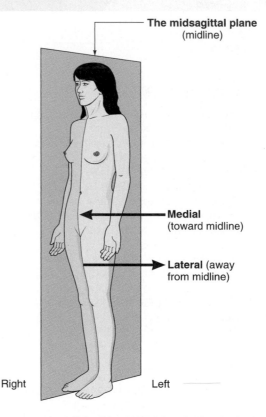

FIGURE 2.1 The midsagittal plane divides the body from top to bottom into equal left and right halves.

- A **sagittal plane** (**SADJ**-ih-tal) is any vertical plane parallel to the midline that divides the body into unequal left and right portions.
- The **coronal plane** (koh-**ROH**-nal) is also known as the **frontal plane** (**coron** means head or crown and **-al** means pertaining to). This is any vertical plane, at right angles to the sagittal plane, that divides the body into anterior (front) and posterior (back) portions (Figure 2.2).

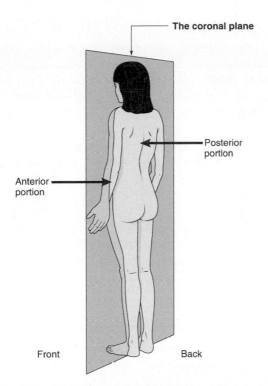

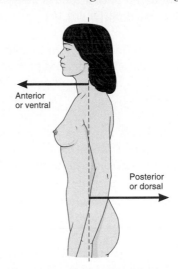

FIGURE 2.2 The coronal plane divides the body into anterior (front) and posterior (back) portions.

Horizontal Planes

● A **horizontal plane** is a flat crosswise line like the horizon.

● The **transverse plane** (trans-**VERSE**), also known as the **horizontal plane**, divides the body into superior (upper) and inferior (lower) portions (Figure 2.3). The transverse plane can be at the waist or at any other level across the body.

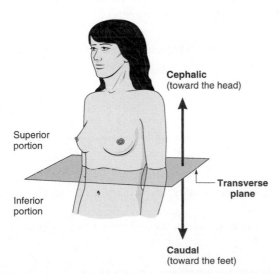

FIGURE 2.3 The transverse plane divides the body into superior (upper) and inferior (lower) portions. This division can be at the waist or at any other level across the body.

BODY DIRECTIONS

The relative location of the whole body or an organ is described through the use of pairs of contrasting body direction terms. These terms are summarized in Table 2.1 and are illustrated in Figures 2.1 through 2.5.

FIGURE 2.4 Body directions. *Anterior* means toward the front, and the front of the body is called the *ventral surface. Posterior* means toward the back, and the back of the body is called the *dorsal surface*.

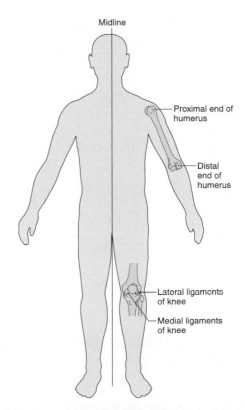

FIGURE 2.5 Body directions. *Proximal* means situated nearest the midline, and *distal* means situated farthest from the midline. *Medial* means toward the midline, and *lateral* means toward the side.

Table 2.1

TERMS USED TO DESCRIBE BODY DIRECTION

Ventral (**VEN**-tral) refers to the front or belly side of the body or organ (**ventr** means belly side of body and **-al** means pertaining to).	**Dorsal** (**DOR**-sal) refers to the back of the body or organ (**dors** means back of body and **-al** means pertaining to).
Anterior (an-**TEER**-ee-or) means situated in the front. It also means on the forward part of an organ (**anter** means front or before and **-ior** means pertaining to). For example, the stomach is located anterior to (in front of) the pancreas. **Anterior** is also used in reference to the ventral surface of the body.	**Posterior** (pos-**TEER**-ee-or) means situated in the back. It is also used in reference to the back part of an organ (**poster** means front or before and **-ior** means pertaining to). For example, the pancreas is located posterior to (behind) the stomach. **Posterior** is also used in reference to the dorsal surface of the body.
Superior means uppermost, above, or toward the head. For example, the lungs are located superior to (above) the diaphragm.	**Inferior** means lowermost, below, or toward the feet. For example, the stomach is located inferior to (below) the diaphragm.
Cephalic (seh-**FAL**-ick) means toward the head (**cephal** means head and **-ic** means pertaining to).	**Caudal** (**KAW**-dal) means toward the lower part of the body (**caud** means tail or lower part of the body and **-al** means pertaining to).
Proximal (**PROCK**-sih-mal) means situated nearest the midline or beginning of a body structure. For example, the proximal end of the humerus (the bone of the upper arm) forms part of the shoulder.	**Distal** (**DIS**-tal) means situated farthest from the midline or beginning of a body structure. For example, the distal end of the humerus forms part of the elbow.
Medial means the direction toward or nearer the midline. For example, the medial ligament of the knee is near the inner surface of the leg.	**Lateral** means the direction toward or nearer the side and away from the midline. For example, the lateral ligament of the knee is near the side of the leg. **Bilateral** means relating to, or having, two sides.

MAJOR BODY CAVITIES

A **body cavity** is a space within the body that contains and protects the internal organs (Figure 2.6).

THE DORSAL CAVITY

The dorsal cavity, which is divided into two parts, protects the structures of the nervous system that coordinate the bodily functions:

- The **cranial cavity,** located within the skull, protects the brain.
- The **spinal cavity,** located within the spinal column, protects the spinal cord.

THE VENTRAL CAVITY

The ventral cavity, which is divided into three parts, contains many of the body organs that maintain homeostasis.

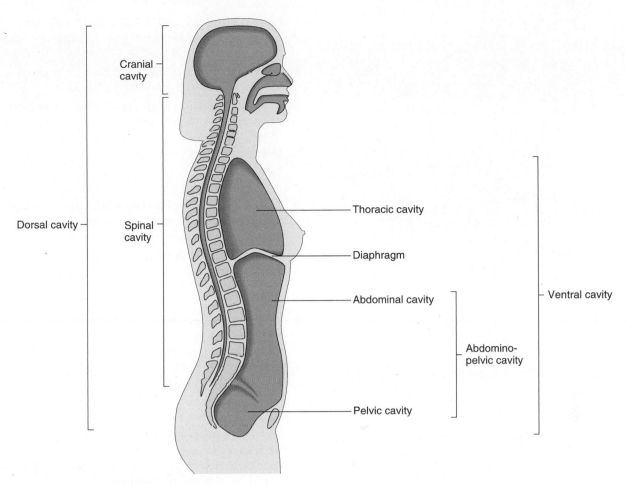

Cranial cavity

Dorsal cavity

Spinal cavity

Thoracic cavity

Diaphragm

Abdominal cavity

Ventral cavity

Abdomino-pelvic cavity

Pelvic cavity

FIGURE 2.6 Major body cavities.

Homeostasis (**hoh**-mee-oh-**STAY**-sis) means maintaining a constant internal environment (**homeo** means constant and **-stasis** means control).

● The **thoracic cavity** (thoh-**RAS**-ick), also known as the **chest cavity,** protects the heart and the lungs. The **diaphragm** is a muscle that separates the thoracic and abdominal cavities.

● The **abdominal cavity** (ab-**DOM**-ih-nal), which contains primarily the major organs of digestion, frequently is referred to simply as the **abdomen** (ab-**DOH**-men *or* **AB**-doh-men).

● The **pelvic cavity** (**PEL**-vick) is the space formed by the pelvic (hip) bones. It contains primarily the organs of the reproductive and excretory systems.

● There is no division between the abdominal and pelvic cavities. Together, they are referred to as the **abdominopelvic cavity** (ab-**dom**-ih-noh-**PEL**-vick).

DIVISIONS OF THE ABDOMEN

Describing where an organ or a pain is located is made easier by dividing the abdomen into four imaginary quadrants (Figure 2.7). (*Quadrant* means divided into four.) These are the

1. Right upper quadrant (RUQ)
2. Left upper quadrant (LUQ)
3. Right lower quadrant (RLQ)
4. Left lower quadrant (LLQ)

REGIONS OF THE THORAX AND ABDOMEN

Another descriptive system divides the abdomen and lower portion of the thorax into nine regions (Figure 2.8):

● The **right** and **left hypochondriac** (**high**-poh-**KON**-dree-ack) **regions** are located on the sides and are covered by the lower ribs. The term **hypochondriac** means below the ribs. It also means an individual with an abnormal and excessive concern about his or her health.

● The **epigastric** (**ep**-ih-**GAS**-trick) **region** is located above the stomach.

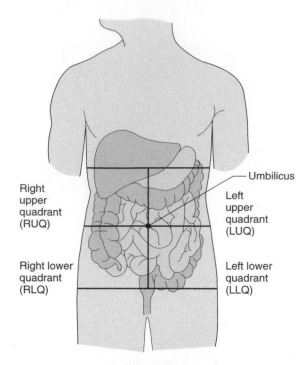

FIGURE 2.7 Division of the abdomen into quadrants.

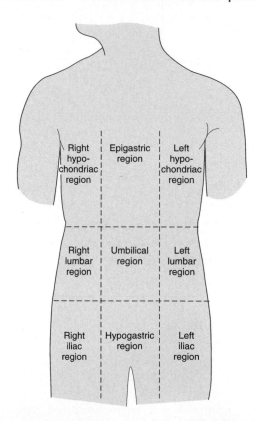

FIGURE 2.8 Regions of the thorax and abdomen.

- The **right** and **left lumbar** (**LUM**-bar) **regions** are located on the sides near the inward curve of the spine.
- The **umbilical** (um-**BILL**-ih-kal) **region** surrounds the **umbilicus** (um-**BILL**-ih-kus). Also known as the

belly button or **navel,** the umbilicus is the pit in the center of the abdominal wall marking the point where the umbilical cord was attached to the fetus.

- The **right** and **left iliac** (**ILL**-ee-ack) **regions** are located on the sides over the hipbones.
- The **hypogastric** (**high**-poh-**GAS**-trick) **region** is located below the stomach. The entire lower region of the abdomen is also referred to as the **groin** or **inguinal** (**ING**-gwih-nal) area.

PERITONEUM

- The **peritoneum** (**pehr**-ih-toh-**NEE**-um) is the membrane that protects and supports (suspends in place) the organs located in the abdominal cavity.
- The **parietal peritoneum** (pah-**RYE**-eh-tal **pehr**-ih-toh-**NEE**-um) is the outer layer of this membrane that lines the abdominal cavity. *Parietal* means cavity wall.
- The **visceral peritoneum** (**VIS**-er-al **pehr**-ih-toh-**NEE**-um) is the inner layer of this membrane that surrounds the organs of the abdominal cavity. *Visceral* means relating to the internal organs.
- The **mesentery** (**MESS**-en-**terr**-ee) is a layer of the peritoneum that suspends parts of the intestine within the abdominal cavity.
- The term **retroperitoneal** (**ret**-roh-**pehr**-ih-toh-**NEE**-al) means located behind the peritoneum of the abdominal cavity (**retro-** means behind, **periton** means peritoneum, and **-eal** means pertaining to).
- **Peritonitis** (**pehr**-ih-toh-**NIGH**-tis) is an inflammation of the peritoneum (**periton** means peritoneum and **-itis** means inflammation).
- **Ascites** (ah-**SIGH**-teez) is an abnormal accumulation of clear or milky serous (watery) fluid in the peritoneal cavity.

LAPAROSCOPIC PROCEDURES

Laparoscopy (**lap**-ah-**ROS**-koh-pee) is the visual examination of the interior of the abdomen with the use of a laparoscope (**lapar/o** means abdomen and **-scopy** means visual examination).

Laparoscopic surgery involves the use of a laparoscope plus instruments inserted into the abdomen through small incisions (Figure 2.9). These are used to

- Explore and examine the interior of the abdomen.
- Take specimens to be biopsied.
- Perform surgical procedures.

CYTOLOGY

Cells are the basic structural units of the body that are specialized and grouped together to form the tissues and organs (Figure 2.10).

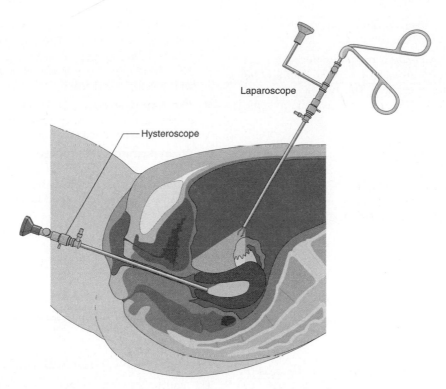

FIGURE 2.9 A laparoscope is used to examine the interior of the abdomen. A hysteroscope is used to examine the interior of the uterus.

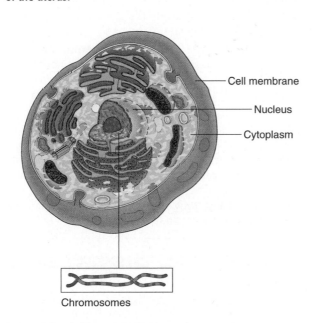

FIGURE 2.10 A diagrammatic representation of basic cell structure.

- **Cytology** (sigh-**TOL**-oh-jee) is the study of the formation, structure, and function of cells (**cyt** means cell and **-ology** means study of).

- The **cell membrane** is the structure that surrounds and protects the cell. A **membrane** (**MEM**-brain) is a thin layer of tissue that covers a surface, lines a cavity, or divides a space or organ.

- **Cytoplasm** (**SIGH**-toh-plazm) is the material within the cell membrane that is *not* part of the nucleus (**cyt/o** means cell and **-plasm** means formative material of cells).

- The **nucleus** (**NEW**-klee-us) (plural, **nuclei**), which is surrounded by the nuclear membrane, is a structure within the cell that has two important functions: (1) It controls the activities of the cell; and (2) it helps the cell divide.

CHROMOSOMES

- The nucleus of each cell contains 46 **chromosomes** (**KROH**-moh-sohmes) arranged into 23 pairs. There are 22 identical pairs plus the single pair (XX or XY) that determines the sex of the child.

- **Sex cells** (sperm and ovum), also known as **gametes** (**GAM**-eets), are the only cells that do not have 46 chromosomes. Instead, each mature sex cell has 23 single chromosomes. When a sperm and ovum join to form a new life, the embryo receives half of its chromosomes from each parent.

DNA

- Chromosomes are organized as two long, coiled molecules of **deoxyribonucleic acid** (dee-**ock**-see-**rye**-boh-new-**KLEE**-ick), which are commonly referred to as **DNA**.

- **Genes** are the functional units of heredity. Each gene is a segment of DNA that is located in a specific site on a chromosome. Each chromosome contains about 100,000 genes.

- The genes in DNA create a unique pattern for each individual. That pattern can be used to identify the source of a tissue specimen. The unique nature of this pattern makes DNA evidence useful in some court cases.

TERMS RELATED TO GENETICS

- **Genetics** is the study of how genes are transferred from the parents to their children and the role of genes in health and disease (**gene** means producing and **-tics** means pertaining to).
- A specialist in the field of genetics is known as a **geneticist** (jeh-**NET**-ih-sist).
- **Genetic engineering** is research to identify defective genes and to develop gene therapy to treat or replace these faulty genes.
- The term **genetic mutation** describes changes that occur within genes.
- **Somatic cell mutation** is change within the cells of the body. These changes affect the individual but cannot be transmitted to the next generation.
- **Gametic cell mutation** is change within the genes found in the gametes (sperm or ovum) that can be transmitted by parents to their children.

GENETIC DISORDERS

Genetic disorders, also known as **hereditary disorders,** are diseases or conditions caused by a defective gene. Although these genes were transmitted from the parents, a genetic disorder may be manifested at any time in life.

There are more than 2,000 known genetic disorders affecting all of the body systems. The following are examples. Additional genetic disorders also are described throughout the text.

- **Cystic fibrosis,** which is discussed in Chapter 7, is a genetic disorder of the exocrine glands. (Exocrine glands are explained later in this chapter in the section titled "Glands.")
- **Down syndrome,** also known as **trisomy 21,** is a genetic syndrome characterized by varying degrees of mental retardation and multiple physical abnormalities. *Note:* Down's syndrome is an alternative spelling. However, the preferred spelling is Down syndrome without the apostrophe and the *s*.)
- **Hemophilia** (**hee**-moh-**FILL**-ee-ah) is a group of hereditary bleeding disorders in which one of the factors needed to clot the blood is missing. Genetic transmission is from a mother to her son.
- **Huntington's disease (HD),** also known as **Huntington's chorea (HC),** is a hereditary disorder with symptoms that first appear in midlife and cause

the irreversible and progressive loss of muscle control and mental ability. The HD gene, which can be detected through genetic testing, is a dominant gene. This means that 50 percent of persons inheriting it will develop the disease.

- **Muscular dystrophy** (**DIS**-troh-fee) (**MD**) is a group of genetic diseases characterized by progressive weakness of muscle fibers (see Chapter 4).
- **Phenylketonuria** (**fen**-il-**kee**-toh-**NEW**-ree-ah) (**PKU**) is a genetic disorder in which an essential digestive enzyme is missing. PKU can be detected by a blood test at birth. If not detected and treated early, PKU causes severe mental retardation.
- **Sickle cell anemia,** which is discussed in Chapter 5, is a serious genetic disorder caused by genes that produce abnormal hemoglobin in the red blood cells.
- **Tay-Sachs disease,** also known as **TSD,** is a hereditary disease marked by progressive physical degeneration, mental retardation, and early death.

GENETIC COUNSELING

The transmission of genetic disorders is a complex "game of chance," and genetic counseling is a valuable tool for persons concerned about genetic disorders. The following example describes the possibilities of transmitting sickle cell anemia:

- An individual with **sickle cell anemia** has only genes for abnormal hemoglobin. If both parents have this disorder, they will both pass this gene to their children and the children will also have sickle cell anemia.
- An individual with **sickle cell trait** does *not* have the disease sickle cell anemia. However, he or she does have one gene for sickle cell anemia and one gene for normal hemoglobin. As shown in Figure 2.11, although the potential parents with sickle cell trait are healthy, they are carriers and can transmit the disease to their children.

CONGENITAL DISORDERS

A **congenital disorder** (kon-**JEN**-ih-tahl) is an abnormal condition that exists at the time of birth and may be caused by a developmental disorder before birth, prenatal influences, premature birth, or injuries during birth:

- A **developmental disorder** may result in an anomaly or malformation such as the absence of a limb or the presence of an extra toe at birth. An **anomaly** (ah-**NOM**-ah-lee) is a deviation from what is regarded as normal.
- **Prenatal influences** are the mother's health and the care she receives before delivery. For example, maternal alcohol consumption during pregnancy can cause the congenital disorder **fetal alcohol syndrome,** which is also known as **FAS.** FAS is charac-

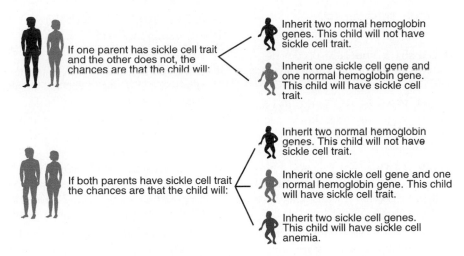

FIGURE 2.11 The genetic probabilities that parents with sickle cell trait will transmit sickle cell anemia to their children.

terized by prenatal and postnatal physical and behavior traits including growth deficiencies and abnormalities, mental retardation, brain damage, and socialization difficulties.

- **Birth injuries** are congenital disorders that were not present before the events surrounding the time of birth. As an example, **cerebral palsy (CP),** which is discussed in Chapter 10, may be caused by premature birth or be due to inadequate oxygen to the brain during birth.

HISTOLOGY

A tissue is a group or layer of similarly specialized cells that join together to perform certain specific functions. **Histology** (hiss-**TOL**-oh-jee) is the study of the structure, composition, and function of tissues (**hist** means tissue and **-ology** means a study of). A **histologist** (hiss-**TOL**-oh-jist) is a specialist in the study of cells and microscopic tissues.

STEM CELLS

- **Stem cells,** also known as **precursor cells,** are cells with the ability to divide without limit and to give rise to specialized cells. Stem cells are abundant in a fetus and in the cord blood of a newborn. These cells are present in limited quantities in adults.

- Each type of tissue has its own stem cells, and when implanted into the appropriate type of tissue the stem cells can regenerate the full range of cell types normally found there. The research goal is to discover how to use stem cells as a source for organ and tissue regeneration. Some applications, such as bone marrow transplants, are already in use (see Chapter 3).

TYPES OF TISSUE

The four main types of tissue are epithelial, connective, muscle, and nerve.

Epithelial Tissues

- **Epithelial tissues** (**ep**-ih-**THEE**-lee-al) form a protective covering for all of the internal and external surfaces of the body.

- **Epithelium** (**ep**-ih-**THEE**-lee-um) is the specialized epithelial tissue that forms the epidermis of the skin and the surface layer of mucous membranes. The skin is discussed further in Chapter 12.

- **Endothelium** (**en**-doh-**THEE**-lee-um) is the specialized epithelial tissue that lines the blood and lymph vessels, body cavities, glands, and organs.

- Glands are made up of specialized epithelial tissues that are capable of producing secretions.

Connective Tissues

Connective tissues support and connect organs and other body tissues.

- Bone, cartilage and other **dense connective tissues** are discussed in Chapter 3.

- **Adipose tissue** (**AD**-ih-pohs), also known as **fat,** provides protective padding, insulation, and support and acts as a nutrient reserve (**adip** means fat and **-ose** means pertaining to).

- **Loose connective tissue** surrounds various organs and supports both nerve cells and blood vessels.

- Blood and lymph, which are discussed in Chapters 5 and 6, are **liquid connective tissues.**

Muscle Tissue

- **Muscle tissue,** which is discussed in Chapter 4, contains cell material with the specialized ability to contract and relax.

Nerve Tissue

- **Nerve tissue,** which is discussed in Chapter 10, contains cells with the specialized ability to react to stimuli and conduct electrical impulses.

PATHOLOGY OF TISSUE FORMATION

- **Aplasia** (ah-**PLAY**-zee-ah) is the lack of development of an organ or tissue (**a-** means without and **-plasia** means formation).
- **Hypoplasia** (**high**-poh-**PLAY**-zee-ah) is the incomplete development of an organ or tissue, but it is less severe in degree than aplasia (**hypo-** means deficient and **-plasia** means formation).
- **Hyperplasia** (**high**-per-**PLAY**-zee-ah) is an abnormal increase in the number of normal cells in normal arrangement in a tissue (**hyper-** means excessive and **-plasia** means formation).
- **Dysplasia** (dis-**PLAY**-see-ah) is the abnormal development or growth, especially of cells (**dys-** means bad and **-plasia** means formation).
- **Anaplasia** (**an**-ah-**PLAY**-zee-ah) is a change in the structure of cells and in their orientation to each other (**ana-** means excessive and **-plasia** means formation). These abnormal cells are characteristic of malignancy and are discussed in Chapter 6. (A *malignancy* is a life-threatening tumor that tends to spread to distant body sites.)

GLANDS

A gland is a group of specialized epithelial cells that form secretions. A **secretion** is the substance produced by a gland. The two types of glands are exocrine and endocrine glands (Figure 2.12):

- **Exocrine glands** (**ECK**-soh-krin), such as sweat glands, secrete their chemical substances into ducts that lead either to other organs or out of the body (**exo-** means out of and **-crine** means to secrete).
- **Endocrine glands** (**EN**-doh-krin), which secrete hormones, do *not* have ducts (**endo-** means within and **-crine** means to secrete). These secretions flow directly into the bloodstream for transportation to organs and other structures throughout the body. (The endocrine system is discussed further in Chapter 13.)

PATHOLOGY AND PROCEDURES OF THE GLANDS

- **Adenectomy** (**ad**-eh-**NECK**-toh-mee) is the surgical removal of a gland (**aden** means gland and **-ectomy** means surgical removal).
- **Adenitis** (ad-eh-**NIGH**-tis) is the inflammation of a gland (**aden** means gland and **-itis** means inflammation).
- An **adenoma** (ad-eh-**NOH**-mah) is a benign tumor in which the cells form recognizable glandular structures (**aden** means gland and **-oma** means tumor). (*Benign* means not life threatening.)
- **Adenomalacia** (ad-eh-noh-mah-**LAY**-shee-ah) is the abnormal softening of a gland (**aden/o** means gland and **-malacia** means abnormal softening).
- **Adenosclerosis** (ad-eh-noh-skleh-**ROH**-sis) is the abnormal hardening of a gland (**aden/o** means gland and **-sclerosis** means abnormal hardening).
- **Adenosis** (ad-eh-**NOH**-sis) is any disease condition of a gland (**aden** means gland and **-osis** means an abnormal condition).

ORGANS AND BODY SYSTEMS

An **organ** is a somewhat independent part of the body that performs a special function or functions.

The tissues and organs of the body are organized into systems that perform specialized functions (Figure 2.13). These systems are outlined in Table 2.2.

PATHOLOGY

- **Pathology** (pah-**THOL**-oh-jee) is the study of structural and functional changes caused by disease (**path/o** and **-pathy** mean disease; however, they also mean suffering, feeling, and emotion). Pathology also means a condition caused by disease.
- A **pathologist** (pah-**THOL**-oh-jist) specializes in the laboratory analysis of tissue samples removed at

(continues)

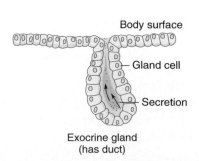

Exocrine gland
(has duct)

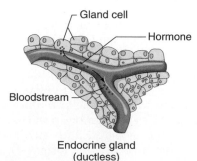

Endocrine gland
(ductless)

FIGURE 2.12   Exocrine glands secrete their chemical substances into ducts that lead either to other organs or out of the body. Endocrine glands pour their secretions directly into the bloodstream.

LEVEL

EXAMPLES

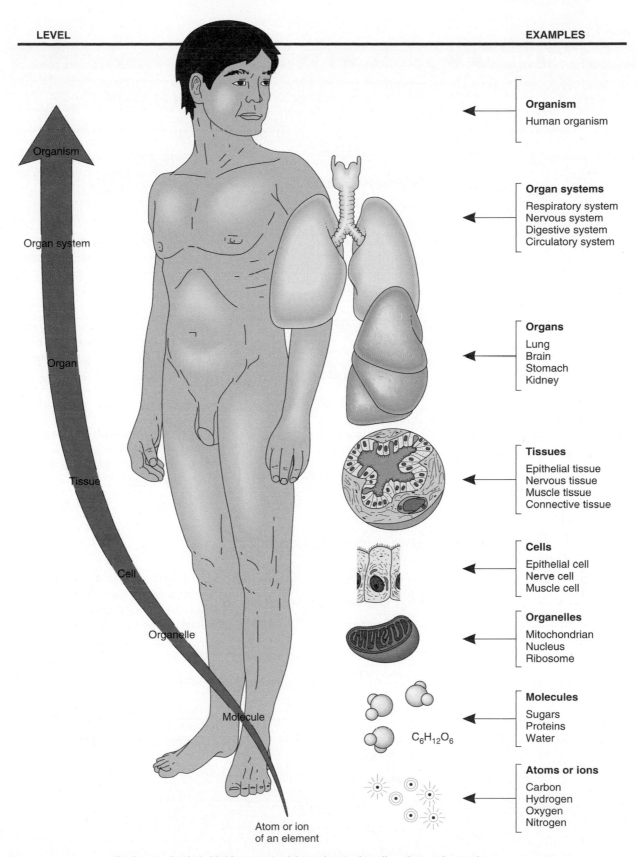

Organism
Human organism

Organ systems
Respiratory system
Nervous system
Digestive system
Circulatory system

Organs
Lung
Brain
Stomach
Kidney

Tissues
Epithelial tissue
Nervous tissue
Muscle tissue
Connective tissue

Cells
Epithelial cell
Nerve cell
Muscle cell

Organelles
Mitochondrian
Nucleus
Ribosome

Molecules
Sugars
Proteins
Water

$C_6H_{12}O_6$

Atoms or ions
Carbon
Hydrogen
Oxygen
Nitrogen

Organism

Organ system

Organ

Tissue

Cell

Organelle

Molecule

Atom or ion
of an element

FIGURE 2.13 The human body is highly organized from the single cell to the total organism.

Table 2.2

MAJOR BODY SYSTEMS

Body System	Major Structures and Related Word Parts	Major Functions
Skeletal System	bones (**oste/o**) cartilage (**chondr/o**) joints (**arthr/o**)	Supports and shapes the body. Protects the internal organs. Forms some blood cells and stores minerals.
Muscular System	fascia (**fasci/o**) muscles (**my/o**) tendons (**ten/o, tend/o, tendin/o**)	Holds the body erect. Makes movement possible. Moves body fluids and generates body heat.
Cardiovascular System	arteries (**arteri/o**) blood (**hem/o, hemat/o**) heart (**card/o, cardi/o**) veins (**phleb/o, ven/o**)	Pumps blood that carries oxygen and nutrients throughout the body. Carries liquid waste to the lungs and kidneys.
Lymphatic and Immune Systems	lymph, lymph vessels, and lymph nodes (**lymph/o**) specialized blood cells spleen (**splen/o**) thymus (**thym/o**) tonsils (**tonsill/o**)	Protects the body from harmful substances. Brings oxygen and nutrients to cells. Removes waste from the cells.
Respiratory System	larynx (**laryng/o**) lungs (**pneum/o, pneumon/o**) nose (**nas/o**) pharynx (**pharyng/o**) trachea (**trache/o**)	Brings oxygen into the body for transportation to the cells. Removes carbon dioxide and some water waste from the body.
Digestive System	esophagus (**esophag/o**) large intestines (**col/o**) liver (**hepat/o**) mouth (**or/o**) pancreas (**pancreat/o**) small intestines (**enter/o**) stomach (**gastr/o**)	Digests ingested food so it can be absorbed into the bloodstream. Eliminates solid wastes.

Body System	Major Structures and Related Word Parts	Major Functions
Urinary System	kidneys (**nephr/o, ren/o**) ureters (**ureter/o**) urethra (**urethr/o**) urinary bladder (**cyst/o, vesic/o**)	Filters blood to remove waste. Maintains the electrolyte and fluid balance within the body.
Nervous System	brain (**encephal/o**) ears (**acoust/o, ot/o**) eyes (**ocul/o, ophthalm/o**) nerves (**neur/o**) spinal cord (**myel/o**)	Coordinates the reception of stimuli. Transmits messages throughout the body.
Integumentary System	sebaceous glands (**seb/o**) skin (**cutane/o, dermat/o, derm/o**) sweat glands (**hidr/o**)	Protects the body against invasion by bacteria. Regulates the body temperature and water content.
Endocrine System	adrenals (**adren/o**) gonads **gonad/o** pancreas (**pancreat/o**) parathyroids (**parathyroid/o**) pineal (**pineal/o**) pituitary (**pituit/o**) thymus (**thym/o**) thyroid (**thyroid/o**)	Integrates all body functions.
Reproductive System	**Male:** testicles (**orch/o, orchid/o**) **Female:** ovaries (**oophor/o, ovari/o**) uterus (**hyster/o, metr/o, metri/o, uter/o**)	Produces new life.

operations and postmortem (after death) examinations to confirm or establish a diagnosis (**path** means disease and **-ologist** means specialist). A postmortem examination is also known as an **autopsy** (**AW**-top-see).

- **Etiology** (**ee**-tee-**OL**-oh-jee) is the study of the causes of diseases (**eti-** means cause and **-ology** means study of). The organisms that cause diseases are discussed further in Chapter 6.

- Terms used to describe different types of diseases are summarized in Table 2.3.

DISEASE TRANSMISSION

- A **communicable disease** (kuh-**MEW**-nih-kuh-bul), also known as a **contagious disease,** is any disease transmitted from one person to another either by

Table 2.3

TYPES OF DISEASES

An **infectious disease** (in-**FECK**-shus) is an illness caused by a pathogenic organism.

An **idiopathic disorder** (id-ee-oh-**PATH**-ick) is an illness without known cause.

In an **organic disorder** (or-**GAN**-ick), there are pathologic, physical changes that explain the symptoms being experienced by the patient. For example, a gastric ulcer is an organic disorder (see Chapter 8).

In a **functional disorder**, there are no detectable physical changes to explain the symptoms that are being experienced by the patient. For example, a panic attack is a functional disorder (see Chapter 10).

An **iatrogenic illness** (eye-**at**-roh-**JEN**-ick) is a problem, such as a side effect or an unfavorable response, arising from a prescribed medical treatment.

A **nosocomial infection** (nos-oh-**KOH**-mee-al) is an infection acquired in a hospital setting that was not present on admission but appears 72 hours or more after hospitalization.

direct contact or indirectly by contact with contaminated objects.

- **Contaminated** means the possible presence of an infectious agent. Contamination may occur through a lack of proper hygiene standards such as handwashing or taking proper precautions.
- **Bloodborne transmission** is through contact with blood or body fluids that are contaminated with blood. Examples include acquired immunodeficiency syndrome (AIDS) and hepatitis. Bloodborne diseases are also transmitted through sexual contact. These disorders are discussed in Chapters 5 and 6.
- **Sexually transmitted diseases,** also known as **STDs** and **venereal diseases,** require direct person-to-person contact or contact with lesions. These disorders are discussed in Chapter 14.
- **Airborne transmission** occurs through respiratory droplets such as contact with material from a cough or a sneeze. Examples include tuberculosis, influenza, colds, and measles. These disorders are discussed in Chapter 7.
- **Foodborne and waterborne transmission,** also known as **fecal/oral transmission,** is caused by eating or drinking contaminated food or water that

has not been prepared properly to kill the contamination. These disorders are discussed in Chapter 8.

OUTBREAKS OF DISEASES

- An **epidemiologist** (**ep**-ih-**dee**-mee-**OL**-oh-jist) specializes in the study of outbreaks of disease within a population group.
- **Endemic** (en-**DEM**-ick) refers to the ongoing presence of a disease within a population, group, or area. For example, the common cold is endemic because it is always present within the population.
- An **epidemic** (**ep**-ih-**DEM**-ick) is a sudden and widespread outbreak of a disease within a population group or area. For example, a sudden widespread outbreak of measles is an epidemic.
- **Pandemic** (pan-**DEM**-ick) refers to an outbreak of a disease occurring over a large geographic area, possibly worldwide. For example, AIDS is pandemic.

Career Opportunities

In addition to medical specialties requiring advanced graduate degrees, such as an MD, there are many interesting health occupations to consider. Some specialists work primarily with one body system, such as a dental assistant or a respiratory therapist. (These are listed at the end of each of the body system chapters following this one.) Others treat the patient's general healthcare needs, including:

- **Medical assistant:** prepares patients for examination, takes vital signs and medical history, performs basic laboratory tests, and cleans and maintains equipment; may also fill an administrative role such as receptionist or office manager
- **Nurse assistant, nurse's aide, patient care technician (PCT),** or **orderly:** provides basic and essential patient care such as bathing, bed making, and feeding
- **Registered nurse (RN), licensed practical nurse (LPN),** and **licensed vocational nurse (LVN):** state licensed to provide and manage patient care. An RN is authorized to provide specialized services, including administering medications, teaching, and supervising other staff members. An LPN or LVN provides for patients' needs under the supervision of an RN or physician. There are many nursing specialties, including:

Community health nurse	IV therapy nurse
Critical care nurse	Nurse anesthetist
Flight nurse	Private duty nurse
Hospice nurse	School nurse
Infectious disease nurse	Surgery scrub nurse

- **Nurse practitioner (NP):** an RN with advanced training in the diagnosis and treatment of illness. An NP provides primary care for patients, often in collaboration with a physician, and in some states NPs may write prescriptions.
- **Physician's assistant (PA):** performs routine medical examinations and diagnostic tests and treats minor injuries and diseases under the supervision of a physician. In many states, a PA may prescribe medications.
- **Medical translator:** provides bilingual assistance for accurate communications between healthcare providers and non-English-speaking patients. A medical translator must know medical terminology in English and a second language.

STUDY BREAK

What is the most common infectious disease on the earth? Hint: You would have to live in a small, very isolated community, or perhaps in the frozen wastelands of Antarctica to avoid it, and yet no one has found a cure.

Answer: the **common cold.** We do know that this contagious condition is usually caused by one of more than 100 types of rhinovirus (*rhino* = nose, plus *virus*) and that it is spread through sneezing, coughing, and inadequate hand washing.

The common cold is sometimes confused with the flu, or influenza, which can be fatal. In fact, in the deadliest flu outbreak on record, more than 21 million people died worldwide in just two years (1918 and 1919). The flu is a viral infection characterized by a fever in addition to coldlike symptoms. It is very contagious and usually occurs in epidemics rather than isolated cases. An annual vaccination with inactivated flu virus strains helps the body develop antibodies to protect against infection.

Health Occupation Profile: EMERGENCY ROOM TECHNICIAN

Vicky Edwards is an emergency room technician at a hospital in St. Louis. "My years of working for doctors in their offices (ENT, internal medicine, general surgery) gave me a good background for the interesting and intense work I do at the hospital. My duties include aiding with triage (screening patients to determine the priority of treatment), head-to-toe patient assessment, phlebotomy (taking blood), and all point-of-care procedures such as inserting catheters and taking blood sugar tests, EKGs, and vital signs. Emergency trauma situations are frequent in a big city hospital, and it is exhilarating when we are able to save a life. But caring for all our patients and giving them that little extra TLC are just as important."

Review Time

Write the answers to the following questions on a separate piece of paper or in your notebook. In addition, be prepared to take part in the classroom discussion.

1. **Written assignment:** Using terms a layperson would understand, state the differences between **congenital** and **genetic disorders** and give an example of each.

    Discussion assignment: How do you think genetic counseling would affect a young couple who are at risk for transmitting cystic fibrosis to their children?

2. **Written assignment:** What is the difference between an **organic disorder** and a **functional disorder?**

    Discussion assignment: Give examples of organic and functional disorders.

3. **Written assignment:** What is the difference between an **iatrogenic illness** and a **nosocomial infection?**

    Discussion assignment: What are potential causes of each type of condition?

4. **Written assignment:** Using your own words, describe the differences between **sagittal, coronal,** and **transverse planes.**

    Discussion assignment: Where is each of these planes located?

5. **Written assignment:** Identify the **two dorsal** and **three ventral body cavities.**

    Discussion assignment: How would you describe to a patient which organs are protected by each cavity?

Optional Internet Activity

*The goal of this activity is to help you learn more about medical terminology while improving your Internet skills. Select **one** of these two options and follow the instructions.*

1. **Internet Search:** Search for information about **Down syndrome.** Write a brief (one- or two-paragraph) report on something new that you learned here and include the address of the web site where you found this information.

2. **Web Site:** To learn more about diseases that can be treated with **cord blood,** go to this web address: **http://www.americancordblood.com** and look under FAQs. Write a brief (one- or two-paragraph) report on something new you learned here.

The Human Touch: Critical Thinking Exercise

The following story and questions are designed to stimulate critical thinking through class discussion or as a brief essay response. There are no right or wrong answers to these questions.

Tabriah and Justise Brown have three wonderful children. The oldest is in her second year at the community college. The middle one plays third base for his high school varsity team, and the youngest is a freshman with an eye on the tennis team. The Browns are looking forward to planning weddings and spoiling grandbabies. But then, at age 44, Tabriah discovers she is pregnant.

Her obstetrician, Dr. Makay, suggests performing genetic testing using amniotic fluid gathered by a procedure called amniocentesis. He tells her, "Technical advances allow a glimpse into the womb to discover genetic anomalies. Because of your age, Tabriah, I am concerned about Down syndrome." He waits, gauging her reaction, then continues.

"This genetic disorder causes various degrees of mental retardation and physical defects. Severe cases produce a child unable to feed or care for itself. Life-threatening physical defects may require expensive, painful surgical procedures. Although they do exhibit the typical Down facial appearance, some of these children display only marginal symptoms and function within societal norms."

Dr. Makay discusses choices the Browns would need to make if genetic testing indicates Down syndrome. Finally he says, "We can detect its presence, but not the degree or severity. Don't decide now. Go home, talk with your family, and call me soon with your decision."

Tabriah, Justise, and their children discuss the possibilities that amniocentesis presents. They talk late into the night. The decision is difficult, but in the morning Tabriah calls Dr. Makay to...

Suggested Discussion Topics

1. Discuss the challenges a Down syndrome child would present to the Brown family.
2. Genetic testing can determine gender, negative and positive genetic characteristics, and whether a fetus will grow up to have a high risk of certain diseases (such as breast cancer). Discuss how this type of information could be used by parents, healthcare providers, and insurance companies.
3. Discuss the options available to Tahriah if the genetic test is positive for Down syndrome.
4. If you were aware that you carried a gene that gave you a 50-50 chance of having a child with a severe birth defect, would you still plan to have children? Why or why not?
5. Children with severe handicaps require expensive care whether they live at home or in an institution. Who should pay for this burden and why?

Student Workbook and Student Activity CD-ROM

1. Go to your **Student Workbook** and complete the Learning Exercises for this chapter and the **Word Part Review** activities.
2. Go to the **Student Activity CD-ROM** and have fun with the exercises and games for this chapter.

3 The Skeletal System

● Overview of Structures, Word Parts, and Functions of the Skeletal System

MAJOR STRUCTURES	RELATED WORD ROOTS	PRIMARY FUNCTIONS
Bones	**oss/e, oss/i, oste/o, ost/o**	Act as the framework for the body, protect the internal organs, and store the mineral calcium.
Bone Marrow	**myel/o** *(also means spinal cord)*	Forms some blood cells.
Cartilage	**chondr/o**	Creates a smooth surface for motion within the joints and protects the ends of the bones.
Joints	**arthr/o**	Work with the muscles to make a variety of motions possible.
Ligaments	**ligament/o**	Connect one bone to another.
Synovial Membrane	**synovi/o, synov/o**	Forms the lining of synovial joints and secretes synovial fluid.
Synovial Fluid	**synovi/o, synov/o**	Lubricant that makes smooth joint movements possible.
Bursa	**burs/o**	Cushions areas subject to friction during movement.

Vocabulary Related to the Skeletal System

Terms marked with the ❖ symbol are pronounced on the Student Activity CD-ROM that accompanies this text.

KEY WORD PARTS

- [ ] ankyl/o
- [ ] arthr/o
- [ ] chondr/o
- [ ] cost/o
- [ ] crani/o
- [ ] -desis
- [ ] kyph/o
- [ ] lord/o
- [ ] -lysis
- [ ] myel/o
- [ ] oss/e, oss/i, ost/o, oste/o
- [ ] -poietic
- [ ] scoli/o
- [ ] spondyl/o
- [ ] -um

KEY MEDICAL TERMS

- [ ] **allogenic** (**al**-oh-**JEN**-ick) ❖
- [ ] **ankylosing spondylitis**
      (**ang**-kih-**LOH**-sing **spon**-dih-**LYE**-tis) ❖
- [ ] **ankylosis** (**ang**-kih-**LOH**-sis) ❖
- [ ] **arthrocentesis** (**ar**-throh-sen-**TEE**-sis) ❖
- [ ] **arthrodesis** (**ar**-throh-**DEE**-sis) ❖
- [ ] **arthrolysis** (**ar**-**THROL**-ih-sis) ❖
- [ ] **arthroplasty** (**AR**-throh-**plas** tee) ❖
- [ ] **arthrosclerosis** (**ar**-throh-skleh-**ROH**-sis) ❖
- [ ] **arthroscopic** (**ar**-throh-**SKOP**-ick)
- [ ] **arthroscopy** (**ar**-**THROS**-koh-pee) ❖
- [ ] **autologous** (aw-**TOL**-uh-guss) ❖
- [ ] **bursectomy** (ber-**SECK**-toh-mee) ❖
- [ ] **bursitis** (ber-**SIGH**-tis) ❖
- [ ] **callus** (**KAL**-us) ❖
- [ ] **chondroma** (kon-**DROH**-mah) ❖
- [ ] **chondromalacia** (**kon**-droh-mah-**LAY**-shee-ah) ❖
- [ ] **chondroplasty** (**KON**-droh-**plas**-tee) ❖
- [ ] **comminuted** (**KOM**-ih-**newt**-ed) ❖
- [ ] **craniectomy** (**kray**-nee-**EK**-toh-mee) ❖
- [ ] **cranioplasty** (**KRAY**-nee-oh-**plas**-tee) ❖
- [ ] **crepitation** (**krep**-ih-**TAY**-shun)
- [ ] **crepitus** (**KREP**-ih-tus) ❖
- [ ] **cruciate** (**KROO**-shee-ayt)
- [ ] **Ewing's sarcoma** (**YOU**-ingz sar-**KOH**-mah) ❖
- [ ] **exostosis** (**eck**-sos-**TOH**-sis) ❖
- [ ] **fontanel** (**fon**-tah-**NELL**)
- [ ] **gouty arthritis** (**GOW**-tee ar-**THRIGH**-tis) ❖
- [ ] **hallux valgus** (**HAL**-ucks **VAL**-guss) ❖
- [ ] **hematopoietic** (**hee**-mah-toh-poi-**ET**-ick *or* **hem**-ah-toh-poi-**ET**-ick)

- [ ] **kyphosis** (kye-**FOH**-sis) ❖
- [ ] **laminectomy** (**lam**-ih-**NECK** toh mee) ❖
- [ ] **lordosis** (lor-**DOH**-sis) ❖
- [ ] **lumbago** (lum-**BAY**-goh) ❖
- [ ] **luxation** (luck-**SAY**-shun) ❖
- [ ] **maxillary** (**MACK**-sih-**ler**-ee)
- [ ] **myeloma** (**my**-eh-**LOH**-mah) ❖
- [ ] **orthopedist** (**or**-thoh-**PEE**-dist) ❖
- [ ] **orthotics** (or-**THOT**-icks) ❖
- [ ] **ostectomy** (oss-**TECK**-toh-mee)
- [ ] **osteitis** (**oss**-tee-**EYE**-tis) ❖
- [ ] **osteitis deformans**
      (**oss**-tee-**EYE**-tis dee-**FOR**-manz)
- [ ] **osteoarthritis** (**oss**-tee-oh-ar-**THRIGH**-tis) ❖
- [ ] **osteochondroma**
      (**oss**-tee-oh-kon-**DROH**-mah) ❖
- [ ] **osteoclasis** (**oss**-tee-**OCK**-lah-sis) ❖
- [ ] **osteomalacia** (**oss**-tee-oh-mah-**LAY**-shee-ah) ❖
- [ ] **osteomyelitis** (**oss**-tee-oh-**my**-eh-**LYE**-tis) ❖
- [ ] **osteonecrosis** (**oss**-tee-oh-neh-**KROH**-sis) ❖
- [ ] **osteoplasty** (**OSS**-tee-oh-**plas**-tee) ❖
- [ ] **osteoporosis** (**oss**-tee-oh-poh-**ROH**-sis) ❖
- [ ] **osteorrhaphy** (**oss**-tee-**OR**-ah-fee) ❖
- [ ] **osteotomy** (**oss**-tee-**OT**-oh-mee) ❖
- [ ] **Paget's** (**PAJ**-its) ❖
- [ ] **patella** (pah-**TEL**-ah)
- [ ] **percutaneous diskectomy**
      (**per**-kyou-**TAY**-nee-us dis-**KECK**-toh-mee) ❖
- [ ] **periosteotomy** (**pehr**-ee-**oss**-tee-**OT**-oh-mee) ❖
- [ ] **periosteum** (**pehr**-ee-**OSS**-tee-um)
- [ ] **periostitis** (**pehr**-ee-oss-**TYE**-tis) ❖
- [ ] **podiatrist** (poh-**DYE**-ah-trist) ❖
- [ ] **popliteal** (pop-**LIT**-ee-al)
- [ ] **rheumatoid arthritis**
      (**ROO**-mah-toyd ar-**THRIGH**-tis) ❖
- [ ] **rheumatologist** (roo-mah-**TOL**-oh-jist) ❖
- [ ] **rickets** (**RICK**-ets) ❖
- [ ] **sacroiliac** (**say**-kroh-**ILL**-ee-ack)
- [ ] **scoliosis** (**skoh**-lee-**OH**-sis) ❖
- [ ] **spina bifida** (**SPY**-nah **BIF**-ih-dah) ❖
- [ ] **spondylitis** (spon-dih-**LYE**-tis) ❖
- [ ] **spondylolisthesis** (**spon**-dih-loh-liss-**THEE**-sis) ❖
- [ ] **spondylosis** (**spon**-dih-**LOH**-sis) ❖
- [ ] **subluxation** (**sub**-luck-**SAY**-shun)
- [ ] **synovectomy** (sin-oh-**VECK**-toh-mee) ❖
- [ ] **synovitis** (sin-oh-**VYE**-tiss) ❖
- [ ] **talipes** (**TAL**-ih-peez) ❖
- [ ] **vertebrae** (**VER**-teh-bray *or* **VER**-teh-bree) ❖
- [ ] **vertebral** (**VER**-tee-bral *or* **VER**-teh-bral)

Objectives

Upon completion of this chapter, you should be able to:

1. Identify and describe the major functions and structures of the skeletal system.

2. Describe three types of joints.

3. Differentiate between the axial and appendicular skeletons.

4. Identify the medical specialists who treat disorders of the skeletal system.

5. Recognize, define, spell, and pronounce terms related to the pathology and diagnostic and treatment procedures of the skeletal system.

FUNCTIONS OF THE SKELETAL SYSTEM

The skeletal system has many important functions:

● Bones act as the framework of the body.

● Bones support and protect the internal organs.

● Joints, in conjunction with muscles, ligaments, and tendons, make possible the wide variety of body movements.

● Calcium required for normal nerve and muscle function is stored in bones.

● Red bone marrow, which is located in spongy bone, has an important function in the formation of blood.

STRUCTURES OF THE SKELETAL SYSTEM

The structures of the skeletal system include bones, cartilage, ligaments, joints, and bursa.

THE STRUCTURE OF BONES

Bone is a form of connective tissue and is almost the hardest tissue in the human body (only dental enamel is harder).

THE TISSUES OF BONE

Although it is very hard and dense, bone is a living structure that changes and is capable of healing itself. The tissues that make up a bone are summarized in Table 3.1.

BONE MARROW

● **Red bone marrow,** located within the spongy bone, is hematopoietic and manufactures red blood cells, hemoglobin, white blood cells, and megakaryocytes that produce thrombocytes. These types of blood cells are discussed in Chapter 5. *Caution*: The word part **myel/o** means either bone marrow *or* spinal cord.

● **Hematopoietic** (**hee**-mah-toh-poi-**ET**-ick *or* **hem**-ah-toh-poi-**ET**-ick) means pertaining to the formation of blood cells (**hemat/o** means blood and **-poietic** means pertaining to formation). The term **hemopoietic** (**hee**-moh-poy-**ET**-ick) also means pertaining to the formation of blood cells (**hem/o** means blood and **-poietic** means pertaining to formation).

● **Yellow bone marrow,** found in the medullary cavity, is composed chiefly of fat cells and functions as a fat storage area.

Table 3.1

TISSUES OF A BONE	
Periosteum (pehr-ee-**OSS**-tee-um)	The tough, fibrous tissue that forms the outermost covering of bone (**peri-** means surrounding, **oste** means bone, and **-um** is a noun ending).
Compact Bone	The hard, dense, and very strong bone that forms the outer layer of the bones.
Spongy Bone	Lighter and not as strong as compact bone, it is commonly found in the ends and inner portions of long bones such as the femur. Red bone marrow is located within this spongy bone.
Medullary Cavity (MED-you-**lehr**-ee)	Located in the shaft of a long bone, the medullary cavity is surrounded by compact bone. It is lined with **endosteum** (en-**DOS**-tee-um) and contains yellow bone marrow.

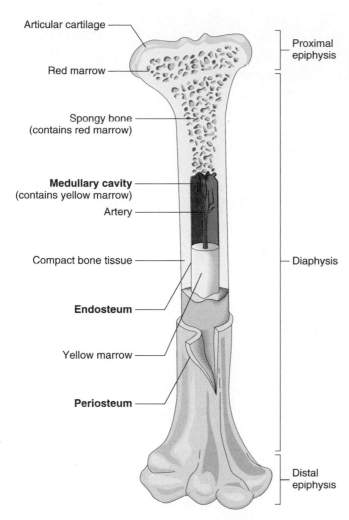

FIGURE 3.1 Anatomic features of a typical long bone.

CARTILAGE

● **Cartilage** (**KAR**-tih-lidj) is the smooth, rubbery blue-white connective tissue that acts as a shock absorber between bones. Cartilage, which is more elastic than bone, makes up the flexible parts of the skeleton such as the outer ear and the tip of the nose.

● **Articular cartilage** (ar-**TICK**-you-lar **KAR**-tih-lidj) covers the surfaces of bones that form joints to make smooth joint movement possible and to protect the bones from rubbing against each other (see Figure 3.1 [on the proximal epiphysis] and Figure 3.5).

● The **meniscus** (meh-**NIS**-kus) is the curved fibrous cartilage found in some joints such as the knee and the temporomandibular joint of the jaw (see Figure 3.4).

ANATOMIC LANDMARKS OF A BONE

● The **diaphysis** (dye-**AF**-ih-sis) is the shaft of a long bone (see Figure 3.1).

● The **epiphysis** (eh-**PIF**-ih-sis), which is covered with articular cartilage, is the wide end of a long bone.

● The **proximal epiphysis** is the end of the bone that is located nearest to the midline of the body.

● The **distal epiphysis** is the end of the bone that is located farthest away from the midline.

● A **foramen** (foh-**RAY**-men) (plural **foramina**) is an opening in a bone through which blood vessels, nerves, and ligaments pass. For example, the spinal cord runs through the vertebral foramen shown in Figure 3.13.

● A **process** is a normal projection on the surface of a bone that serves as attachments for muscles and tendons. For example, the mastoid process is a bony projection located on each temporal bone just behind the ear (see Figure 3.9).

JOINTS

Joints, also known as **articulations,** are connections between bones.

● As used here, the term **articulate** (ar-**TICK**-you-late) means to join or come together in a manner that allows motion between the parts.

● Articulate also means to speak clearly.

TYPES OF JOINTS

Different types of joints make a wide range of motions possible. These include sutures, symphyses, and synovial joints.

Sutures

● A **suture** is the jagged line where bones join and form a joint that does not move. (*Suture* also means to stitch.) Figure 3.2 shows the coronal and sagittal sutures across the top of the skull in an adult.

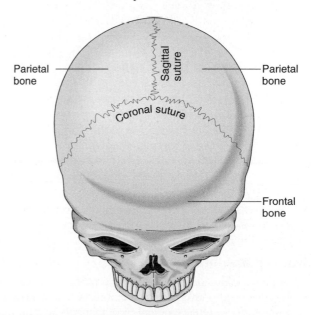

FIGURE 3.2 Bones and sutures of the adult skull as viewed from above.

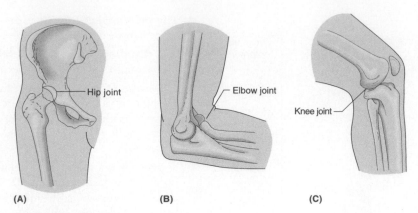

FIGURE 3.3 Examples of synovial joints. (A) Ball and socket joint of the hip. (B) Hinge joint of the elbow. (C) Hinge joint of the knee.

- On a baby's head the **fontanel** (**fon**-tah-**NELL**), also known as the **soft spot,** is where the sutures between the frontal and parietal bones have not yet closed. This spot disappears as the child grows and the sutures close. (This is also spelled **fontanelle**.)

Symphysis

- A **symphysis** (**SIM**-fih-sis) (plural, **symphyses**), also known as a **cartilaginous joint** (**kar**-tih-**LADJ**-ih-nus), is where two bones join and are held firmly together so that they function as one bone. The pubic symphysis is shown in Figure 3.15.

Synovial Joints

- **Synovial joints** (sih-**NOH**-vee-al) are the movable joints of the body. Although these joints are described in simple terms, they are actually very complex structures (Figure 3.3).
- **Ball and socket joints,** such as the hips and shoulders, are synovial joints that allow a wide range of movement in many directions (Figure 3.3A).
- **Hinge joints,** such as the knees and elbows, are synovial joints that allow movement primarily in one direction or plane (Figure 3.3B and 3.3C).

STRUCTURES OF SYNOVIAL JOINTS

Ligaments

- A **ligament** (**LIG**-ah-ment) is a band of fibrous connective tissue that connects one bone to another bone (Figure 3.4).
- Be careful not to confuse ligaments and tendons. **Tendons,** which attach muscles to bones, are discussed in Chapter 4.

Synovial Membrane and Fluid

- Synovial joints are surrounded by a fibrous capsule and are lined with synovial membrane. The synovial membrane secretes synovial fluid that acts as a lubricant to make the smooth movement of the joint possible (Figure 3.5).

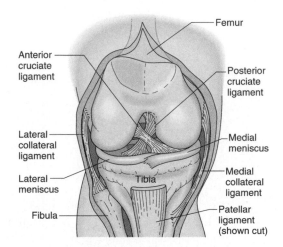

FIGURE 3.4 Major ligaments of the knee. This anterior schematic representation of the knee, with the patella removed, shows the complex system of ligaments that makes knee movements possible.

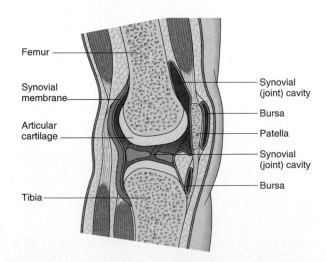

FIGURE 3.5 Structures of a synovial joint and bursa. (This is a lateral view of the knee.)

Bursa

● A **bursa** (**BER**-sah) (plural, **bursae**) is a fibrous sac that is lined with a synovial membrane and contains synovial fluid. A bursa acts as a cushion to ease movement in areas that are subject to friction such as in shoulder, elbow, and knee joints where a tendon passes over a bone (see Figures 3.5 and 4.16).

THE SKELETON

The 206 bones in the adult human body are shown in Figures 3.6, 3.7, and 3.8. For descriptive purposes, the skeleton is divided into the axial and appendicular skeletal systems.

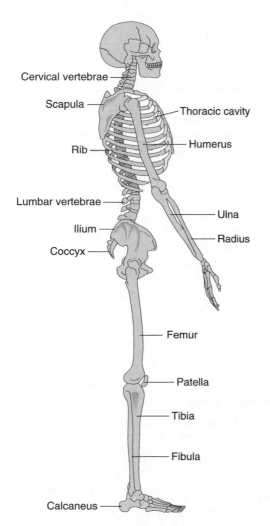

FIGURE 3.6 Lateral view of the adult human skeleton.

AXIAL SKELETON

● The **axial skeleton** (80 bones) protects the major organs of the nervous, respiratory, and circulatory systems. The term *axial* refers to an imaginary line or axis that runs through the center of the body.

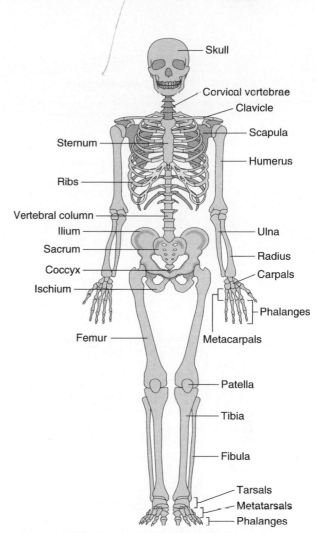

FIGURE 3.7 Anterior view of the adult human skeleton.

● The axial skeleton consists of the skull, spinal (vertebral) column, ribs, and sternum.

APPENDICULAR SKELETON

● The **appendicular skeleton** (126 bones) makes body movement possible and also protects the organs of digestion, excretion, and reproduction. The term *appendicular* means referring to an appendage, which is anything that is attached to a major part of the body.

● The appendicular skeleton is organized into the **upper extremities** (shoulders, arms, forearms, wrists, and hands) and the **lower extremities** (hips, thighs, legs, ankles, and feet).

BONES OF THE SKULL

As you study the following bones of the skull, refer to Figures 3.9 and 3.10.

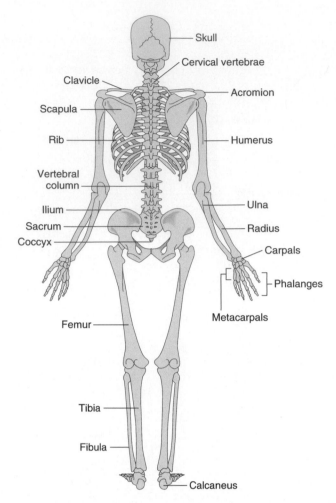

Skull
Cervical vertebrae
Clavicle
Acromion
Scapula
Rib
Humerus
Vertebral column
Ilium
Ulna
Sacrum
Radius
Coccyx
Carpals
Phalanges
Metacarpals
Femur
Tibia
Fibula
Calcaneus

FIGURE 3.8 Posterior view of the adult human skeleton.

Bones of the Cranium

- The **cranium (KRAY**-nee-um) is the portion of the skull that encloses the brain (**crani** means skull and **-um** is a noun ending). The cranium is made up of the following bones:

  - The **frontal bone** forms the forehead.

  - The **parietal bones** (pah-**RYE**-eh-tal) form most of the roof and upper sides of the cranium.

  - The **occipital bone** (ock-**SIP**-ih-tal) forms the posterior floor and walls of the cranium. The spinal cord passes through the **foramen magnum** of the occipital bone.

  - The **temporal bones** form the sides and base of the cranium.

  - The **sphenoid bone** (**SFEE**-noid) forms part of the base of the skull and parts of the floor and sides of the orbit. The *orbit* is the bony socket that surrounds and protects the eyeball.

  - The **ethmoid bone** (**ETH**-moid) forms part of the nose, the orbit, and the floor of the cranium.

Auditory Ossicles

- The **auditory ossicles** (**OSS**-ih-kulz), which are the bones of the middle ear, are discussed in Chapter 11.

- The **external auditory meatus** (mee-**AY**-tus), which is the external opening of the ear, is located in the temporal bone.

Bones of the Face

- The **zygomatic bones** (zye-goh-**MAT**-ick), also known as the **cheekbones,** articulate with the frontal bones.

- The **maxillary bones** (**MACK**-sih-**ler**-ee) form most of the upper jaw.

- The **palatine bones** (**PAL**-ah-tine) form part of the hard palate of the mouth and the floor of the nose.

- The **lacrimal bones** (**LACK**-rih-mal) make up part of the orbit at the inner angle of the eye.

- The **inferior conchae** (**KONG**-kee *or* **KONG**-kay) are the thin, scroll-like bones that form part of the interior of the nose (singular, **concha**).

- The **vomer bone** (**VOH**-mer) forms the base for the nasal septum. The **nasal septum** is the cartilage structure that divides the two nasal cavities and forms the base of the nose.

- The **mandible** (**MAN**-dih-bul), also known as the **lower jawbone,** is the only movable bone of the skull. The mandible is attached to the skull at the **temporomandibular joint** (tem-poh-roh-man-**DIB**-you-lar), which is also known as the **TMJ.**

- The **hyoid bone** (**HIGH**-oid) is unique in that it does not articulate with any other bone. Instead, it is suspended between the mandible and the laryngopharynx (see Figure 7.5).

THORACIC CAVITY, RIBS, AND STERNUM

Thoracic Cavity

- The **thoracic cavity** (thoh-**RAS**-ick) is made up of the ribs, sternum, and thoracic vertebrae (see Figure 3.6). Also known as the **rib cage,** this structure protects the heart and lungs.

Ribs

- There are 12 pairs of ribs, called **costals** (**KOSS**-tulz), which attach posteriorly to the thoracic vertebrae (**cost** means rib, and **-al** means pertaining to).

- The first seven pairs of ribs, called **true ribs,** are attached anteriorly to the sternum (Figure 3.11).

- The next three pairs of ribs, called **false ribs,** are attached anteriorly to cartilage that joins with the sternum.

- The last two pairs of ribs, called **floating ribs,** are not attached anteriorly.

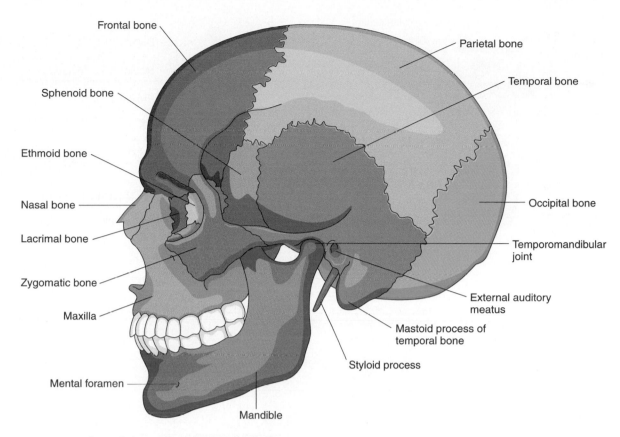

FIGURE 3.9   Lateral view of the adult human skull.

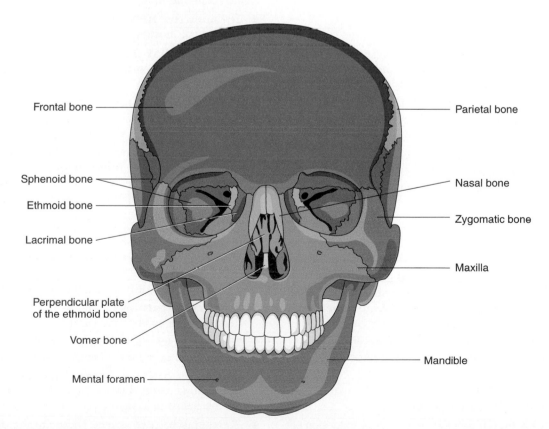

FIGURE 3.10   Anterior view of the adult human skull.

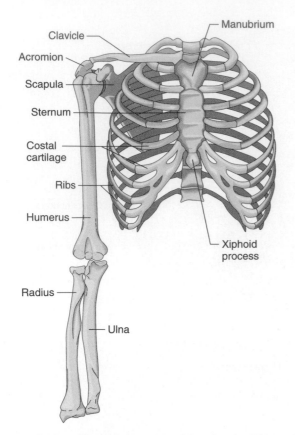

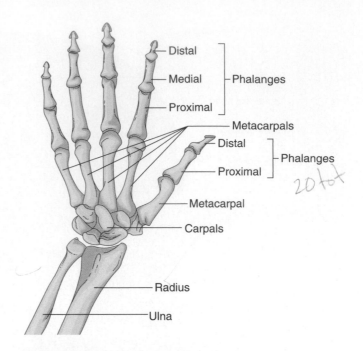

FIGURE 3.12 Dorsal view of the bones of the lower left arm, wrist, and hand.

FIGURE 3.11 Anterior view of the ribs, shoulder, and arm. (Cartilage structures are shown in blue.)

Sternum

● The **sternum** (**STER**-num), also known as the **breastbone,** forms the middle of the front of the rib cage. It is divided into three parts (see Figure 3.11).

● The **manubrium** (mah-**NEW**-bree-um), which is bone, is the upper portion of the sternum.

● The **body** of the sternum, which is bone, is the middle portion of the sternum.

● The **xiphoid process** (**ZIF**-oid), which is cartilage, is the lower portion of the sternum.

SHOULDERS

As you study the bones of the shoulder, refer to Figures 3.8 and 3.11.

● The shoulders form the **pectoral girdle** (**PECK**-toh-rahl), which is also known as the **shoulder girdle,** that supports the arms and hands. As used here, the term *girdle* means a structure that encircles the body.

● The **clavicle** (**KLAV**-ih-kul), also known as the **collar bone,** is a slender bone that connects the sternum to the scapula.

● The **scapula** (**SKAP**-you-lah) is also known as the **shoulder blade** (plural, **scapulae**).

● The **acromion** (ah-**KROH**-mee-on) is an extension of the scapula that forms the high point of the shoulder.

ARMS

As you study the following bones of the arms, refer to Figures 3.11 and 3.12.

● The **humerus** (**HEW**-mer-us) is the bone of the upper arm (plural, **humeri**).

● The **radius** (**RAY**-dee-us) is the smaller bone in the forearm. The radius runs up the thumb side of the forearm.

● The **ulna** (**ULL**-nah) is the larger bone of the forearm. It articulates with the humerus to form the elbow joint.

● The **olecranon process** (oh-**LEK**-rah-non), commonly known as the **funny bone,** is a large projection on the upper end of the ulna that forms the point of the elbow that tingles when struck.

WRISTS AND HANDS

As you study the following bones of the wrists and hands, refer to Figure 3.12.

● The **carpals** (**KAR**-palz) are the bones of the wrist.

● The **metacarpals** (met-ah-**KAR**-palz) are the bones that form the palm of the hand.

● The **phalanges** (fah-**LAN**-jeez) are the bones of the fingers (and of the toes) (singular, **phalanx**).

● Each finger has three bones. These are the **distal** (outermost), **medial** (middle), and **proximal** (nearest the hand) phalanges.

● The thumb has two bones. These are the **distal** and **proximal** phalanges.

SPINAL COLUMN

- The **spinal column** is also known as the **vertebral column** (**VER**-teh-bral *or* **VER**-tee-bral).
- This vertebral column consists of 26 **vertebrae** (**VER**-teh-bray *or* **VER**-teh-bree) (singular, **vertebra**).
- The functions of the spinal column are to support the head and body and to protect the spinal cord.

Structures of Vertebrae

- The **body** is the solid anterior portion of a vertebra (Figure 3.13).

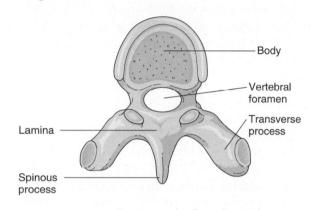

FIGURE 3.13 Structures of a thoracic vertebra.

- A **lamina** (**LAM**-ih-nah) is the posterior portion of a vertebra (plural, **laminae**). Several **processes** extend from this area.
- The **vertebral foramen** is the opening in the middle of the vertebra. The spinal cord passes through this opening.

Types of Vertebrae

- The **cervical vertebrae** (**SER**-vih-kal) are the first set of seven vertebrae that form the neck. They are also known as **C1** through **C7** (Figure 3.14). (*Cervical* means pertaining to the neck.)
- The **thoracic vertebrae** (thoh-**RASS**-ick) make up the second set of 12 vertebrae. They form the outward curve of the spine and are known as **T1** through **T12**.
- The **lumbar vertebrae** (**LUM**-bar) make up the third set of five vertebrae. They are known as **L1** through **L5**. The lumbar vertebrae are the largest and strongest of the vertebrae and form the inward curve of the spine.

Intervertebral Disks

- The **intervertebral disks** (**in**-ter-**VER**-teh-bral), which are made of cartilage, separate and cushion the vertebrae from each other. These disks act as the shock absorbers and allow for movement of the spinal column (see Figure 3.21A).

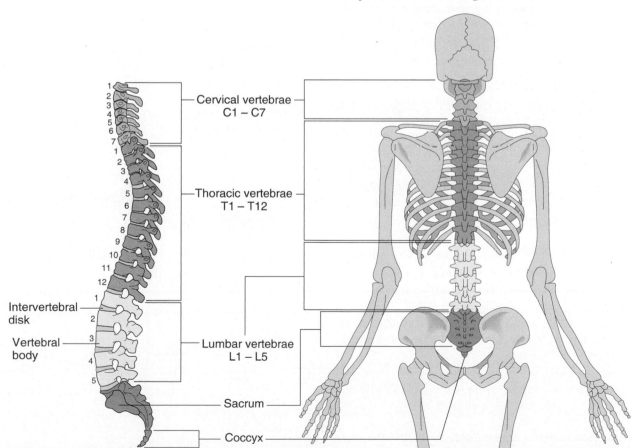

FIGURE 3.14 Lateral and posterior views of the spinal column.

Sacrum

● The **sacrum** (**SAY**-krum) is a slightly curved, triangular-shaped bone near the base of the spine (Figure 3.15). At birth it is composed of five separate sacral bones; however, in the young child they fuse together to form a single bone.

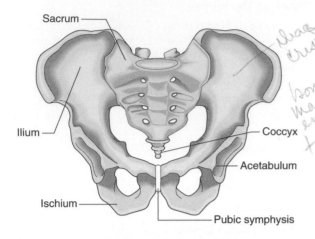

Sacrum

Ilium

Coccyx

Acetabulum

Ischium

Pubic symphysis

FIGURE 3.15 Anterior view of the pelvis.

Coccyx

● The **coccyx** (**KOCK**-sicks), also known as the **tailbone,** forms the end of the spine and is made up of four small vertebrae fused together (see Figure 3.15).

PELVIC GIRDLE

● The **pelvic girdle,** also known as the **hips** or **pelvic bone,** protects internal organs and supports the lower extremities. This structure is made up of three bones fused together (see Figure 3.15).

● The **ilium** (**ILL**-ee-um) is the upper, blade-shaped part of the hip on each side of the pelvic girdle.

● The **sacroiliac** (**say**-kroh-**ILL**-ee-ack) is the slightly movable articulation between the sacrum and the ilium.

● The **ischium** (**ISS**-kee-um) is the lower and posterior portion of the pelvic girdle.

● The **pubis** (**PEW**-bis) is the anterior portion of the pelvic girdle.

● These three bones, which are also known as the **pubic bones,** fuse together, and in the posterior they fuse with the sacrum.

● The two pubic bones join at the anterior midline to form the **pubic symphysis** (**PEW**-bick **SIM**-fih-sis). This is a cartilaginous joint that holds the bones firmly together.

● The **acetabulum** (**ass**-eh-**TAB**-you-lum), the large socket in the pelvic bones, forms the hip socket for the head of the femur.

LEGS AND KNEES

As you study the following bones, refer to Figures 3.16 and 3.17.

Femur

● The **femur** (**FEE**-mur) is the upper leg bone (see Figure 3.16). Also known as the **thigh bone,** it is the largest bone in the body.

● The **head** of the femur articulates with the acetabulum (hip socket).

● The **femoral neck** (**FEM**-or-al) is the narrow area just below the head of the femur.

● The **trochanter** (tro-**KAN**-ter) is one of the two large bony projections on the upper end of the femur just below the femoral neck.

Knees

● The **patella** (pah-**TEL**-ah) is the bony anterior portion of the kneecap.

● The term **popliteal** (pop-**LIT**-ee-al) refers to the posterior surface of the knee and is used to describe the space, ligaments, vessels, and muscles in this area.

● The **anterior cruciate ligament (ACL)** and **posterior cruciate ligament (PCL),** which are shown in Figure 3.4, make possible the movements of the knee. These are known as **cruciate ligaments** (**KROO**-shee-ayt) because they are shaped like a cross.

Lower Leg

● The **tibia** (**TIB**-ee-ah), also known as the **shinbone,** is the larger weight-bearing bone in the anterior of the lower leg.

● The **fibula** (**FIB**-you-lah) is the smaller of the two bones of the lower leg.

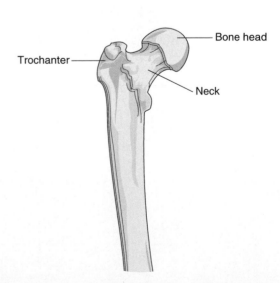

Bone head

Trochanter

Neck

FIGURE 3.16 Structures of the proximal end of the femur.

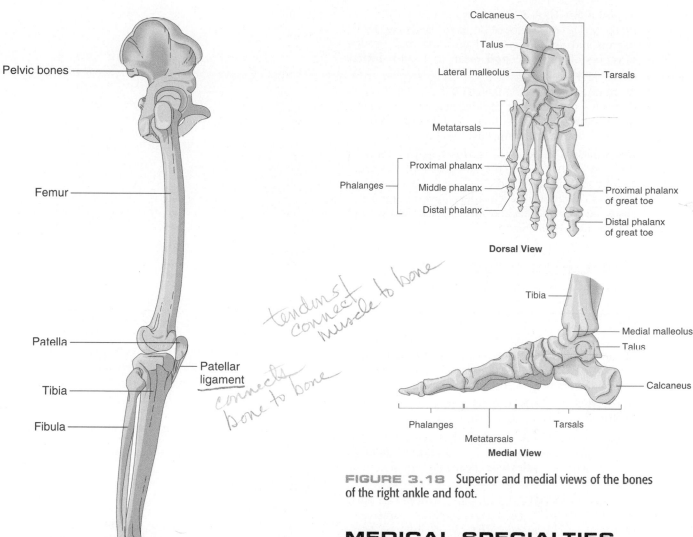

FIGURE 3.18 Superior and medial views of the bones of the right ankle and foot.

FIGURE 3.17 Lateral view of bones of the lower extremity.

ANKLES AND FEET

- The **tarsals** (**TAHR**-salz) are the bones that make up the ankles (Figure 3.18).

- The **malleolus** (mal-**LEE**-oh-lus) is the rounded bony protuberance on each side of the ankle (plural, **malleoli**).

- The **talus** (**TAY**-luss) is the anklebone that articulates with the tibia and fibula (see Figure 3.17).

- The **calcaneus** (kal-**KAY**-nee-uss), or **heel bone,** is the largest of the tarsal bones (see Figure 3.18).

- The **metatarsals** (**met**-ah-**TAHR**-salz) are the bones of the foot.

- The **phalanges** (fah-**LAN**-jeez) are the bones of the toes (and of the fingers) (singular, **phalanx**).

MEDICAL SPECIALTIES RELATED TO THE SKELETAL SYSTEM

- A **chiropractor** (**KYE**-roh-**prack**-tor) holds a Doctor of Chiropractic (DC) degree and specializes in manipulative treatment of disorders originating from misalignment of the spine.

- An **orthopedic surgeon**, also known as an **orthopedist** (**or** thoh **PEE**-dist), specializes in diagnosing and treating diseases and disorders involving the bones, joints, and muscles.

- **Orthotics** (or-**THOT**-icks) is the field of knowledge relating to the making and fitting of orthopedic appliances, such as a brace or splint to support, align, prevent, or correct deformities or to improve the function of movable parts of the body.

- **Osteopathic physicians** (**oss**-tee-oh-**PATH**-ick) hold a Doctor of Osteopathy (DO) degree and specialize in treating health problems by manipulation (changing the positions of the bones). They may also use traditional forms of medical treatment. The term **osteopathy** (**oss**-tee-**OP**-ah-thee) also refers to any bone disease.

- A **podiatrist** (poh-**DYE**-ah-trist) holds a Doctor of Podiatry (DP) or Doctor of Podiatric Medicine (DPM) degree and specializes in diagnosing and treating disorders of the foot (**pod** mean foot, and **-iatrist** means specialist).

- A **rheumatologist** (roo-mah-**TOL**-oh-jist) is a physician who specializes in the diagnosis and treatment of rheumatic diseases that are characterized by inflammation in the connective tissues.

- **Rheumatism** (**ROO**-mah-tizm) is a general term for a variety of acute and chronic conditions characterized by inflammation and deterioration of connective tissues. This group of disorders includes joint diseases such as arthritis and muscle disorders such as fibromyalgia (see Chapter 4).

PATHOLOGY OF THE SKELETAL SYSTEM

JOINTS

- **Ankylosis** (**ang**-kih-**LOH**-sis) is the loss or absence of mobility in a joint due to disease, an injury, or a surgical procedure (**ankyl** means crooked, bent, or stiff and **-osis** means abnormal condition).

- **Arthralgia** (ar-**THRAL**-jee-ah) is pain in a joint (**arthr** means joint and **-algia** means pain).

- **Arthrosclerosis** (**ar**-throh-skleh-**ROH**-sis) is stiffness of the joints, especially in the elderly (**arthr/o** means joint and **-sclerosis** means abnormal hardening).

- **Bursitis** (ber-**SIGH**-tis) is an inflammation of a bursa that is typically caused by repetitive movements (**burs** means bursa and **-itis** means inflammation). Repetitive stress disorders are discussed in Chapter 4.

- A **chondroma** (kon-**DROH**-mah) is a slow-growing benign tumor derived from cartilage cells (**chondr** means cartilage and **-oma** means tumor).

- **Chondromalacia** (**kon**-droh-mah-**LAY**-shee-ah) is the abnormal softening of the cartilage (**chondr/o** means cartilage and **-malacia** means abnormal softening).

- **Hallux valgus** (**HAL**-ucks **VAL**-guss), commonly known as a **bunion,** is an abnormal enlargement of the joint at the base of the great toe (**hallux** means big toe and **valgus** means bent). This shift in the joint creates pressure on the other toes because the great toe is forced laterally (Figure 3.19).

- **Luxation** (luck-**SAY**-shun), also known as **dislocation,** is the dislocation or displacement of a bone from its joint. **Subluxation** (**sub**-luck-**SAY**-shun) is the partial displacement of a bone from its joint.

- **Synovitis** (sin-oh-**VYE**-tiss) is inflammation of the synovial membrane that results in swelling and pain (**synov** means synovial membrane and **-itis** means inflammation). It may be caused by an injury, infection, or irritation produced by damaged cartilage.

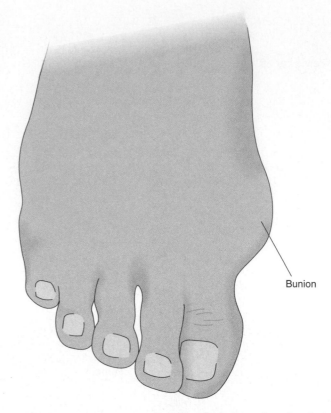

FIGURE 3.19 Superior view of a hallux valgus (bunion).

ARTHRITIS

- **Arthritis** (ar-**THRIGH**-tis) is an inflammatory condition of one or more joints (**arthr** means joint, and **-itis** means inflammation). There are many different forms and causes of arthritis (plural, **arthritides**).

- **Osteoarthritis** (**oss**-tee-oh-ar-**THRIGH**-tis), also known as **wear-and-tear arthritis** or **OA** (**oste/o** means bone, **arthr** means joint, and **-itis** means inflammation), a **degenerative joint disease (DJD)** that is most commonly associated with aging (Figure 3.20).

- **Gouty arthritis** (**GOW**-tee ar-**THRIGH**-tis), also known as **gout,** is a type of arthritis associated with the formation of uric acid crystals in the joint as the result of hyperuricemia (excess uric acid concentrations in the blood).

Rheumatoid Arthritis

- **Rheumatoid arthritis** (**ROO**-mah-toyd ar-**THRIGH**-tis), also known as **RA,** is an autoimmune disorder. In contrast to osteoarthritis, the symptoms are generalized and usually more severe. In RA, the synovial membranes are inflamed and thickened. Other tissues are also attacked, causing the joints to become swollen, painful, and immobile.

- **Ankylosing spondylitis** (**ang**-kih-**LOH**-sing **spon**-dih-**LYE**-tis) is a form of rheumatoid arthritis characterized by progressive stiffening of the spine caused by fusion of the vertebral bodies.

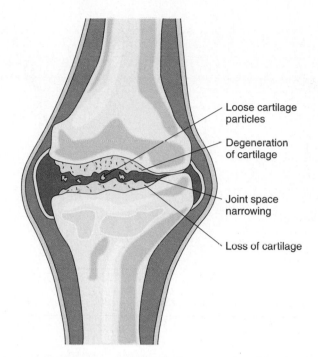

FIGURE 3.20 Damage to the knee caused by osteoarthritis.

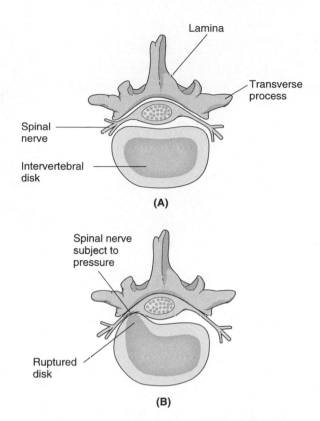

FIGURE 3.21 (A) Normal intervertebral disk. (B) Ruptured disk causing pressure on a spinal nerve.

● **Juvenile rheumatoid arthritis** affects children. Symptoms include pain and swelling in the joints, skin rash, fever, slowed growth, and fatigue.

SPINAL COLUMN

● A **herniated disk** (**HER**-nee-**ayt**-ed), also known as a **ruptured disk,** is a rupture of the intervertebral disk that results in pressure on spinal nerve roots (Figure 3.21B).

● **Lumbago** (lum-**BAY**-goh), also known as **low back pain,** is pain of the lumbar region (**lumb** means lumbar and **-ago** means diseased condition).

● **Spondylitis** (**spon**-dih-**LYE**-tis) is an inflammation of the vertebrae (**spondyl** means vertebrae and **-itis** means inflammation).

● **Spondylolisthesis** (**spon**-dih-loh-liss-**THEE**-sis) is the forward movement of the body of one of the lower lumbar vertebra on the vertebra below it or on the sacrum (**spondyl/o** means vertebrae and **-listhesis** means slipping).

● **Spondylosis** (**spon**-dih-**LOH**-sis) is any degenerative condition of the vertebrae (**spondyl** means vertebrae and **-osis** means abnormal condition).

Spina Bifida

● **Spina bifida** (**SPY**-nah **BIF**-ih-dah) is the congenital defect that occurs during early pregnancy in which the spinal canal fails to close around the spinal cord (**spina** means pertaining to the spine and **bifida** means split). Many cases of spina bifida are caused by a lack of folic acid (a vitamin) during the early stages of pregnancy.

Curvatures of the Spine

● **Kyphosis** (kye-**FOH**-sis) is an abnormal increase in the outward curvature of the thoracic spine as viewed from the side (**kyph** means hump and **-osis** means abnormal condition). This condition is also known as **humpback** or **dowager's hump** (Figure 3.22A).

● **Lordosis** (lor-**DOH**-sis) is an abnormal increase in the forward curvature of the lower or lumbar spine (**lord** means bent backward and **-osis** means abnormal condition). This condition is also known as **swayback** (see Figure 3.22B).

● **Scoliosis** (skoh-lee-**OH**-sis) is an abnormal lateral (sideways) curvature of the spine (**scoli** means curved, and **-osis** means abnormal condition). (See Figure 3.22C).

BONES

● An **exostosis** (**eck**-sos-**TOH**-sis) is a benign growth on the surface of a bone (**ex-** means outside, **ost** means bone, and **-osis** means abnormal condition).

● **Ostealgia** (oss-tee-**AL**-jee-ah) is any pain linked to an abnormal condition within a bone (**oste** means bone and **-algia** means pain).

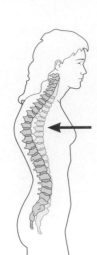
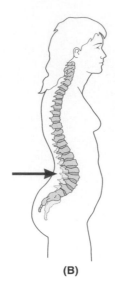
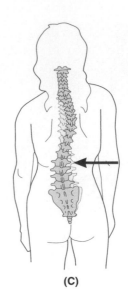

(A)   **(B)**   **(C)**

FIGURE 3.22 Abnormal curvatures of the spine. (A) Kyphosis. (B) Lordosis. (C) Scoliosis. (Normal curvatures are shown in shadow.)

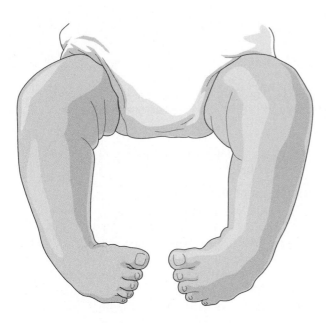

FIGURE 3.23 Talipes, also known as clubfoot, with the feet turned inward.

- **Osteitis** (**oss**-tee-**EYE**-tis) is an inflammation of bone (**oste** means bone and **-itis** means inflammation).

- **Osteomalacia** (**oss**-tee-oh-mah-**LAY**-shee-ah) is the abnormal softening of bones due to disease (**oste/o** means bone and **-malacia** means abnormal softening).

- **Osteomyelitis** (**oss**-tee-oh-**my**-eh-**LYE**-tis) is an inflammation of the bone and bone marrow (**oste/o** means bone, **myel** means bone marrow, and **-itis** means inflammation).

- **Osteonecrosis** (**oss**-tee-oh-neh-**KROH**-sis) is the destruction and death of bone tissue caused by an insufficient blood supply, infection, malignancy, or trauma (**oste/o** means bone and **-necrosis** means tissue death).

- **Paget's disease** (**PAJ**-its), also known as **osteitis deformans** (**oss**-tee-**EYE**-tis dee-**FOR**-manz), is a disease of unknown cause that is characterized by extensive bone destruction followed by abnormal bone repair. As the disease progresses, the bones become deformed and weakened and may bend or break easily.

- **Periostitis** (**pehr**-ee-oss-**TYE**-tis) is an inflammation of the periosteum (**peri-** means surrounding, **ost** means bone, and **-itis** means inflammation).

- **Rickets** (**RICK**-ets), which is caused by calcium and vitamin D deficiencies in early childhood, results in demineralized bones and related deformities.

- **Talipes** (**TAL**-ih-peez), also known as **clubfoot,** is a congenital deformity in which the foot may be turned outward or inward as shown in Figure 3.23.

Tumors of Bones

- **Ewing's sarcoma** (**YOU**-ingz sar-**KOH**-mah), also known as **Ewing's family of tumors,** is a group of cancers that most frequently affects children or adolescents. A *sarcoma* is a malignant tumor of connective tissue, and in Ewing's sarcoma they usually occur in the diaphyses (shaft) of long bones in the arms and legs and then may spread rapidly to other body sites.

- A **myeloma** (**my**-eh-**LOH**-mah) is a malignant tumor composed of cells derived from blood-forming tissues of the bone marrow. Myeloma is usually progressive, may cause pathologic fractures, and is often fatal (**myel** means bone marrow and **-oma** means tumor).

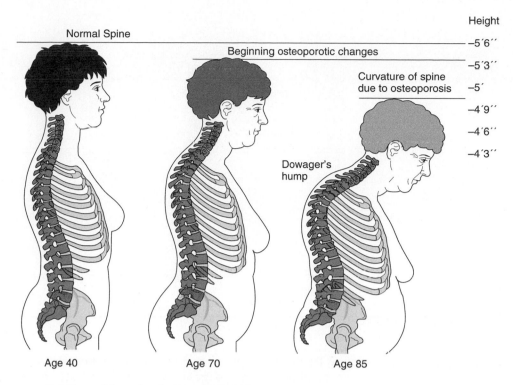

FIGURE 3.24 Curvature of the spine due to osteoporosis.

- An **osteochondroma** (oss-tee-oh-kon-**DROH**-mah) is the most common benign bone tumor (**oste/o** means bone, **chondr** means cartilage, and **-oma** means tumor). These tumors are growths on the surface of a bone that protrude as hard lumps covered with a cap of cartilage.

OSTEOPOROSIS

Osteoporosis (oss-tee-oh-poh-**ROH**-sis) is a marked loss of bone density and an increase in bone porosity frequently associated with aging (**oste/o** means bone and **-porosis** means porous condition). Osteoporosis is primarily responsible for three types of fractures:

- **Vertebral crush fractures**, also known as **compression fractures** of the spine, occur when one or more of the vertebrae become so weak that they collapse spontaneously or under minimal stress. This results in pain, loss of height, and development of the spinal curvature known as **dowager's hump**. These changes in the spine cause the loss of height, crowding of the internal organs, and reduced lung capacity (Figure 3.24).

- **Colles' fracture**, also known as a **fractured wrist,** is a fracture of the lower end of the radius. This occurs when a person tries to break a fall by landing on his or her hands and the trauma causes the weakened bone to break (Figure 3.25).

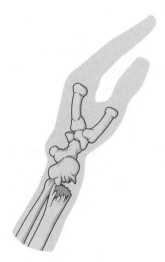

FIGURE 3.25 A Colles' fracture of the left wrist.

- An **osteoporotic hip fracture** (oss-tee-oh-pah-**ROT**-ick), also known as a **broken hip,** can occur spontaneously or as the result of a fall. Complications from these fractures may result in death or the loss of function, mobility, and independence.

FRACTURES

- A **fracture,** which is abbreviated as **Fx,** is a broken bone. Fractures are described in terms of their complexity (Figure 3.26):

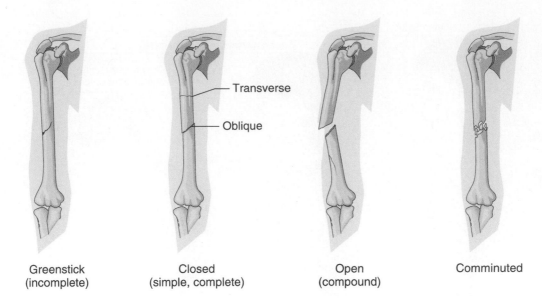

Transverse

Oblique

Greenstick
(incomplete)

Closed
(simple, complete)

Open
(compound)

Comminuted

FIGURE 3.26 Types of bone fractures.

- A **greenstick fracture,** or **incomplete fracture,** is one in which the bone is partially bent and only partially broken. This type of fracture is usually longitudinal and occurs primarily in children.

- A **closed fracture,** also known as a **simple** or **complete fracture,** is one in which the bone is broken but there is no open wound in the skin (see Figure 3.26). A **transverse fracture** is straight across the bone. An **oblique fracture** is at an angle.

- An **open fracture,** also known as a **compound fracture,** is one in which the bone is broken and there is an open wound in the skin.

- A **comminuted fracture** is one in which the bone is splintered or crushed. **Comminuted** (**KOM**-ih-newt-ed) means crushed into small pieces.

- A **compression fracture** occurs when the bone is pressed together (compressed) on itself (see osteoporosis).

- A **spiral fracture** is a fracture in which the bone has been twisted apart. This occurs as the result of a severe twisting motion as in a sports injury.

- A **stress fracture** is a small crack in bones that often develops from chronic, excessive impact. These fractures are usually due to a sports injury.

- A **fat embolus** (**EM**-boh-lus) may form when a long bone is fractured and fat cells from yellow bone marrow are released into the blood. (An **embolus** is any foreign matter circulating in the blood that may become lodged and block the blood vessel. Emboli are discussed in Chapter 5.)

- **Crepitation** (krep-ih-**TAY**-shun), also known as **crepitus** (**KREP**-ih-tus), is the crackling sensation that is felt and heard when the ends of a broken bone move together.

- As the bone heals, a **callus** (**KAL**-us) forms a bulging deposit around the area of the break. This tissue eventually becomes bone.

DIAGNOSTIC PROCEDURES OF THE SKELETAL SYSTEM

- **Arthrocentesis** (**ar**-throh-sen-**TEE**-sis) is a surgical puncture of the joint space to remove synovial fluid for analysis (**arthr/o** means joint and **-centesis** means a surgical puncture to remove fluid).

- **Arthroscopy** (ar-**THROS**-koh-pee) is the visual examination of the internal structure of a joint (**arthro** means joint and **-scopy** means visual examination) using an **arthroscope** (see Figure 15.18).

- **Bone density testing (BDT),** also known as **bone mass measurement** or **densitometry,** is the use of several types of radiation tests to determine bone density. These tests are indicated for conditions such as osteoporosis, osteomalacia, and Paget's disease.

- A **bone marrow biopsy (BMB)** is performed by inserting a sharp needle into the hipbone or sternum and removing bone marrow cells. It is performed as a diagnostic test to determine why blood cells are abnormal. It is also performed to find a donor match for a bone marrow transplant.

- A **bone scan** is the use of nuclear medicine to detect bone cancer and osteomyelitis before these pathologies become visible on traditional radiographs (see Chapter 15 and Figure 15.29).

- **Dual x-ray absorptiometry** (ab-**sorp**-shee-**OM**-eh-tree) **(DXA)** is a low-exposure radiographic measurement that is most often used to detect early signs of osteoporosis.

- **Ultrasonic bone density testing**, called a **bone sonometer**, uses sound waves to take measurements of the heel bone. This is a screening test for osteoporosis or other conditions that cause a loss of bone mass. If the test indicates risks, more definitive testing is indicated.

- **Magnetic resonance imaging (MRI)** is used to image soft tissue structures such as the interior of complex joints and spinal disorders. It is not the most effective method of imaging hard tissues such as bone.

- **Radiographs,** also known as **x-rays,** are used to visualize fractured bones (Figure 3.27).

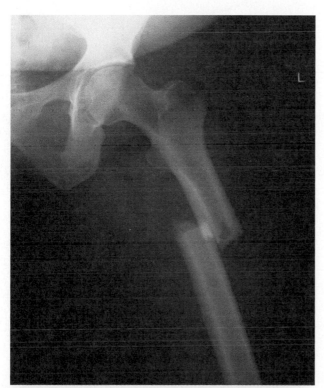

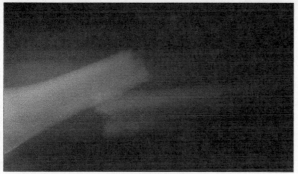

FIGURE 3.27 Radiographs (x-rays) of a simple fracture of the femur. The top picture is an anterior posterior (AP) view. The bottom picture is a lateral view that more exactly locates the fractured ends of the bone.

TREATMENT PROCEDURES OF THE SKELETAL SYSTEM

MEDICATIONS

- **Nonsteroidal anti-inflammatory drugs,** also known as **NSAIDs,** are administered to control pain and to reduce inflammation and swelling. Aspirin is a NSAID. Medications in this group also may thin the blood and attack the stomach lining.

- **Acetaminophen** also controls pain but without the side effects of NSAIDs. However, it does not have the ability to reduce inflammation and swelling.

- Aspirin and acetaminophen are also used as antipyretics. An **antipyretic** (**an**-tih-pye-**RET**-ick) reduces or relieves fever.

- **COX-2 inhibitors,** a newer class of medications, control the pain and inflammation of osteoarthritis and rheumatoid arthritis while greatly reducing the side effects of NSAIDs. These medications are named for the two *cyclooxygenase* (COX) enzymes that are associated with arthritic pain and inflammation.

BONE MARROW TRANSPLANTS

A **bone marrow transplant (BMT)**, also known as a **stem cell transplant,** is used to treat certain types of cancers, such as leukemia and lymphomas, that affect bone marrow. These cancers are discussed in Chapters 5 and 6.

- In this treatment, both the cancer and the patient's bone marrow are destroyed with high-intensity radiation and chemotherapy.

- Next, healthy bone marrow cells are transfused into the recipient's blood. These cells migrate to the spongy bone, where they grow into cancer-free red bone marrow.

Autologous Transplants

- Most frequently, the BMT is an **autologous transplant,** using some of the patient's own bone marrow that was harvested before treatment began. (**Autologous** (aw-**TOL**-uh-guss) means originating within an individual.)

Allogenic Transplants

- If the patient's own marrow cannot be used, an **allogenic transplant,** using bone marrow from a donor, may be a possibility. However, unless this is a perfect match, there is the danger that the recipient's body will reject the transplant. (**Allogenic** (**al**-oh-**JEN**-ick) means originating within another.)

Cord Blood

- **Cord blood,** which is collected from the umbilical cord immediately after birth, is a rich source of stem

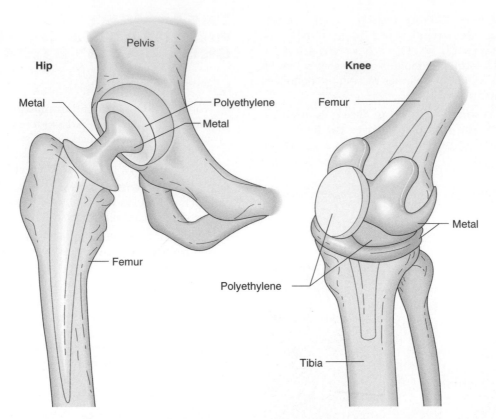

FIGURE 3.28 Components of a total hip replacement and a total knee replacement. Polyethylene, a smooth tough plastic, makes smooth movement possible.

cells and has the potential of being an alternative to bone marrow transplants. (Stem cells are discussed further in Chapter 2.)

JOINTS

- **Arthroscopic surgery** (ar-throh-**SKOP**-ick) is the treatment of the interior of a joint, such as the removal of torn cartilage, with the use of an arthroscope and instruments inserted through small incisions (see Figure 15.18).

- A **bursectomy** (ber-**SECK**-toh-mee) is the surgical removal of a bursa (**burs** means the bursa and **-ectomy** means surgical removal).

- **Chondroplasty** (**KON**-droh-**plas**-tee) is the surgical repair of cartilage (**chondr/o** means cartilage and **-plasty** means surgical repair).

- A **synovectomy** (sin-oh-**VECK**-toh-mee) is the surgical removal of a synovial membrane from a joint (**synov** means synovial membrane and **-ectomy** means surgical removal). This procedure is performed to repair a joint damaged by rheumatoid arthritis.

- **Arthrodesis** (ar-throh-**DEE**-sis), also known as **fusion** or **surgical ankylosis,** is a surgical procedure to stiffen a joint, such as a hip, or to join spinal

vertebrae (**arthr/o** means joint and **-desis** means surgical fixation of bone or joint).

- **Arthrolysis** (ar-**THROL**-ih-sis) is the surgical loosening of an ankylosed joint (**arthr/o** means joint and **-lysis** means loosening or setting free). *Note:* The suffix **-lysis** also means breaking down or destruction and may indicate either a pathologic state or a therapeutic procedure.

- A **periosteotomy** (**peer**-ee-**oss**-tee-**OT**-oh-mee) is an incision through the periosteum (**peri-** means surrounding, **oste** means bone, and **-otomy** means surgical incision).

JOINT REPLACEMENT

- **Arthroplasty** (**AR**-throh-**plas**-tee) is any surgical repair of a damaged joint (**arthr/o** means joint and **-plasty** means surgical repair); however, this term has come to mean the surgical replacement of a joint. These procedures are named for the involved joint and the amount of the joint that is replaced.

- The replacement part is called a **prosthesis** (pros-**THEE**-sis) or an **implant** (Figure 3.28). The broader definition of prosthesis is a substitute for a diseased or missing part of the body (plural, **prostheses**).

- A **laminectomy** (**lam**-ih-**NECK**-toh-mee) is the surgical removal of a lamina from a vertebra.
- **Spinal fusion** is a technique to immobilize part of the spine by joining together (fusing) two or more vertebrae. This may be performed with a diskectomy or laminectomy.

BONES

- A **craniectomy** (**kray**-nee-**EK**-toh-mee) is the surgical removal of a portion of the skull (**crani** means skull and **-ectomy** means surgical removal).
- A **craniotomy** (**kray**-nee-**OT**-oh-mee) is also known as a **bone flap** (**crani** means skull and **-otomy** means a surgical incision). This procedure is a surgical incision or opening into the skull that is performed to gain access to part of the brain (Figure 3.30).

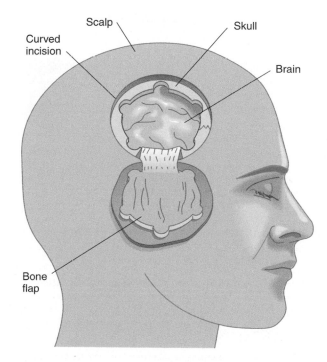

Scalp   Skull

Curved incision

Brain

Bone flap

FIGURE 3.30 A craniotomy is performed to gain access to a portion of the brain.

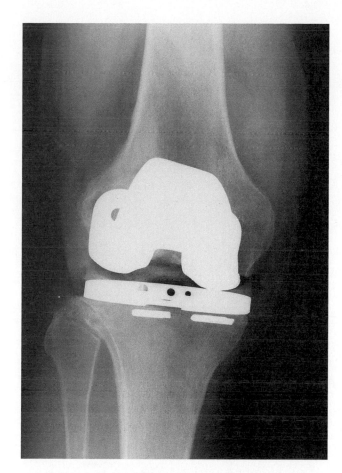

FIGURE 3.29 Radiograph (x-ray) of a total knee replacement. The metallic components are brighter than the bone.

- A **total knee replacement (TKR)** means that all of the parts of the knee were replaced (Figures 3.28 and 3.29).
- A **partial knee replacement (PKR)** means that only part of the knee was replaced.
- A **total hip replacement (THR)** consists of two components. The thigh component is a metal shaft fitted into the femur with a metal ball at the top end. The ball fits into a plastic lined cup-shaped socket that replaces the acetabulum within the hipbone.
- **Revision surgery** is the replacement of a worn or failed implant.

SPINAL COLUMN

- **Diskectomy** (dis-**KECK**-toh-mee) is the surgical removal of an intervertebral disk.
- In a **percutaneous diskectomy** (**per**-kyou-**TAY**-nee-us dis-**KECK**-toh-mee), a thin tube is inserted through the skin of the back to suction out the ruptured disk or to vaporize it with a laser. *Percutaneous* means through the skin.

- A **cranioplasty** (**KRAY**-nee-oh-**plas**-tee) is the surgical repair of the skull (**crani/o** means skull and **-plasty** means surgical repair).
- **Osteoclasis** (**oss**-tee-**OCK**-lah-sis) is the surgical fracture of a bone to correct a deformity (**oste/o** means bone and **-clasis** means to break).
- An **ostectomy** (oss-**TECK**-toh-mee) is the surgical removal of bone (**ost** means bone and **-ectomy** means the surgical removal). (Notice that the root word **ost** is used to avoid having two **e**s together when it joins the suffix **-ectomy**.)

- **Osteoplasty** (OSS-tee-oh-**plas**-tee) is the surgical repair of bones (**oste/o** means bone and **-plasty** means surgical repair).

- **Osteorrhaphy** (oss-tee-**OR**-ah-fee) is the suturing or wiring together of bones (**oste/o** means bone and **-rrhaphy** means to suture).

- **Osteotomy** (oss-tee-**OT**-oh-mee) is a surgical incision or sectioning of a bone (**oste** means bone and **-otomy** means a surgical incision). This procedure may be performed to realign a joint damaged by arthritis.

TREATMENT OF FRACTURES

- **Manipulation,** also known as **closed reduction,** is the attempted realignment of the bone involved in a fracture or joint dislocation. The affected bone is returned to its normal anatomic alignment by manually applied forces and then is usually immobilized to maintain the realigned position (Figure 3.31).

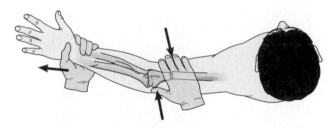

FIGURE 3.31 Closed reduction of a fractured left humerus.

- **Traction** is a pulling force exerted on a limb in a distal direction in an effort to return the bone or joint to normal alignment.

- **Immobilization,** also known as **stabilization,** is the act of holding, suturing, or fastening the bone in a fixed position with strapping or a cast.

External Fixation

- **External fixation** is a fracture treatment procedure in which pins are placed through the soft tissues and bone so that an external appliance can be used to hold the pieces of bone firmly in place during healing. When healing is complete, the appliance is removed (Figure 3.32).

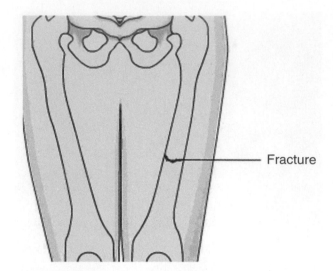

Fracture

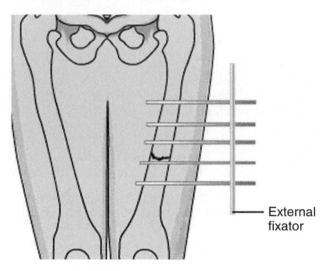

External fixator

FIGURE 3.32 External fixation. (A) Fracture of the epiphysis of a femur. (B) External fixation stabilizes the bone and is removed after the bone has healed.

Internal Fixation

- **Internal fixation,** which is also known as **open reduction internal fixation (ORIF),** is a fracture treatment procedure in which pins or a plate are placed directly into the bone to hold the broken pieces in place. This form of fixation is *not* usually removed after the fracture has healed (Figure 3.33).

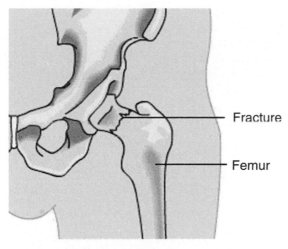

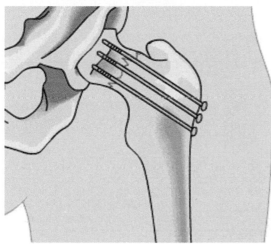

FIGURE 3.33 Internal fixation. (A) Fracture of the femoral neck. (B) Internal fixation pins are placed to stabilize the bone. These are not removed.

Fracture

Femur

Career Opportunities

In addition to the medical specialties already discussed, some of the health occupations involving the treatment of the skeletal system are:

- **Emergency medical technician (EMT):** provides emergency treatment of injuries, such as bones broken in accidents or falls, as well as many other medical crises. The work of EMTs involves the speedy treatment of a wide variety of problems and taking action to protect the patient from further injury if in a dangerous situation.

- **Paramedic (EMT-P):** an EMT with additional training who is authorized to provide advanced treatment such as in-depth patient assessment, EKG interpretation, and drug administration

- **Prosthetist:** creates artificial substitutions for body parts such as a limb, eye, or tooth

- **Pedorthist:** trained to fit or create orthotics (orthopedic appliances) and other therapeutic footwear

- **Podiatric medical assistant:** makes castings of feet, takes x-rays, and assists the podiatrist in surgery

- **Orthopedic assistant:** works under the supervision of a physician or therapist in the field of sports medicine or orthopedics, performing diagnostic tests such as x-rays and assisting with injury treatment such as bandaging, casting, and rehabilitation exercises

Health Occupation Profile: PARAMEDIC

Pat Terry, 46, is a firefighter/paramedic (EMT-P) with the Madison, Wisconsin, Fire Department. She joined the force 15 years ago as a firefighter, and after a few years decided to take the additional training necessary to become a paramedic. "I'd always been interested in medicine, in problem solving, and in helping people. As a firefighter, I'd received basic EMT training, but I wanted to do more. In addition to responding to fires, the paramedics respond to accidents and distress calls. I love my work, although it can be stressful and physically draining. At an accident scene, we stabilize injured patients with equipment such as back boards. We perform many of the same procedures as emergency room staff, such as starting IV medications, using defibrillators, and administering CPR, but often we perform these tasks in a very challenging environment. Many of our ambulance calls are from individuals suffering from cardiac arrests, diabetic emergencies, and asthma attacks. I love being able to calm patients down and to get them the help they need in time."

STUDY BREAK

Do you know anyone who can bend his or her thumbs back to the wrist? Who can lie flat on the floor with both knees bent backward? We would usually say that such persons are *double jointed*, although of course they don't have two joints instead of one. This small percentage of people just have limb and finger joints that are much more flexible than most people's joints. The medical term *hypermobility*, made up of the word part **hyper-** (excessive) added to the word *mobility*, is sometimes used to describe this syndrome.

However, being double-jointed is not really "excessive" or really even a syndrome. It simply means that a person naturally has a greater range of joint movement than most others. Some people are born with a tendency toward hypermobility. This tendency can either be ignored (except for showing off at parties) or strengthened through exercise and stretching for certain types of gymnastic and dance performances.

Review Time

Write the answers to the following questions on a separate piece of paper or in your notebook. In addition, be prepared to take part in the classroom discussion.

1. **Written assignment:** Describe the primary characteristics of these **three types of joints:** (1) sutures, (2) symphyses, and (3) synovial joints.

   Discussion assignment: Give examples of the location of each type of joint and the motion that each permits.

2. **Written assignment:** Describe the three types of fractures that are commonly associated with **osteoporosis.**

   Discussion assignment: How would you explain to a patient's family why the patient fractured a bone in a very minor fall?

3. **Written assignment:** Use your own words to describe the differences between **internal fixation** and **external fixation.**

   Discussion assignment: How would you explain to a patient what to expect with each type of fixation?

4. Max has leukemia and requires a **bone marrow transplant.** However, his bone marrow is not suitable.

   Written assignment: Describe the alternative type of bone marrow transplant that could be used in Max's case.

   Discussion assignment: What would some benefits be of using Max's own bone marrow?

5. Mrs. Valdez fell and broke her hip, and her physician said she needs a **THR.**

   Written assignment: Explain this procedure in terms that Mrs. Valdez and her family will understand.

   Discussion assignment: How is a total hip replacement designed to function like a natural hip?

Optional Internet Activity

*The goal of this activity is to help you learn more about medical terminology while improving your Internet skills. Select **one** of these two options and follow the instructions.*

1. **Internet Search:** Search for information about **osteoporosis.** Write a brief (one- or two-paragraph) report on the prevention of this disorder and include the address of the web site where you found this information.

2. **Web Site:** To learn more about the 100 forms of **arthritis,** go to this web address: **http://www. arthritis.org/.** Click first on Resources and then on Disease Center. Write a brief (one- or two-paragraph) report on at least two forms of arthritis that are not mentioned in your text.

The Human Touch: Critical Thinking Exercise

The following story and questions are designed to stimulate critical thinking through class discussion or as a brief essay response. There are no right or wrong answers to these questions.

Dr. Johnstone didn't like what he saw. The x-rays of Gladys Gwynn's hip showed a fracture of the femoral neck and severe osteoporosis of the hip. Mrs. Gwynn had been admitted to the orthopedic ward of Hamilton Hospital after a fall that morning at Sunny Meadows, an assisted-living facility. The accident had occurred when Sheri Smith, a new aide, lost her grip while helping Mrs. Gwynn in the shower.

A frail but alert and cheerful woman of 85, Gladys Gwynn has osteoarthritis and osteoporosis, which have forced her to rely on a walker. She has been living at Sunny Meadows since her husband's death four years ago. Dr. Johnstone knew that she didn't have any relatives in the area, and he did not think that she had signed a healthcare power of attorney designating someone to help with medical decisions like this.

A total hip replacement (THR) would be the logical treatment for a younger patient because it could restore some of her lost mobility. However, for a frail patient like Mrs. Gwynn, internal fixation of the fracture might be the treatment of choice. This would repair the break but not improve her mobility.

Dr. Johnstone needed to make a decision soon, but Mrs. Gwynn was still groggy from the pain medication. With one more look at the x-ray, Dr. Johnstone sighed and walked toward Mrs. Gwynn's room.

Suggested Discussion Topics

1. Gladys Gwynn has no children or other relatives in the area and is unable to speak for herself. Who should decide which surgery should be performed?

2. Do you think Sheri Smith or Sunny Meadows should be held responsible for Mrs. Gwynn's accident? If so, who should be held responsible?

3. A total hip replacement is more expensive than the internal fixation procedure and has a longer, more strenuous recovery period. Given the patient's condition and the limited dollars available for health care, which procedure should be performed?

4. How would you have answered Question 3 if Mrs. Gwynn were your mother?

5. If Mrs. Gwynn's recovery does not go well and she is no longer able to get around by herself, will she be allowed to continue living at Sunny Meadows?

Student Workbook and Student Activity CD-ROM

1. Go to your **Student Workbook** and complete the Learning Exercises for this chapter.

2. Go to the **Student Activity CD-ROM** and have fun with the exercises and games for this chapter.

4

The Muscular System

● **Overview of Structures, Word Parts, and Functions of the Muscular System**

MAJOR STRUCTURES	RELATED WORD ROOTS	PRIMARY FUNCTIONS
Muscles	my/o, myos/o	Make body movement possible, hold body erect, move body fluids, and produce body heat.
Fascia	fasci/o	Cover, support, and separate muscles.
Tendons	ten/o, tend/o, tendin/o	Attach muscle to bone.

Vocabulary Related to the Muscular System

Terms marked with the ❖ symbol are pronounced on the Student Activity CD-ROM that accompanies this text.

KEY WORD PARTS

- [ ] bi-
- [ ] -cele
- [ ] -desis
- [ ] fasci/o
- [ ] -ia
- [ ] -ic
- [ ] kinesi/o
- [ ] -lysis
- [ ] my/o
- [ ] -plegia
- [ ] -rrhexis
- [ ] tax/o
- [ ] ten/o, tend/o, tendin/o
- [ ] ton/o
- [ ] tri-

KEY MEDICAL TERMS

- [ ] **abduction** (ab-**DUCK**-shun)
- [ ] **Achilles tendinitis** (ten-dih-**NIGH**-tis) ❖
- [ ] **adduction** (ah-**DUCK**-shun)
- [ ] **adhesion** (ad-**HEE**-zhun) ❖
- [ ] **anticholinergic** (**an**-tih-**koh**-lin-**ER**-jik)
- [ ] **ataxia** (ah-**TACK**-see-ah) ❖
- [ ] **atonic** (ah-**TON**-ick) ❖
- [ ] **atrophy** (**AT**-roh-fee) ❖
- [ ] **atropine** (**AT**-roh-peen)
- [ ] **Becker's muscular dystrophy** (**BECK**-urz) ❖
- [ ] **bradykinesia** (**brad**-ee-kih-**NEE**-zee-ah *or* **brad**-ee-kih-**NEE**-zhuh) ❖
- [ ] **cardioplegia** (**kar**-dee-oh-**PLEE**-jee-ah)
- [ ] **carpal tunnel syndrome** (**KAR**-pul) ❖
- [ ] **cervical radiculopathy** (rah-**dick**-you-**LOP**-ah-thee) ❖
- [ ] **circumduction** (**ser**-kum-**DUCK**-shun)
- [ ] **claudication** (**klaw**-dih-**KAY**-shun) ❖
- [ ] **contracture** (kon-**TRACK**-chur) ❖
- [ ] **dorsiflexion** (**dor**-sih-**FLECK**-shun)
- [ ] **Duchenne's muscular dystrophy** (doo-**SHENZ**) ❖
- [ ] **dyskinesia** (**dis**-kih-**NEE**-zee-ah) ❖
- [ ] **dystaxia** (dis-**TACK**-see-ah) ❖
- [ ] **dystonia** (dis-**TOH**-nee-ah) ❖
- [ ] **electromyography** (ee-**leck**-troh-my-**OG**-rah-fee) ❖
- [ ] **electroneuromyography** (ee-**leck**-troh-**new**-roh-my-**OG**-rah-fee) ❖
- [ ] **epicondylitis** (**ep**-ih-**kon**-dih-**LYE**-tis) ❖
- [ ] **ergonomics** (er-goh-**NOM**-icks) ❖
- [ ] **fasciitis** (fas-ee-**EYE**-tis) ❖
- [ ] **fascioplasty** (**FASH**-ee-oh-**plas**-tee) ❖
- [ ] **fasciotomy** (**fash**-ee-**OT**-oh-mee) ❖

- [ ] **fibromyalgia syndrome** (**figh**-broh-my-**AL**-jee-ah) ❖
- [ ] **hemiparesis** (**hem**-ee-pah-**REE**-sis)
- [ ] **hemiplegia** (hem-ee-**PLEE**-jee-ah) ❖
- [ ] **hyperkinesia** (**high**-per-kye-**NEE**-zee-ah) ❖
- [ ] **hypertonia** (**high**-per-**TOH**-nee-ah) ❖
- [ ] **hypokinesia** (**high**-poh-kye-**NEE**-zee-ah) ❖
- [ ] **hypotonia** (**high**-poh-**TOH**-nee-ah) ❖
- [ ] **impingement syndrome** (im-**PINJ**-ment) ❖
- [ ] **kinesiology** (kih-**nee**-see-**OL**-oh-jee) ❖
- [ ] **muscular dystrophy** (**DIS**-troh-fee) ❖
- [ ] **myalgia** (my-**AL**-jee-ah) ❖
- [ ] **myasthenia** (**my**-as-**THEE**-nee-ah) ❖
- [ ] **myasthenia gravis** (**my**-as-**THEE**-nee-ah **GRAH**-vis) ❖
- [ ] **myectomy** (my-**ECK**-toh-mee)
- [ ] **myocele** (**MY**-oh-seel) ❖
- [ ] **myoclonus** (**my**-oh-**KLOH**-nus *or* my-**OCK**-loh-nus) ❖
- [ ] **myofascial** (**my**-oh-**FASH**-ee-ahl) ❖
- [ ] **myolysis** (my-**OL**-ih-sis) ❖
- [ ] **myomalacia** (**my**-oh-mah-**LAY**-shee-ah) ❖
- [ ] **myoparesis** (**my**-oh-**PAR**-eh-sis)
- [ ] **myoplasty** (**MY**-oh-**plas**-tee) ❖
- [ ] **myorrhaphy** (my-**OR**-ah-fee) ❖
- [ ] **myorrhexis** (**my**-oh-**RECK**-sis) ❖
- [ ] **myositis** (**my**-oh-**SIGH**-tis) ❖
- [ ] **myotonia** (**my**-oh-**TOH**-nee-ah) ❖
- [ ] **oblique** (oh-**BLEEK**)
- [ ] **paraplegia** (**par**-ah-**PLEE**-jee-ah) ❖
- [ ] **polymyositis** (**pol**-ee-**my**-oh-**SIGH**-tis) ❖
- [ ] **pronation** (proh-**NAY**-shun)
- [ ] **quadriplegia** (**kwad**-rih-**PLEE**-jee-ah) ❖
- [ ] **rectus** (**RECK**-tus)
- [ ] **singultus** (sing-**GUL**-tus) ❖
- [ ] **spasmodic torticollis** (spaz-**MOD**-ick **tor**-tih-**KOL**-is) ❖
- [ ] **sphincter** (**SFINK**-ter)
- [ ] **supination** (**soo**-pih-**NAY**-shun)
- [ ] **tardive dyskinesia** (**TAHR**-div **dis**-kih-**NEE**-zee-ah) ❖
- [ ] **tenalgia** (ten-**AL**-jee-ah) ❖
- [ ] **tendinitis** (**ten**-dih-**NIGH**-tis) ❖
- [ ] **tendonitis** (**ten**-doh-**NIGH**-it-is) ❖
- [ ] **tenectomy** (teh-**NECK**-toh-mee) ❖
- [ ] **tenodesis** (ten-**ODD**-eh-sis) ❖
- [ ] **tenolysis** (ten-**OL**-ih-sis) ❖
- [ ] **tenonectomy** (**ten**-oh-**NECK**-toh-mee) ❖
- [ ] **tenoplasty** (**TEN**-oh-**plas**-tee) ❖
- [ ] **tenorrhaphy** (ten-**OR**-ah-fee) ❖
- [ ] **tenotomy** (teh-**NOT**-oh-mee) ❖

Upon completion of this chapter, you should be able to:

1. Describe the functions and structures of the muscular system including muscle fibers, fascia, tendons, and the three types of muscle.

2. Recognize, define, spell, and pronounce the terms related to muscle movements and explain how the muscles are named.

3. Recognize, define, pronounce, and spell the terms related to the pathology and diagnostic and treatment procedures of the muscular system.

FUNCTIONS OF THE MUSCULAR SYSTEM

- Muscles hold the body erect and make movement possible.

- Muscle movement generates nearly 85 percent of the heat that keeps the body warm.

- Muscles move food through the digestive system (see Chapter 8).

- Muscle movement, such as walking, aids the flow of blood through veins as it returns to the heart (see Chapter 5).

- Muscle action moves fluids through the ducts and tubes associated with other body systems.

STRUCTURES OF THE MUSCULAR SYSTEM

The body has more than 600 muscles, which make up about 40 percent to 45 percent of the body's weight. These muscles are made up of fibers, are covered with fascia, and are attached to bones by tendons.

MUSCLE FIBERS

- The muscles are composed of long, slender cells known as **muscle fibers.** (A fiber is a threadlike structure.) Each muscle consists of a group of fibers that are held together by connective tissue and enclosed in a fibrous sheath.

FASCIA

- **Fascia** (**FASH**-ee-ah) is the sheet or band of fibrous connective tissue that covers, supports, and separates muscle (plural, **fasciae** or **fascias**).

TENDONS

- A **tendon** is a narrow band of nonelastic, dense, fibrous connective tissue that attaches a muscle to a bone (Figure 4.1).

- For example, the **Achilles tendon** attaches the gastrocnemius muscle (the major muscle of the calf of the leg) to the heel bone (see Figure 4.8).

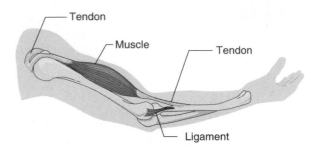

FIGURE 4.1 Tendons attach muscle to bone. Ligaments join bone to bone.

- Be careful not to confuse tendons with ligaments. As shown in Figure 4.1, ligaments connect one bone to another bone. Ligaments are discussed further in Chapter 3.

APONEUROSIS

- An **aponeurosis** (**ap**-oh-new-**ROH**-sis) is a flat fibrous sheet of connective tissue that is very similar to a tendon. However, an aponeurosis attaches a muscle to bone *or* to other tissues (plural, **aponeuroses**). As an example, the abdominal aponeurosis can be seen in Figure 4.7.

TYPES OF MUSCLE TISSUE

The three types of muscle tissue are skeletal, smooth, and cardiac (Figure 4.2). These types are described according to their appearance and function.

SKELETAL MUSCLES

- **Skeletal muscles** attach to the bones of the skeleton and are the muscles that make possible body motions such as walking and smiling.

- Skeletal muscles are also known as **striated** (**STRYE**-ayt-ed) muscles because the dark and light bands in the muscle fibers create a striped (striated) appearance (see Figure 4.2A).

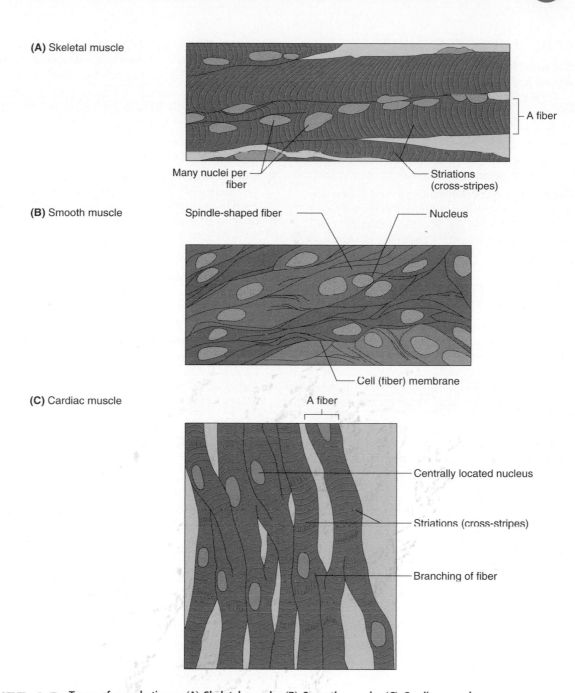

(A) Skeletal muscle

A fiber

Many nuclei per fiber

Striations (cross-stripes)

(B) Smooth muscle

Spindle-shaped fiber

Nucleus

Cell (fiber) membrane

(C) Cardiac muscle

A fiber

Centrally located nucleus

Striations (cross-stripes)

Branching of fiber

FIGURE 4.2   Types of muscle tissue. (A) Skeletal muscle. (B) Smooth muscle. (C) Cardiac muscle.

● Skeletal muscles are also known as **voluntary muscles** because we have conscious (voluntary) control over these muscles.

SMOOTH MUSCLES

● **Smooth muscles** are located in the walls of internal organs such as the digestive tract, blood vessels, and ducts leading from glands. Their function is to move and control the flow of fluids through these structures.

● Smooth muscles are also known as **unstriated muscles** because they do *not* have the dark and light bands that produce the striped (striated) appearance seen in striated muscles (see Figure 4.2B).

● Smooth muscles are also known as **involuntary muscles** because they are under the control of the autonomic nervous system and are not under voluntary control.

● Smooth muscles are also known as **visceral muscles** (**VIS**-er-al) because they are found in the large internal organs (except the heart) and in hollow structures such as those of the digestive and urinary systems.

CARDIAC MUSCLE

- **Cardiac muscle**, also known as **myocardial muscle** (**my**-oh-**KAR**-dee-al), forms the muscular wall of the heart (**my/o** means muscle, **cardi** means heart, and **-al** means pertaining to). The heart is discussed further in Chapter 5.

- This muscle is also known as the **myocardium** (**my**-oh-**KAR**-dee-um) (**my/o** means muscle, **card** means heart, and **-ium** means tissue).

- **Cardiac muscle** is specialized tissue that is like striated muscle in appearance but like smooth muscle in its action (see Figure 4.2C). It is the contraction and relaxation of this muscle that causes the heartbeat.

CHARACTERISTICS OF MUSCLES

Kinesiology (kih-**nee**-see-**OL**-oh-jee) is the study of muscular activity and the resulting movement of body parts (**kinesi** means movement and **-ology** means the study of).

ANTAGONISTIC MUSCLE PAIRS

- The muscles are arranged in antagonistic pairs. **Antagonistic** means to work in opposition to each other.

- In an antagonistic pair, one muscle produces movement in one direction, and the other muscle produces movement in the opposite direction.

CONTRACTION AND RELAXATION

- Muscles are made up of specialized cells that can change length or shape by contracting and relaxing. These contrasting actions make motion possible.

- **Contraction** is the tightening of a muscle. As the muscle contracts, it becomes shorter and thicker, causing the belly (center) of the muscle to enlarge.

- **Relaxation** occurs when a muscle returns to its original form. As the muscle relaxes, it becomes longer and thinner and its belly is no longer enlarged.

- When one muscle of a pair contracts, the other usually relaxes (Figure 4.3).

- **Muscle tone,** also known as **tonus** (**TOH**-nus), is the normal state of balanced muscle tension (contraction and relaxation) that is required to hold the body in an awake position.

MUSCLE INNERVATION

- **Muscle innervation** (**in**-err-**VAY**-shun) is the stimulation of the muscle by an impulse transmitted by a motor nerve. This stimulation causes the muscle to contract. When the stimulation stops, the muscle relaxes.

- **Neuromuscular** (**new**-roh-**MUS**-kyou-lar) means pertaining to the relationship between nerve and muscle. If the nerve impulse is interrupted because of injury or pathology of the nervous system, the muscle is paralyzed and cannot contract.

RANGE OF MOTION

Range of motion (ROM) is the change in joint position that is produced by muscle movements. These muscle motions, which occur as pairs of opposites, are described in the following text, contrasted in Table 4.1, and illustrated in Figures 4.4 through 4.6.

ABDUCTION AND ADDUCTION

- **Abduction** (ab-**DUCK**-shun) is movement away from the midline of the body (Figure 4.4). For example, during abduction the arm moves outward, away from the side of the body.

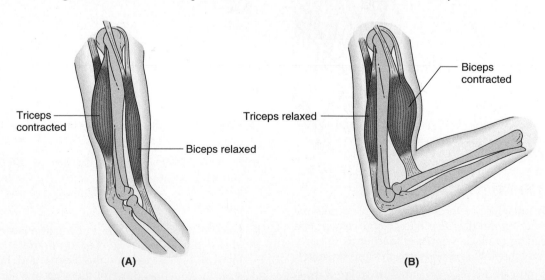

Triceps contracted

Biceps relaxed

Biceps contracted

Triceps relaxed

(A)

(B)

FIGURE 4.3 An antagonistic muscle pair of the upper arm. (A) During extension of the elbow, the triceps is contracted and the biceps is relaxed. (B) During flexion of the elbow, the triceps is relaxed and the biceps is contracted.

Table 4.1

CONTRASTING MUSCLE MOTIONS

Abduction moves away from the midline.	**Adduction** moves toward the midline.
Flexion (bending) decreases an angle as in bending a joint.	**Extension** (straightening) increases an angle as in straightening a joint.
Elevation raises a body part.	**Depression** lowers a body part.
Rotation turns a bone on its own axis.	**Circumduction** turns at the far end.
Supination turns the palm upward or forward.	**Pronation** turns the palm downward or backward.
Dorsiflexion bends the foot upward at the ankle.	**Plantar flexion** bends the foot downward at the ankle.

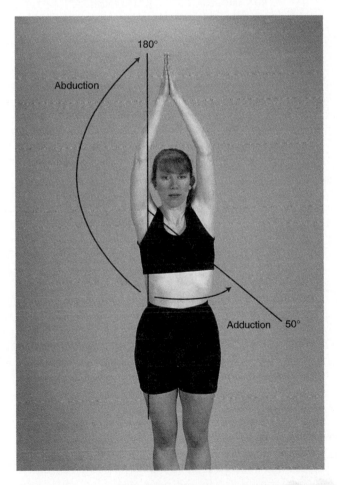

FIGURE 4.4 Abduction moves the arm away from the body. Adduction moves the arm toward the body.

- An **abductor** is a muscle that moves a part away from the midline.
- **Adduction** (ah-**DUCK**-shun) is movement toward the midline of the body (Figure 4.4). For example, during adduction the arm moves inward, toward the side of the body.

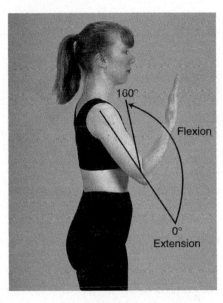

FIGURE 4.5 Extension increases the angle of the elbow. Flexion decreases the angle of the elbow.

- An **adductor** is a muscle that moves a part toward the midline.

FLEXION AND EXTENSION

- **Flexion** (**FLECK**-shun) means decreasing the angle between two bones or bending a limb at a joint (Figure 4.5). During flexion of the arm, the elbow is bent and the lower arm is brought upward. During flexion of the leg, the knee is bent and the lower leg is brought backward.
- A **flexor** is a muscle that bends a limb at a joint.
- **Extension** means increasing the angle between two bones or straightening out a limb (Figure 4.5). During extension of the arm, the elbow is straightened and the lower syrm is brought downward. During extension of the leg, the knee is straightened and the lower leg brought forward.

- An **extensor** is a muscle that straightens a limb at a joint.
- **Hyperextension** is the extreme or overextension of a limb or body part beyond its normal limit. For example, movement of the head far backward or far forward beyond the normal range of motion causes hyperextension of the muscles of the neck.

ELEVATION AND DEPRESSION

- **Elevation** is the act of raising or lifting a body part, such as raising the ribs when breathing in.
- A **levator** (lee-**VAY**-tor) is a muscle that raises a body part. For example, the *levator anguli oris* raises the corner of the mouth (*anguli* means angle and *oris* means mouth).
- **Depression** is the act of lowering a body part such as lowering the ribs when breathing out.
- A **depressor** is a muscle that lowers a body part. For example, the *depressor anguli oris* lowers the corner of the mouth.

ROTATION AND CIRCUMDUCTION

- **Rotation** is a circular movement around an axis. Turning the head as when saying no is an example of rotation.
- A **rotator muscle** turns a body part on its axis. (An *axis* is the central line of the body or any of its parts.) For example, the head of the humerus (upper arm bone) rotates within the shoulder joint.
- The **rotator cuff** is the group of muscles that hold the head of the humerus securely in place as it rotates within the shoulder joint (see Figure 4.12).
- **Circumduction** (ser-kum-**DUCK**-shun) is the circular movement of a limb at the far end. An example of circumduction is the swinging motion of the far end of the arm when throwing a ball.

SUPINATION AND PRONATION

- **Supination** (soo-pih-**NAY**-shun) is the act of rotating the arm or the leg so that the palm of the hand or sole of the foot is turned forward or upward (Figure 4.6).
- **Pronation** (proh-**NAY**-shun) is the act of rotating the arm or leg so that the palm of the hand or sole of the foot is turned downward or backward (Figure 4.6).

DORSIFLEXION AND PLANTAR FLEXION

toes to the nose

- **Dorsiflexion** (dor-sih-**FLECK**-shun) bends the foot upward at the ankle. Pointing the toes and foot

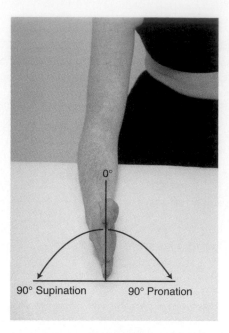

FIGURE 4.6 Supination is turning the arm so that the palm of the hand is turned upward. Pronation is turning the arm so that the palm of the hand is turned downward.

upward narrows the angle between the top of the foot and the front of the leg.

- **Plantar flexion** (**PLAN**-tar **FLECK**-shun) bends the foot downward at the ankle (*plantar* means pertaining to the sole of the foot). Pointing the toes and foot downward increases the angle between the top of the foot and the front of the leg.

HOW MUSCLES ARE NAMED

As you study this section, refer to Figures 4.7 through 4.11.

ORIGIN AND INSERTION

Some muscles are named by joining the name of the place of origin to the name of the place of insertion.

- **Muscle origin** is the place where the muscle begins (originates). This is the more fixed attachment or the end of the muscle nearest the midline of the body.
- **Muscle insertion** is the place where the muscle ends (inserts). It is the more moveable end or the portion of the muscle farthest from the midline of the body.
- For example, the **sternocleidomastoid** (ster-noh-kly-doh-**MASS**-toid) muscle, which helps flex the neck and rotate the head is named for its origin and insertion (Figure 4.9). This muscle, which has two

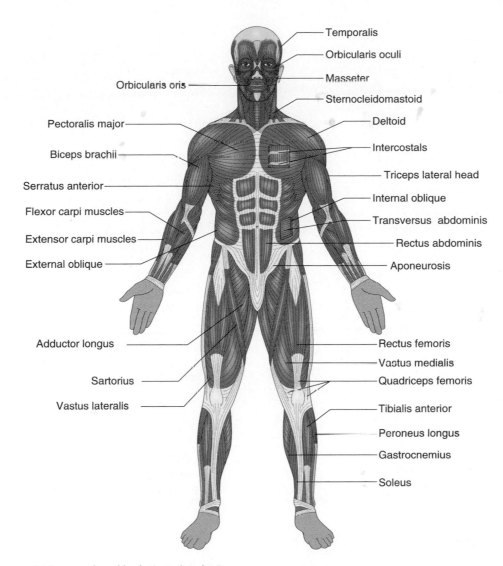

FIGURE 4.7 Major muscles of body (anterior view).

origins, begins near the midline from the sternum (breastbone) and clavicle (collar bone). It inserts away from the midline into the mastoid process of the temporal bone (located just behind the ear).

MUSCLES NAMED FOR THEIR ACTION

Some muscles are named for their action, such as flexing or extending. For example, the **flexor carpi muscles** work with the **extensor carpi muscles** to make possible the flexion and extension motions of the wrist (Figure 4.7).

MUSCLES NAMED FOR THEIR LOCATION

Some muscles are named for their location on the body or the organ they are near:

- The **pectoralis major** is an important muscle of the chest, and **pectoral** (**PECK**-toh-rahl) means relating to the chest (see Figure 4.7).

- Other muscles, such as **vastus lateralis** and **vastus medialis,** indicate their location by including *lateral* (toward the side) and *medial* (toward the midline) in their names (see Figures 4.7 and 4.8).

- Some muscles indicate their location by including *external* (near the surface) and *internal* (deeper location) in their names: Examples are the **external oblique** and **internal oblique** muscles (see Figures 4.7 and 4.10).

MUSCLES NAMED FOR FIBER DIRECTION

Some muscles are named for the direction in which their fibers run.

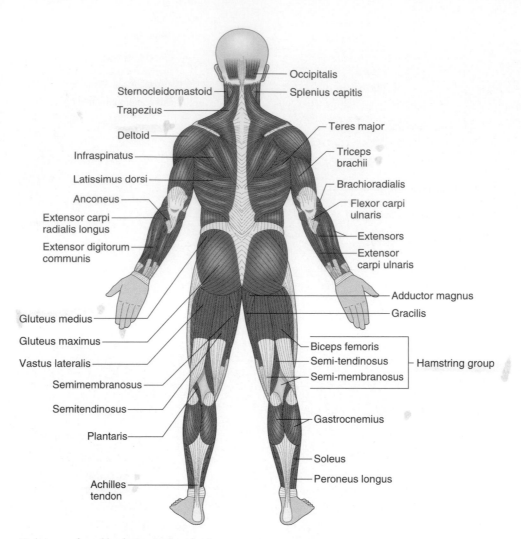

FIGURE 4.8 Major muscles of body (posterior view).

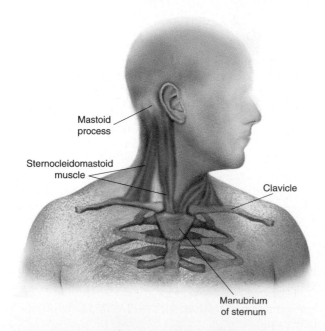

FIGURE 4.9 The sternocleidomastoid muscle is named for its origins and insertion.

- **Rectus** (**RECK**-tus) means straight. For example, **rectus abdominis** is an abdominal muscle in straight alignment with the vertical axis of the body (see Figures 4.7 and 4.10).

- **Oblique** (oh-**BLEEK**) means slanted or at an angle. For example, the **external abdominal oblique** is an abdominal muscle that slants outward, at an oblique angle, away from the midline.

- **Transverse** means in a crosswise direction. For example, the **transverse abdominis** is an abdominal muscle with a crosswise alignment.

- A **sphincter** (**SFINK**-ter) is a ringlike muscle that tightly constricts the opening of a passageway. A sphincter is named for the passage involved. For example, the **anal sphincter** closes the anus.

MUSCLES NAMED FOR NUMBER OF DIVISIONS

Muscles may be named according to the number of divisions forming them (see Figure 4.11).

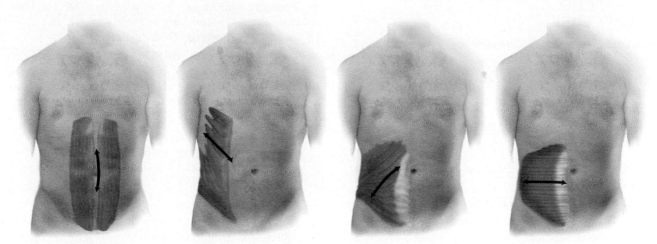

FIGURE 4.10 Examples of muscles named for their direction.

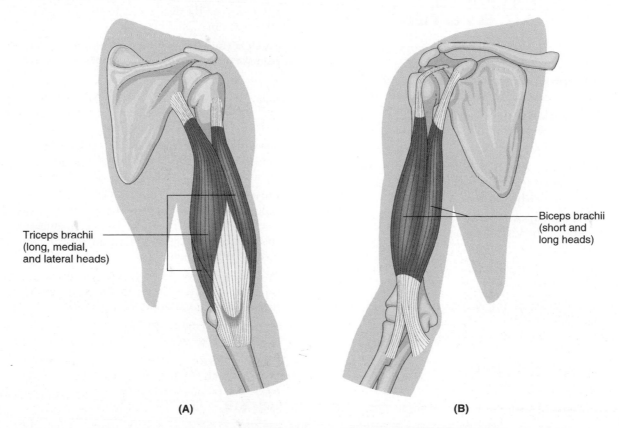

Triceps brachii
(long, medial,
and lateral heads)

Biceps brachii
(short and
long heads)

(A)   (B)

FIGURE 4.11 Muscles named for the number of divisions. (A) Posterior view. (B) Anterior view.

● The **biceps brachii** (**BRAY**-kee-eye), also known as the **biceps** muscle, is formed from two divisions (**bi-** means two and **-ceps** means head). This is the muscle of the anterior upper arm that flexes the elbow.

● The **triceps brachii** (**BRAY**-kee-eye), also known as the **triceps** muscle, is formed from three divisions (**tri-** means three and **-ceps** means head). This is the

muscle of the posterior upper arm that extends the elbow.

● The **quadriceps femoris** (**FEM**-or-iss) is formed from four muscle divisions (**quadri** means four and **-ceps** means head). This large muscle, which is located on the anterior thigh, assists in extending the femur (bone of the upper leg).

MUSCLES NAMED FOR THEIR SIZE

Some muscles are named because they are broad or narrow, or large or small.

- The **gluteus maximus** (**GLOO**-tee-us) is the largest muscle of the buttock (see Figure 4.10).

MUSCLES NAMED FOR THEIR SHAPE

Other muscles are named because they are shaped like a familiar object.

- The **deltoid muscle**, which forms the muscular shoulder cap, is shaped like an inverted triangle or the Greek letter delta (see Figures 4.7 and 4.8).

MEDICAL SPECIALTIES RELATED TO THE MUSCULAR SYSTEM

SKELETAL MUSCLE DISORDERS

- An **orthopedic surgeon** treats injuries and disorders involving bones, joints, muscles, and tendons.
- A **rheumatologist** (roo-mah-**TOL**-oh-jist) treats disorders that involve the inflammation of connective tissues including muscles.
- A **neurologist** (new-**ROL**-oh-jist) treats the cause of paralysis and similar muscular disorders in which there is a loss of function.
- A specialist in **sports medicine** treats sports-related injuries of the bones, joints, and muscles.

SMOOTH MUSCLE DISORDERS

- Smooth muscles are a key component in most body systems. The specialist who treats the involved body system also cares for any involved muscles.

CARDIAC MUSCLE DISORDERS

- A **cardiologist** treats disorders of the cardiac muscles. These disorders are discussed in Chapter 5.

PATHOLOGY OF THE MUSCULAR SYSTEM

Herni orapy surgical procedure

FIBERS, FASCIA, AND TENDONS

- **Fasciitis** (**fas**-ee-**EYE**-tis) is inflammation of a fascia (**fasci** means fascia and **-itis** means inflammation). This term is spelled correctly with two Is next to each other, but fascitis is also an acceptable spelling.

- **Tenalgia** (ten-**AL**-jee-ah) is pain in a tendon (**ten** means tendon and **-algia** means pain). It is also known as **tenodynia** (ten-oh-**DIN**-ee-ah).
- **Tendinitis** (ten-dih-**NIGH**-tis) is an inflammation of the tendons caused by excessive or unusual use of the joint (**tendin** means tendon and **-itis** means inflammation). It is also known as **tendonitis** (ten-doh-**NIGH**-it-is).
- **Overuse tendinitis** is an inflammation of tendons caused by excessive or unusual use of a joint.

MUSCLES

- An **adhesion** (ad-**HEE**-zhun) is a band of fibrous tissue that holds structures together abnormally. Adhesions may form in muscles and internal organs as the result of an injury or surgery.
- **Muscle atrophy** (**AT**-roh-fee) is the weakness and wasting away of muscle tissue. It may be caused by pathology or by disuse of the muscle over a long period of time.
- **Myalgia** (my-**AL**-jee-ah) means muscle tenderness or pain (**my** means muscle and **-algia** means pain).
- **Myolysis** (my-**OL**-ih-sis) is the degeneration (breaking down) of muscle tissue (**my/o** means muscle and **-lysis** means destruction or breaking down in disease).
- **Myositis** (my-oh-**SIGH**-tis) is inflammation of a muscle tissue, especially skeletal muscles (**myos** means muscle and **-itis** means inflammation).
- **Polymyositis** (**pol**-ee-**my**-oh-**SIGH**-tis) is a chronic, progressive disease affecting the skeletal muscles that is characterized by muscle weakness and atrophy (**poly-** means many, **myos** means muscle, and **-itis** means inflammation).
- **Myomalacia** (**my**-oh-mah-**LAY**-shee-ah) is abnormal softening of muscle tissue (**my/o** means muscle, and **-malacia** means abnormal softening).
- **Myorrhexis** (my-oh-**RECK**-sis) is the rupture of a muscle (**my/o** means muscle and **-rrhexis** means rupture).
- **Myosclerosis** (my-oh-skleh-**ROH**-sis) is abnormal hardening of muscle tissue (**my/o** means muscle and **-sclerosis** means abnormal hardening).

Hernias

- A **hernia** (**HER**-nee-ah) is the protrusion of a part or structure through the tissues normally containing it.
- A **myocele** (**MY**-oh-seel) is the protrusion of a muscle through its ruptured sheath or fascia (**my/o** means muscle and **-cele** means hernia).

Muscle Tone

- **Atonic** (ah-**TON**-ick) means the lack of normal muscle tone (**a-** means without, **ton** means tone, and **-ic** means pertaining to).

- **Dystonia** (dis-**TOH**-nee-ah) is a condition of abnormal muscle tone (**dys-** means bad, **ton** means tone, and **-ia** means condition).

- **Hypertonia** (**high**-per-**TOH**-nee-ah) is a condition of excessive tone of the skeletal muscles with an increased resistance of muscle to passive stretching (**hyper-** means excessive, **ton** means tone, and **-ia** means condition).

- **Hypotonia** (**high**-poh-**TOH**-nee-ah) is a condition of diminished tone of the skeletal muscles with decreased resistance of muscle to passive stretching (**hypo-** means deficient, **ton** means tone, and **-ia** means condition).

- **Myotonia** (**my**-oh-**TOH**-nee-ah) is the delayed relaxation of a muscle after a strong contraction (**my/o** means muscle, **ton** means tone, and **-ia** means condition).

Voluntary Muscle Movement

- **Ataxia** (ah-**TACK**-see-ah) is an inability to coordinate the muscles in the execution of voluntary movement (**a-** means without, **tax** means coordination, and **-ia** means condition).

- **Dystaxia** (dis-**TACK**-see-ah), also known as **partial ataxia,** is difficulty in controlling voluntary movement (**dys-** means bad, **tax** means coordination, and **-ia** means condition).

- A **contracture** (kon-**TRACK**-chur) is an abnormal shortening of muscle tissues, making the muscle resistant to stretching.

- **Intermittent claudication** (klaw-dih-**KAY**-shun) is a complex of symptoms including cramplike pain of the leg muscles caused by poor circulation. It may be an indication of a larger cardiovascular problem.

- A **spasm,** also known as a **cramp,** is a sudden, violent, involuntary contraction of a muscle or a group of muscles.

- **Spasmodic torticollis** (spaz-**MOD**-ick **tor**-tih-**KOL**-is), also known as **wryneck,** is a stiff neck due to spasmodic contraction of the neck muscles that pull the head toward the affected side.

Muscle Function

- **Bradykinesia** (**brad**-ee-kih-**NEE**-zee-ah *or* **brad**-ee-kih-**NEE**-zhuh) means extreme slowness in movement (**brady-** means slow, **kines** means movement, and **-ia** means condition).

- **Dyskinesia** (**dis**-kih-**NEE**-zee-ah) means distortion or impairment of voluntary movement as in a tic or spasm (**dys-** means bad, **kines** means movement, and **-ia** means condition).

- **Hyperkinesia** (**high**-per-kye-**NEE**-zee-ah), also known as **hyperactivity,** means abnormally increased motor function or activity (**hyper-** means excessive, **kines** means movement, and **-ia** means condition).

- **Hypokinesia** (**high**-poh-kye-**NEE**-zee-ah) is abnormally decreased motor function or activity (**hypo-** means deficient, **kines** means movement, and **-ia** means condition).

- **Tardive dyskinesia** (**TAHR**-div **dis**-kih-**NEE**-zee-ah) is the late appearance of dyskinesia as a side effect of long-term treatment with certain antipsychotic drugs. (*Tardive* means lateness in appearance.)

Myoclonus

- **Myoclonus** (**my**-oh-**KLOH**-nus *or* **my**-**OCK**-loh-nus) is a spasm or twitching of a muscle or group of muscles (**my/o** means muscle, **clon** mean violent action, and **-us** is a singular noun ending).

- **Nocturnal myoclonus** (nock-**TER**-nal **my**-oh-**KLOH**-nus *or* **my**-**OCK**-loh-nus) is jerking of the limbs that may occur normally as a person is falling asleep. (*Nocturnal* means pertaining to night.)

- **Singultus** (sing-**GUL**-tus), also known as **hiccups,** is myoclonus of the diaphragm that causes the characteristic hiccup sound with each spasm. (The diaphragm is the muscle separating the chest and abdomen.)

Myasthenia Gravis

- **Myasthenia** (**my**-as-**THEE**-nee-ah) is muscle weakness from any cause (**my** means muscle, and **-asthenia** means weakness or lack of strength).

- **Myasthenia gravis** (**my**-as-**THEE**-nee-ah **GRAH**-vis), also known as **MG,** is a chronic autoimmune disease in which there is an abnormality in the neuromuscular function causing episodes of muscle weakness. MG most frequently affects the muscles that control eye movements, eyelids, chewing, swallowing, coughing, and facial expression.

Muscular Dystrophy

- **Muscular dystrophy** (**DIS**-troh-fee) is a group of inherited muscle disorders that cause muscle weakness without affecting the nervous system. The most common forms, which affect only males, are Duchenne's muscular dystrophy (DMD) and Becker's muscular dystrophy (BMD).

- **Duchenne's muscular dystrophy** (doo-**SHENZ**) appears from two to six years of age and progresses slowly. However, survival is rare beyond the late twenties.

- **Becker's muscular dystrophy** (**BECK**-urz) is a less severe illness and does not appear until early adolescence or adulthood. The progression is slower, with survival well into middle to late adulthood.

Fibromyalgia Syndrome

- **Fibromyalgia syndrome** (**figh**-broh-my-**AL**-jee-ah) is a chronic disorder of unknown cause, characterized by widespread aching pain, tender points, and fatigue (**fibr/o** means fibrous connective tissue, **my** means muscle, and **-algia** means pain). Also known as **FMS,** this syndrome does not cause joint deformity, is not progressive, and is not crippling.

ROTATOR CUFF

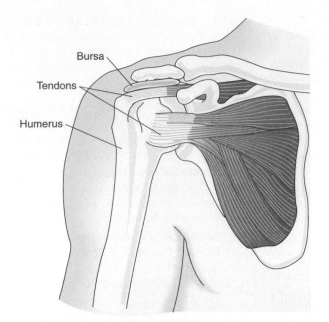

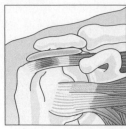

Overuse
tendinitis

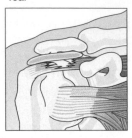

Tear

FIGURE 4.12 The rotator cuff in health (left) and with injuries (right).

- **Tender points,** which are abnormal localized areas of soreness, are important diagnostic indicators of FMS. These points occur at predictable locations at the base of the neck, along the backbone, in front of the hip and elbow, and at the rear of the knee and shoulder.

REPETITIVE STRESS DISORDERS

- **Repetitive stress disorders** have symptoms caused by repetitive motions that involve muscles, tendons, nerves, and joints. These conditions most commonly occur as workplace or sports injuries.

- **Ergonomics** (er-goh-**NOM**-icks) is the study of human factors that affect the design and operation of tools and the work environment (**erg/o** means work, **nom** means control, and **-ics** means pertaining to). The term *ergonomic* is also applied to the design of sports equipment.

- **Overuse injuries** are minor tissue injuries that have not been given time to heal. Such injuries may be caused by spending hours at the keyboard or by lengthy sports training sesions.

Myofascial Damage

- **Myofascial damage** (**my**-oh-**FASH**-ee-ahl), which can be caused by overworking the muscles, results in tenderness and swelling of the muscles and their surrounding tissues (**my/o** means muscle, **fasci** means fascia, and **-al** means pertaining to).

Rotator Cuff Injuries

- **Rotator cuff tendinitis** (ten-dih-**NIGH**-tis) is an inflammation of the tendons of the rotator cuff (Figure

4.12). This condition is often named for the cause, such as **tennis shoulder** or **pitcher's shoulder.**

- **Impingement syndrome** (im-**PINJ**-ment) occurs when the tendons become inflamed and get caught in the narrow space between the bones within the shoulder joint.

- **Calcium deposits** may form within the tendons of the rotator cuff. These deposits cause chronic irritation of the tendons.

- If left untreated, or if the overuse continues, the irritated tendon may weaken and tear, becoming a **torn tendon.**

Carpal Tunnel Syndrome

- The **carpal tunnel** (**KAR-pul**) is a narrow bony passage under the carpal ligament located 1/4 inch below the inner surface of the wrist (Figure 4.13). The median nerve and the tendons that bend the fingers pass through this tunnel. (*Carpal* means pertaining to the wrist.)

- **Carpal tunnel syndrome** occurs when the tendons passing through the carpal tunnel are chronically overused and become inflamed and swollen. This swelling creates compression (pressure) on the median nerve as it passes through the carpal tunnel. This causes pain, burning, and paresthesia (tingling) in the fingers and hand.

Cervical Radiculopathy

- **Cervical radiculopathy** (rah-**dick**-you-**LOP**-ah-thee) is nerve pain caused by pressure on the spinal nerve roots in the neck region (**cervical** means neck,

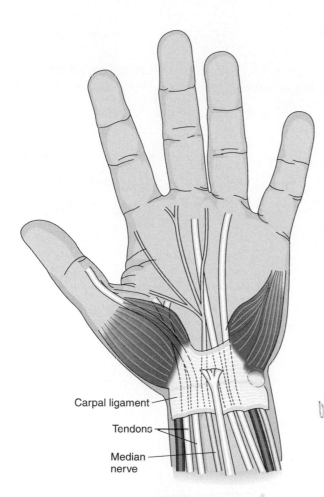

Carpal ligament

Tendons

Median
nerve

FIGURE 4.13 Carpal tunnel syndrome.

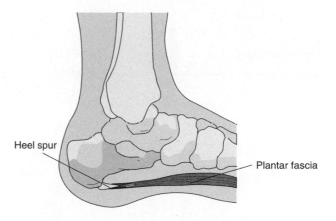

Heel spur

Plantar fascia

FIGURE 4.14 Plantar fasciitis and heel spur.

SPORTS INJURIES

- A **sprain** is an injury to a joint such as ankle, knee, or wrist. Frequently caused by overuse, a sprain frequently involves a stretched or torn ligament.

- A **strain** is an injury to the body of the muscle or attachment of the tendon. Strains usually are associated with overuse injuries that involve a stretched or torn muscle or tendon attachment.

- Although *sprain* and *strain* have different meanings, these terms are frequently used interchangeably.

- A **shin splint** is pain caused by the muscle tearing away from the tibia, which is also known as the **shinbone.** Shin splints can develop in the anterolateral (front and side) muscles or in the posteromedial (back and side) muscles of the lower leg (see Figures 4.7 and 4.8). This type of injury is usually caused by repeated stress to the lower leg.

- A **hamstring injury** may be a strain or tear of the posterior femoral muscles. (*Hamstring* refers to the three muscles on the posterior of the thigh that straighten the hip and bend the knee, as shown in Figure 4.10.) These injuries usually cause sudden pain in the back of the thigh as these muscles contract suddenly.

- **Achilles tendinitis** (ten-dih-**NIGH**-tis) is a painful inflammation of the Achilles tendon caused by excessive stress being placed on the tendon.

PARALYSIS

- **Myoparesis** (**my**-oh-**PAR**-eh-sis) is a weakness or slight paralysis of a muscle (**my/o** means muscle and **-paresis** means partial or incomplete paralysis).

- **Hemiparesis** (**hem**-ee-pah-**REE**-sis) means slight paralysis of one side of the body (**hemi-** means half and **-paresis** means partial or incomplete paralysis).

- **Paralysis** (pah-**RAL**-ih-sis) is the loss of sensation and voluntary muscle movements through disease or injury to its nerve supply. Damage may be either temporary or permanent (plural, **paralyses**).

radicul/o means nerve root, and **-pathy** means disease). This pressure may caused by muscle spasms due to repetitive motions or by compression of cervical vertebral disks.

Epicondylitis

- **Epicondylitis** (**ep**-ih-**kon**-dih-**LYE**-tis) is inflammation of the tissues surrounding the elbow.

- **Lateral epicondylitis,** with pain on the outer side of the arm of the forearm, is also known as **tennis elbow.**

- **Medial epicondylitis,** with pain on the palm-side of the forearm, is also known as **golfer's elbow.**

Plantar Fasciitis

- **Plantar fasciitis** is an inflammation of the plantar fascia causing foot or heel pain when walking or running. A **heel spur** is a thickening on the surface of the calcaneus bone that causes severe pain when standing (Figure 4.14).

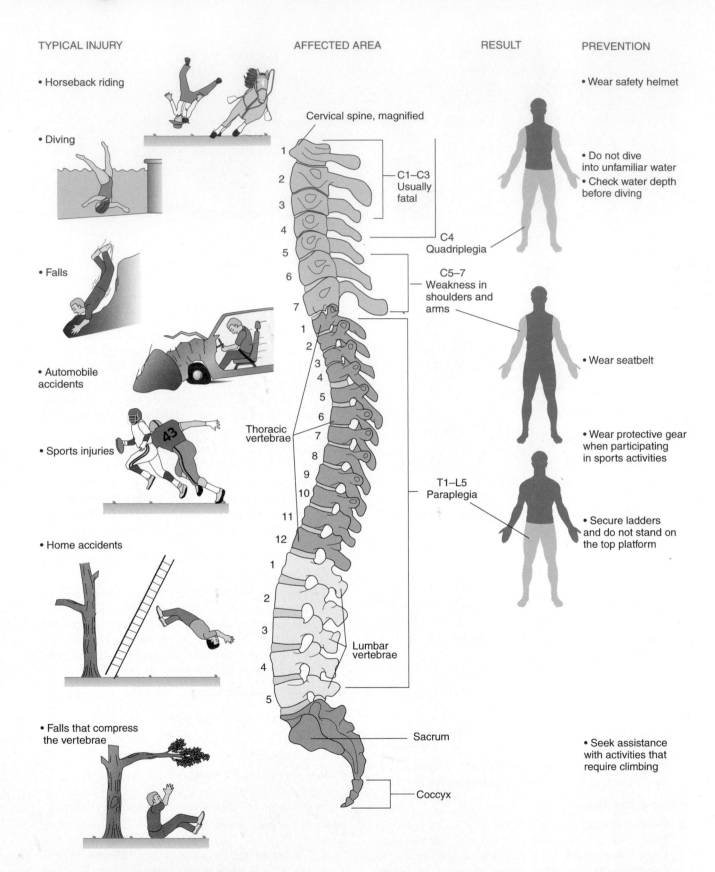

TYPICAL INJURY

• Horseback riding

• Diving

• Falls

• Automobile accidents

• Sports injuries

• Home accidents

• Falls that compress the vertebrae

AFFECTED AREA

Cervical spine, magnified

1
2
3
4
5
6
7

C1–C3
Usually
fatal

C4
Quadriplegia

C5–7
Weakness in
shoulders and
arms

Thoracic
vertebrae

1
2
3
4
5
6
7
8
9
10
11
12

T1–L5
Paraplegia

Lumbar
vertebrae

1
2
3
4
5

Sacrum

Coccyx

RESULT

PREVENTION

• Wear safety helmet

• Do not dive into unfamiliar water
• Check water depth before diving

• Wear seatbelt

• Wear protective gear when participating in sports activities

• Secure ladders and do not stand on the top platform

• Seek assistance with activities that require climbing

FIGURE 4.15 Spinal cord injuries.

- A **spinal cord injury (SCI)** often causes paralysis because nerve impulses cannot be carried below the level of the injury (Figure 4.15).

- **Paraplegia** (**par**-ah-**PLEE**-jee-ah) is the paralysis of both legs and the lower part of the body. An individual affected with paraplegia is known as a **paraplegic.** An SCI below the cervical vertebrae results in paraplegia.

- **Quadriplegia** (**kwad**-rih-**PLEE**-jee-ah) is the paralysis of all four extremities (**quadri** means four and **-plegia** means paralysis). An SCI involving the cervical vertebrae causes quadriplegia. If the injury is above C5, it also affects respiration.

- **Hemiplegia** (**hem**-ee-**PLEE**-jee-ah) is the total paralysis of one side of the body (**hemi-** means half and **-plegia** means paralysis). This form of paralysis is usually associated with a stroke or brain damage. Damage to one side of the brain causes paralysis on the opposite side of the body.

- **Cardioplegia** (**kar**-dee-oh-**PLEE**-jee-ah) is paralysis of the muscles of the heart (**cardi/o** means heart and **-plegia** means paralysis).

DIAGNOSTIC PROCEDURES OF THE MUSCULAR SYSTEM

- **Deep tendon reflexes (DTR)** are tested with a reflex hammer used to strike the tendon. Figure 4.16 shows reflex testing on the kneecap (patellar reflex) and Achilles tendon (calcaneus reflex). No response or an abnormal response may indicate a disruption of the nerve supply to the involved muscles. Reflexes also are lost in deep coma or because of medication such as heavy sedation.

- **Electromyography** (ee-**leck**-troh-my-**OG**-rah-fee), also known as an **EMG**, records the strength of muscle contractions as the result of electrical stimulation. The resulting record is called an **electromyogram** (**electr/o** means electricity, **my/o** means muscle, and **-gram** means record). This test may be helpful in determining the cause of pain, numbness, tingling, or weakness in the muscles or nerves.

- **Electroneuromyography** (ee-**leck**-troh-**new**-roh-my-**OG**-rah-fee), also known as **nerve conduction studies,** is a procedure for testing and recording neuromuscular activity by the electric stimulation of the nerve trunk that carries fibers to and from the muscle (**electr/o** means electricity, **neur/o** means nerve, **my/o** means muscle, and **-graphy** means the process of recording).

- **Range of motion testing (ROM)** is a diagnostic procedure to evaluate joint mobility and muscle strength (see Figure 4.17).

TREATMENT PROCEDURES OF THE MUSCULAR SYSTEM
MEDICATIONS

- An **anti-inflammatory,** such as ibuprofen (Motrin), acts as an analgesic (relieves pain) and as an anti-inflammatory (relieves inflammation).

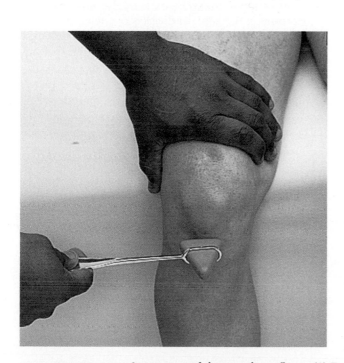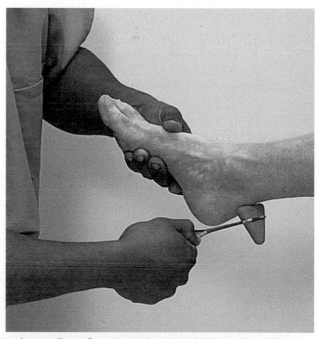

FIGURE 4.16 Assessment of deep tendon reflexes. (A) Testing the patellar reflex. (B) Testing the Achilles tendon reflex.

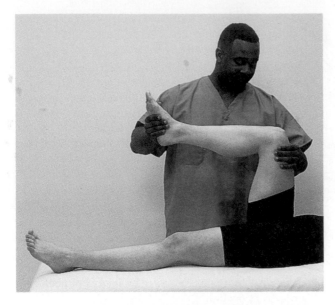

FIGURE 4.17 Range of motion (ROM) exercises aid in restoring joint mobility and muscle strength.

- An **antispasmodic,** also known as an **anticholinergic drug** (an-tih-**koh**-lin-**ER**-jik), acts to control spasmodic activity of the smooth muscles such as those of the intestine.
- **Atropine** (**AT**-roh-peen) is an antispasmodic that may be administered preoperatively to relax smooth muscles.
- A **muscle relaxant,** such as diazepam (Valium), acts on the central nervous system to relax muscle tone and relieve spasms. Many of these medications also relieve anxiety and tension.

PHYSICAL THERAPY

- **Physical therapy (PT)** is treatment to prevent disability or to restore functioning through the use of exercise, heat, massage, and other methods to improve circulation, flexibility, and muscle strength.
- **Range of motion exercises (ROM)** are one form of PT. The goal of these therapeutic measures is to increase strength, flexibility, and mobility (Figure 4.17).

Activities of Daily Living

The minimum goal of therapy is to restore the individual to the level of self-help known as **activities of daily living.** Also known as **ADL,** these activities include

- personal hygiene
- dressing
- grooming
- eating
- toileting

FASCIA

- A **fasciotomy** (fash-ee-**OT**-oh-mee) is a surgical incision of a fascia (**fasci** means fascia and **-otomy** means a surgical incision).
- **Fascioplasty** (**FASH**-ee-oh-**plas**-tee) is the surgical repair of a fascia (**fasci/o** means fascia and **-plasty** means surgical repair).

TENDONS

- **Carpal tunnel release** is the surgical enlargement of the carpal tunnel or cutting of the carpal ligament to relieve nerve pressure. This treatment is used to relieve the pressure on tendons and nerves in severe cases of carpal tunnel syndrome.
- A **tenectomy** (teh-**NECK**-toh-mee) is the surgical removal of a lesion from a tendon or tendon sheath (**ten** means tendon and **-ectomy** means surgical removal).
- **Tenodesis** (ten-**ODD**-eh-sis) means to suture the end of a tendon to bone (**ten/o** means tendon and **desis** means to bind or tie together).
- **Tenolysis** (ten-**OL**-ih-sis) means to free a tendon from adhesions (**ten/o** means tendon, and **-lysis** means to set free).
- A **tenonectomy** (ten-oh-**NECK**-toh-mee) is the surgical removal of part of a tendon for the purpose of shortening it (**tenon** means tendon and **-ectomy** means surgical removal). (Notice that *tenectomy* and *tenonectomy* are similar in spelling but different in meaning.)
- A **tenotomy** (teh-**NOT**-oh-mee), also known as **tendotomy,** is the surgical division of a tendon for relief of a deformity caused by the abnormal shortening of a muscle such as strabismus (crossed eyes).
- **Tenoplasty** (**TEN**-oh-**plas**-tee), also known as **tendoplasty,** is the surgical repair of a tendon (**ten/o** means tendon and **-plasty** means surgical repair).
- **Tenorrhaphy** (ten-**OR**-ah-fee) is the suturing of a divided tendon (**ten/o** means tendon and **-rrhaphy** means to suture).

MUSCLES

- A **myectomy** (my-**ECK**-toh-mee) is the surgical removal of a portion of a muscle (**my** means muscle and **-ectomy** means surgical removal).
- **Myoplasty** (**MY**-oh-**plas**-tee) is the surgical repair of a muscle (**my/o** means muscle and **-plasty** means surgical repair).
- **Myorrhaphy** (my-**OR**-ah-fee) means to suture a muscle wound (**my/o** means muscle and **-rrhaphy** means to suture).

Career Opportunities

In addition to the medical specialties already discussed, some of the health occupations involving the treatment of the muscular system include

- **Physical therapist (PT):** provides treatment to improve mobility and prevent or limit permanent disability of patients with injuries or diseases. PTs plan, implement, and evaluate their patients' physical therapy programs. Some of their specialties are

  Cardiopulmonary physical therapy

  Clinical electrophysiology (therapeutic use of electric currents)

  Geriatric physical therapy

  Neurological physical therapy

  Orthopedic physical therapy

  Pediatric physical therapy

  Sports physical therapy

- **Physical therapy assistant (PTA)** or **aide:** helps carry out plans of treatment prescribed by the physical therapist. PTAs also maintain equipment and accessories.

- **Massage therapist:** uses bodywork or therapeutic touch to provide pain relief and encourage healing

- **Athletic trainer (AT):** works to prevent and treat athletic injuries and provides rehabilitative services to athletes who have been hurt. ATs provide massage, corrective exercises, diet supervision, and equipment fittings. An ATC is a certified athletic trainer.

- **Kinesiotherapist:** works under the supervision of a physician to provide rehabilitation exercise programs designed to reverse or minimize the debilitation of patients undergoing medical treatment. Kinesiotherapists' specialties include aquatic therapy, prosthetic or orthotic training, and geriatric rehabilitation.

- **Occupational therapist (OT):** treats people with mental, physical, developmental, and emotional disabilities, helping them develop or maintain daily living skills

- **Occupational therapist, assistant,** or **aide:** works under the supervision of an OT to help patients with prescribed exercises and activities

Health Occupation Profile: PHYSICAL THERAPIST

Barb Park is a physical therapist with many years of varied work experience. "I chose to study physical therapy because I liked science and working with people. I knew that PTs could find work in many settings including hospitals, rehabilitation centers, schools, clinics, and institutions. I started out in a rehab setting helping patients who had suffered strokes, amputations, and spinal cord injuries. My work there included helping people increase mobility skills such as relearning how to walk. I then got a chance to work in hospitals with people with a wide variety of problems including back pain, orthopedic problems, and burns. For the last 30 years I've worked in an institution with severely developmentally disabled adults and children, making a real difference in their lives by helping them learn very basic skills, such as head control, and helping design wheelchairs for their comfort and optimal function."

STUDY BREAK

Singultus, better known as the *hiccups,* are the result of an involuntary, spasmodic contraction of the diaphragm followed by the closing of the throat. Although hiccups usually eventually disappear on their own, an Iowa man is known to have hiccuped for more than 60 years!

Thousands of folk "cures" for singultus have been proposed, including

- Drinking water from the far side of a glass with your head upside down
- Sucking on a lemon

- Blowing into and out of a paper bag
- Drinking water while pinching your nose closed
- Pulling on your forefingers
- Standing on your head
- Eating sugar

However, a few unlucky, frequent hiccups sufferers require a physician's care because continuous hiccups are curtailing their work opportunities, sleep, and social life.

Review Time

Write the answers to the following questions on a separate piece of paper or in your notebook. In addition, be prepared to take part in the classroom discussion.

1. **Written assignment:** Identify four ways in which **muscles can be named.**

   Discussion assignment: Give an example of the muscles in each of the four categories.

2. **Written assignment:** Use your own words to describe the difference between **Duchenne's muscular dystrophy** and **Becker's muscular dystrophy.**

   Discussion assignment: What do you think will be the emotional impact on a family that has just received a diagnosis of either condition?

3. Hilda has been a "wiz" on the computer keyboard for years. Recently, she has complained of pain and a burning sensation in her fingers.

   Written assignment: Describe what happens within the wrist to cause **carpal tunnel syndrome.**

   Discussion assignment: How would you explain this condition to Hilda?

4. In the ER, Dr. Woo performed a **myorrhaphy** on the gluteus maximus of a young stabbing victim.

   Written assignment: Describe the procedure performed by Dr. Woo.

   Discussion assignment: How do these word parts work together to form this term, and is a combining vowel used?

5. Jennifer is on the tennis team and is experiencing pain when she serves. Dr. Hendrix performed several tests, including ROM, and established a diagnosis of **tennis elbow.**

   Written assignment: Use terms a physician would understand to describe this condition.

   Discussion assignment: How would you present this diagnosis to Jennifer in terms she can understand?

Optional Internet Activity

*The goal of this activity is to help you learn more about medical terminology while improving your Internet skills. Select **one** of these two options and follow the instructions.*

1. **Internet Search:** Search for information about the prevention of **carpal tunnel syndrome.** Write a brief (one- or two-paragraph) report on something new you learned here and include the address of the web site where you found this information.

2. **Web Site:** To have fun while learning about sports injuries go to this web address: **http://www.medfacts.com/**. Click first on Sports Doc and then on Play Doctor. Write a brief (one- or two-paragraph) report on a patient you treated and be honest as to whether your diagnosis was accurate.

The Human Touch: Critical Thinking Exercise

The following story and questions are designed to stimulate critical thinking through class discussion or as a brief essay response. There are no right or wrong answers to these questions.

"Leg muscles save back muscles. . . . Mandatory OSHA meeting Tuesday at noon. Bring lunch," states the company memo. Sandor Padilla, a 28-year-old cargo loader, sighs. "Third meeting this year, and it's not even June yet!" He only has two minutes to reach the tarmac. "Oh well, cargo waits for no man," he thinks as he jogs off to work.

Sandor enjoys his job. It keeps him fit but lets his mind follow more creative avenues. Today, his thoughts stray to his daughter Reina's fifth birthday party, just two weeks away. "A pony or a clown? Hot dogs or tacos?" he muses. Single parenting has its moments. As he is busy thinking of other things, the heavy crate slips, driving him into a squatting position that injures his thigh muscles. His cry of pain brings Janet Wilson, his supervisor, running to help.

The first aid station ices his leg to reduce swelling and pain. After the supervisor completes the incident report, she drives Sandor to the emergency room. Dr. Basra, the orthopedic specialist on call, diagnoses myorrhexis of the left rectus femoris with myoparesis. A myotomy with myorrhaphy is performed. After four days in the hospital, Sandor is sent home with a Vicodin prescription for pain and orders for physical therapy sessions three times a week. He is not expected to return to work for at least 90 days.

AirFreight Systems receives the first report of injury and compares it with the supervisor's incident report. Ruling: Safety Violation. No Liability. Return to work in 30 days or dismissal.

Suggested Discussion Topics

1. On what basis do you think AirFreight determined that this was a safety violation?
2. Who do you think should be liable for Sandor's accident and the cost of his medical care? Why?
3. Do you think the air freight company can take away Sandor's job if he does not return in 30 calendar days?
4. What do you think are Sandor's options if he cannot return to work at the airport within 30 calendar days?
5. Use your knowledge of medical terminology to describe the extent of Sandor's injury, diagnosis, and treatment to someone with no medical background.

Student Workbook and Student Activity CD-ROM

1. Go to your **Student Workbook** and complete the Learning Exercises for this chapter.
2. Go to the **Student Activity CD-ROM** and have fun with the exercises and games for this chapter.

The Cardiovascular System

● Overview of Structures, Word Parts, and Functions of the Cardiovascular System

MAJOR STRUCTURES	RELATED WORD ROOTS	PRIMARY FUNCTIONS
Heart	card/o, cardi/o	Pumps blood into the arteries.
Arteries	arteri/o	Transport blood to all body parts.
Capillaries	capill/o	Exchange nutrients and waste products with cells.
Veins	phleb/o, ven/o	Return blood to the heart.
Blood	hem/o, hemat/o	Brings oxygen and nutrients to all cells and carries away waste. Plays several important roles in the immune and endocrine systems.

Vocabulary Related to the Cardiovascular System

Terms marked with the ❖ symbol are pronounced on the Student Activity CD-ROM that accompanies this text.

KEY WORD PARTS

- [ ] angi/o
- [ ] aort/o
- [ ] arteri/o
- [ ] ather/o
- [ ] brady-
- [ ] cardi/o
- [ ] coron/o
- [ ] -emia
- [ ] erythr/o
- [ ] hem/o, hemat/o
- [ ] leuk/o
- [ ] phleb/o
- [ ] tachy-
- [ ] thromb/o
- [ ] ven/o

KEY MEDICAL TERMS

- [ ] **aneurysm** (**AN**-you-rizm) ❖
- [ ] **aneurysmectomy** (an-you-riz-**MECK**-toh-mee) ❖
- [ ] **aneurysmorrhaphy** (an-you-riz-**MOR**-ah-fee) ❖
- [ ] **angiitis** (an-je-**EYE**-tis) ❖
- [ ] **angina** (an-**JIGH**-nah *or* **AN**-jih-nuh) ❖
- [ ] **angiocardiography** (an-jee-oh-**kar**-dee-**OG**-rah-fee) ❖
- [ ] **angiography** (an-jee-**OG**-rah-fee)
- [ ] **angionecrosis** (an-jee-oh-neh-**KROH**-sis)
- [ ] **angiostenosis** (**AN**-jee-oh-steh-**NOH**-sis)
- [ ] **antiarrhythmic** (an-tih-ah-**RITH**-mick) ❖
- [ ] **anticoagulant** (an-tih-koh-**AG**-you-lant) ❖
- [ ] **antihypertensive** (an-tih-**high**-per-**TEN**-siv) ❖
- [ ] **aplastic anemia** (ay-**PLAS**-tick ah-**NEE**-mee-ah) ❖
- [ ] **arrhythmia** (ah-**RITH**-mee-ah) ❖
- [ ] **arteriectomy** (ar-teh-ree-**ECK**-toh-mee) ❖
- [ ] **arteriosclerosis** (ar-**tee**-ree-oh-skleh-**ROH**-sis) ❖
- [ ] **arteritis** (ar-teh-**RYE**-tis)
- [ ] **atherectomy** (ath-er-**ECK**-toh-mee)
- [ ] **atheroma** (ath-er-**OH**-mah) ❖
- [ ] **athcrosclcrosis** (ath-cr-oh-sklch-**ROH**-sis) ❖
- [ ] **basophils** (**BAY**-soh-fills)
- [ ] **bradycardia** (brad-ee-**KAR**-dee-ah) ❖
- [ ] **cardiac catheterization** (**KAR**-dee-ack **kath**-eh-ter-eye-**ZAY**-shun) ❖
- [ ] **cholesterol** (koh-**LES**-ter-ol) ❖
- [ ] **defibrillation** (dee-**fib**-rih-**LAY**-shun) ❖
- [ ] **diastolic** (dye-ah-**STOL**-ick) ❖
- [ ] **dyscrasia** (dis-**KRAY**-zee-ah) ❖
- [ ] **echocardiography** (eck-oh-**kar**-dee-**OG**-rah-fee) ❖
- [ ] **electrocardiogram** (ee-**leck**-troh-**KAR**-dee-oh-**gram**) ❖

- [ ] **embolism** (**EM**-boh-lizm) ❖
- [ ] **embolus** (**EM**-boh-lus) ❖
- [ ] **endarterectomy** (**end**-ar-ter-**ECK**-toh-mee) ❖
- [ ] **endocarditis** (en-doh-kar-**DYE**-tis) ❖
- [ ] **eosinophils** (ee-oh-**SIN**-oh-fills)
- [ ] **erythrocytes** (eh-**RITH**-roh-sights)
- [ ] **fibrillation** (fih-brih-**LAY**-shun) ❖
- [ ] **hemangioma** (hee-**man**-jee-**OH**-mah) ❖
- [ ] **hemochromatosis** (hee-moh-**kroh**-mah-**TOH**-sis) ❖
- [ ] **hemoglobin** (**hee**-moh-**GLOH**-bin)
- [ ] **hemolytic anemia** (hee-moh-**LIT**-ick ah-**NEE**-mee-ah) ❖
- [ ] **hemostasis** (hee-moh-**STAY**-sis) ❖
- [ ] **homocysteine** (hoh-moh-**SIS**-teen) ❖
- [ ] **hypoperfusion** (high-poh-per-**FYOU**-zhun) ❖
- [ ] **ischemia** (iss-**KEE**-me-ah) ❖
- [ ] **leukemia** (loo-**KEE**-me-ah) ❖
- [ ] **leukocytes** (**LOO**-koh-sites)
- [ ] **leukopenia** (loo-koh-**PEE**-nee-ah) ❖
- [ ] **lymphocytes** (**LIM**-foh-sights)
- [ ] **megaloblastic anemia** (**MEG**-ah-loh-**blas**-tick ah-**NEE**-mee-ah) ❖
- [ ] **monocytes** (**MON**-oh-sights)
- [ ] **myocardial infarction** (my-oh-**KAR**-dee-al in-**FARK**-shun) ❖
- [ ] **myocarditis** (my-oh-kar-**DYE**-tis) ❖
- [ ] **neutrophils** (**NEW**-troh-fills)
- [ ] **palpitation** (pal-pih-**TAY**-shun) ❖
- [ ] **pericarditis** (pehr-ih-kar-**DYE**-tis) ❖
- [ ] **pernicious anemia** (per-**NISH**-us ah-**NEE**-mee-ah) ❖
- [ ] **phlebitis** (fleh-**BYE**-tis) ❖
- [ ] **phlebography** (fleh-**BOG**-rah-fee) ❖
- [ ] **plaque** (**PLACK**)
- [ ] **polyarteritis** (pol-ee-ar-teh-**RYE**-tis) ❖
- [ ] **Raynaud's** (ray-**NOHZ**) ❖
- [ ] **septicemia** (sep-tih-**SEE**-mee-ah) ❖
- [ ] **systolic** (sis-**TOL**-ick) ❖
- [ ] **tachycardia** (tack-ee-**KAR**-dee-ah) ❖
- [ ] **thrombocytes** (**THROM**-boh-sights)
- [ ] **thrombocytopenia** (throm-boh-**sigh**-toh-**PEE**-nee-ah) ❖
- [ ] **thrombolytic** (throm-boh-**LIT**-ick) ❖
- [ ] **thrombosis** (throm-**BOH**-sis) ❖
- [ ] **thrombus** (**THROM**-bus) ❖
- [ ] **triglycerides** (try-**GLIS**-er-eyeds) ❖
- [ ] **valvoplasty** (**VAL**-voh-**plas**-tee) ❖
- [ ] **valvulitis** (val-view-**LYE**-tis) ❖
- [ ] **valvuloplasty** (**VAL**-view-loh-**plas**-tee) ❖
- [ ] **varicose veins** (**VAR**-ih-kohs **VAYNS**) ❖
- [ ] **vasculitis** (vas-kyou-**LYE**-tis) ❖

Objectives

Upon completion of this chapter, you should be able to:

1. Describe the heart in terms of chambers, valves, blood flow, heartbeat, blood supply, and heart sounds.

2. Differentiate among the three different types of blood vessels and describe the major function of each.

3. Identify the major components of blood and the major functions of each.

4. State the difference between pulmonary and systemic circulation.

5. Recognize, define, spell, and pronounce the terms related to the pathology, diagnostic, and treatment procedures of the cardiovascular system.

FUNCTIONS OF THE CARDIOVASCULAR SYSTEM

The term **cardiovascular** means pertaining to the heart and the blood vessels (**cardi/o** means heart, **vascul** means blood vessels, and **-ar** means pertaining to). These structures work together as an efficient pumping system to supply all body tissues with oxygen and nutrients and to transport cellular waste products to the appropriate organs for removal from the body.

● In addition, the blood cells play important roles in the immune system (see Chapter 6) and endocrine system (see Chapter 13).

STRUCTURES OF THE CARDIOVASCULAR SYSTEM

The major structures of the cardiovascular system are the heart, blood vessels, and blood.

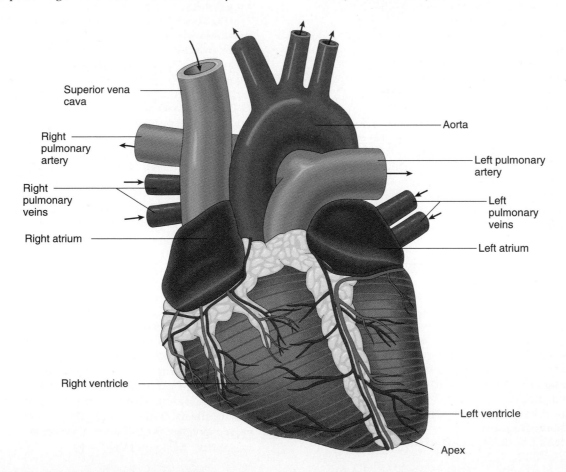

FIGURE 5.1 External view of the heart.

Labels in figure:
- Superior vena cava
- Right pulmonary artery
- Right pulmonary veins
- Right atrium
- Right ventricle
- Aorta
- Left pulmonary artery
- Left pulmonary veins
- Left atrium
- Left ventricle
- Apex

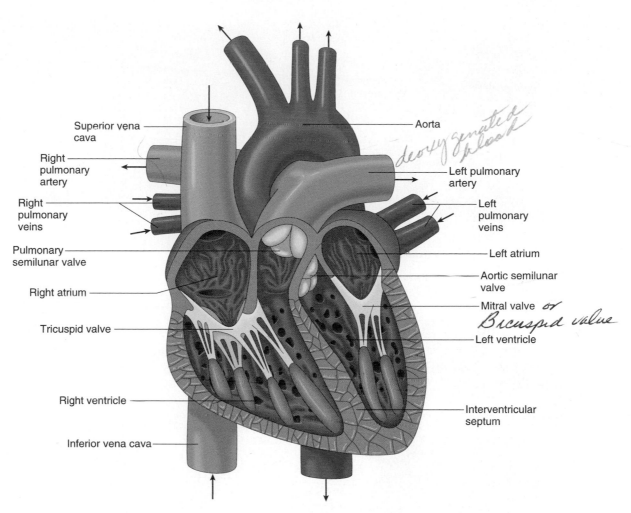

Superior vena cava

Right pulmonary artery

Right pulmonary veins

Pulmonary semilunar valve

Right atrium

Tricuspid valve

Right ventricle

Inferior vena cava

Aorta

deoxygenated blood

Left pulmonary artery

Left pulmonary veins

Left atrium

Aortic semilunar valve

Mitral valve *or*
Bicuspid value

Left ventricle

Interventricular septum

FIGURE 5.2 Cross section of the heart.

THE HEART

The heart, which is a hollow muscular organ located between the lungs and above the diaphragm, is a very effective pump that furnishes the power to maintain blood flow throughout both the pulmonary and systemic circulatory systems (Figures 5.1 and 5.2).

THE PERICARDIUM

● The **pericardium** (pehr-ih-**KAR**-dee-um) is the double-walled membranous sac that encloses the heart.

● **Pericardial fluid** between the layers prevents friction when the heart beats.

THE WALLS OF THE HEART

The walls of the heart are made up of three layers: the epicardium, myocardium, and endocardium (Figure 5.3).

● The **epicardium** (ep-ih-**KAR**-dee-um) is the external layer of the heart and also is part of the inner layer of the pericardial sac.

● The **myocardium** (my-oh-**KAR**-dee-um), which is the middle and thickest of the three layers, consists of the cardiac muscle. (See Cardiac Muscle in Chapter 4.)

● The **endocardium** (en-doh-**KAR**-dee-um), which is the lining of the heart, forms the inner surface that comes in direct contact with blood being pumped through the heart.

THE BLOOD SUPPLY TO THE MYOCARDIUM

● The myocardium is specialized muscle that beats constantly and *must* have a continuous supply of oxygen and nutrients and prompt removal of waste.

● The **coronary arteries and veins** supply the blood needs of the myocardium. If this blood supply is disrupted, the myocardium in the affected area dies (Figure 5.4).

THE HEART CHAMBERS

The heart is divided into left and right sides. Each side is subdivided, thus forming four chambers (see Figure 5.2).

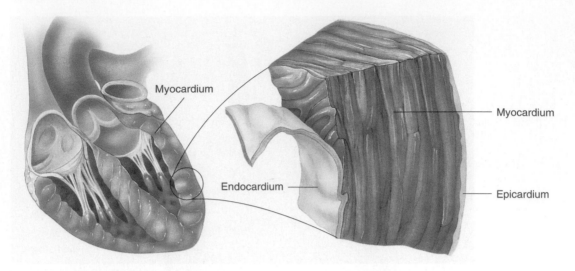

FIGURE 5.3 Schematic of the tissues of the walls of the heart.

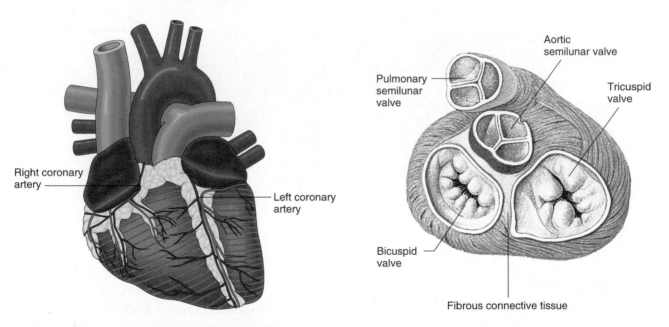

FIGURE 5.4 The coronary arteries supply blood to the myocardium.

FIGURE 5.5 The valves of the heart. This is a superior view with the atria removed.

- The **atria** (**AY**-tree-ah), the two upper chambers of the heart, are the receiving chambers. All blood vessels coming into the heart enter here (singular, **atrium**).

- The atria are separated by the **interatrial septum.** A **septum** (**SEP**-tum) is a separating wall or partition.

- The two **ventricles** (**VEN**-trih-kuhls) are the lower chambers of the heart. All vessels leaving the heart emerge from the ventricles. (The term *ventricle* refers to the ventricles of both the heart and the brain.)

- The ventricles, separated by the **interventricular septum,** are the pumping chambers. The ventricular walls are thicker than the atrial walls because the ventricles pump blood longer distances.

- The narrow tip of the heart is called the **cardiac apex** (see Figure 5.1).

THE HEART VALVES

The flow of blood through the heart is controlled by the tricuspid, pulmonary semilunar, mitral, and aortic semilunar valves. If any of these valves is not working correctly, blood does not flow properly through the heart and cannot be pumped effectively to all parts of the body (see Figures 5.2 and 5.5).

- The **tricuspid valve** (try-**KUS**-pid) **(TV)** controls the opening between the right atrium and the right ventricle. (Tricuspid means having three points or cusps and this valve is shaped with three points.)

- The **pulmonary semilunar valve** (**sem**-ee-**LOO**-nar) is located between the right ventricle and the pulmonary artery. (Semilunar means half-moon, and this valve is shaped like a half-moon.)
- The **mitral valve** (**MY**-tral), also known as the **MV** or **bicuspid valve,** is located between the left atrium and left ventricle. (Bicuspid means having two points and this valve is shaped with two points.)
- The **aortic semilunar valve** (ay-**OR**-tick **sem**-ee-**LOO**-nar) is located between the left ventricle and the aorta.

SYSTEMIC AND PULMONARY CIRCULATION

The flow of blood through the heart is summarized in Table 5.1. The red arrows indicate **oxygenated** (oxygen-rich) blood and blue arrows indicate **deoxygenated** (oxygen-poor) blood. This flow travels through both the systemic and pulmonary circulation systems. Together these systems allow blood to bring oxygen to the cells and remove waste products (Figure 5.6).

Systemic Circulation

- **Systemic circulation** includes blood flow to all parts of the body *except* the lungs.
- Oxygenated blood flows out of the heart from the left ventricle into arterial circulation.
- Deoxygenated blood returns to the heart through the veins and flows into the right atrium.

Pulmonary Circulation

- **Pulmonary circulation** is the flow of blood between the heart and lungs.
- Blood flows out of the heart from the right ventricle and through the pulmonary arteries to the lungs. This is the only place in the body where arteries carry oxygen-poor blood.
- In the lungs, waste material (carbon dioxide) from the body is exchanged for oxygen from the inhaled air.
- The pulmonary veins carry the oxygen-rich blood into the left atrium of the heart. This is the only place in the body where veins carry oxygen-rich blood.

THE HEARTBEAT

- To pump blood effectively throughout the body, the contraction and relaxation (beating) of the heart must occur in exactly the correct sequence.
- The rate and regularity of the heartbeat is determined by **electrical impulses** from nerves that stimulate the myocardium of the chambers of the heart.
- Also known as the **conduction system,** these electrical impulses are controlled by the sinoatrial (S-A) node, atrioventricular (A-V) node, and bundle of His (Figure 5.7).

Table 5.1

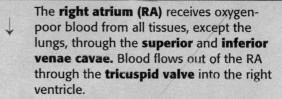

BLOOD FLOW THROUGH THE HEART

↓ The **right atrium (RA)** receives oxygen-poor blood from all tissues, except the lungs, through the **superior** and **inferior venae cavae.** Blood flows out of the RA through the **tricuspid valve** into the right ventricle.

↓ The **right ventricle (RV)** pumps the oxygen-poor blood through the **pulmonary semilunar valve** and into the **pulmonary artery,** which carries it to the lungs.

↓ The **left atrium (LA)** receives oxygen-rich (oxygenated) blood from the lungs through the **four pulmonary veins.** The blood flows out of the LA, through the **mitral valve,** and into the left ventricle.

↓ The **left ventricle (LV)** receives oxygen-rich blood from the left atrium. Blood flows out of the LV through the **aortic semilunar valve** and into the **aorta,** which carries it to all parts of the body, except the lungs.

↓ Oxygen-poor blood is returned by the venae cavae to the right atrium and the cycle continues.

The Sinoatrial Node

- The **sinoatrial node** (**sigh**-noh-**AY**-tree-ahl), also known as the **S-A node,** is located in the posterior wall of the right atrium near the entrance of the superior vena cava.
- Because the S-A node establishes the basic rhythm of the heartbeat, it is called the **natural pacemaker** of the heart.
- Electrical impulses from the S-A node start each wave of muscle contraction in the heart.
- The impulse in the right atrium spreads over the muscles of both atria, causing them to contract simultaneously.
- This contraction forces blood into the ventricles.

The Atrioventricular Node

- The impulses from the S-A node also travel to the **atrioventricular node** (**ay**-tree-oh-ven-**TRICK**-you-lahr).
- Also known as the **A-V node,** it is located on the floor of the right atrium near the interatrial septum.

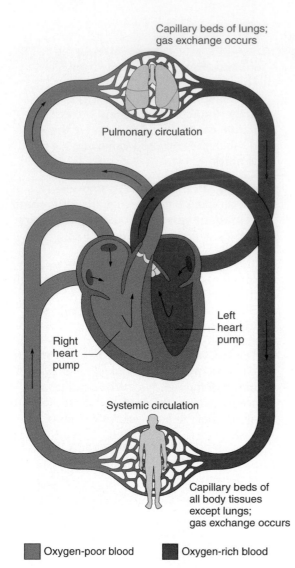

Capillary beds of lungs;
gas exchange occurs

Pulmonary circulation

Left
heart
pump

Right
heart
pump

Systemic circulation

Capillary beds of
all body tissues
except lungs;
gas exchange occurs

■ Oxygen-poor blood   ■ Oxygen-rich blood

FIGURE 5.6 Systemic and pulmonary circulation.

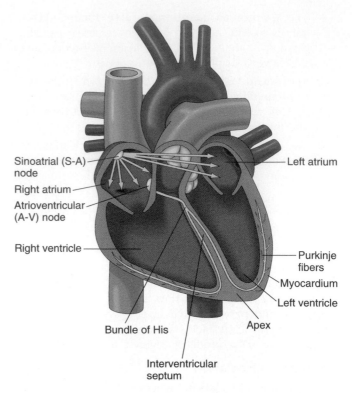

Sinoatrial (S-A)
node

Right atrium

Atrioventricular
(A-V) node

Right ventricle

Left atrium

Purkinje
fibers

Myocardium

Left ventricle

Apex

Bundle of His

Interventricular
septum

FIGURE 5.7 The electrical conduction system of the heart.

- The A-V node transmits the electrical impulses on to the bundle of His.

The Bundle of His

- The **bundle of His (HISS),** named for Wilhelm His Jr., a nineteenth-century Swiss physician, is located within the interventricular septum.
- Branches of the bundle of His carry the impulses to the right and left ventricles and the **Purkinje fibers.**
- Stimulation of the **Purkinje fibers,** named for Johannes Purkinje, a nineteenth-century physiologist, causes the ventricles to contract simultaneously forcing blood into the aorta and pulmonary arteries.

Electrical Waves

The activities of the electrical conduction system of the heart can be visualized as wave movements on a monitor or an electrocardiogram (Figure 5.8).

- The **P wave** is due to the contraction (stimulation) of the atria.
- The **QRS complex** shows the contraction (stimulation) of the ventricles. The atria relax as the ventricles contract.
- The **T wave** is the relaxation (recovery) of the ventricles.

HEART SOUNDS

When a stethoscope is used to listen to the heartbeat, two distinct sounds are heard. They are called the "lubb dupp" sounds.

- Heard first is the **lubb sound.** This is caused by the tricuspid and mitral valves closing between the atria and the ventricles.
- Heard next is the **dupp sound,** which is shorter and higher pitched. It is caused by the closing of the semilunar valves in the aorta and pulmonary arteries as blood is pumped out of the heart.

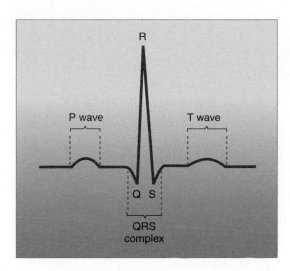

FIGURE 5.8 The waves of contraction and relaxation of the heart can be visualized on a monitor or on an ECG.

THE BLOOD VESSELS

There are three major types of blood vessels in the body: arteries, capillaries, and veins.

● The **lumen** (**LOO**-men) is the opening within these vessels through which the blood flows.

THE ARTERIES

The arteries are the large blood vessels that carry blood away from the heart to all regions of the body. It is the high oxygen content that gives arterial blood its bright red color (Figure 5.9).

● The term **endarterial** (**end**-ar-**TEE**-ree-al) means pertaining to the interior or lining of an artery (**end-** means within, **arteri** means artery, and **-al** means pertaining to).

● The walls of the arteries are composed of three layers. This structure makes them both muscular and elastic so they can expand and contract with the pumping beat of the heart. It is this contraction and expansion that causes blood to spurt out when an artery is cut.

● The **aorta** (ay-**OR**-tah) is the main trunk of the arterial system and begins from the left ventricle of the heart (see Figure 5.1).

● The **coronary artery** (**KOR**-uh-**nerr**-ee) branches from the aorta and supplies blood to the myocardium (see Figure 5.4).

● The **arterioles** (ar-**TEE**-ree-ohlz), which are the smaller thinner branches of arteries, carry blood to the capillaries.

THE CAPILLARIES

● **Capillaries** serve as the anatomic units connecting the arterial and venous circulatory systems. The cap-

illaries, which are only one epithelial cell in thickness, are the smallest vessels in the body.

● Blood flows rapidly along the arteries and veins. However, this flow is much slower through the expanded vascular bed provided by the network of capillaries.

● This slower flow allows time for the exchange of oxygen, nutrients, and waste materials between the tissue fluids and the surrounding cells.

THE VEINS

The veins form a low-pressure collecting system to return the waste-filled blood to the heart (Figures 5.10 and 5.11).

● Veins have thinner walls and are less elastic than the arteries. Contractions of the skeletal muscles cause the blood to flow through the veins toward the heart.

● Veins have valves that enable blood to flow only toward the heart but prevent it from flowing away from the heart.

● **Venules** (**VEN**-youls) are small veins that join to form the larger veins.

The Venae Cavae

● The **venae cavae** (**VEE**-nee **KAY**-vee) are the two large veins that enter the heart (singular, **vena cava**).

● The **superior vena cava** (**VEE**-nah **KAY**-vah) **(SVC)** brings blood from the upper portion of the body (see Figure 5.1).

● The **inferior vena cava (IVC)** brings blood from the lower portion of the body (see Figure 5.2).

THE PULSE AND BLOOD PRESSURE

● The **pulse** is the rhythmic expansion and contraction of an artery produced by the pressure of the blood moving through the artery (see Chapter 15).

● **Blood pressure** is a measurement of the amount of pressure exerted against the walls of the vessels.

● **Systolic pressure** (sis-**TOL**-ick), which occurs when the ventricles contract, is the highest pressure against the walls of the blood vessels.

● **Diastolic pressure** (dye-ah-**STOL**-ick), which occurs when the ventricles are relaxed, is the lowest pressure against the walls of the blood vessels.

● Blood pressure is recorded as systolic over diastolic. A normal blood pressure reading for a seated adult is about 130/84 mm Hg. (*Hg* is the abbreviation for mercury.)

THE BLOOD

Blood is composed of 55 percent liquid plasma and 45 percent formed elements (Figure 5.12). The **formed elements,** also known as **blood corpuscles,** include the red blood cells, white blood cells, and platelets.

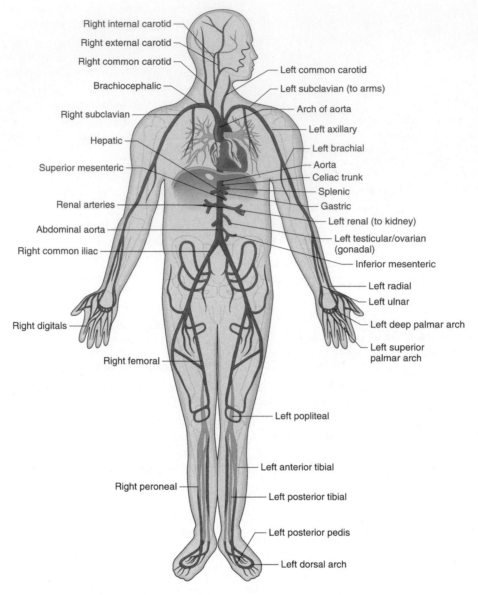

Right internal carotid
Right external carotid
Right common carotid
Brachiocephalic
Right subclavian
Hepatic
Superior mesenteric
Renal arteries
Abdominal aorta
Right common iliac

Right digitals

Right femoral

Right peroneal

Left common carotid
Left subclavian (to arms)
Arch of aorta
Left axillary
Left brachial
Aorta
Celiac trunk
Splenic
Gastric
Left renal (to kidney)
Left testicular/ovarian (gonadal)
Inferior mesenteric
Left radial
Left ulnar
Left deep palmar arch
Left superior palmar arch

Left popliteal

Left anterior tibial

Left posterior tibial

Left posterior pedis

Left dorsal arch

FIGURE 5.9 Arterial circulation.

PLASMA

- **Plasma** (**PLAZ**-mah) is a straw-colored fluid that contains nutrients, hormones, and waste products. Plasma is 91 percent water. The remaining 9 percent consists mainly of proteins including the clotting proteins.

- **Fibrinogen** (figh-**BRIN**-oh-jen) and **prothrombin** (proh-**THROM**-bin) are clotting proteins found in plasma. They have an important role in clot formation to control bleeding.

- **Serum** (**SEER**-um) is plasma with these clotting proteins removed.

ERYTHROCYTES

- **Erythrocytes** (eh-**RITH**-roh-sights), which are also known as **red blood cells (RBCs)**, are mature red blood cells (**erythr/o** means red and **-cytes** means cells).

- These cells, which are produced by the red bone marrow, are shaped like a doughnut with a thin central portion instead of a hole (see Figure 5.12).

- **Hemoglobin** (**hee**-moh-**GLOH**-bin), which is the iron-containing pigment of the erythrocytes, transports oxygen from the lungs to the tissues of the body.

- A **reticulocyte** (reh-**TICK**-you-loh-**site**) is an immature erythrocyte that is characterized by a meshlike pattern of threads.

- The normal life span of an RBC is about 120 days. After this, **macrophages** in the spleen, liver, and bone marrow destroy erythrocytes that are no longer useful.

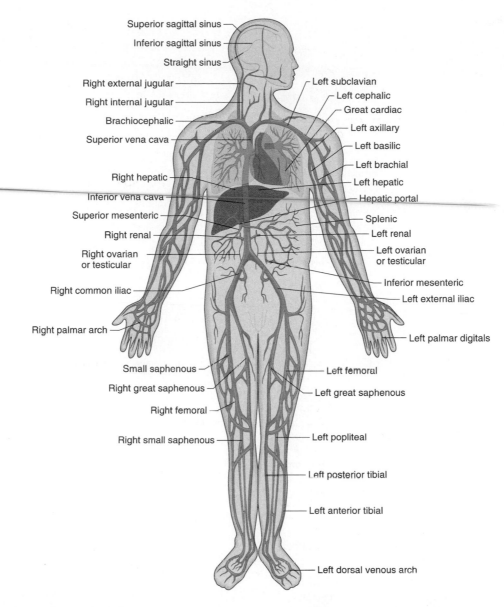

Superior sagittal sinus
Inferior sagittal sinus
Straight sinus
Right external jugular
Right internal jugular
Brachiocephalic
Superior vena cava
Right hepatic
Inferior vena cava
Superior mesenteric
Right renal
Right ovarian or testicular
Right common iliac
Right palmar arch
Small saphenous
Right great saphenous
Right femoral
Right small saphenous

Left subclavian
Left cephalic
Great cardiac
Left axillary
Left basilic
Left brachial
Left hepatic
Hepatic portal
Splenic
Left renal
Left ovarian or testicular
Inferior mesenteric
Left external iliac
Left palmar digitals
Left femoral
Left great saphenous
Left popliteal
Left posterior tibial
Left anterior tibial
Left dorsal venous arch

FIGURE 5.10 Venous circulation.

LEUKOCYTES

● **Leukocytes** (**LOO**-koh-sites), also known as **white blood cells (WBCs),** protect the body against harmful invaders such as bacteria (**leuk/o** means white and **-cytes** means cells). The following are the major groups of leukocytes.

● **Neutrophils** (**NEW**-troh-fills), which are formed in red bone marrow, are the most prevalent type of WBC. These cells fight infection by phagocytosis. **Phagocytosis** (**fag**-oh-sigh-**TOH**-sis) is the process of engulfing and swallowing germs (**phag/o** means to eat or swallow, **cyt** means cell, and **-osis** means abnormal condition). An elevated neutrophil count indicates a bacterial infection.

● **Basophils** (**BAY**-soh-fills), which are formed in red bone marrow, promote the inflammatory response.

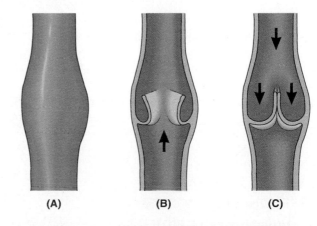

(A) (B) (C)

FIGURE 5.11 Veins contain valves to prevent the backward flow of blood. (A) External view of the vein shows wider area of valve. (B) Internal view with the valve open as blood flows through. (C) Internal view with the valve closed.

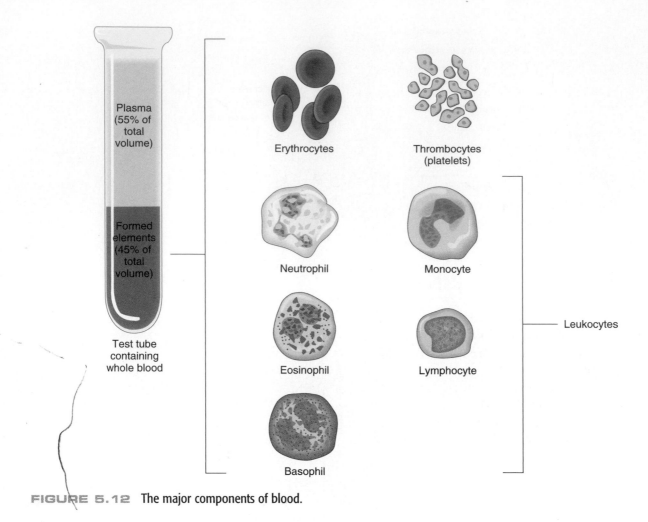

FIGURE 5.12   The major components of blood.

An elevated basophil count may indicate an allergic condition.

- **Eosinophils** (**ee**-oh-**SIN**-oh-fills), which are formed in red bone marrow, increase in response to allergic reactions. An elevated eosinophil count indicates an allergic condition.

- **Lymphocytes** (**LIM**-foh-sights) are formed in red bone marrow, lymph nodes, and the spleen. These cells have an important role in protecting the body against disease (see Chapter 6).

- **Monocytes** (**MON**-oh-sights) are formed in red bone marrow, lymph nodes, and the spleen. They also are important in protecting against disease and an elevated monocyte count usually indicates a chronic infection.

THROMBOCYTES

- **Thrombocytes** (**THROM**-boh-sights), also known as **platelets,** are the smallest formed elements of the blood. They are not cells but are fragments of specialized large bone marrow cells known as megakaryocytes.

- Thrombocytes play an important role in the clotting of blood. When the blood vessel is damaged, platelets are activated. Once activated, the platelets become sticky and clump together to form a clot.

BLOOD TYPES

The four major types of blood are A, AB, B, and O. These groups are based on the presence of the A and/or B antigens on red blood cells. In type O, both antigens are absent. Table 5.2 explains how these types interact in terms of donating and receiving blood.

- The safe administration of blood from donor to recipient requires careful typing and cross-matching to ensure a correct match.

- A patient receiving blood incompatible with his or her own can experience serious and possibly fatal reactions.

THE RH FACTOR

In addition to having antigens A or B, or both, red blood cells also contain the Rh antigen. Because this was first found in Rhesus monkeys, this factor was named for

Table 5.2

BLOOD TYPES AS DONORS AND RECIPIENTS		
Blood Type	**Can Donate To**	**Can Receive From**
A	A or AB only	A or O only
B	B or AB only	B or O only
AB (the universal recipient)	AB only	A, B, AB, O
O (the universal donor)	A, B, AB, O	O only

them. Each individual is either positive or negative for the **Rh factor.**

● About 85 percent of Americans are **Rh positive (Rh+).** This means that they *have* the Rh antigen.

● The remaining 15 percent are **Rh negative (Rh-).** This means that they *do not have* the Rh antigen.

● The Rh factor is an important consideration in cross-matching blood for transfusions.

● The Rh factor also causes difficulties when an Rh-positive infant is born to an Rh-negative mother (see Chapter 14).

BLOOD GASES

A **blood gas** is a gas that is dissolved in the liquid part of the blood. The major blood gases are **oxygen** (O_2), **carbon dioxide** (CO_2), and **nitrogen** (N_2).

MEDICAL SPECIALTIES RELATED TO THE CARDIOVASCULAR SYSTEM

● A **cardiologist** (**kar**-dee-**OL**-oh-jist) specializes in diagnosing and treating abnormalities, diseases, and disorders of the heart (**cardi** means heart and **-ologist** means specialist).

● A **hematologist** (**hee**-mah-**TOL**-oh-jist *or* **hem**-ah-**TOL**-oh-jist) specializes in diagnosing and treating diseases and disorders of the blood and blood-forming tissues (**hemat** means blood and **-ologist** means specialist).

PATHOLOGY OF THE CARDIOVASCULAR SYSTEM

CORONARY ARTERY DISEASE

● **Coronary artery disease (CAD)** is atherosclerosis of the coronary arteries that may cause angina pec-

toris, myocardial infarction, and sudden death (Figure 5.13).

● **End-stage coronary artery disease,** which is the final phase of CAD, is characterized by unrelenting angina pain and a severely limited lifestyle.

● **Atherosclerosis** (**ath**-er-oh-skleh-**ROH**-sis) is hardening and narrowing of the arteries due to a buildup of cholesterol plaques (**ather/o** means plaque or fatty substance and **-sclerosis** means abnormal hardening) (see Figures 5.13 and 5.14).

● An **atheroma** (**ath**-er-**OH**-mah), which is characteristic of atherosclerosis, is a plaque (fatty deposit) within the arterial wall (**ather** means plaque and **-oma** means tumor).

● This type of **plaque (PLACK)** is similar to the buildup of rust inside a pipe, and it may protrude outward into the opening of the vessel or move inward into the wall of the vessel. (Compare this with dental plaque, which is discussed in Chapter 8.)

● **Ischemia** (iss-**KEE**-mee-ah) is a deficiency in blood supply due to either the constriction or the obstruction of a blood vessel (**isch** means to hold back and **-emia** means blood).

● **Ischemic heart disease** (iss-**KEE**-mick) **(IHD)** is a group of cardiac disabilities resulting from an insufficient supply of oxygenated blood to the heart that is usually associated with CAD.

● **Angina pectoris** (an-**JIGH**-nah *or* **AN**-jih-nuh **PECK**-toh-riss) is severe episodes of spasmodic choking or suffocating chest pain. This is usually due to interference with, but not complete blockage of, the supply of oxygen to the myocardium.

● A **myocardial infarction** (**my**-oh-**KAR**-dee-al in-**FARK**-shun), also known as a **heart attack** or **MI,** is the occlusion (closing off) of a coronary artery resulting in an infarct of the affected myocardium. Damage to the myocardium impairs the heart's ability to pump blood throughout the body.

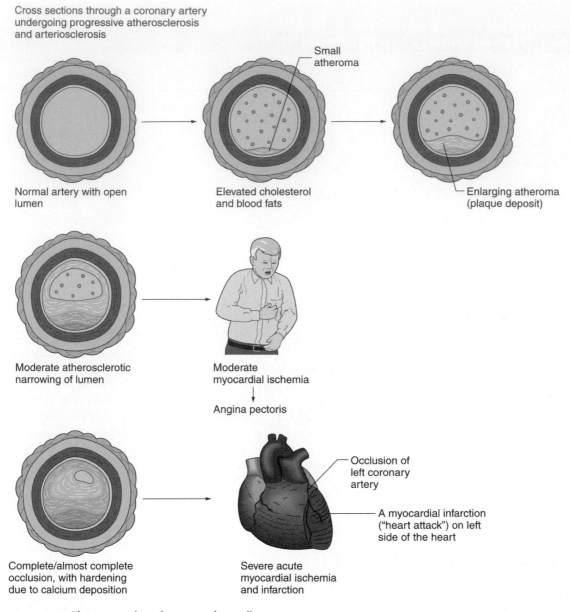

Cross sections through a coronary artery undergoing progressive atherosclerosis and arteriosclerosis

Small atheroma

Normal artery with open lumen

Elevated cholesterol and blood fats

Enlarging atheroma (plaque deposit)

Moderate atherosclerotic narrowing of lumen

Moderate myocardial ischemia

Angina pectoris

Complete/almost complete occlusion, with hardening due to calcium deposition

Severe acute myocardial ischemia and infarction

Occlusion of left coronary artery

A myocardial infarction ("heart attack") on left side of the heart

FIGURE 5.13 The progression of coronary heart disease.

- An **infarct** (**IN**-farkt) is a localized area of necrosis (tissue death) caused by an interruption of the blood supply.

CONGESTIVE HEART FAILURE

- **Congestive heart failure (CHF)** is a syndrome in which the heart is unable to pump enough blood to meet the body's needs for oxygen and nutrients. In response to the reduced blood flow, the kidneys retain more fluid within the body and this fluid accumulates in the legs, ankles, and lungs. The term *congestive* refers to this fluid buildup (Figure 5.15).

FORMS OF CARDITIS

- The term **carditis** (kar-**DYE**-tis) means an inflammation of the heart (**card** means heart and **-itis** means inflammation). *Note the spelling of carditis:* **cardi/o** and **card/o** both mean heart. In this term, the word root **card/o** is used to avoid having a double *i* when it is joined with the suffix **-itis**.

- **Endocarditis** (**en**-doh-kar-**DYE**-tis) is an inflammation of the inner layer of the heart (**endo-** means within, **card** means heart, and **-itis** means inflammation).

- **Bacterial endocarditis** is an inflammation of the lining or valves of the heart caused by bacteria.

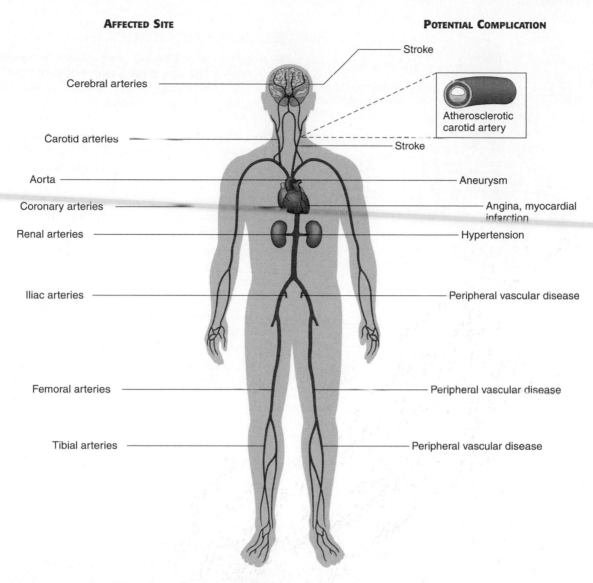

AFFECTED SITE — POTENTIAL COMPLICATION

- Stroke
- Cerebral arteries
- Atherosclerotic carotid artery
- Carotid arteries
- Stroke
- Aorta — Aneurysm
- Coronary arteries — Angina, myocardial infarction
- Renal arteries — Hypertension
- Iliac arteries — Peripheral vascular disease
- Femoral arteries — Peripheral vascular disease
- Tibial arteries — Peripheral vascular disease

FIGURE 5.14 The risks of atherosclerosis. (Left) Affected sites. (Right) Potential complications.

- **Myocarditis** (**my**-oh-kar-**DYE**-tis) is an inflammation of the myocardium (**my/o** means muscle, **card** means heart, and **-itis** means inflammation).

- **Pericarditis** (**pehr**-ih-kar-**DYE**-tis) is an inflammation of the pericardium (**peri-** means surrounding, **card** means heart, and **-itis** means inflammation).

HEART VALVES

- **Valvulitis** (**val**-view-**LYE**-tis) is an inflammatory condition of a heart valve (**valvul** means valve, and **-itis** means inflammation).

- **Mitral valve prolapse** is an abnormal protrusion of the mitral value that results in the incomplete closure of the valve. (*Prolapse* means falling down.)

- **Mitral stenosis** (steh-**NOH**-sis) is an abnormal narrowing of the opening of the mitral valve. **Tricuspid stenosis** is an abnormal narrowing of the opening of the tricuspid valve.

- A valve that does not function properly may allow blood to flow back into the heart chamber. The sound of this abnormal flow is called a **heart murmur.**

ARRHYTHMIAS

- **Cardiac arrhythmia** (ah-**RITH**-mee-ah), also known as **dysrhythmia** (dis-**RITH**-mee-ah), is an irregularity or the loss of normal rhythm of the heartbeat.

- **Bradycardia** (**brad**-ee-**KAR**-dee-ah) is an abnormally slow heartbeat (**brady-** means slow, **card** means heart, and **-ia** means abnormal condition). This term is usually applied to rates less than 60 beats per minute. (Compare this with tachycardia.)

- A **flutter** is a cardiac arrhythmia in which the atrial contractions are rapid but regular. (Compare this with atrial fibrillation.)

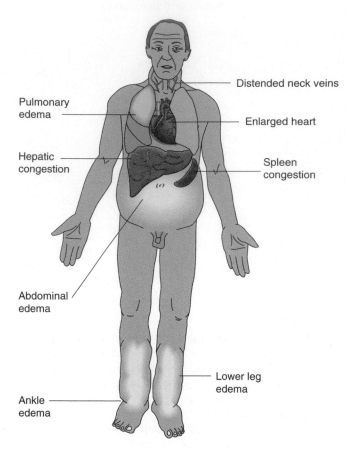

Pulmonary edema

Hepatic congestion

Abdominal edema

Ankle edema

Distended neck veins

Enlarged heart

Spleen congestion

Lower leg edema

FIGURE 5.15 Signs of congestive heart failure.

- **Palpitation** (**pal**-pih-**TAY**-shun) is a pounding or racing heart with or without irregularity in rhythm. This is associated with certain heart disorders, or it may be a response accompanying a panic attack (see Chapter 10).
- **Tachycardia** (**tack**-ee-**KAR**-dee-ah) is an abnormally fast heartbeat (**tachy-** means rapid, **card** means heart, and **-ia** means abnormal condition). This term is usually applied to rates greater than 100 beats per minute. (Compare this with bradycardia.)
- **Paroxysmal tachycardia** is a fast heartbeat of sudden onset. *Paroxysm* (**PAR**-ock-sizm) means a sudden convulsion, seizure, or spasm.

FIBRILLATION

- **Fibrillation** (**fih**-brih-**LAY**-shun) is rapid, random, and ineffective contractions of the heart.
- In **atrial fibrillation (AF),** also known as **A fib,** the atria beat faster than the ventricles. This condition produces an irregular quivering action of the atria and a very rapid ventricular heartbeat.
- **Ventricular fibrillation,** also known as **V fib,** is the result of irregular contractions of the ventricles and is fatal unless reversed by electric defibrillation.

BLOOD VESSELS

- **Angiitis** (an-je-**EYE**-tis), also known as **vasculitis** (**vas**-kyou-**LYE**-tis), is the inflammation of a blood or lymph vessel (**angi** means vessel and **-itis** means inflammation). *Note:* This term is spelled with a double **i.**
- **Angionecrosis** (**an**-jee-oh-neh-**KROH**-sis) is the necrosis (death) of the walls of the blood vessels (**angi/o** means vessel and **-necrosis** means tissue death).
- An **angiospasm** (**AN**-jee-oh-**spazm**) is a spasmodic contraction of the blood vessels (**angi/o** means vessel and **-spasm** means tightening or cramping).
- **Angiostenosis** (**AN**-jee-oh-steh-**NOH**-sis) is the narrowing of a blood vessel (**angi/o** means vessel and **stenosis** means abnormal narrowing).
- A **hemangioma** (hee-**man**-jee-**OH**-mah) is a benign tumor made up of newly formed blood vessels (**hemangi** means blood vessel and **-oma** means tumor). (See also Chapter 12.)
- **Hypoperfusion** (**high**-poh-per-**FYOU**-zhun) is a deficiency of blood passing through an organ or body part. *Perfusion* (per-**FYOU**-zuhn) means the flow of blood through the vessels of an organ.

ARTERIES

- An **aneurysm** (**AN**-you-rizm) is a localized weak spot or balloon-like enlargement of the wall of an artery. Most aneurysms occur in large blood vessels and are named for the involved blood vessels such as an aortic aneurysm. If an aneurysm ruptures, it is often fatal because of the rapid loss of blood.
- **Arteritis** (ar-teh-**RYE**-tis) is inflammation of an artery (**arter** means artery and **-itis** means inflammation).
- **Polyarteritis** (pol-ee-ar-teh-**RYE**-tis) is an inflammation involving several arteries (**poly-** means many, **arter** means artery, and **-itis** means inflammation).
- **Arteriosclerosis** (ar-**tee**-ree-oh-skleh-**ROH**-sis) is the hardening of the arteries, which reduces the flow of blood through these vessels (**arteri/o** means artery and **-sclerosis** means abnormal hardening).
- **Raynaud's phenomenon** (ray-**NOHZ**) consists of intermittent attacks of pallor (paleness), cyanosis (blue color), and redness of the fingers and toes. These symptoms are due to arterial and arteriolar contraction and are usually caused by cold or emotion.

VEINS

- **Phlebitis** (fleh-**BYE**-tis) is the inflammation of a vein (**phleb** means vein and **-itis** means inflammation).
- **Varicose veins** (**VAR**-ih-kohs **VAYNS**) are abnormally swollen veins usually occurring in the legs (Figure 5.16). A *varicosity* (**var**-ih-**KOS**-ih-tee) is one area of swelling (plural, *varices*).

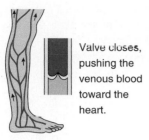

Valve closes, pushing the venous blood toward the heart.

(A) Normal veins

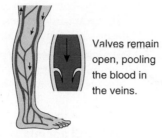

Valves remain open, pooling the blood in the veins.

(B) Varicose veins

FIGURE 5.16 Normal veins and varicose veins compared.

THROMBOSES AND EMBOLISMS

- A **thrombosis** (throm-**BOH**-sis) is an abnormal condition in which a thrombus develops within a blood vessel (**thromb** means clot and **-osis** means abnormal condition) (plural, **thromboses**).

- A **thrombus** (**THROM**-bus) is a blood clot attached to the interior wall of a vein or artery (**thromb** means clot and **-us** is a singular noun ending).

- A **thrombotic occlusion** (throm-**BOT**-ick ah-**KLOO**-zhun) is the blocking of an artery by a clot (**thromb/o** means clot and **-tic** means pertaining to). As used here, *occlusion* means a blockage in a canal, vessel, or passageway in the body.

- A **coronary thrombosis** (**KOR**-uh-**nerr**-ee throm-**BOH**-sis) is damage to the heart caused by a thrombus blocking a coronary artery.

- An **embolus** (**EM**-boh-lus) is a foreign object, such as a blood clot, quantity of air or gas, or a bit of tissue or tumor that is circulating in the blood (**embol** means something inserted and **-us** is a singular noun ending) (plural, **emboli**).

- An **embolism** (**EM**-boh-lizm) is the blockage of a vessel by an embolus. An embolism occurs when the embolus is larger than the blood vessel and blocks

the flow of blood (**embol** means something inserted and **-ism** means condition).

BLOOD DISORDERS

- **Dyscrasia** (dis-**KRAY**-zee-ah) is any abnormal or pathologic condition of the blood (**dys** means bad, and **-crasia** means a mixture or blending).

- **Hemochromatosis** (**hee**-moh-**kroh**-mah-**TOH**-sis) is also known as **iron overload disease** (**hem/o** means blood, **chromat** means color, and **-osis** means abnormal condition). This is a genetic disorder in which the intestines absorb too much iron. The excess iron enters the bloodstream and accumulates in organs where it causes damage.

- **Septicemia** (**sep**-tih-**SEE**-mee-ah), also known as **blood poisoning,** is the presence of pathogenic microorganisms or their toxins in the blood.

Cholesterol

- **Cholesterol** (koh-**LES**-ter-ol) consists of lipids (fatty substances) that travel in the blood in packages called **lipoproteins.** The presence of cholesterol at certain levels is normal and essential for good health. A pathologic condition is present when these fats are present in excessive amounts. Table 5.3 shows the desirable levels of each substance for people without heart disease. These are expressed as milligrams per deciliter (mg/dl).

- **Low-density lipoprotein cholesterol** is also known as **LDL** or **bad cholesterol** because excess quantities contribute to plaque buildup in the arteries.

- **High-density lipoprotein cholesterol** is also known as **HDL** or **good cholesterol** because it carries unneeded cholesterol back to the liver for processing and does not contribute to plaque buildup.

- **Triglycerides** (try-**GLIS**-er-eyeds) are combinations of fatty acids attached to glycerol that are also found normally in the blood in limited quantities.

Table 5.3

BLOOD LIPOPROTEIN LEVELS			
Test	**Desirable (mg/dl)**	**Borderline (mg/dl)**	**Undesirable (mg/dl)**
Total cholesterol	Below 200	200–239	Above 240
LDL cholesterol	Below 130	130–159	Below 160
HDL cholesterol	Above 45	35–45	Below 35
Triglycerides	Below 150	150–199	Above 200–499

- **Homocysteine** (**hoh**-moh-**SIS**-teen) is an amino acid normally found in the blood and used by the body to build and maintain tissues. However when present in elevated levels of more than 12 micromoles per liter, homocysteine can damage arterial walls and increase the risk of coronary artery disease. Such increases may be caused by a diet severely lacking in several B vitamins.
- **Hyperlipidemia** (**high**-per-**lip**-ih-**DEE**-mee-ah), also known as **hyperlipemia** (**high**-per-lye-**PEE**-mee-ah), is a general term for elevated plasma concentrations of cholesterol, triglycerides, and lipoproteins. The levels of each of these substances can be measured by a blood test.

BLOOD CELLS

- **Erythrocytosis** (eh-**rith**-roh-sigh-**TOH**-sis) is an abnormal increase in the number of circulating red blood cells (**erythr/o** means red, **cyt** means cell, and **-osis** means abnormal condition).
- **Thrombocytopenia** (**throm**-boh-**sigh**-toh-**PEE**-nee-ah), also known as **thrombopenia,** is an abnormal decrease in the number of platelets (**thromb/o** means clot, **cyt/o** means cell, and **-penia** means a deficiency of).
- **Leukopenia** (**loo**-koh-**PEE**-nee-ah) is an abnormal decrease in the number of white blood cells. It may affect one or all kinds of white blood cells (**leuk/o** means white and **-penia** means a deficiency of).
- **Leukemia** (loo-**KEE**-mee-ah) is a malignancy characterized by a progressive increase of abnormal leukocytes (**leuk** means white and **-emia** means blood condition).

ANEMIAS

- **Anemia** (ah-**NEE**-mee-ah) is a disorder characterized by lower than normal levels of red blood cells in the blood (**an-** means without or less than and **-emia** means blood condition).
- **Aplastic anemia** (ay-**PLAS**-tick ah-**NEE**-mee-ah) is marked by an absence of *all* formed blood elements (**a-** means without, **plast** means growth, and **-ic** means pertaining to). This is caused by the failure of blood cell production in the bone marrow.
- In **hemolytic anemia** (**hee**-moh-**LIT**-ick ah-**NEE**-mee-ah), red blood cells are destroyed faster than the bone marrow can replace them (**hem/o** means relating to blood and **-lytic** means to destroy).
- **Iron-deficiency anemia** develops if not enough iron is available to bone marrow to make hemoglobin. It may be caused by inadequate iron intake, malabsorption of iron, pregnancy and lactation, or chronic blood loss.
- In **megaloblastic anemia** (**MEG**-ah-loh-**blas**-tick ah-**NEE**-mee-ah), the bone marrow produces megaloblasts.

These are large abnormal red blood cells with a reduced capacity to carry oxygen. This type of anemia is almost always caused by a vitamin deficiency.

- **Pernicious anemia** (per-**NISH**-us ah-**NEE**-mee-ah) is an autoimmune disorder in which the red blood cells are abnormally formed, due to an inability to absorb vitamin B_{12}. (*Pernicious* means destructive, fatal, or harmful.)
- **Sickle cell anemia** is a genetic disorder that causes abnormal hemoglobin, resulting in the red blood cells assuming an abnormal sickle shape. This abnormal shape interferes with normal blood flow, resulting in damage to most of the body systems.
- **Thalassemia** (thal-ah-**SEE**-mee-ah), also known as **Cooley's anemia,** is a group of genetic disorders characterized by short-lived red blood cells that lack the normal ability to produce hemoglobin.

HYPERTENSION

- **Essential hypertension,** also known as **primary hypertension** or **idiopathic hypertension,** is consistently elevated blood pressure of unknown origin. (*Idiopathic* means of unknown cause.) The classifications of blood pressure for adults are summarized in Table 5.4.
- **Secondary hypertension** is caused by a different medical problem such as a kidney disorder or a tumor on the adrenal glands. When the other problem is cured, the secondary hypertension should be resolved.
- **Malignant hypertension** is characterized by the sudden onset of severely elevated blood pressure. It can be life-threatening and commonly damages small vessels in the brain, retina, heart, and kidneys.

DIAGNOSTIC PROCEDURES OF THE CARDIOVASCULAR SYSTEM

- **Blood tests** are discussed in Chapter 15.
- A **pulse oximeter** is an external monitor that is placed on the patient's finger to measure the amount of oxygenated blood in the circulatory system. In a normal reading, 96 percent to 100 percent of the blood is saturated by oxygen. The levels of other blood gases are measured with a blood test.
- **Angiography** (**an**-jee-**OG**-rah-fee) is a radiographic (x-ray) study of the blood vessels after the injection of a contrast medium (**angi/o** means blood vessel and **-graphy** means the process of recording). The resulting film is an **angiogram** (Figure 5.17). This procedure is frequently performed in conjunction with cardiac catheterization.

Table 5.4

BLOOD PRESSURE CLASSIFICATIONS FOR ADULTS		
Category	**Systolic (mm Hg)**	**Diastolic (mm Hg)**
Optimal	less than 120	less than 80
Normal	less than 130	less than 85
High-normal	130–139	85–89
Hypertension	higher than 140	higher than 90

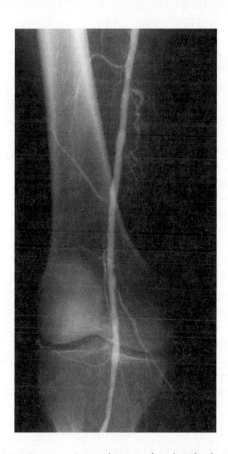

FIGURE 5.17 An angiogram showing the femoral arteries. The use of a contrast medium makes the arteries visible.

- **Angiocardiography** (an-jee-oh-**kar**-dee-**OG**-rah-fee) uses a contrast medium and chest x-rays to visualize the dimensions of the heart and large blood vessels (**angi/o** means blood vessel, **cardi/o** means heart and **-graphy** means the process of recording). The contrast medium, which appears white on the film, is used to make these soft tissue structures visible on the resulting **angiocardiogram.**

- **Cardiac catheterization** (**KAR**-dee-ack **kath**-eh-ter-eye-**ZAY**-shun) (**CC**) is a procedure in which a catheter is passed into a vein or artery and is guided into the heart. When the catheter is in place, a contrast medium is introduced to produce an angiogram to determine how well the heart is working. This procedure is also used for treatment purposes (see Clearing Blocked Arteries).

- **Phlebography** (fleh-**BOG**-rah-fee) is the technique of preparing an x-ray image of veins injected with a contrast medium (**phleb/o** means vein and **-graphy** means the process of recording). The resulting film is a **phlebogram.**

ELECTROCARDIOGRAPHY

- An **electrocardiogram** (ee-**leck**-troh-**KAR**-dee-oh-**gram**), also known as **ECG** or **EKG,** is a record of the electrical activity of the myocardium (see Figure 5.8). **Electrocardiography** (ee-**leck**-troh-kar-dee-**OG**-rah-fee) is the process of recording this activity (**electr/o** means electric, **cardi/o** means heart, and **-graphy** means the process of recording).

- A **Holter monitor** is a portable ECG that is worn by an ambulatory patient to continuously monitor the heart rates and rhythms over a 24-hour period.

- **Stress tests** are ECGs used to assess cardiovascular health and function during and after the application of stress such as exercise on a treadmill.

- In a **thallium stress test** (**THAL**-ee-um), the flow of blood through the heart during activity is assessed through the use of thallium (a radiopharmaceutical) during a stress test. Radiopharmaceuticals are discussed further in Chapter 15.

ULTRASONIC DIAGNOSTIC PROCEDURES

- **Echocardiography** (eck-oh-**kar**-dee-**OG**-rah-fee) (**ECHO**) is an ultrasonic diagnostic procedure used to evaluate the structures and motion of the heart (**ech/o** means sound, **cardi/o** means heart, and **-graphy** means the process of recording). The resulting record is an **echocardiogram.**

- **Transesophageal echocardiography** (**trans**-eh-**sof**-ah-**JEE**-al **eck**-oh-**kar**-dee-**OG**-rah-fee) **(TEE)** is an ultrasonic procedure that images the heart from inside the esophagus. Because the esophagus is so close to the heart, this technique produces clearer images than those obtained with echocardiography.

TREATMENT PROCEDURES OF THE CARDIOVASCULAR SYSTEM

Antihypertensive Medications

An **antihypertensive** (**an**-tih-**high**-per-**TEN**-siv) is administered to lower blood pressure. The following are medications used for this purpose:

- **ACE inhibitors** (angiotensin-converting-enzyme inhibitors), which are used to treat hypertension and congestive heart failure (CHF), interfere with the action of the kidney hormone renin that causes the heart muscles to squeeze.
- **Beta-blockers** slow the heartbeat.
- **Calcium channel blockers** reduce the contraction of the muscles that squeeze blood vessels tight. These medications are used to treat hypertension, angina, and arrhythmia.
- **Diuretics** (**dye**-you-**RET**-icks), which increase urine secretion to rid the body of excess sodium and water, are administered to treat hypertension and CHF.

Additional Medications

- **Statins,** a type of **cholesterol lowering drug,** are used to reduce LDL (bad) cholesterol and triglycerides or to raise HDL (good) cholesterol.
- **Digoxin** (dih-**JOCK**-sin) also known as **digitalis** (**dij**-ih-**TAL**-is), slows and strengthens the heart muscle contractions and is used in the treatment of atrial fibrillation and CHF.
- **Nitroglycerin,** a vasodilator, is used to relieve the pain of angina. It may be administered sublingually (under the tongue), through the skin (by a patch), or orally as a spray.
- An **anticoagulant** (**an**-tih-koh-**AG**-you-lant), also known as a **thrombolytic** (**throm**-boh-**LIT**-ick) agent, slows blood clotting (coagulation) and prevents new clots from forming.
- An **antiarrhythmic** (**an**-tih-ah-**RITH**-mick) is administered to control irregularities of the heartbeat.
- **Tissue plasminogen activator** (**TISH**-you plaz-**MIN**-oh-jen **ACK**-tih-**vay**-tor) **(TPA)** is a clot-dissolving enzyme used for the immediate treatment of heart attack victims.

- A **vasoconstrictor** (**vas**-oh-kon-**STRICK**-tor) constricts (narrows) the blood vessels.
- A **vasodilator** (**vas**-oh-dye-**LAYT**-or) dilates (expands) the blood vessels.

CLEARING BLOCKED ARTERIES

- **Percutaneous transluminal coronary angioplasty** (**AN**-jee-oh-**plas**-tee) is also called **PTCA** or **balloon angioplasty** (Figure 5.18). In this procedure, a small balloon on the end of a catheter is used to open a partially blocked coronary artery by flattening the plaque deposit and stretching the lumen. After the plaque has been flattened, the balloon is deflated and the catheter and balloon are removed.
- **Percutaneous** (**per**-kyou-**TAY**-nee-us) means through the skin (**per-** means through, **cutane** means skin, and **-ous** means pertaining to). *Transluminal* means within the lumen of an artery.
- In a similar technique, a **stent** is implanted in a coronary artery to provide support to the arterial wall to prevent restenosis (Figure 5.19). **Restenosis** describes the condition when an artery that has been opened by angioplasty closes again (**re-** means again and **-stenosis** means narrowing).
- An **atherectomy** (**ath**-er-**ECK**-toh-mee) is the surgical removal of plaque from the interior lining of an artery (**ather** means plaque and **-ectomy** means surgical removal). After the catheter and balloon are in place, the balloon is inflated and a cutting tool is used to shave off pieces of the plaque buildup (Figure 5.20).
- An **endarterectomy** (**end**-ar-ter-**ECK**-toh-mee) is the surgical removal of the lining of an artery that is clogged with plaque (**end-** means within, **arter** means artery, and **-ectomy** means surgical removal).
- A **carotid endarterectomy** is the surgical removal of the lining of a portion of a clogged carotid artery leading to the brain. The artery may be reinforced with a piece of vein taken from the leg. This procedure is performed to reduce the risk of stroke by ensuring the blood flow to the brain.

CORONARY ARTERY BYPASS GRAFT

- **Coronary artery bypass graft (CABG)** is also known as **bypass surgery** (Figure 5.21). In this surgery, which requires opening the chest, a piece of vein from the leg is implanted on the heart to bypass a blockage in the coronary artery and to improve the flow of blood to the heart.
- A **minimally invasive direct coronary artery bypass (MIDCAB),** also known as a **keyhole** or **buttonhole bypass,** is an alternative technique for some bypass cases. This procedure is performed with the aid of a fiberoptic camera through small openings between the ribs.

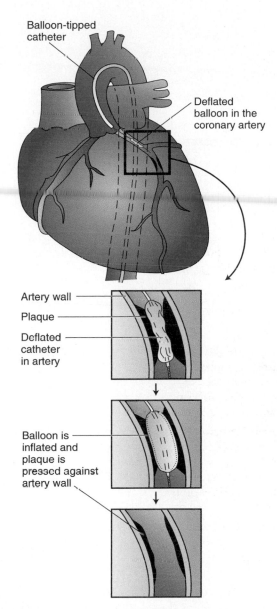

FIGURE 5.18 Balloon angioplasty is used to reopen a blocked coronary artery.

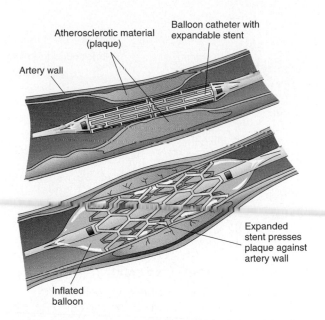

FIGURE 5.19 A stent is placed to prevent restenosis of the treated artery.

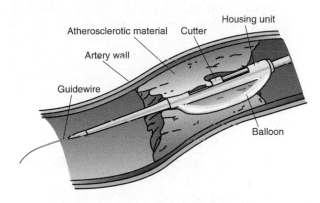

FIGURE 5.20 A cutting instrument is used to remove plaque from the artery wall.

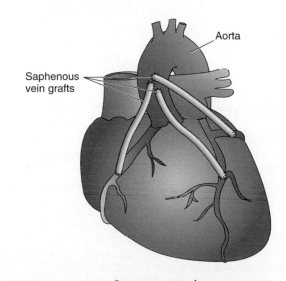

FIGURE 5.21 Coronary artery bypass surgery.

HEART

● **Defibrillation** (dee-**fib**-rih-**LAY**-shun), also known as **cardioversion** (**kar**-dee-oh-**VER**-zhun), is the use of electrical shock to restore the heart's normal rhythm. This can be performed externally as an emergency procedure or a device may be implanted to control severe arrhythmias.

● **Valvoplasty** (**VAL**-voh-**plas**-tee), also known as **valvuloplasty** (**VAL**-view-loh-**plas**-tee), is the surgical repair of a heart valve (**valv/o** means valve and **-plasty** means surgical repair). This term also describes the surgical replacement of a heart valve.

● A **pacemaker** is an electronic device that may be attached externally or implanted under the skin, with

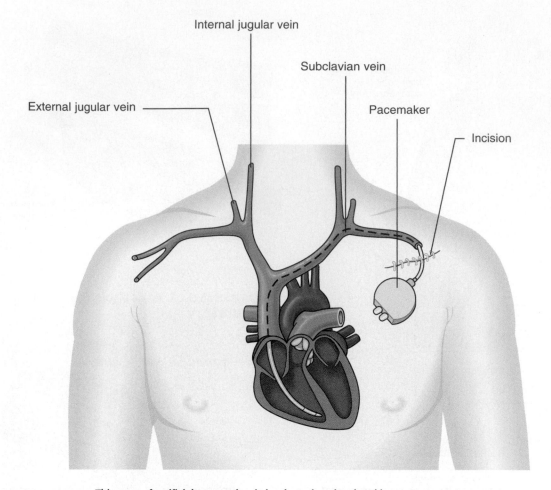

Internal jugular vein

Subclavian vein

External jugular vein

Pacemaker

Incision

FIGURE 5.22 This type of artificial pacemaker is implanted under the skin.

connections leading into the heart to regulate the heartbeat (Figure 5.22). Pacemakers are used primarily as treatment for bradycardia or atrial fibrillation.

● **Cardiopulmonary resuscitation (CPR),** is an emergency procedure for life support consisting of artificial respiration and manual external cardiac compression.

BLOOD VESSELS, BLOOD, AND BLEEDING

● An **aneurysmectomy** (**an**-you-riz-**MECK**-toh-mee) is the surgical removal of an aneurysm (**aneurysm** means aneurysm and **-ectomy** means surgical removal).

● **Aneurysmorrhaphy** (**an**-you-riz-**MOR**-ah-fee) means to suture an aneurysm (**aneurysm/o** means aneurysm and **-rrhaphy** means to suture).

● An **arteriectomy** (**ar**-teh-ree-**ECK**-toh-mee) is the surgical removal of part of an artery (**arteri** means artery and **-ectomy** means surgical removal).

● **Hemostasis** (**hee**-moh-**STAY**-sis) means to control bleeding (**hem/o** means blood and **-stasis** means stopping or controlling).

● **Plasmapheresis** (**plaz**-mah-feh-**REE**-sis) is a procedure in which the plasma is removed from donated blood, and the remaining components, mostly RBCs, are returned to the donor. This is performed to reduce or eliminate harmful substances present in the plasma.

● A **transfusion** is the introduction of whole blood or blood components into the bloodstream of the recipient. Unless the blood for transfusion has been carefully typed and cross-matched, the patient may suffer a severe transfusion reaction. Donated blood is also tested to prevent the transmission of bloodborne diseases such as the human immunodeficiency virus (HIV) and hepatitis.

Career Opportunities

In addition to the medical specialties already discussed, some of the health occupations involving the treatment of the cardiovascular system include

- **Phlebotomist,** or **venipuncture technician:** takes patient blood samples and prepares them for testing
- **Perfusionist:** operates a heart-lung machine during coronary bypass surgery
- **Cardiovascular technologist:** assists with cardiac catheterization procedures and angioplasty, monitors patients during open-heart surgery and the implantation of pacemakers, and performs tests to check circulation
- **Electrocardiograph (ECG** or **EKG) technician:** a cardiovascular technologist who operates electrocardiograph machines and Holter monitors and performs other specialized cardiac tests

STUDY BREAK

Have you ever taken a big bite of a Popsicle or a mouthful of an ice-cold drink and felt a sudden pain in your head? The not-very-scientific term *ice cream headache* is sometimes used to describe this phenomenon as are the alarming (and inaccurate) terms *brain freeze* and *frozen brain syndrome.* An ice cream headache occurs when a really cold food or beverage comes into contact with the roof of the mouth; it usually lasts only about 30 seconds.

The cause of the pain is the dilation of blood vessels in the head. This dilation is probably caused by a reaction in the nerve center located above the roof of your mouth. When this nerve center gets cold, it seems to overreact and tries to heat your brain with warm blood. The *carotid arteries,* which carry blood to the brain, send a sudden surge of blood to all the blood vessels in the forehead and face, causing a temporary but painful buildup of pressure.

About one out of every three people experience ice cream headaches from time to time. The best way to avoid them is to keep icy cold foods and beverages away from the roof of the mouth or to cool the mouth down gradually by taking small bites or sips if you are really hot.

Health Occupation Profile: CARDIAC SONOGRAPHER

Michael C. Foster, 34, is a cardiac sonographer. "I take pictures (still and moving) of people's hearts using ultrasound. As a runner, I've always been fascinated by the heart and how it works, how it acquires disease, and how it is repaired. I completed the two-year cardiovascular technology program at our local community college and now have a great job at Duke University Medical Center. It's my job to make a 'movie' that will inform the doctor about the patient's heart function. I do this by using a handheld probe placed on the patient's chest. The study usually takes about 30 minutes, and I see 8 to 10 patients a day. Since my skills center on diagnosis, I'm often the first person to have an idea of what might be wrong with a patient's heart. I work closely with doctors to identify the cardiac problem. My work helps the medical team plan the patient's care. I like my job because my specialized skills help solve important medical problems and often make people's quality of life significantly better."

Review Time

Write the answers to the following questions on a separate piece of paper or in your notebook. In addition, be prepared to take part in the classroom discussion.

1. **Written assignment:** Identify the arteries that carry only **deoxygenated** (oxygen-poor) blood and the veins that carry only **oxygenated** (oxygen-rich) blood.

   Discussion assignment: Which heart chambers pump deoxygenated blood to the lungs and which chambers receive oxygenated blood from the lungs?

2. **Written assignment:** Explain the meaning of the abbreviation **CHF.** Include with your explanation some of the symptoms that the patient with this condition experiences.

   Discussion assignment: How would you explain this condition in terms that a patient's family might understand?

3. Mike Muldoon's **blood pressure** is 160/90. **Written assignment:** Describe what each number indicates.

   Discussion assignment: How could you explain to Mr. Muldoon the risks of not controlling his blood pressure?

4. James has been diagnosed with **high cholesterol,** and he is confused about the difference between LDL and HDL.

   Written assignment: Describe the differences between LDL and HDL.

   Discussion assignment: How would you explain to James why one is considered good and the other is considered bad?

5. Mrs. Warren requires an **artificial pacemaker.**

   Written assignment: Identify which structure is known as the natural pacemaker and list two conditions that might make this surgery necessary.

   Discussion assignment: How would you explain to Mrs. Warren how the artifical pacemaker will work in her body?

Optional Internet Activity

*The goal of this activity is to help you learn more about medical terminology while improving your Internet skills. Select **one** of these two options and follow the instructions.*

1. **Internet Search:** Search for information about **blood cancers** such as leukemia and lymphoma. Write a brief (one- or two-paragraph) report on something new you learned here and include the address of the web site where you found this information.

2. **Web Site:** To learn more about **heart attack symptoms** go to this web address: **http://www.heartinfo.org/**. Write a brief (one- or two-paragraph) report on something new you learned here.

The Human Touch: Critical Thinking Exercise

The following story and questions are designed to stimulate critical thinking through class discussion or as a brief essay response. There are no right or wrong answers to these questions.

Randi Marchant, a 42-year-old waitress, was vacuuming the family room when she felt that painful squeezing in her chest again. Third time today, but this one really hurt. She sat down to catch her breath and stubbed out the cigarette smoldering in the half-filled ashtray by the couch. Her husband, Jimmy, and stepdaughter Melonie had pestered her until she finally had taken time off work to see her doctor. Dr. Harris found that her blood pressure was 168/98—probably owing to the noon rush stress at work, she rationalized. At least her cholesterol test was only 30 points above average this time. It had been slowly coming down, even though she cheated on her diet.

Another wave of pain tightened its icy fingers around her heart, and the pain moved up into both sides of her jaw. Randi remembered the doctor's words: "Probably just a little heartburn. Women have less risk for heart attack than men." This didn't feel like heartburn, but the pain didn't radiate down her left arm so it couldn't be her heart, could it?

"Don't think about the pain," she told herself. "Think of something else.... Melonie's prom dress ... needs altering ... " Randi fell to the floor, clutching her chest, just as Melonie walked in. She saw her stepmother slumped on the floor and screamed, "Oh my God! Help, somebody help!"

Suggested Discussion Topics

1. What information in the story indicates that Randi might be a candidate for heart disease?
2. Discuss why you think Dr. Harris didn't consider Randi a candidate for heart attack.
3. What can Melonie do immediately to save Randi's life?
4. Discuss why it is important that Randi receive appropriate treatment immediately.
5. What steps should someone at risk for heart disease take to help prevent the problem from becoming more serious?

Student Workbook and Student Activity CD-ROM

1. Go to your **Student Workbook** and complete the Learning Exercises for this chapter.

2. Go to the **Student Activity CD-ROM** and have fun with the exercises and games for this chapter.

6 The Lymphatic and Immune Systems

Overview of Structures, Word Parts, and Functions of the Lymphatic and Immune Systems

MAJOR STRUCTURES	RELATED WORD ROOTS	PRIMARY FUNCTIONS
Lymph Fluid and Vessels	lymph/o	Return cellular waste and tissue fluid to the circulatory system.
Lymph Nodes	lymph/o, aden/o	Produce lymphocytes and filter harmful substances from lymph.
Tonsils and Adenoids	tonsill/o, adenoid/o	Protect the entry into the respiratory system.
Spleen	splen/o	Filters foreign materials from the blood. Stores red blood cells and maintains the appropriate balance between cells and plasma in the blood. Destroys old worn-out blood cells, acts as a blood reservoir, and stores platelets.
Bone Marrow	myel/o	Produces blood cells (see Chapters 3 and 5).
Lymphocytes	lymph/o, -cyte	Play an important role in immune reactions.
Thymus	thym/o	Produces T lymphocytes for the immune system.
Immune System	immun/o	Defends the body against harmful substances such as pathogenic microorganisms, allergens, toxins, and malignant cells.

Vocabulary Related to the Lymphatic and Immune Systems

Terms marked with the ❖ symbol are pronounced on the Student Activity CD-ROM that accompanies this text.

KEY WORD PARTS

- [ ] blast/o
- [ ] carcin/o
- [ ] cervic/o
- [ ] -cide
- [ ] -genesis
- [ ] immun/o
- [ ] -lytic
- [ ] neo-
- [ ] -oma
- [ ] onc/o
- [ ] phag/o
- [ ] -plasm
- [ ] sarc/o
- [ ] splen/o
- [ ] -tic

KEY MEDICAL TERMS

- [ ] acquired immunodeficiency syndrome
- [ ] allergen (**AL**-er-jen) ❖
- [ ] anaphylaxis (**an**-ah-fih-**LACK**-sis) ❖
- [ ] antibody
- [ ] antigen (**AN**-tih-jen)
- [ ] antiviral (**an**-tih-**VYE**-ral) ❖
- [ ] aspergillosis (**ass**-per-jil-**OH**-sis) ❖
- [ ] autoimmune disorder (**aw**-toh-ih-**MYOUN**) ❖
- [ ] axillary lymph nodes (**AK**-sih-**lar**-ee) ❖
- [ ] bacilli (bah-**SILL**-eye) ❖
- [ ] bacteria (back-**TEER**-ree-ah) ❖
- [ ] bactericide (back-**TEER**-ih-sighd)
- [ ] bacteriostatic (bac-**tee**-ree-oh-**STAT**-ick)
- [ ] brachytherapy (**brack**-ee-**THER**-ah-pee) ❖
- [ ] carcinoma (**kar**-sih-**NOH**-mah) ❖
- [ ] cervical lymph nodes (**SER**-vih-kal) ❖
- [ ] complement (**KOM**-pleh-ment)
- [ ] cytomegalovirus (**sigh**-toh-**meg**-ah-loh-**VYE**-rus) ❖
- [ ] cytotoxic (**sigh**-toh-**TOK**-sick) ❖
- [ ] ductal carcinoma in situ
- [ ] ELISA
- [ ] herpes zoster (**HER**-peez **ZOS**-ter) ❖
- [ ] Hodgkin's disease (**HODJ**-kinz) ❖
- [ ] human immunodeficiency virus
- [ ] immunodeficiency disorder (**im**-you-noh-deh-**FISH**-en-see) ❖
- [ ] immunoglobulin (**im**-you-noh-**GLOB**-you-lin) ❖
- [ ] immunologist (**im**-you-**NOL**-oh-jist) ❖
- [ ] immunosuppressant (**im**-you-noh-soo-**PRES**-ant) ❖
- [ ] immunosuppression (**im**-you-noh-sup-**PRESH**-un)
- [ ] immunotherapy (ih-**myou**-noh-**THER**-ah-pee) ❖
- [ ] infectious mononucleosis (**mon**-oh-**new**-klee-**OH**-sis) ❖
- [ ] infiltrating ductal carcinoma
- [ ] infiltrating lobular carcinoma
- [ ] inguinal lymph nodes (**ING**-gwih-nal) ❖
- [ ] interferon (in-ter-**FEAR**-on) ❖
- [ ] Kaposi's sarcoma (**KAP**-oh-seez sar-**KOH**-mah) ❖
- [ ] lumpectomy (lum-**PECK**-toh-mee) ❖
- [ ] lymphadenitis (lim-**fad**-eh-**NIGH**-tis) ❖
- [ ] lymphadenopathy (lim-**fad**-eh-**NOP**-ah-thee) ❖
- [ ] lymphangiogram (lim-**FAN**-jee-oh-**gram**) ❖
- [ ] lymphangioma (lim-**fan**-jee-**OH**-mah) ❖
- [ ] lymphedema (**lim**-feh-**DEE**-mah) ❖
- [ ] lymphocytes (**LIM**-foh-sights) ❖
- [ ] lymphokines (**LIM**-foh-kyens) ❖
- [ ] lymphoma (lim-**FOH**-mah) ❖
- [ ] macrophage (**MACK**-roh-fayj) ❖
- [ ] metastasis (meh **TAS** tah sis) ❖
- [ ] metastasize (meh-**TAS**-tah-sighz) ❖
- [ ] moniliasis (mon-ih-**LYE**-ah-sis) ❖
- [ ] myoma (my-**OH**-mah) ❖
- [ ] myosarcoma (**my**-oh-sahr-**KOH**-mah) ❖
- [ ] neoplasm (**NEE**-oh-plazm) ❖
- [ ] neuroblastoma (**new**-roh-blas-**TOH**-mah) ❖
- [ ] non-Hodgkin's lymphoma (non-**HODJ**-kinz lim-**FOH**-mah) ❖
- [ ] oncologist (ong-**KOL**-oh-jist) ❖
- [ ] oncology (ong-**KOL**-oh-jee) ❖
- [ ] opportunistic infection (**op**-ur-too-**NIHS**-tick) ❖
- [ ] osteosarcoma (**oss**-tee-oh-sar-**KOH**-mah) ❖
- [ ] parasite (**PAR**-ah-sight) ❖
- [ ] pathogen (**PATH**-oh-jen) ❖
- [ ] phagocyte (**FAG**-oh-sight) ❖
- [ ] phagocytosis (**fag**-oh-sigh-**TOH**-sis) ❖
- [ ] rabies (**RAY**-beez) ❖
- [ ] retinoblastoma (**ret**-ih-noh-blas-**TOH**-mah) ❖
- [ ] rickettsia (rih-**KET**-see-ah) ❖
- [ ] rubella (roo-**BELL**-ah) ❖
- [ ] sarcoma (sar-**KOH**-mah) ❖
- [ ] spirochetes (**SPY**-roh-keets) ❖
- [ ] splenomegaly (splee-noh-**MEG**-ah-lee) ❖
- [ ] splenorrhagia (splee-noh-**RAY**-jee-ah) ❖
- [ ] staphylococci (staf-ih-loh-**KOCK**-sigh) ❖
- [ ] streptococci (strep-toh-**KOCK**-sigh) ❖
- [ ] teletherapy (tel-eh-**THER**-ah-pee) ❖
- [ ] thymus (**THIGH**-mus)
- [ ] Western blot test

Upon completion of this chapter, you should be able to:

1. Describe the major functions and structures of the lymphatic and immune systems.
2. Recognize, define, spell, and pronounce the major terms related to pathology and diagnostic and treatment procedures of the lymphatic and immune systems.
3. Recognize, define, spell, and pronounce terms related to oncology.

MEDICAL SPECIALTIES RELATED TO THE LYMPHATIC AND IMMUNE SYSTEMS

● An **allergist** (**AL**-er-jist) specializes in diagnosing and treating conditions of altered immunologic reactivity such as allergic reactions.

● A **hematologist** (**hee**-mah-**TOL**-oh-jist *or* **hem**-ah-**TOL**-oh-jist) specializes in diagnosing and treating diseases and disorders of the blood and blood-forming tissues (**hemat** means blood, and **-ologist** means specialist).

● An **immunologist** (**im**-you-**NOL**-oh-jist) is a specialist in the study, diagnosis, and treatment of disorders of the immune system (**immun** means protected and **-ologist** means specialist).

● An **oncologist** (ong-**KOL**-oh-jist) is a specialist in diagnosing and treating malignant disorders such as tumors and cancer (**onc** means tumor, and **-ologist** means specialist).

FUNCTIONS AND STRUCTURES OF THE LYMPHATIC SYSTEM

FUNCTIONS OF THE LYMPHATIC SYSTEM

The lymphatic system has three primary functions. These are to:

● Absorb fats and fat-soluble vitamins from the digestive system and transport them to the cells.

● Return cellular waste products and excess fluid from the tissues to the circulatory system.

● Serve as an important part of the immune system.

STRUCTURES OF THE LYMPHATIC SYSTEM

The major structures of the lymphatic system are **lymph fluid, lymph vessels, lymph nodes, tonsils, spleen, thymus,** and **lymphocytes** (these specialized white blood cells [WBCs] are discussed with the immune system).

Lymph Fluid

● **Intercellular fluid,** also known as **interstitial fluid** (**in**-ter-**STISH**-al) or **tissue fluid,** is plasma that flows out of the capillaries of the circulatory system into the spaces between the cells. This fluid carries food, oxygen, and hormones to the cells (Figure 6.1).

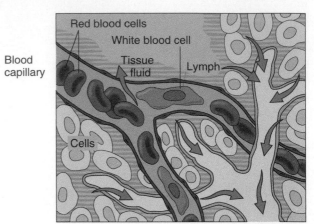

FIGURE 6.1 Lymph circulation showing the interaction of blood vessels, lymph, tissue cells, and lymph capillaries.

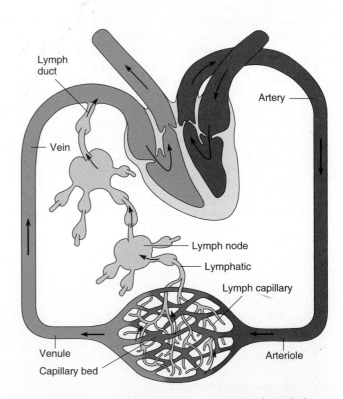

FIGURE 6.2 Fluids that leave circulation through the capillaries are returned to venous circulation by the lymphatic system.

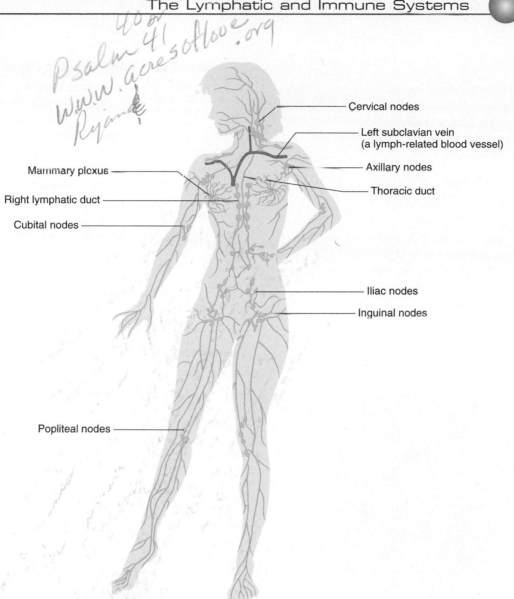

Cervical nodes

Left subclavian vein
(a lymph-related blood vessel)

Axillary nodes

Thoracic duct

Mammary plexus

Right lymphatic duct

Cubital nodes

Iliac nodes

Inguinal nodes

Popliteal nodes

FIGURE 6.3 Lymphatic circulation and major lymph node locations.

- **Lymph fluid,** usually referred to simply as **lymph,** is intercellular fluid as it returns to the venous circulatory system. Lymph, which removes waste products from the cells, must be filtered by the lymph nodes before it reenters the circulatory system (Figure 6.2).

Lymph Vessels

- **Lymph capillaries**, which are microscopic thin-walled tubes located just under the skin, carry lymph fluid from the tissues to the larger **lymphatic vessels** (Figure 6.3).

- Like veins, lymphatic vessels have valves to prevent the backward flow of fluid, and lymph always flows *toward* the thoracic cavity.

- The **right lymphatic duct** and the **thoracic duct** empty lymph into veins in the upper thoracic region.

- **Lacteals** (**LACK**-tee-ahls) are specialized lymph capillaries located in the villi of the small intestine. There

fats and fat-soluble vitamins are absorbed and carried into the bloodstream.

Lymph Nodes

- Lymph nodes are small bean-shaped structures located in lymph vessels that provide a site for lymphocyte production (see Figures 6.2 and 6.3 and Table 6.1).

- These nodes filter lymph to remove harmful substances such as bacteria, viruses, and malignant cells as lymph flows through the node. Because of this function, swollen lymph nodes are often an indication of a disease process.

The Tonsils

The **tonsils** (**TON**-sils) are masses of lymphatic tissue that form a protective ring around the nose and upper throat (Figure 6.4 and Table 6.2).

Table 6.1

MAJOR LYMPH NODE SITES

Cervical lymph nodes (**SER**-vih-kal) are located in the neck (**cervic** means neck and **-al** means pertaining to).

Axillary lymph nodes (**AK**-sih-**lar**-ee) are located under the arms (**axill** means armpit and **-ary** means pertaining to).

Inguinal lymph nodes (**ING**-gwih-nal) are located in the inguinal (groin) area of the lower abdomen (**inguin** means groin and **-al** means pertaining to).

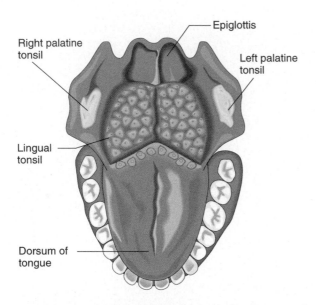

Right palatine tonsil

Epiglottis

Left palatine tonsil

Lingual tonsil

Dorsum of tongue

FIGURE 6.4 The tonsils form a protective ring around the entrance to the respiratory system.

Table 6.2

LOCATIONS OF THE TONSILS

The **adenoids** (**AD**-eh-noids), also known as the **nasopharyngeal tonsils** (nay-zoh-fah-**RIN**-jee-al), are located in the nasopharynx.

The **palatine tonsils** (**PAL**-ah-tine) are located in the portion of the throat that is visible through the mouth.

The **lingual tonsils** (**LING**-gwal) are located at the base of the tongue.

The Vermiform Appendix and Peyer's Patches

The vermiform appendix and Peyer's patches protect against the entry of invaders through the digestive system.

- The **vermiform appendix** is lymphatic tissue that hangs from the lower portion of the cecum of the large intestine (see Figure 6.6).
- **Peyer's patches** are small bundles of lymphatic tissue located on the walls of the ileum of the small intestine.

The Spleen

The spleen is a saclike mass of lymphatic tissue located in the left upper quadrant of the abdomen, just inferior to (below) the diaphragm and posterior to (behind) the stomach (Figure 6.5).

- The spleen filters microorganisms and other foreign material from the blood.
- The spleen forms lymphocytes and monocytes, which are specialized WBCs with roles in the immune system.
- The spleen is **hemolytic** (**hee**-moh-**LIT**-ick). This means it removes and destroys worn-out red blood cells (**hem/o** means blood and **-lytic** means to destroy).
- The spleen stores extra erythrocytes and maintains the appropriate balance between the red blood cells and plasma in the circulation.

The Thymus

The **thymus** (**THIGH**-mus) is located superior to (above) the heart (see Figure 6.6). Although it is composed largely of lymphatic tissue, the thymus plays important roles in the endocrine (see Chapter 13) and immune systems.

PATHOLOGY AND DIAGNOSTIC PROCEDURES OF LYMPHATIC STRUCTURES

- **Lymphadenitis** (lim-**fad**-eh-**NIGH**-tis), also known as **swollen glands,** is an inflammation of the lymph nodes (**lymphaden** means lymph node and **-itis** means inflammation).
- **Lymphadenopathy** (lim-**fad**-eh-**NOP**-ah-thee) is any disease process usually involving enlargement of the lymph nodes (**lymphaden/o** means lymph node and **-pathy** means disease).
- **Persistent generalized lymphadenopathy (PGL)** is the continued presence of enlarged lymph nodes. PGL is often an indication of the presence of a malignancy or deficiency in immune system function.
- A **lymphangiogram** (lim-**FAN**-jee-oh-**gram**) is a radiographic study of the lymphatic vessels and nodes with the use of a contrast medium to make these structures visible (**lymphangi/o** means lymph vessel and **-gram** means resulting record).

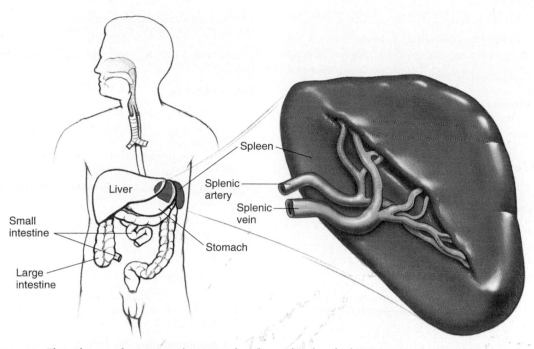

FIGURE 6.5 The spleen performs many important functions related to the immune system.

- A **lymphangioma** (lim-**fan**-jee-**OH**-mah) is a benign abnormal collection of lymphatic vessels forming a mass (**lymphangi** means lymph vessel and **-oma** means tumor).

- **Lymphedema** (**lim**-feh-**DEE**-mah) is an abnormal accumulation of lymphatic fluid that causes swelling usually in the arms or legs (**lymph** means lymph and **-edema** means swelling). Compare with lipedema in Chapter 12.

- **Primary lymphedema,** which is a hereditary disorder, may occur at any time in life. It can affect any of the limbs.

- **Secondary lymphedema** is caused by identifiable factors such as the surgical removal or radiation of the lymph nodes in the treatment of cancer. This affects the limb nearest the treatment.

- **Splenomegaly** (**splee**-noh-**MEG**-ah-lee) is an enlargement of the spleen (**splen/o** means spleen and **-megaly** means abnormal enlargement). Notice that the word root for spleen is spelled with only one *e*.

- **Splenorrhagia** (**splee**-noh-**RAY**-jee-ah) is bleeding from the spleen (**spleen/o** means spleen and **-rrhagia** means bleeding).

FUNCTIONS AND STRUCTURES OF THE IMMUNE SYSTEM

FUNCTIONS OF THE IMMUNE SYSTEM

The functions of the immune system are to protect the body from harmful substances including pathogens

(disease-producing microorganisms), allergens (substances producing an allergic reaction), toxins (poisons), and malignant cells.

STRUCTURES OF THE IMMUNE SYSTEM

Unlike other body systems, the immune system is not contained within a single set of organs or vessels. Instead, it depends on structures from several other body systems (Figure 6.6).

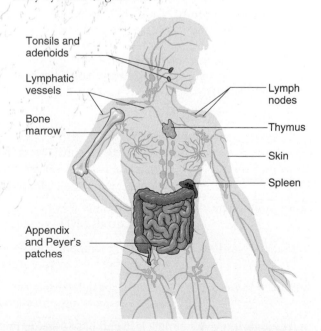

FIGURE 6.6 The immune system involves structures from many body systems.

THE FIRST LINES OF DEFENSE

The first role of the immune system is to prevent foreign substances from entering the body. However, several other body systems make up this important first line of defense.

- **Intact skin** wraps the body in a physical barrier that prevents invading organisms from entering the body. (*Intact* means there are no cuts, scrapes, or open sores.)

- The **respiratory system** traps breathed-in foreign matter with nose hairs and the moist mucous membranes that line the respiratory system. Coughing and sneezing help expel foreign matter from the respiratory system.

- The **digestive system** uses the acids and enzymes produced by the stomach to destroy invaders that are swallowed or consumed with food.

- The **lymphatic system** structures and cells are essential components in fighting invaders once they have entered the body.

THE IMMUNE RESPONSE

When infectious microorganisms enter the body, one way in which the immune system destroys them is through antigen-antibody reactions.

- An **antigen** (**AN**-tih-jen) **(Ag)** is any substance such as a virus, bacterium, toxin, or tissue that the body regards as foreign. As foreign substances, antigens stimulate an immune response.

- An **antibody (Ab)** is a disease-fighting protein created by the immune system in response to the presence of that specific antigen. (These are discussed further under immunoglobulin.)

- The **antigen-antibody reaction,** also known as the **immune reaction,** involves binding these foreign antigens to antibodies to form antigen-antibody complexes. This tags the potentially dangerous antigen so that it can be recognized and destroyed by other cells of the immune system.

SPECIALIZED CELLS OF THE IMMUNE REACTIONS

The immune response requires the actions of many specialized cells.

Lymphocytes

- **Lymphocytes** (**LIM**-foh-sights) are WBCs that specialize so they can attack specific microorganisms. All lymphocytes are formed in bone marrow as stem cells. These cells undergo further maturation and differentiation in lymphatic tissue throughout the body including the lymph nodes, spleen, thymus, tonsils, and Peyer's patches.

- The two major classes of lymphocytes are B cells and T cells.

B Cells

- Each **B cell,** also known as a **B lymphocyte,** is designed to make only one specific antibody against a specific antigen. B cells are most effective against viruses and bacteria circulating in the blood.

- **Immunoglobulin** (**im**-you-noh-**GLOB**-you-lin) **(Ig)** is a synonym for antibody. The classes of immunoglobulins, which are secreted only by B cells, are summarized in Table 6.3.

- When confronted with this type of antigen, B cells are transformed into plasma cells. **Plasma cells** produce and secrete antibodies coded to match the antigen. This process enables the body to destroy the antigen in the antigen-antibody response.

- **Complement** (**KOM**-pleh-ment) is a complex series of proteins that normally circulate in the blood in an inactive form. They are activated on contact with an antigen and aid the antibodies by puncturing the cell membrane of the antigen. (*Memory aid:* These proteins "complement" the work of antibodies in destroying bacteria.)

T Cells

- **T cells,** also known as **T lymphocytes,** are small circulating lymphocytes that have traveled to the thy-

Table 6.3

IMMUNOGLOBULINS	
Immunoglobulin M	IgM is the first immunoglobulin the body produces when challenged by an antigen and is found in circulating fluids.
Immunoglobulin G	IgG is the most common type of antibody found in the plasma. It is formed after a second exposure to an antigen.
Immunoglobulin A	IgA is the major antibody that protects against invasion through the mucous membranes and is found primarily in body fluids such as tears, saliva, and mucus.
Immunoglobulin E	IgE provides defenses against environmental antigens. It also is the antibody that causes acute allergic reactions such as hay fever.
Immunoglobulin D	IgD is found in small amounts in serum and is thought to play a role in B cell activation and differentiation.

mus. There they mature as a result of their exposure to thymosin (the hormone secreted by the thymus).

- T cells contribute to the immune defense in two major ways. Regulatory T cells coordinate immune defenses. Cytotoxic T cells kill infected cells on contact.

- **Interferon** (**in**-ter-**FEAR**-on), which is produced by the T cells, is a family of proteins released by cells when invaded by a virus. Interferon causes the non-infected cells to form an antiviral protein that slows or stops viral multiplication. Interferons are grouped into three categories: alpha, beta, and gamma.

- **Lymphokines** (**LIM**-foh-kyens), which are produced by the T cells, direct the immune response by signaling between the cells of the immune system. Lymphokines attract macrophages to the infected site and prepare them to attack.

- A **macrophage** (**MACK**-roh-fayj), which is a type of phagocyte, protects the body by ingesting (eating) invading cells and by interacting with the other cells of the immune system (**macro-** means large and **-phage** means a cell that eats).

- A **phagocyte** (**FAG**-oh-sight) is a large WBC that can ingest (eat) and destroy substances such as cell debris, dust, pollen, and pathogens (**phag/o** means to eat or swallow and **-cyte** means cell). This process is known as **phagocytosis** (**fag**-oh-sigh-**TOH**-sis).

IMMUNITY

Immunity is the state of being resistant or not susceptible to a specific disease.

- **Natural immunity** is passed from mother to fetus before birth. Immediately after birth, additional immunity is passed from mother to child through breast milk.

- **Acquired immunity** is obtained by the development of antibodies during an attack of an infectious disease. As an example, after having chickenpox antibodies are present against it.

- **Artificial immunity,** which is also known as **immunization,** is immunity that was acquired through **vaccination.** Examples of currently available vaccines include chickenpox, diphtheria, hepatitis B, influenza (some types), measles, meningitis, mumps, pertussis (whooping cough), pneumonia (some types), poliomyelitis, smallpox, tetanus, and typhoid.

IMMUNE SYSTEM RESPONSE FACTORS

Important factors that influence the immune system's ability to respond are health, age, and heredity.

- **Health.** The better the individual's general health, the more likely that the immune system can respond effectively. Disease strikes more easily when general health, and in particular the functioning of the immune system, is compromised.

- **Age.** Older individuals usually have more acquired immunity. However, their immune systems tend to respond less quickly and effectively to new challenges.

- **Heredity.** Genes and genetic disorders shape the makeup of antibodies and other immune cells. These factors influence the body's ability to respond (see Chapter 2).

- An **opportunistic infection** (**op**-ur-too-**NIIIS**-tick) is a pathogen that normally does not cause disease but is able to cause illness in a weakened host whose resistance has been decreased by a different disorder.

PATHOLOGY AND DIAGNOSTIC PROCEDURES OF THE IMMUNE SYSTEM

Allergic Reactions

- An **allergy,** also known as **hypersensitivity,** is an overreaction by the body to a particular antigen.

- An allergic reaction occurs when the body's immune system reacts to a harmless allergen, such as pollen, food, or animal dander, as if it were a dangerous invader. An **allergen** (**AL**-er-jen) is an antigen that is capable of inducing an allergic response.

- In a **cellular response,** also known as a **localized** or **delayed allergic response,** the body does not react the first time it is exposed to the allergen. However, sensitivity is established and future contacts cause symptoms that include itching, erythema (redness of the skin), and large hives. As an example, contact dermatitis is a skin reaction caused by a localized allergic response (see Chapter 12).

- A **systemic reaction,** also described as **anaphylaxis** (**an**-ah-fih-**LACK**-sis), is a severe response to a foreign substance such as a drug, food, insect venom, or chemical. Symptoms develop very quickly and include swelling, blockage of air passages, and a drop in blood pressure. Without appropriate care, the patient may die within minutes.

- A **scratch test** is a diagnostic test to identify commonly troublesome allergens such as tree pollen and ragweed. Swelling and itching indicate an allergic reaction (Figure 6.7).

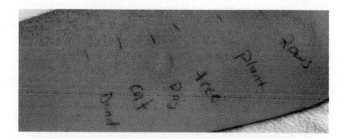

FIGURE 6.7 In scratch tests, allergens are placed on the skin, the skin is scratched, and the allergen is labeled. Reactions usually occur within 20 minutes. Pictured is a reaction to ragweed.

Table 6.4

EXAMPLES OF AUTOIMMUNE DISORDERS AND AFFECTED BODY SYSTEMS

Disease	Affected Area
Crohn's disease	Intestines, the ileum, or the colon (see Chapter 8)
Diabetes mellitus, type 1	Insulin-producing pancreatic cells (see Chapter 13)
Graves' disease	Thyroid gland (see Chapter 13)
Hashimoto's thyroiditis	Thyroid gland (see Chapter 13)
Lupus erythematosus	Skin and other body systems (see Chapter 12)
Myasthenia gravis	Nerve/muscle synapses (see Chapter 4)
Multiple sclerosis	Brain and spinal cord (see Chapter 10)
Psoriasis	Skin (see Chapter 12)
Rheumatoid arthritis	Connective tissue (see Chapter 3)
Scleroderma	Skin and other tissues (see Chapter 12)

- **Antihistamines** are medications administered to block and control allergic reactions.

Autoimmune Disorders

An **autoimmune disorder** (**aw**-toh-ih-**MYOUN**) is a condition in which the immune system misreads normal antigens and creates antibodies and directs T cells against the body's own tissues. Many of these disorders appear to be genetically transmitted and they affect most body systems (Table 6.4). For reasons that are not understood, 75 percent of these diseases occur most frequently in women during the childbearing years.

Immunodeficiency

- An **immunodeficiency disorder** (**im**-you-noh-deh-**FISH**-en-see) is a condition that occurs when one or more parts of the immune system are deficient or missing.

- When the immune system is weakened, it is also described as being **compromised.**

- Some immunodeficiency disorders, such as **congenital immunodeficiency,** are hereditary. Other forms are caused by pathogens.

- The **human immunodeficiency virus,** also known as **HIV** (pronounced **H-I-V**), is a bloodborne pathogen that invades and then progressively impairs or kills cells of the immune system.

- **Acquired immunodeficiency syndrome,** also known as **AIDS,** describes the advanced stages of an HIV infection (Figure 6.8).

- **ELISA,** which is the abbreviation for **enzyme-linked immunosorbent assay,** is a blood test used to screen for the presence of HIV antibodies. However, this test may produce a false-positive result. (A *false positive* is an inaccurate test result indicating the presence of HIV when it is not true.)

- When the results of the ELISA test are positive, a **Western blot test** is performed to confirm the diagnosis. The Western blot test, which detects the presence of specific viral proteins, produces more accurate results.

TREATMENT PROCEDURES OF THE IMMUNE SYSTEM

Immunotherapy

- **Immunotherapy** (ih-**myou**-noh-**THER**-ah-pee) is a treatment of disease either by enhancing or repressing the immune response.

- In the treatment of allergies, immunotherapy is used to repress the immune response.

- In the treatment of cancers, immunotherapy is used to stimulate the immune response.

Antibody Therapy

- **Synthetic immunoglobulins,** also known as **immune serum,** are used as a postexposure preventive measure against certain viruses including rabies and some types of hepatitis.

- **Synthetic interferon** is used in the treatment of multiple sclerosis and some cancers.

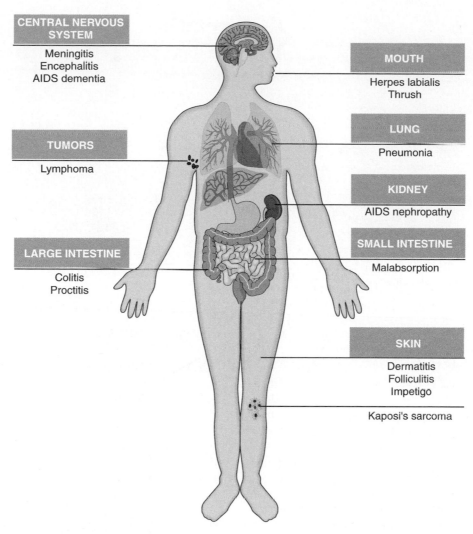

CENTRAL NERVOUS SYSTEM

Meningitis
Encephalitis
AIDS dementia

TUMORS

Lymphoma

LARGE INTESTINE

Colitis
Proctitis

MOUTH

Herpes labialis
Thrush

LUNG

Pneumonia

KIDNEY

AIDS nephropathy

SMALL INTESTINE

Malabsorption

SKIN

Dermatitis
Folliculitis
Impetigo

Kaposi's sarcoma

FIGURE 6.8 Pathologies associated with AIDS.

- **Monoclonal antibodies (MAbs)** are antibodies produced in the laboratory. Currently, MAbs are used in laboratory research, medical tests, and the treatment of some non-Hodgkin's lymphoma, melanoma, and breast and colon cancers.

Immunosuppression

- **Immunosuppression** (**im**-you-noh-sup-**PRESH**-un) is treatment used to interfere with the ability of the immune system to respond to stimulation by antigens.

- An **immunosuppressant** (**im**-you-noh-soo-**PRES**-ant) is a drug that prevents or reduces the body's normal reactions to invasion by disease or by foreign tissues. Immunosuppressants are used to prevent the rejection of donor tissue or to depress autoimmune disorders.

- A **corticosteroid drug** is a hormone-like preparation used primarily as an anti-inflammatory and as an immunosuppressant.

- A **cytotoxic drug** (**sigh**-toh-**TOK**-sick) kills or damages cells (**cyt/o** means cell, **tox** means poison and **-ic** means pertaining to). It is used as an immunosuppressant and as an antineoplastic.

- An **antineoplastic** (**an**-tih-nee-oh-**PLAS**-tick) blocks the growth of neoplasms and is used to treat cancer.

PATHOGENIC ORGANISMS

A **pathogen** (**PATH**-oh-jen) is a microorganism that causes a disease (Figure 6.9). A **microorganism** is a living organism that is so small it can be seen only with the aid of a microscope.

BACTERIA

Bacteria (back-**TEER**-ree-ah) are a group of one-celled microscopic organisms (singular, **bacterium**). The pathogenic types of bacteria include bacilli, rickettsia, spirochetes, staphylococci, and streptococci.

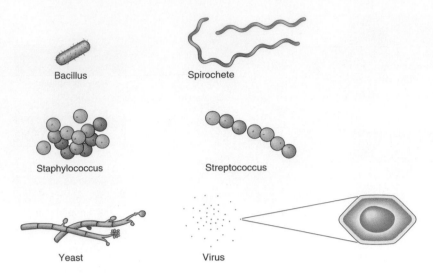

Bacillus   Spirochete

Staphylococcus   Streptococcus

Yeast   Virus

FIGURE 6.9 Types of pathogens.

- **Bacilli** (bah-**SILL**-eye) are rod-shaped spore-forming bacteria (singular, **bacillus**) (see Figure 6.9). **Tetanus** and **tuberculosis** are caused by bacilli.

- A **rickettsia** (rih-**KET**-see-ah) is a small bacterium that lives in lice, fleas, ticks, and mites (plural, **rickettsiae**). **Rocky Mountain spotted fever,** which is caused by *Rickettsia rickettsii,* is transmitted to humans by the bite of an infected tick.

- **Spirochetes** (**SPY**-roh-keets) are spiral-shaped bacteria that have flexible walls and are capable of movement (see Figure 6.9). **Lyme disease,** which is caused by the spirochete *Borrelia burgdorferi,* is transmitted to humans by the bite of an infected deer tick.

- **Staphylococci** (**staf**-ih-loh-**KOCK**-sigh) are bacteria that form irregular groups or clusters (singular, **staphylococcus**) (see Figure 6.9). **Bacterial pneumonia** is caused by *Streptococcus pneumoniae.*

- **Streptococci** (**strep**-toh-**KOCK**-sigh) are bacteria that form a chain (singular, **streptococcus**) (see Figure 6.9). *Group A streptococci* cause the form of severe **pharyngitis** (**far**-in-**JIGH**-tis) that is commonly known as a **strep throat.**

FUNGUS, YEAST, AND PARASITES

- A **fungus** (**FUNG**-gus) is a simple parasitic plant. Some of these plants are harmless to humans and others are pathogenic (plural, **fungi**). **Aspergillosis** (**ass**-per-jil-**OH**-sis), which is an infection caused by a fungus of the genus *Aspergillus,* may cause inflammation and lesions on or in any organ.

- **Yeast** is a type of fungus (see Figure 6.9). **Moniliasis** (mon-ih-**LYE**-ah-sis), which is caused by the pathogenic yeast *Candida albicans,* is an infection of the skin or mucous membranes. These infections are usually localized in the mouth or the vagina.

- A **parasite** (**PAR**-ah-sight) is a plant or animal that lives on or within another living organism at the expense of that organism. **Malaria** (mah-**LAY**-ree-ah), which is caused by a parasite that lives within certain mosquitoes, is transferred to humans by the bite of an infected mosquito.

VIRUSES

- **Viruses** (**VYE**-rus-ez) are very small infectious agents that live only by invading cells (singular, **virus**) (see Figure 6.9). Within the cell, the virus reproduces and then breaks the cell wall. The newly formed viruses are released so they can spread to other cells.

Viral Infections

- **Chickenpox,** also known as **varicella** or **VZV,** is an acute highly contagious viral disease that is characterized by fever and pustules. It is caused by the herpes virus *Varicella zoster* and is transmitted by respiratory droplets or direct contact with sores.

- **Cytomegalovirus** (**sigh**-toh-**meg**-ah-loh-**VYE**-rus) **(CMV)** is an infection caused by a group of large herpes-type viruses with a wide variety of disease effects.

- **Herpes zoster** (**HER**-peez **ZOS**-ter) **(HZ),** also known as **shingles,** is an acute viral infection characterized by painful skin eruptions that follow the underlying route of the inflamed nerve. This inflammation, which is caused by the chickenpox virus that remained dormant in a nerve, is reactivated years later when the immune system is compromised.

- **Infectious mononucleosis** (**mon**-oh-**new**-klee-**OH**-sis), which is caused by the Epstein-Barr virus (one of the herpesviruses), is characterized by fever, a sore throat, and enlarged lymph nodes.

- **Measles** is an acute, highly contagious viral disease transmitted by respiratory droplets. It is characterized first by the appearance of Koplik's spots and then followed by a spreading skin rash. **Koplik's spots** are small red spots with blue-white centers that appear on the lining of the mouth. (Compare measles with rubella.)

- **Mumps** is an acute viral disease characterized by the swelling of the parotid glands. (The parotid glands are salivary glands located on the face just in front of the ears.)

- **Rabies** (RAY-beez) is an acute viral infection that may be transmitted to humans by the blood, tissue, or saliva of an infected animal.

- **Rubella** (roo-BELL-ah), also known as **German measles** or **3-day measles,** is a viral infection characterized by fever and a diffuse, fine, red rash. If the mother has rubella during the early stages of pregnancy, the disease may cause congenital abnormalities in the infant. (Compare rubella with measles.)

MEDICATIONS TO CONTROL INFECTIONS

- An **antibiotic** is a chemical substance capable of inhibiting growth or killing pathogenic microorganisms (**anti-** means against, **bio** means life, and **-tic** means pertaining to). Antibiotics are used to combat bacterial infections.

- A **bactericide** (back-TEER-ih-sighd) is a substance that causes the death of bacteria (**bacteri** means bacteria and **-cide** means causing death). Bactericides include primarily the antibiotic groups of **penicillins** and **cephalosporins.**

- A **bacteriostatic** (bac-tee-ree-oh-STAT-ick) is an agent that inhibits, slows, or retards the growth of bacteria. These include primarily the antibiotic groups of **tetracyclines, sulfonamides,** and **erythromycin.**

- An **antiviral drug** (an-tih-VYE-ral), such as acyclovir, is used to treat viral infections or to provide temporary immunity (**anti-** means against, **vir** means virus, and **-al** means pertaining to). Antibiotics are not effective against viruses.

ONCOLOGY

Oncology (ong-KOL-oh-jee) is the study of the prevention, causes, and treatment of tumors and cancer (**onc** means tumor and **-ology** means study of).

The term **cancer** is used to describe over 200 different kinds of malignancies. Cancer attacks all body systems and is the second leading cause of death in the United States. Most cancers are named for the part of the body where the cancer first starts.

TERMS RELATED TO TUMORS

- A **tumor,** also known as a **neoplasm** (NEE-oh-plazm), is a new and abnormal tissue formation (**neo-** means new or strange and **-plasm** means formation).

- Through a process known as **angiogenesis** (an-jee-oh-JEN-eh-sis), the tumor supports its growth by creating its own blood supply (**angi/o** means vessel and **-genesis** means reproduction). **Antiangiogenesis** is a form of treatment being developed that will cut off this blood supply to the tumor (**anti-** means against, **angi/o** means vessel, and **-genesis** means reproduction).

- Within a tumor, the multiplication of cells is uncontrolled, more rapid than normal, and progressive. A **tumor** may be either benign or malignant.

Benign

Benign means not recurring, nonmalignant, and with a favorable chance for recovery. For example, a **myoma** (my-OH-mah) is a benign neoplasm made up of muscle tissue (**my** means muscle, and **-oma** means tumor). Although, not malignant, these tumors can cause problems through pressure on adjacent structures. (*Memory aid:* Benign sounds like *be nice!)*

Malignant

- **Malignant** means harmful, tending to spread, becoming progressively worse, and life threatening. Malignant tumors tend to spread to distant body sites. (*Memory aid:* Malignant sounds like *malicious or mean!)*

- The term **carcinoma in situ (CIS)** describes a malignant tumor in its original position that has not yet disturbed or invaded the surrounding tissues.

- An **invasive malignancy** grows and spreads into healthy adjacent tissue. Figure 6.10 shows the progression as colorectal cancer invades the surrounding tissues.

- **Metastasize** (meh-TAS-tah-sighz) is the verb that describes the process by which cancer spreads from one place to another. The cancer starts at the primary site and spreads to a secondary site.

- A **metastasis** (meh-TAS-tah-sis) is the new cancer site that results from the spreading process (**meta-** means beyond and **-stasis** means stopping). The metastasis may be within the same body system or in another body system at a distance from the primary site (plural, **metastases**).

STAGING

Staging is the process of classifying tumors with respect to how far the disease has progressed, the potential for its responding to therapy, and the patient's prognosis. Specific staging systems are used for different types of cancer (for examples, see Tables 6.5 and 6.6).

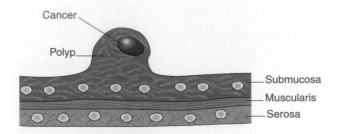

Cancer
Polyp
Submucosa
Muscularis
Serosa

Class A colorectal cancer

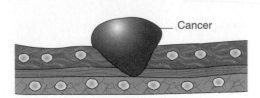

Cancer

Class B colorectal cancer

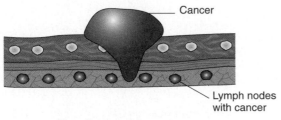

Cancer

Lymph nodes
with cancer

Class C colorectal cancer

FIGURE 6.10 Stages of colorectal cancer. *Class A:* The polyp has form but has not yet invaded the surrounding tissue. *Class B:* The cancer has invaded the underlying tissue. *Class C:* The cancer has spread to surrounding lymph nodes.

CARCINOMAS

- A **carcinoma** (**kar**-sih-**NOH**-mah), also known as **CA** or **Ca,** is a malignant tumor that occurs in epithelial tissue (**carcin** means cancer and **-oma** means tumor). Epithelial tissue covers the internal and external surfaces of the body (Figure 6.11).

- These cancers tend to infiltrate and produce metastases that may affect any organ or part of the body.

- For example, an **adenocarcinoma** (**ad**-eh-noh-**kar**-sih-**NOH**-mah) is any one of a large group of carcinomas derived from glandular tissue (**aden/o** means gland, **carcin** means cancer, and **-oma** means tumor).

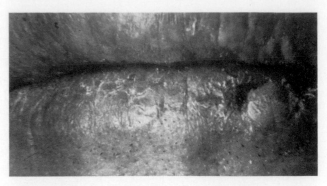

FIGURE 6.11 Carcinoma of the lip. *(Courtesy of Dr. Joseph Konzelman, School of Dentistry, Medical College of Georgia.)*

SARCOMAS

- A **sarcoma** (sar-**KOH**-mah) is a malignant tumor that arises from connective tissue (**sarc** means flesh and **-oma** means tumor) (plural, **sarcomas** or **sarcomata**). Tissues affected by sarcomas include bones, the bladder, kidneys, liver, lungs, muscles, and spleen.

- Hard-tissue sarcomas arise from bone or cartilage (see also Chapter 3). For example, **osteosarcoma** (**oss**-tee-oh-sar-**KOH**-mah) is a malignant tumor usually involving the upper shaft of long bones, the pelvis, or knee (**oste/o** means bone, **sarc** means flesh, and **-oma** means tumor).

- Soft-tissue sarcomas arise from tissues such as fat, muscle, and nerves. As an example, a **myosarcoma** (**my**-oh-sahr-**KOH**-mah) is a malignant tumor derived from muscle tissue (**myo** means muscle, **sarc** means flesh, and **oma** means tumor).

- **Kaposi's sarcoma** (**KAP**-oh-seez sar-**KOH**-mah) **(KS)** is an opportunistic infection frequently associated with HIV. It may affect the skin, mucous membranes, lymph nodes, and internal organs.

LYMPHOMAS

- **Lymphoma** (lim-**FOH**-mah) is a general term applied to malignancies that develop in the lymphatic system (**lymph** means lymph and **-oma** means tumor). The two most common types are Hodgkin's disease and non-Hodgkin's lymphoma.

Hodgkin's Disease

- **Hodgkin's disease** (**HODJ**-kinz), also known as **Hodgkin's lymphoma (HL),** is distinguished by the presence of *Reed-Sternberg cells.* These are large cancerous lymphocytes that are identified by microscopic examination of a biopsy specimen taken from an enlarged lymph node. The staging system to describe this disease is shown in Table 6.5.

Table 6.5

STAGING FOR HODGKIN'S DISEASE

Stage	Has Spread to	15-Year Cure Rate
I	Limited to lymph nodes in one area of the body such as one side of the neck.	95% plus
II	Involves lymph nodes in two or more areas on the same side of the diaphragm (either above or below).	90%
III	Involves lymph nodes above and below the diaphragm.	80%
IV	Involves lymph nodes plus other tissues including bone marrow, lungs, or liver.	60% to 70%

Non-Hodgkin's Lymphomas

- The term **non-Hodgkin's lymphomas** (non-**HODJ**-kinz lim-**FOH**-mah) **(NHL)** is used to describe all lymphomas *other than* Hodgkin's lymphoma.

- In NHL, the cells of the lymphatic system divide and grow without any order or control. This causes tumors to develop in different locations on the body and these cancer cells can also spread to other organs.

- The disease is described as low-grade (growing slowly), intermediate-grade (growing moderately), and high-grade (growing rapidly).

- Treatment depends on the type and stage of NHL and usually includes chemotherapy, radiation therapy, and possibly a bone marrow transplant (see Chapter 3).

BLASTOMAS

- A **blastoma** (blas-**TOH**-mah) is a neoplasm composed chiefly or entirely of immature undifferentiated cells (**blast** means immature or embryonic and **-oma** means tumor). Blastomas are frequently named for the tissues involved.

- A **neuroblastoma** (**new**-roh-blas-**TOH**-mah) is a sarcoma of nervous system origin (**neur/o** means nerve, **blast** means immature or embryonic, and **-oma** means tumor).

- A **retinoblastoma** (ret-ih-noh-blas-**TOH**-mah) is a malignant tumor of childhood arising from cells of the retina of the eye and usually occurring before the third year of life (**retin/o** means retina, **blast** means immature or embryonic, and **-oma** means tumor).

BREAST CANCER

Breast cancer is a malignant tumor that develops from the cells of the breast and may spread to adjacent lymph nodes and other body sites (Figure 6.12).

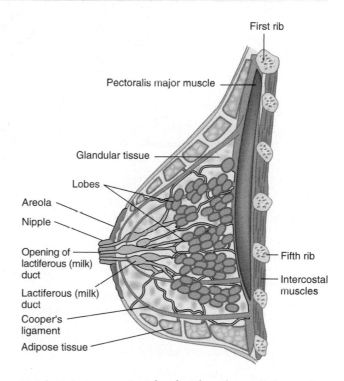

FIGURE 6.12 Invasive ductal carcinoma is the most common form of all breast cancers.

Types of Breast Cancer

- **Invasive ductal carcinoma,** also known as **infiltrating ductal carcinoma (IDC),** starts in the milk duct, breaks through the wall of that duct, and invades fatty breast tissue. IDC accounts for the majority of all breast cancers.

- **Ductal carcinoma in situ (DCIS)** is breast cancer at its earliest stage (stage 0) before the cancer has broken through the wall of the duct. At this stage, the cure rate is nearly 100 percent.

- **Invasive lobular carcinoma,** also known as **infiltrating lobular carcinoma (ILC),** is cancer that starts in the milk glands (lobules), breaks through the wall of the gland, and invades the fatty tissue of the breast. Once the cancer reaches the lymph nodes, it can rapidly spread to distant parts of the body.

- **Male breast cancer** can occur in the small amount of breast tissue that is normally present in men. The types of cancers are similar to those occurring in women.

Detection of Breast Cancer

Early detection is possible through **breast self-examination (BSE), mammograms,** and professional palpation. Diagnosis is confirmed by biopsy. These are discussed further in Chapter 14.

A **biopsy** is the removal of tissue to confirm a diagnosis. After a diagnosis has been established, treatment is then based on the stage of the cancer (Table 6.6).

Treatment of Breast Cancer

- A **lumpectomy** is the surgical removal of only the cancerous tissue and a margin (rim) of normal tissue (Figure 6.13).

- A **mastectomy** is the surgical removal of an entire breast (**mast** means breast and **-ectomy** means surgical removal.

- A **modified radical mastectomy** is the surgical removal of the entire breast and axillary lymph nodes under the adjacent arm (Figure 6.14).

CANCER TREATMENTS

The three most common forms of cancer treatments are surgery, chemotherapy, and radiation therapy.

Surgery

When possible, cancer surgery involves removing the malignancy plus a margin of normal surrounding tissue.

Table 6.6

STAGING BREAST CANCER

Stage	Explanation
I	The cancer is no larger than two centimeters (about one inch) and has not spread outside the breast.
II	Any of the following may be true:
	The cancer is no larger than two centimeters but has spread to the axillary lymph nodes.
	The cancer is between two and five centimeters (from one to two inches) and may or may not have spread to the axillary lymph nodes.
	The cancer is larger than five centimeters (greater than two inches) but has not spread to the axillary lymph nodes.
IIIA	Either of the following is true:
	The cancer is smaller than five centimeters and has spread to the axillary lymph nodes and the lymph nodes are attached to each other or to other structures.
	The cancer is larger than five centimeters and has spread to the axillary lymph nodes.
IIIB	Either of the following is true:
	The cancer has spread to tissues near the breast (skin or chest wall, including the ribs and muscles of the chest).
	The cancer has spread to lymph nodes inside the chest wall along the breastbone.
IV	The cancer has spread to other organs of the body, most often the bones, lungs, liver, or brain. Or, the cancer has spread locally to the skin and lymph nodes inside the neck, near the collarbone.

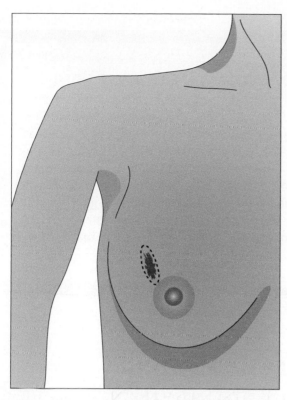

FIGURE 6.13 A lumpectomy is the removal of the cancerous tissue plus a margin of healthy tissue.

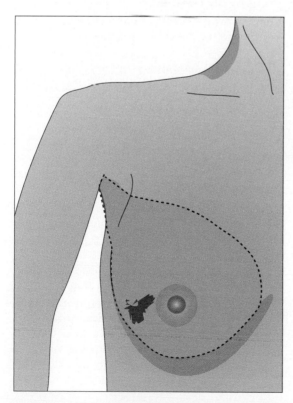

FIGURE 6.14 A modified radical mastectomy is the removal of the entire breast and the adjacent lymph nodes.

Chemotherapy

Chemotherapy is the use of chemical agents and drugs in combinations selected to effectively destroy malignant cells and tissues.

Radiation Therapies

- **Radiation therapy** is the treatment of cancers through the use of x-rays. The goal of these therapies is to destroy the cancer while sparing healthy tissues.
- **Brachytherapy** (**brack**-ee-**THER**-ah-pee) is the use of radioactive materials in contact with, or implanted into, the tissues to be treated (**brachy-** means short and **-therapy** means treatment).
- **Teletherapy** (**tel**-eh-**THER**-ah-pee) is radiation therapy administered at a distance from the body (**tele-** means distant and **-therapy** means treatment). With three-dimensional computer imaging, it is possible to aim doses more precisely.

Career Opportunities

In addition to the medical specialties already discussed, some of the health occupations involving the treatment of the lymphatic and immune systems include:

- **Cytotechnologist:** a clinical laboratory technologist who examines human cell samples under a microscope for signs of cancer
- **Lymphedema therapist:** provides decongestive lymphatic therapy, including skin care, manual lymphatic massage, bandaging, exercises, and instruction in self care to lymphedema patients

STUDY BREAK

Very few scientists are lucky enough to be immortalized by having a body part carry their name. It's obvious that **Peyer's patches** is an eponym (named after a person), so you're probably wondering who Dr. Peyer was—and why the small areas of lymphatic tissue on the walls of the large intestine are named after him.

Johann Conrad Peyer was a Swiss anatomist who lived from 1653 to 1712. He was born into a wealthy family and studied medicine in Switzerland and Paris. In addition to working as a physician, he taught rhetoric, logic, and medicine and conducted scientific experiments. In 1682, he was the first person to describe the lymphatic nodules on the walls of the ileum that now bear his name.

Humans are not the only species with lymphatic tissue called Peyer's patches. Johann Conrad Peyer also lives on in veterinary studies, where all students learning about the intestines of cows, dogs, rats, and other mammals must remember his name.

Health Occupation Profile: LYMPHEDEMA THERAPIST

Joanna Burgess, 39, is a registered nurse specializing in working with patients with lymphedema. "The treatment of lymphedema utilizing Combined Decongestive Therapy is a European approach that has been used in the United States since about 1990. This work enables me to utilize my traditional nursing experience as well as other skills. I assess patients, formulate treatment plans, establish patient goals, perform CDT massage, apply compression aids, and provide patient education. This type of work also enables me to utilize alternative medical approaches through lymphatic massage therapy and lymphatic exercises. It is an area of nursing in which one can establish a private practice. I am currently the clinical coordinator for a private lymphedema clinic that I established in partnership with an occupational therapist."

Review Time

Write the answers to the following questions on a separate piece of paper or in your notebook. In addition, be prepared to take part in the classroom discussion.

1. **Written assignment:** Use terms a physician would understand to describe the primary characteristic that differentiates **Hodgkin's lymphoma** from **non-Hodgkin's lymphoma.**

    Discussion assignment: How would you explain to a patient the process of "staging" Hodgkin's disease and the prognosis at each stage?

2. **Written assignment:** Define **autoimmune disorder** and explain what happens within the immune system.

    Discussion assignment: How would you explain an autoimmune disorder to a patient who had just been diagnosed with having one?

3. **Written assignment:** Identify three major functions of the **lymphatic system.**

    Discussion assignment: What role does the lymphatic system play in the immune system?

4. **Written assignment:** Identify at least three parts of the first lines of defense of the **immune system.**

    Discussion assignment: What is the role of each of these defenses?

5. **Written assignment:** Use terms a patient would understand to describe the role of **immunosuppression.**

    Discussion assignment: What is the role of immunosuppressants in preventing the rejection of a transplanted organ?

Optional Internet Activity

*The goal of this activity is to help you learn more about medical terminology while improving your Internet skills. Select **one** of these two options and follow the instructions.*

1. **Internet Search:** Search for information about **autoimmune disorders.** Write a brief (one- or two-paragraph) report on something new you learned here and include the address of the web site where you found this information.

2. **Web Site**: To learn more about **lymphedema** go to this web address: **http://lymphnet.org/.** Explore the site and then write a brief (one- or two-paragraph) report on something new you learned here.

The Human Touch: Critical Thinking Exercise

The following story and questions are designed to stimulate critical thinking through class discussion or as a brief essay response. There are no right or wrong answers to these questions.

Hernani Fermin, a 35-year-old married father, was diagnosed HIV positive two years ago. He is a sales representative for a nationally recognized pharmaceutical company, and his hectic travel schedule was beginning to take a toll on his health. A few weeks ago, his doctor suggested he rethink his career goals. "You know, stress and this disease don't mix," Dr. Wettstein reminded him. "Why don't you look for something closer to home?"

That evening over lasagna his wife, Emily, suggested teaching. Hernani had enjoyed sharing the challenging concepts of math and science with seventh graders during the six years he had taught in a rural school upstate. It was only the financial demands of Kim and Kili's birth seven years ago that had tempted him into the better paying field of pharmaceuticals.

He sent out resumes for the next five weeks. Finally one was well received by South Hills Middle School. They had an opening in their math department, plus a need for someone to coach after-school athletics, and they wanted to meet with him. He hadn't interviewed since the twins were born. He thought about the questions normally asked—would there be some about his health? Being HIV positive shouldn't have any bearing on his ability to teach, but parents might be concerned. And it might disqualify him for the school's health insurance policy. Hernani believed in honesty, but what would happen to his family if he revealed his HIV status?

Suggested Discussion Topics

1. Do you think Hernani should reveal his HIV status to South Hills Middle School? If so, why? If not, why not?

2. Do you think South Hills Middle School would hire Hernani if they knew he was HIV positive? Why or why not?

3. How would you feel if your child were on one of the teams Hernani would be coaching? Why?

4. Discuss the insurance problems Hernani might encounter by changing jobs.

5. Confidentiality is an important physician-patient issue. Discuss whether it would be Dr. Wettstein's duty to reveal Hernani's HIV status if asked about it.

Student Workbook and Student Activity CD-ROM

1. Go to your **Student Workbook** and complete the Learning Exercises for this chapter.

2. Go to the **Student Activity CD-ROM** and have fun with the exercises and games for this chapter.

The Respiratory System

Overview of Structures, Word Parts, and Functions of the Respiratory System

MAJOR STRUCTURES	RELATED WORD PARTS	PRIMARY FUNCTIONS
Nose	**nas/o**	Exchanges air during inhaling and exhaling; warms, moisturizes, and filters inhaled air.
Sinuses	**sinus/o**	Provides mucus, makes bones of the skull lighter, aids in sound production.
Epiglottis	**epiglott/o**	Closes off the trachea during swallowing.
Pharynx	**pharyng/o**	Transports air to and from the nose to the trachea.
Larynx	**laryng/o**	Makes speech possible.
Trachea	**trache/o**	Transports air to and from the pharynx to the bronchi.
Bronchi	**bronch/o, bronchi/o**	Transports air from the trachea into the lungs.
Alveoli	**alveol/o**	Air sacs that exchange gases with the pulmonary capillary blood.
Lungs	**pneum/o, pneumon/o**	Brings oxygen into the body and removes carbon dioxide and some water waste from the body.

Vocabulary Related to the Respiratory System

Terms marked with the ❖ symbol are pronounced on the Student Activity CD-ROM that accompanies this text.

KEY WORD PARTS

- ☐ atel/o
- ☐ bronch/o, bronchi/o
- ☐ cyan/o
- ☐ -ectasis
- ☐ laryng/o
- ☐ ox/i, ox/o, ox/y
- ☐ pharyng/o
- ☐ phon/o
- ☐ pleur/o
- ☐ -pnea
- ☐ pneum/o, pneumon/o, pneu-
- ☐ pulm/o, pulmon/o
- ☐ tachy-
- ☐ thorac/o, -thorax
- ☐ trache/o

KEY MEDICAL TERMS

- ☐ **anoxia** (ah-**NOCK**-see-ah)
- ☐ **anthracosis** (**an**-thrah-**KOH**-sis)
- ☐ **aphonia** (ah-**FOH**-nee-ah)
- ☐ **apnea** (**AP**-nee-ah *or* ap-**NEE**-ah) ❖
- ☐ **asbestosis** (**ass**-beh-**STOH**-sis)
- ☐ **asphyxia** (ass-**FICK**-see-ah)
- ☐ **asphyxiation** (ass-**fick**-see-**AY**-shun) ❖
- ☐ **asthma** (**AZ**-mah) ❖
- ☐ **atelectasis** (at-ee-**LEK**-tah-sis) ❖
- ☐ **bradypnea** (**brad**-ihp-**NEE**-ah *or* brad-ee-**NEE**-ah) ❖
- ☐ **bronchiectasis** (**brong**-kee-**ECK**-tah-sis) ❖
- ☐ **bronchoconstrictor** (**brong**-koh-kon-**STRICK**-tor)
- ☐ **bronchodilator** (**brong**-koh-dye-**LAY**-tor)
- ☐ **bronchopneumonia** (**brong**-koh-new-**MOH**-nee-ah) ❖
- ☐ **bronchorrhagia** (**brong**-koh-**RAY**-jee-ah) ❖
- ☐ **bronchorrhea** (**brong**-koh-**REE**-ah) ❖
- ☐ **bronchoscopy** (**brong**-**KOS**-koh-pee) ❖
- ☐ **Cheyne-Stokes respiration** (**CHAYN**-**STOHKS**) ❖
- ☐ **croup** (**KROOP**) ❖
- ☐ **cystic fibrosis** (**SIS**-tick figh-**BROH**-sis) ❖
- ☐ **diphtheria** (dif-**THEE**-ree-ah) ❖
- ☐ **dysphonia** (dis-**FOH**-nee-ah) ❖
- ☐ **dyspnea** (**DISP**-nee-ah) ❖
- ☐ **emphysema** (em-fih-**SEE**-mah) ❖
- ☐ **empyema** (em-pye-**EE**-mah) ❖
- ☐ **endotracheal intubation** (en-doh-'**TRAY**-kee-al in-too-**BAY**-shun)
- ☐ **epiglottis** (ep-ih-**GLOT**-is)
- ☐ **epistaxis** (ep-ih-**STACK**-sis) ❖

- ☐ **hemoptysis** (hee-**MOP**-tih-sis) ❖
- ☐ **hemothorax** (**hee**-moh-**THOH**-racks) ❖
- ☐ **hyperpnea** (**high**-perp-**NEE**-ah) ❖
- ☐ **hyperventilation** (**high**-per-ven-tih-**LAY**-shun) ❖
- ☐ **hypopnea** (**high**-poh-**NEE**-ah) ❖
- ☐ **hypoxia** (high-**POCK**-see-ah) ❖
- ☐ **influenza** (**in**-flew-**EN**-zah) ❖
- ☐ **inhalation** (**in**-hah-**LAY**-shun)
- ☐ **laryngectomy** (**lar**-in-**JECK**-toh-mee) ❖
- ☐ **laryngitis** (**lar**-in-**JIGH**-tis) ❖
- ☐ **laryngoplasty** (lah-**RING**-goh-**plas**-tee) ❖
- ☐ **laryngoplegia** (**lar**-ing-goh-**PLEE**-jee-ah) ❖
- ☐ **laryngoscopy** (**lar**-ing-**GOS**-koh-pee) ❖
- ☐ **laryngospasm** (lah-**RING**-goh-spazm) ❖
- ☐ **mediastinum** (**mee**-dee-as-**TYE**-num)
- ☐ **mycoplasma pneumonia** (**my**-koh-**PLAZ**-mah new **MOH**-nee-ah) ❖
- ☐ **nasopharyngitis** (**nay**-zoh-**far**-in-**JIGH**-tis) ❖
- ☐ **otolaryngologist** (**oh**-toh-**lar**-in-**GOL**-oh-jist) ❖
- ☐ **otorhinolaryngologist** (**oh**-toh-**rye**-noh-**lar**-in-**GOL**-oh-jist) ❖
- ☐ **pertussis** (per-**TUS**-is) ❖
- ☐ **pharyngitis** (**far**-in-**JIGH**-tis)
- ☐ **pharyngoplasty** (fah-**RING**-goh-**plas**-tee)
- ☐ **pharyngorrhagia** (**far**-ing-goh-**RAY**-jee-ah) ❖
- ☐ **pharyngorrhea** (**far**-ing-goh-**REE**-ah) ❖
- ☐ **pleuralgia** (ploor-**AL**-jee-ah) ❖
- ☐ **pleurectomy** (ploor-**ECK**-toh-mee) ❖
- ☐ **pleurisy** (**PLOOR**-ih-see) ❖
- ☐ **pneumoconiosis** (**new**-moh-**koh**-nee-**OH**-sis) ❖
- ☐ ***Pneumocystis carinii* pneumonia** (**new**-moh-**SIS**-tis kah-**RYE**-nee-eye new-**MOH**-nee-ah) ❖
- ☐ **pneumonectomy** (**new**-moh-**NECK**-toh-mee) ❖
- ☐ **pneumorrhagia** (**new**-moh-**RAY**-jee-ah) ❖
- ☐ **pneumothorax** (**new**-moh-**THOR**-racks) ❖
- ☐ **pulmonologist** (**pull**-mah-**NOL**-oh-jist) ❖
- ☐ **pyothorax** (**pye**-oh-**THOH**-racks) ❖
- ☐ **rhinorrhea** (**rye**-noh-**REE**-ah)
- ☐ **sinusitis** (**sigh**-nuh-**SIGH**-tis) ❖
- ☐ **sinusotomy** (**sigh**-nuhs-**OT**-oh-mee) ❖
- ☐ **spirometry** (spy-**ROM**-eh-tree) ❖
- ☐ **tachypnea** (**tack**-ihp-**NEE**-ah) ❖
- ☐ **thoracentesis** (**thoh**-rah-sen-**TEE**-sis) ❖
- ☐ **thoracostomy** (**thoh**-rah-**KOS**-toh-mee) ❖
- ☐ **thoracotomy** (**thoh**-rah-**KOT**-oh-mee) ❖
- ☐ **tracheitis** (**tray**-kee-**EYE**-tis) ❖
- ☐ **tracheoplasty** (**TRAY**-kee-oh-**plas**-tee) ❖
- ☐ **tracheostomy** (**tray**-kee-**OS**-toh-mee) ❖
- ☐ **tracheotomy** (**tray**-kee-**OT**-oh-mee) ❖
- ☐ **tuberculosis** (too-**ber**-kew-**LOH**-sis)

FUNCTIONS OF THE RESPIRATORY SYSTEM

The functions of the respiratory system are to

- Bring oxygen-rich air into the body for delivery to the blood cells.

- Expel waste products (carbon dioxide and water) that have been returned to the lungs by the blood.

- Produce the air flow through the larynx that makes speech possible.

STRUCTURES OF THE RESPIRATORY SYSTEM

For descriptive purposes, the respiratory system is divided into upper and lower tracts (Figure 7.1).

- The **upper respiratory tract** consists of the nose, mouth, pharynx, epiglottis, larynx, and trachea (Figure 7.2).

- The **lower respiratory tract** consists of the bronchial tree and lungs. These structures are protected by the thoracic cavity.

THE NOSE

- Air enters the body through the nose and passes through the **nasal cavity.**

- The **nasal septum** (**NAY**-zal **SEP**-tum) is a wall of cartilage that divides the nose into two equal sections.

- **Mucous membrane** (**MYOU**-kus) is the specialized form of epithelial tissue that lines the nose and respiratory system.

- **Mucus** (**MYOU**-kus), which is secreted by the mucous membranes, helps to moisten, warm, and filter the air as it enters the nose. *Notice the different spellings:* Mucous is the name of the tissue; mucus is the secretion that flows from the tissue.

- **Cilia** (**SIL**-ee-ah), the thin hairs located just inside the nostrils, filter incoming air to remove debris.

- The **olfactory receptors** (ol-**FACK**-toh-ree), the receptors for the sense of smell, are nerve endings located in the mucous membrane in the upper part of the nasal cavity.

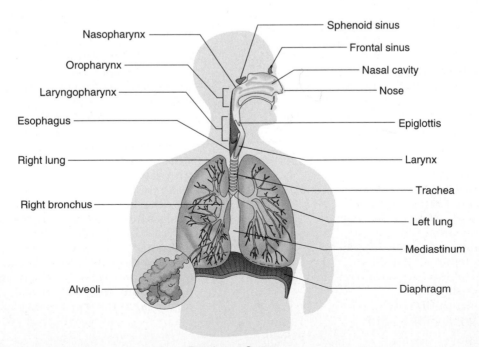

Respiratory System

FIGURE 7.1 Structures of the respiratory system.

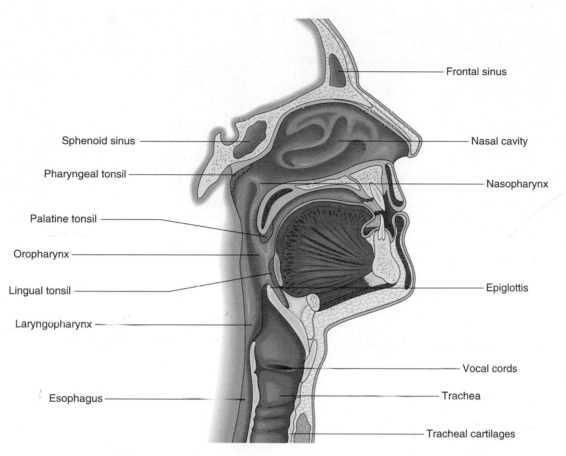

Frontal sinus

Sphenoid sinus

Nasal cavity

Pharyngeal tonsil

Nasopharynx

Palatine tonsil

Oropharynx

Lingual tonsil

Epiglottis

Laryngopharynx

Vocal cords

Trachea

Esophagus

Tracheal cartilages

FIGURE 7.2 Structures of the upper respiratory tract.

THE TONSILS

- The **tonsils,** which have an important function in protecting the body from invading organisms, form a protective circle around the entrance to the respiratory system. Tonsils, which are a type of lymphatic tissue, are discussed in Chapter 6.

THE SINUSES

- A **sinus** is an air-filled cavity within a bone that is lined with mucous membrane.

- The functions of sinuses are (1) to make the bones of the skull lighter, (2) to help produce sound by giving resonance to the voice, and (3) to produce mucus that drains into the nasal cavity.

- The **paranasal sinuses** are located in the bones of the skull (**para-** means near, **nas** means nose, and **-al** means pertaining to). Short ducts connect these sinuses to the nasal cavity.

- The sinuses are named for the bones in which they are located. The paranasal sinuses are summarized in Table 7.1.

Table 7.1

PARANASAL SINUSES

Maxillary sinuses (**MACK**-sih-**ler**-ee), located in the maxillary bones, are the largest of the paranasal sinuses.	**Frontal sinuses** are located in the frontal bone just above the eyebrows.
The **ethmoid sinuses** (**ETH**-moid), located in the ethmoid bones, are irregularly shaped air cells that are separated from the orbital (eye) cavity only by a thin layer of bone.	The **sphenoid sinuses** (**SFEE**-noid), located in the sphenoid bone, are close to the optic nerves. An infection here can damage vision.

THE PHARYNX

- After passing through the nasal cavity, the air reaches the **pharynx** (**FAR**-inks), which is commonly known as the **throat** (see Figure 7.2). The pharynx has three divisions:

- The **nasopharynx** (**nay**-zoh-**FAR**-inks), the first division, is posterior to the nasal cavity and continues downward to behind the mouth.

- The **oropharynx** (**oh**-roh-**FAR**-inks), the second division, is the portion that is visible when looking into the mouth (see Figure 8.2). The oropharynx is shared by the respiratory and digestive systems.

- The **laryngopharynx** (lah-**ring**-goh-**FAR**-inks), the third division, continues downward to the openings of the esophagus and trachea.

Protective Swallowing Mechanisms

The respiratory and digestive systems share part of the pharynx. During swallowing, there is the risk of a blocked airway or pneumonia caused by something entering the lungs instead of traveling into the esophagus.

- Two protective mechanisms act automatically during swallowing to ensure that *only* air goes into the lungs.

- During swallowing, the soft palate, which is the muscular posterior portion of the roof of the mouth, moves up and backward to close off the nasopharynx. This movement prevents food from going up into the nose. (Structures of the mouth are discussed further in Chapter 8.)

- At the same time, the **epiglottis** (**ep**-ih-**GLOT**-is), which is a lidlike structure located at the base of the tongue, swings downward and closes off the laryngopharynx so food does not enter the trachea and the lungs.

THE LARYNX

- The **larynx** (**LAR**-inks), also known as the **voice box,** is a triangular chamber located between the pharynx and the trachea (Figure 7.3).

- The larynx is protected and held open by a series of nine separate cartilages. The **thyroid cartilage** is the largest and its prominent projection is commonly known as the **Adam's apple.**

- The larynx contains the **vocal cords.** During breathing, the cords are separated to let air pass. During speech, they are together, and sound is produced as air is expelled from the lungs, causing the cords to vibrate against each other.

THE TRACHEA

- Air passes from the larynx into the **trachea** (**TRAY**-kee-ah), which is commonly known as the **wind-pipe** (Figure 7.4).

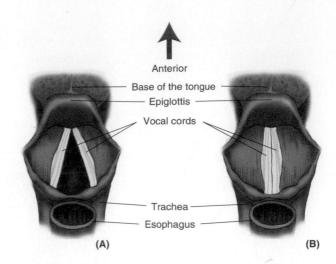

FIGURE 7.3 View of the larynx and vocal cords from above. (A) The vocal cords are open during breathing. (B) The vocal cords vibrate together during speech.

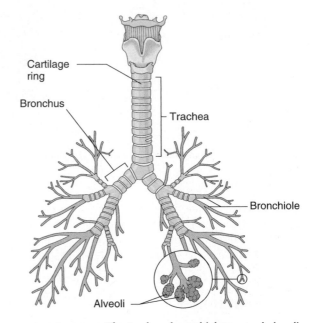

FIGURE 7.4 The trachea, bronchial tree, and alveoli.

- The trachea extends from the neck into the chest, directly in front of the esophagus and is held open by a series of C-shaped cartilage rings. The wall between these rings is elastic, enabling the trachea to adjust to different body positions.

THE BRONCHIAL TREE

- The trachea divides into two branches called **bronchi** (**BRONG**-kye). A branch goes into each lung (singular, **bronchus**).

- Within the lung, the bronchus divides and subdivides into increasingly smaller bronchi. **Bronchioles** (**BRONG**-kee-ohlz) are the smallest branches of the bronchi.

- Because of the similarity of these branching structures to a tree, this is referred to as the **bronchial tree** (see Figure 7.4).

THE ALVEOLI

- **Alveoli** (al-**VEE**-oh-lye), also known as **air sacs,** are the very small grapelike clusters found at the end of each bronchiole (see Figures 7.1 and 7.4) (singular, **alveolus**).
- The thin flexible walls of the alveoli are surrounded by a network of microscopic pulmonary capillaries.
- During respiration, the gas exchange between the alveolar air and the pulmonary capillary blood occurs through the walls of the alveoli.

THE LUNGS

- A **lobe** is a division of the lungs (Figure 7.5).
- The **right lung** has three lobes: the superior, middle, and inferior.
- The **left lung** has two lobes: the superior and inferior.

THE MEDIASTINUM

- The **mediastinum** (**mee**-dee-as-**TYE**-num), also known as the **interpleural space,** is located between the lungs (see Figure 7.1).
- This space contains the thoracic viscera including the heart, aorta, esophagus, trachea, bronchial tubes, and thymus gland.

THE PLEURA

- The **pleura** (**PLOOR**-ah) is a multilayered membrane that surrounds each lung with its blood vessels and nerves (plural, **pleurae**).
- The **parietal pleura** (pah-**RYE**-eh-tal **PLOOR**-ah) is the outer layer of the pleura. It lines the thoracic cavity and forms the sac containing each lung.
- The **visceral pleura** (**VIS**-er-al **PLOOR**-ah) is the inner layer of pleura. It closely surrounds the lung tissue.
- The **pleural space,** also known as the **pleural cavity,** is the airtight space between the folds of the pleural membranes. It contains a watery lubricating fluid that prevents friction when the membranes rub together during respiration.

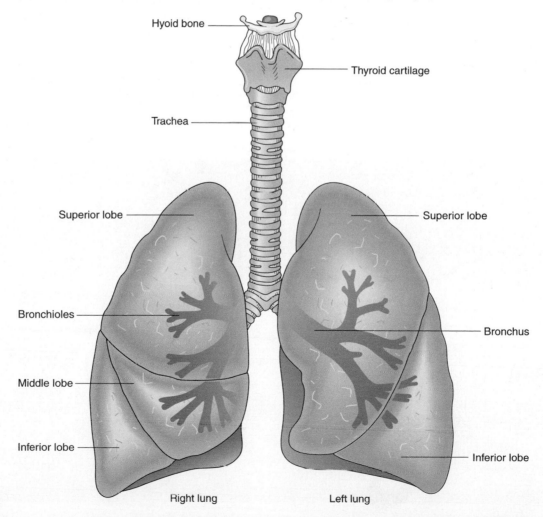

FIGURE 7.5 External view of the lungs. Note the three lobes of the right lung and the two lobes of the left lung.

THE DIAPHRAGM

● The **diaphragm** (**DYE**-ah-fram) is the muscle that separates the thoracic cavity from the abdomen (see Figures 7.1 and 7.6). It is the contraction and relaxation of this muscle that makes breathing possible.

● The **phrenic nerve** (**FREN**-ick) stimulates the diaphragm and causes it to contract (**phren** means diaphragm or mind, and **-ic** means pertaining to).

RESPIRATION

Respiration is the exchange of gases that are essential to life. This occurs in the lungs as external respiration and on a cellular level as internal respiration.

EXTERNAL RESPIRATION

● **Breathing** is the act of bringing air into and out of the lungs.

● **Inhalation** (**in**-hah-**LAY**-shun), also known as **inhaling,** is the act of taking in air as the diaphragm contracts and pulls downward. This action causes the thoracic cavity to expand. This expansion produces a vacuum within the thoracic cavity that draws air into the lungs (Figure 7.6, left photo).

● **Exhalation** (**ecks**-hah-**LAY**-shun) is the act of breathing out. As the diaphragm relaxes, it moves upward, causing the thoracic cavity to become narrower. This action forces air out of the lungs (Figure 7.6, right photo).

The Exchange of Gases within the Lungs

As air moves in and out, there is an **exchange of gases** within the lungs (Figure 7.7A).

● As air is **inhaled** into the alveoli, oxygen (O_2) immediately passes into the surrounding capillaries and is carried by the erythrocytes to all body cells.

● At the same time, the waste product carbon dioxide (CO_2) passes from the capillaries into the airspaces of the lungs to be **exhaled.**

INTERNAL RESPIRATION

● Internal respiration is the exchange of gases within the cells of all the body organs and tissues (Figure 7.7B).

● In this process, oxygen passes from the bloodstream into the tissue cells. At the same time, carbon dioxide passes from the tissue cells into the bloodstream.

MEDICAL SPECIALTIES RELATED TO THE RESPIRATORY SYSTEM

● An **otolaryngologist** (**oh**-toh-**lar**-in-**GOL**-oh-jist), also known as an **otorhinolaryngologist** (**oh**-toh-**rye**-noh-**lar**-in-**GOL**-oh-jist), specializes in diagnosing and treating diseases and disorders of the ears, nose, and throat.

● A **pulmonologist** (**pull**-mah-**NOL**-oh-jist) is a physician who specializes in diagnosing and treating diseases and disorders of the lungs and associated tissues (**pulmon** means lung and **-ologist** means specialist).

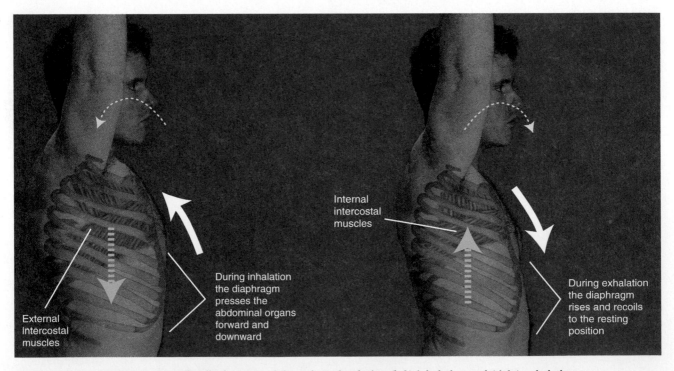

External Intercostal muscles

During inhalation the diaphragm presses the abdominal organs forward and downward

Internal intercostal muscles

During exhalation the diaphragm rises and recoils to the resting position

FIGURE 7.6 Movement of the diaphragm and thoracic cavity during (left) inhalation and (right) exhalation.

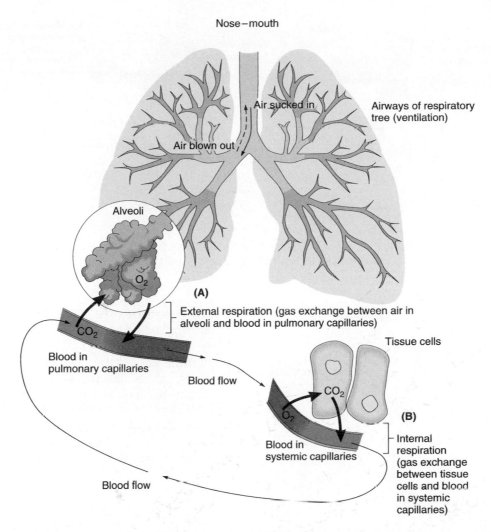

FIGURE 7.7 External and internal respiration compared. (A) External respiration, with the exchange of gases between the lungs and capillaries. (B) Internal respiration, with the exchange between the blood and tissues.

PATHOLOGY OF THE RESPIRATORY SYSTEM

CHRONIC OBSTRUCTIVE PULMONARY DISEASES

- **Chronic obstructive pulmonary disease (COPD)** is a general term used to describe a group of respiratory conditions characterized by chronic airflow limitations.

- **Asthma** (**AZ**-mah) is a chronic allergic disorder characterized by episodes of severe breathing difficulty, coughing, and wheezing (Figure 7.8). Breathing difficulty during an asthma attack is caused by several factors: (1) swelling and inflammation of the lining of the airways, (2) the production of thick mucus, and (3) tightening of the muscles that surround the airways. (For treatment, see **bronchodilator,** under Medications.)

- **Bronchiectasis** (**brong**-kee-**ECK**-tah-sis) is chronic dilation (enlargement) of bronchi or bronchioles resulting from an earlier lung infection that was not cured (**bronchi** means bronchi and **-ectasis** means enlargement) (Figure 7.9).

- **Emphysema** (**em**-fih-**SEE**-mah) is the progressive loss of lung function due to a decrease in the total number of alveoli, the enlargement of the remaining alveoli, and then the progressive destruction of their walls (see Figure 7.10A on page 131). As the alveoli are destroyed, breathing becomes increasingly rapid, shallow, and difficult. In an effort to compensate for the loss of capacity, the lungs expand and the chest assumes an enlarged barrel shape (Figure 7.10B).

- **Smoker's respiratory syndrome (SRS)** is a group of symptoms seen in smokers. These chronic conditions include (1) a cough, (2) wheezing, (3) vocal hoarseness, (4) pharyngitis (sore throat), (5) difficult breathing, and (6) a susceptibility to respiratory infections.

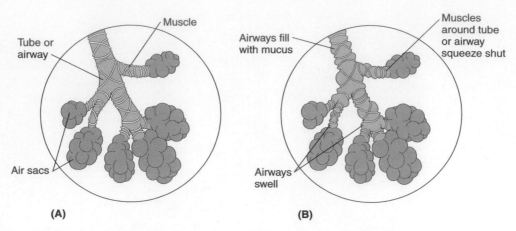

FIGURE 7.8 Changes in the airways during an asthma episode. (A) Before the episode, the muscles are relaxed and the airways are open. (B) During the episode, the muscles tighten and the airways fill with mucus.

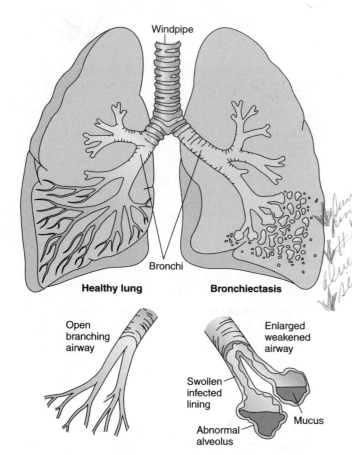

FIGURE 7.9 In bronchiectasis, the bronchi widen and lose their elasticity, thereby allowing mucus to accumulate in the alveoli.

UPPER RESPIRATORY DISEASES

- **Allergic rhinitis** (rye-**NIGH**-tis), commonly referred to as an **allergy,** is an allergic reaction to airborne allergens that causes an increased flow of mucus (**rhin** means nose and **-itis** means inflammation).

- **Croup** (**KROOP**) is an acute respiratory syndrome in children and infants characterized by obstruction of the larynx, hoarseness, and a barking cough.

- **Diphtheria** (dif-**THEE**-ree-ah) is an acute infectious disease of the throat and upper respiratory tract caused by the presence of diphtheria bacteria. Diphtheria can be prevented through immunization.

- **Epistaxis** (ep-ih-**STACK**-sis), also known as a **nosebleed,** is bleeding from the nose, usually caused by an injury, excessive use of blood thinners, or bleeding disorders.

- **Influenza** (in-flew-**EN**-zah), also known as **flu,** is an acute, highly contagious viral respiratory infection, spread by respiratory droplets, that occurs most commonly during the colder months. Some strains of influenza can be prevented by annual immunization.

- **Pertussis** (per-**TUS**-is), also known as **whooping cough,** is a contagious bacterial infection of the upper respiratory tract that is characterized by a paroxysmal cough. *Paroxysmal* (**par**-ock-**SIZ**-mal) means sudden or spasm like. Pertussis can be prevented through immunization.

- **Rhinorrhea** (rye-noh-**REE**-ah), also known as a **runny nose,** is an excessive flow of mucus from the nose (**rhin/o** means nose and **-rrhea** means abnormal flow).

- **Sinusitis** (sigh-nuh-**SIGH**-tis) is an inflammation of the sinuses (**sinus** means sinus and **-itis** means inflammation).

- **Upper respiratory infection (URI)** and **acute nasopharyngitis** (nay-zoh-**far**-in-**JIGH**-tis) are among the terms used to describe the **common cold.**

PHARYNX AND LARYNX

- **Pharyngitis** (**far**-in-**JIGH**-tis), also known as a **sore throat,** is an inflammation of the pharynx (**pharyng** means pharynx and **-itis** means inflammation).

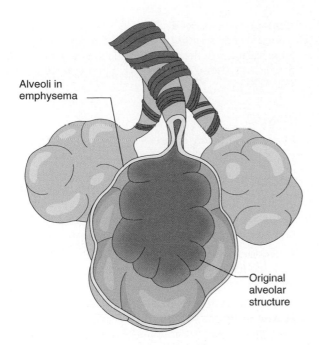

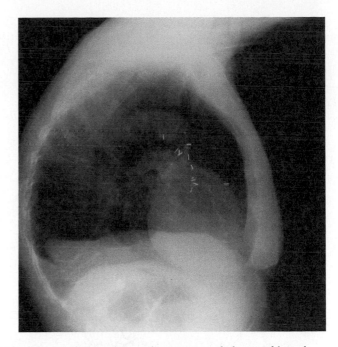

FIGURE 7.10 Emphysema. (A) Changes in the alveoli. (B) Lateral x-ray showing lung enlargement and abnormal barrel chest in emphysema.

epiglottitis — acute emergency may be

- **Pharyngorrhagia** (far-ing-goh-**RAY**-jee-ah) is bleeding from the pharynx (**pharyng/o** means pharynx and **-rrhagia** means bleeding).

- **Pharyngorrhea** (far-ing-goh-**REE**-ah) is a discharge of mucus from the pharynx (**pharyng/o** means pharynx and **-rrhea** means abnormal discharge).

- **Laryngoplegia** (lar-ing-goh-**PLEE**-jee-ah) is paralysis of the larynx (**laryng/o** means larynx and **-plegia** means paralysis).

- A **laryngospasm** (lah-**RING**-goh-spazm) is a sudden spasmodic closure of the larynx (**laryng/o** means larynx and **-spasm** means a sudden involuntary contraction).

Voice Disorders

- **Aphonia** (ah-**FOH**-nee-ah) is the loss of the ability to produce normal speech sounds (**a-** means without, **phon** means voice or sound, and **-ia** means abnormal condition).

- **Dysphonia** (dis-**FOH**-nee-ah) is any voice impairment including hoarseness, weakness, or loss of voice (**dys-** means bad, **phon** means voice or sound, and **-ia** means abnormal condition).

- **Laryngitis** (lar-in-**JIGH**-tis) is an inflammation of the larynx (**laryng** means larynx and **-itis** means inflammation). This term is commonly used to describe voice loss caused by the inflammation.

TRACHEA AND BRONCHI

- **Tracheitis** (tray-kee-**EYE**-tis) is an inflammation of the trachea (**trache** means trachea and **-itis** means inflammation).

- **Tracheorrhagia** (tray-kee-oh-**RAY**-jee-ah) is bleeding from the trachea (**trache/o** means trachea and **-rrhagia** means bleeding).

- **Bronchitis** (brong-**KYE**-tis) is an inflammation of the bronchial walls (**bronch** means bronchus and **-itis** means inflammation). Bronchitis is usually caused by an infection. However, it also may be caused by irritants such as smoking.

- **Bronchorrhagia** (brong-koh-**RAY**-jee-ah) is bleeding from the bronchi (**bronch/o** means bronchus and **-rrhagia** means bleeding).

- **Bronchorrhea** (brong-koh-**REE**-ah) means an excessive discharge of mucus from the bronchi (**bronch/o** means bronchus and **-rrhea** means abnormal flow).

PLEURAL CAVITY

- **Pleurisy** (**PLOOR**-ih-see) is an inflammation of the visceral and parietal pleura in the thoracic cavity.

- **Pleuralgia** (ploor-**AL**-jee-ah) is pain in the pleura or in the side (**pleur** means pleura and **-algia** means pain).

- **Pneumothorax** (new-moh-**THOR**-racks) is an accumulation of air or gas in the pleural space causing the lung to collapse (**pneum/o** means lung or air, and **-thorax** means chest). This may have an external cause such as a stab wound that perforates the chest wall. It also may be caused internally by a perforation in the pleura surrounding the lung that allowed air to leak into the pleural space (Figure 7.11).

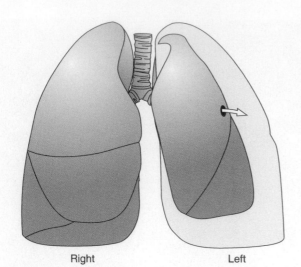

FIGURE 7.11 Pneumothorax is an accumulation of air or gas in the pleural space that causes the lung to collapse. In the left lung, a perforation in the pleura allowed air to escape into the pleural space.

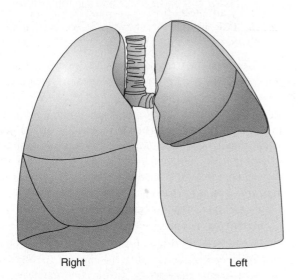

FIGURE 7.12 In pleural effusion, fluid in the pleural cavity prevents the lung from fully expanding.

- **Pleural effusion** (eh-**FEW**-zhun) is the abnormal escape of fluid into the pleural cavity that prevents the lung from fully expanding. (*Effusion* is the escape of fluid from blood or lymphatic vessels into the tissues or a cavity.) (Figure 7.12).

- **Empyema** (**em**-pye-**EE**-mah), also known as **pyothorax** (**pye**-oh-**THOH**-racks), is an accumulation of pus in the pleural cavity. This is usually the result of a primary infection of the lungs. (Empyema is also used to describe pus in other body cavities.)

- **Hemothorax** (**hee**-moh-**THOH**-racks) is an accumulation of blood in the pleural cavity (**hem/o** means blood and **-thorax** means chest).

- **Hemoptysis** (hee-**MOP**-tih-sis) is spitting of blood or blood-stained sputum derived from the lungs or bronchial tubes as the result of a pulmonary or bronchial hemorrhage (**hem/o** means blood and **-ptysis** means spitting).

LUNGS

- **Acute respiratory distress syndrome (ARDS)** is a type of lung failure resulting from many different disorders that cause pulmonary edema. There are many causes of ARDS including severe infection, shock, pneumonia, burns, and injuries.

- **Pulmonary edema** (eh-**DEE**-mah) is an accumulation of fluid in lung tissues. (*Edema* means swelling.)

- **Pneumorrhagia** (**new**-moh-**RAY**-jee-ah) is bleeding from the lungs (**pneum/o** means lungs and **-rrhagia** means bleeding).

- **Atelectasis** (at-ee-**LEK**-tah-sis), also known as a **collapsed lung,** is a condition in which the lung fails to expand because air cannot pass beyond the bronchioles that are blocked by secretions (**atel** means incomplete and **-ectasis** means stretching) (Figure 7.13).

Tuberculosis

- **Tuberculosis** (too-**ber**-kew-**LOH**-sis) **(TB)** is an infectious disease caused by *Mycobacterium tuberculosis.* TB usually attacks the lungs. However, it may also affect other parts of the body. A healthy individual may carry TB but not get the disease. TB most commonly occurs when the immune system is weakened by another condition such as infection with human immunodeficiency virus (HIV).

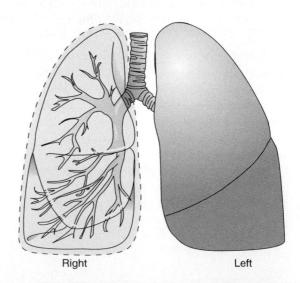

FIGURE 7.13 In atelectasis, as shown here in the right lung, the lung cannot expand because blockage in the bronchioles does not allow air to pass into the lung.

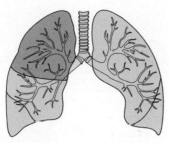
(A) Lobar pneumonia

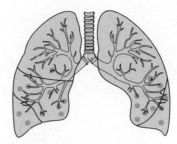
(B) Bronchopneumonia

▉ Affected areas

FIGURE 7.14 Types of pneumonia. (A) Lobar pneumonia affects one or more lobes of a lung. (B) Bronchopneumonia affects the bronchioles. The affected area of each lung is shown in darker pink.

- **Multidrug-resistant tuberculosis (MDR-TB)** is a dangerous form of tuberculosis because the germs have become resistant to the effect of most TB drugs. Resistance may occur if a TB infection has not been adequately treated. MDR-TB can be spread to others just as regular TB is.

Pneumonia

- **Pneumonia** (new-**MOH**-nee-ah) is an inflammation of the lungs in which the air sacs fill with pus and other liquid (**pneumon** means lung or air and **-ia** means abnormal condition). This fluid is known as an **exudate** (**ECKS**-you-dayt), which means accumulated fluid in a cavity that has penetrated through vessel walls into the adjoining tissue.

- The **main causes of pneumonia** are bacteria, viruses, fungi, or inhaled substances such as chemical irritants or vomit.

- **Bacterial pneumonia**, which is commonly caused by *Streptococcus pneumoniae,* is the only form of pneumonia that can be prevented through vaccination.

- **Viral pneumonia** accounts for approximately half of all pneumonias and may be complicated by an invasion of bacteria with all of the symptoms of bacterial pneumonia.

- **Lobar pneumonia** affects one or more lobes of a lung (Figure 7.14A).

- **Bronchopneumonia** (**brong**-koh-new-**MOH**-nee-ah) is a form of pneumonia that begins in the bronchioles (Figure 7.14B).

- **Double pneumonia** involves both lungs.

- **Aspiration pneumonia** may occur when a foreign substance, such as vomit, is inhaled into the lungs. (As used here, *aspiration* (**ass**-pih-**RAY**-shun) means inhaling or drawing a foreign substance, such as food, into the upper respiratory tract. Aspiration also means withdrawal by suction of fluids or gases from a body cavity.)

- **Mycoplasma pneumonia** (**my**-koh-**PLAZ**-mah new-**MOH**-nee-ah), also known as **mycoplasmal** or **walking pneumonia,** is a milder but longer lasting form of the disease caused by the fungus *Mycoplasma pneumoniae.*

- *Pneumocystis carinii* **pneumonia** (**new**-moh-**SIS**-tis kah-**RYE**-nee-eye new-**MOH**-nee-ah) **(PCP)** is caused by an infection with the parasite *Pneumocystis carinii.* PCP is an opportunistic infection that frequently occurs when the immune system is weakened by an HIV infection.

Environmental and Occupational Lung Diseases

- **Pneumoconiosis** (**new**-moh-**koh**-nee-**OH**-sis) is an abnormal condition caused by dust in the lungs that usually develops after years of environmental or occupational contact. This causes cell death and fibrosis (hardening) of the lung tissues. These disorders are named for the causative agents:

  - **Anthracosis** (**an**-thrah-**KOH**-sis), also known as **black lung disease,** is caused by coal dust in the lungs (**anthrac** means coal dust and **-osis** means condition).

  - **Asbestosis** (**ass**-beh-**STOH**-sis) is caused by asbestos particles in the lungs and is found in workers from the shipbuilding and construction trades.

  - **Byssinosis** (**biss**-ih-**NOH**-sis), also known as **brown lung disease,** is caused by cotton, flax, or hemp dust in the lungs.

  - **Silicosis** (**sill**-ih-**KOH**-sis), also known as **grinder's disease,** is caused by silica dust or glass in the lungs.

Pulmonary Fibrosis

- **Pulmonary fibrosis** (figh-**BROH**-sis) is the formation of scar tissue that replaces the pulmonary alveolar walls. (*Fibrosis* means the abnormal formation of fibrous tissue.) This condition may be caused by autoimmune disorders, infections, dust, gases, toxins, and some drugs. This destruction of lung tissue results in decreased lung capacity and increased difficulty in breathing.

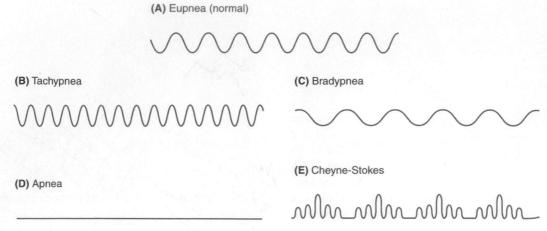

FIGURE 7.15 Respiratory patterns. (A) Eupnea, also known as normal breathing. (B) Tachypnea, also known as abnormally rapid breathing. (C) Bradypnea, also known as abnormally slow breathing. (D) Apnea, is the absence of breathing. (E) Cheyne-Stokes is an alternating series of abnormal patterns.

- **Idiopathic pulmonary fibrosis (IPF)** is a type of pulmonary fibrosis for which a cause cannot be identified. (*Idiopathic* [**id**-ee-oh-**PATH**-ick] means without known cause.)

Cystic Fibrosis

- **Cystic fibrosis** (**SIS**-tick figh-**BROH**-sis) **(CF)** is a genetic disorder in which the lungs are clogged with large quantities of abnormally thick mucus. Antibiotics are administered to control lung infections and daily physical therapy, known as **postural drainage,** is performed to remove excess mucus from the lungs.

- In CF, the digestive system is also impaired by thick gluelike mucus that interferes with digestive juices. Digestive enzymes are administered to aid the digestive system.

BREATHING DISORDERS

Eupnea (youp-**NEE**-ah) is easy or normal breathing (**eu-** means good and **-pnea** means breathing). This is the baseline for judging some breathing disorders (Figure 7.15A).

- **Tachypnea** (**tack**-ihp-**NEE**-ah) is an abnormally rapid rate of respiration usually of more than 20 breaths per minute (**tachy-** means rapid and **-pnea** means breathing). See Figure 7.15B.

- **Bradypnea** (**brad**-ihp-**NEE**-ah *or* **brad**-ee-**NEE**-ah) is an abnormally slow rate of respiration usually of less than 10 breaths per minute (**brady-** means slow and **-pnea** means breathing). See Figure 7.15C.

- **Apnea** (**AP**-nee-ah *or* ap-**NEE**-ah) is the absence of spontaneous respiration (**a-** means without and **-pnea** means breathing). See Figure 7.15D.

- **Sleep apnea syndromes (SAS)** are a group of potentially deadly disorders in which breathing repeatedly stops during sleep for long enough periods to cause a measurable decrease in blood oxygen levels.

- In **Cheyne-Stokes respiration** (**CHAYN-STOHKS**) **(CSR)** there is a pattern of alternating periods of hyperpnea (rapid breathing), hypopnea (slow breathing), and apnea (the absence of breathing). See Figure 7.15E.

- **Dyspnea** (**DISP**-nee-ah), also known as **shortness of breath,** is difficult or labored breathing (**dys-** means painful and **-pnea** means breathing).

- **Hyperpnea** (**high**-perp-**NEE**-ah) is an abnormal increase in the depth and rate of the respiratory movements (**hyper-** means excessive and **-pnea** means breathing).

- **Hypopnea** (**high**-poh-**NEE**-ah) is shallow or slow respiration (**hypo** means decreased and **pnea** means breathing).

- **Hyperventilation** (**high**-per-**ven**-tih-**LAY**-shun) is abnormally rapid deep breathing, resulting in decreased levels of carbon dioxide at the cellular level.

LACK OF OXYGEN

- In an **airway obstruction,** food or a foreign object blocks the airway and prevents air from entering or leaving the lungs. This is a life-threatening emergency requiring immediate action usually by the abdominal (Heimlich) maneuver.

- **Anoxia** (ah-**NOCK**-see-ah) is the absence or almost complete absence of oxygen from inspired gases, arterial blood, or tissues (**an-** means without, **ox** means oxygen, and **-ia** means abnormal condition). If anoxia continues for more than four to six minutes, irreversible brain damage may occur.

- **Asphyxia** (ass-**FICK**-see-ah) describes the pathologic changes caused by a lack of oxygen in air that is breathed in. This produces anoxia and hypoxia.

- **Asphyxiation** (ass-**fick**-see-**AY**-shun), also known as **suffocation,** is any interruption of breathing resulting in the loss of consciousness or death.

Asphyxiation may be caused by an airway obstruction, drowning, smothering, choking, or inhaling gases such as carbon monoxide.

● **Cyanosis** (**sigh**-ah-**NOH**-sis) is a bluish discoloration of the skin caused by a lack of adequate oxygen (**cyan** means blue and **-osis** means abnormal condition).

● **Hypoxia** (high-**POCK**-see ah) is the condition of having subnormal oxygen levels in the cells that is less severe than anoxia (**hypo-** means deficient, **ox** means oxygen, and **-ia** means abnormal condition).

● **Respiratory failure** is a condition in which the level of oxygen in the blood becomes dangerously low or the level of carbon dioxide becomes dangerously high.

SUDDEN INFANT DEATH SYNDROME

● **Sudden infant death syndrome,** also known as **SIDS** and **crib death,** is the sudden and unexplainable death of an apparently healthy infant between the ages of two weeks and one year that typically occurs while the infant is sleeping. This happens more often among babies who sleep on their stomach. For this reason, it is recommended that infants be put down to sleep on the back or side.

DIAGNOSTIC PROCEDURES OF THE RESPIRATORY SYSTEM

● **Respiratory rate (RR)** is an important diagnostic sign. The RR is counted as the number of respirations per minute. A single **respiration** (breath) consists of one inhalation and one exhalation. The normal range for adults is 15 to 20 respirations per minute.

● **Pulmonary function tests (PFTs)** are a group of tests used to measure the capacity of the lungs to hold air as well as their ability to move air in and out and to exchange oxygen and carbon dioxide.

● **Phlegm** (**FLEM**) is the thick mucus secreted by the tissues lining the respiratory passages. When phlegm is ejected through the mouth, it is called **sputum** (**SPYOU**-tum). Sputum may be used for diagnostic purposes.

● **Bronchoscopy** (brong-**KOS**-koh-pee) is the visual examination of the bronchi using a **bronchoscope** (**bronch/o** means bronchus and **-scopy** means direct visual examination). This may also be used for operative procedures such as tissue repair or the removal of a foreign object (Figure 7.16).

● **Laryngoscopy** (**lar**-ing-**GOS**-koh-pee) is the visual examination of the larynx using a **laryngoscope** (**laryng/o** means larynx and **-scopy** means a direct visual examination). This may also be used for operative procedures such as tissue repair or the removal of a foreign object.

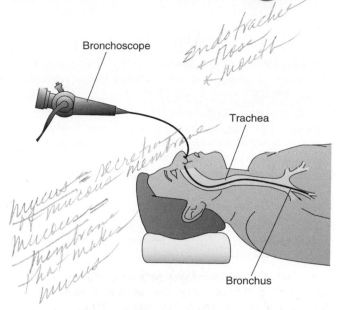

FIGURE 7.16 Bronchoscopy is the visual examination of the bronchi with the use of a bronchoscope.

● **Spirometry** (spy-**ROM**-eh-tree) is a testing method that uses a spirometer to record the volume of air inhaled or exhaled and the length of time each breath takes (**spir/o** means to breathe and **-metry** means to measure).

● **Tuberculin skin testing (TST)**, which is a screening test to detect tuberculosis, can be performed by the **Mantoux method** or the **PPD** (purified protein derivative). In performing the test, the skin of the arm is injected with a small amount of harmless tuberculin protein. A **negative result** (no response) indicates that TB is not present. A **positive result** (hardness within the testing area within two to three days) indicates the possibility of disease and should be followed by additional testing such as a chest x-ray and sputum testing.

● **Chest imaging,** also known as **chest x-rays,** is a valuable tool to show pneumonia, lung tumors, pneumothorax, pleural effusion, tuberculosis, and emphysema (see Figure 7.10B).

TREATMENT PROCEDURES OF THE RESPIRATORY SYSTEM

MEDICATIONS

● A **bronchoconstrictor** (**brong**-koh-kon-**STRICK**-tor) is an agent that narrows the opening of the passages into the lungs.

● A **bronchodilator** (**brong**-koh-dye-**LAY**-tor) is an agent that expands the opening of the passages into the lungs. At the first sign of an asthma attack, the patient uses an inhaler to self-administer a bronchodilator.

NOSE AND THROAT

- **Septoplasty** (**SEP**-toh-**plas**-tee) is the surgical reconstruction of the nasal septum (**sept/o** means septum and **-plasty** means surgical repair).

- A **sinusotomy** (**sigh**-nuhs-**OT**-oh-mee) is a surgical incision into a sinus (**sinus** means sinus and **-otomy** means surgical incision). This procedure is used in the treatment of chronic sinusitis.

- **Functional endoscopic sinus surgery (FSS)** is the surgical enlargement of the opening between the nose and sinus that is used to treat chronic sinusitis.

- **Pharyngoplasty** (fah-**RING**-goh-**plas**-tee) is the surgical repair of the pharynx (**pharyng/o** means pharynx and **-plasty** means surgical repair).

- A **pharyngostomy** (**far**-ing-**GOSS**-toh-mee) is the surgical creation of an artifical opening into the pharynx (**pharyng** means pharynx and **-ostomy** means surgically creating an opening). The resulting opening is called a *pharyngostoma* (**pharyng/o** means pharynx, and **-stoma** means artificial mouth or opening).

- A **pharyngotomy** (**far**-ing-**GOT**-oh-mee) is a surgical incision of the pharynx (**pharyng** means pharynx and **-otomy** means a surgical incision).

- A **laryngectomy** (**lar**-in-**JECK**-toh-mee) is the surgical removal of the larynx (**laryng** means larynx and **-ectomy** means surgical removal).

- **Laryngoplasty** (lah-**RING**-goh-**plas**-tee) is the surgical repair of the larynx (**laryng/o** means larynx and **-plasty** means surgical repair).

- **Endotracheal intubation** (**en**-doh-**TRAY**-kee-al **in**-too-**BAY**-shun) is the passage of a tube through the nose or mouth into the trachea to establish an airway. (*Intubation* is the insertion of a tube, usually for the passage of air or fluids.)

TRACHEA AND BRONCHI

- **Tracheoplasty** (**TRAY**-kee-oh-**plas**-tee) is the surgical repair of the trachea (**trache/o** means trachea and **-plasty** means surgical repair).

- **Tracheorrhaphy** (tray-kee-**OR**-ah-fee) means suturing of the trachea (**trache/o** means trachea and **-rrhaphy** means to suture).

- A **tracheotomy** (tray-kee-**OT**-oh-mee) is usually an emergency procedure in which an incision is made into the trachea to gain access to the airway below a blockage (**trache** means trachea and **-otomy** means surgical incision).

- A **tracheostomy** (tray-kee-**OS**-toh-mee) is creating an opening into the trachea and inserting a tube to facilitate the passage of air or the removal of secretions (**trache** means trachea and **-ostomy** means surgically creating an opening). Placement of this tube may be temporary or permanent. The resulting opening is called a stoma.

- A **stoma** (**STOH**-mah) is an opening on a body surface. A stoma can occur naturally (for example, a pore in the skin) or may be created surgically.

LUNGS, PLEURA, AND THORAX

- A **pneumonectomy** (new-moh-**NECK**-toh-mee) is the surgical removal of all or part of a lung (**pneumon** means lung and **-ectomy** means surgical removal).

- A **lobectomy** (loh-**BECK**-toh-mee) is the surgical removal of a lobe of the lung. This term also is used to describe the removal of a lobe of the liver, brain, or thyroid gland (**lob** means lobe and **-ectomy** means surgical removal).

- A **pleurectomy** (ploor-**ECK**-toh-mee) is the surgical removal of part of the pleura (**pleur** means pleura and **-ectomy** means surgical removal).

- **Thoracentesis** (**thoh**-rah-sen-**TEE**-sis) is the puncture of the chest wall with a needle to obtain fluid from the pleural cavity for diagnostic purposes, to drain pleural effusions, or to reexpand a collapsed lung (Figure 7.17). (*Notice* the spelling of this term. It is *not* a simple combination of familiar word parts.)

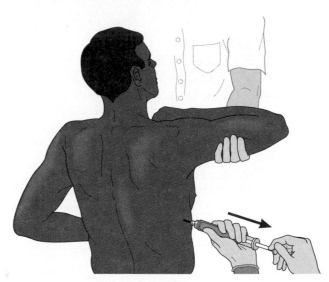

FIGURE 7.17 Fluid being removed from the pleural cavity by means of thoracentesis.

- A **thoracotomy** (**thoh**-rah-**KOT**-toh-mee) is a surgical incision into the wall of the chest (**thorac** means thorax or chest and **-otomy** means surgical incision).

- A **thoracostomy** (**thoh**-rah-**KOS**-toh-mee) is the surgical creation of an opening into the chest (**thorac** means thorax or chest and **-ostomy** means the surgical creation of an opening).

RESPIRATORY THERAPY

- **Supplemental oxygen** may be administered through a nasal canula or rebreather mask to add more oxygen to the air taken in as the patient breathes.

- **Postural drainage** is a procedure in which the patient is tilted and propped at different angles to drain secretions from the lungs.

- A **ventilator** is a mechanical device for artificial ventilation of the lungs that is used to replace or supplement the patient's natural breathing function. The goal is to wean the patient from the ventilator and to resume breathing on his own.

- A **respirator** is a machine used for prolonged artificial respiration. For example, when a spinal cord injury destroys the natural breathing mechanism, the patient can continue to breathe through the use of a respirator.

Career Opportunities

In addition to the medical specialties already discussed, some of the health occupations involving the treatment of the respiratory system include

- **Respiratory therapist (RT):** treats patients with heart or lung problems by administering oxygen, gases, or aerosol medications under a physician's orders. RTs also use exercises to improve patient breathing, perform diagnostic tests, and connect and monitor ventilators.

- **Respiratory therapy technician (RTT):** works under the supervision of an RT to administer respiratory treatment, perform basic diagnostic tests, clean and maintain equipment, and keep records.

STUDY BREAK

We do it when we're bored. We do it when we're sleepy. We sometimes do it because we see someone else do it. We may try not to, but we can't help ourselves. What is it? A yawn. (The word *yawn* doesn't sound like most other medical terms because it comes from the Anglo-Saxon word *geonian* rather than Latin or Greek.)

A yawn is an involuntary *inhalation* of breath, accompanied by an opened mouth. Why do we yawn? Scientists are not entirely sure, but it seems to be a way for the body to get a sudden surge of oxygen into the lungs and to equalize the pressure in the ear. A spasm in the throat muscles opens the mouth so that we try to take in a deep breath.

We may yawn because

- We are drowsy and not breathing deeply enough.
- The body's vital functions are depressed, for example after a *hemorrhage*.
- The pressure in the ear needs to be equalized, such as during a plane landing.
- We see someone else yawn (try this on a group of friends and see how many can resist)!

Health Occupation Profile: RESPIRATORY THERAPIST

Karen Zilles Hickel is a registered respiratory therapist (RT). She specializes in pediatrics, which means she helps children with breathing problems such as asthma and cystic fibrosis. "My job involves giving a variety of treatments including breathing medicines, oxygen, and using small machines to treat diseases of the lung. As a respiratory therapist, I also work in the intensive care unit, where I see children who have had surgery, have been in accidents, or have severe medical problems. When these patients are very sick, they often require a mechanical ventilator or respirator to breathe for them, which is run by an RT. Respiratory therapists are an important part of the hospital's resuscitation team, keeping the patient's airway open and providing oxygen during CPR. I work in a pulmonary clinic, too, where I teach patients and their families how to use devices such as inhalers or nebulizers to treat asthma and encourage them to avoid smoking to keep their lungs healthy. It is very rewarding to help a child breathe more easily!"

Review Time

Write the answers to the following questions on a separate piece of paper or in your notebook. In addition, be prepared to take part in the classroom discussion.

1. **Written assignment:** Identify the four types of **paranasal sinuses** and state the location of each.

   Discussion assignment: What is the role of the sinuses and what are the risks of infection in these cavities?

2. **Written assignment:** Use your own words to describe what occurs within the lungs and chest as **emphysema** progresses.

   Discussion assignment: How would you explain the progressive nature of emphysema to a patient and her family?

3. **Written assignment:** Using terms a physician would understand, describe the difference between **tuberculosis** and **multidrug-resistant tuberculosis.**

   Discussion assignment: Why is tuberculosis a public health threat?

4. **Written assignment:** Using terms the family could understand, describe what happens within the lungs of a child with **cystic fibrosis.**

   Discussion assignment: How is cystic fibrosis transmitted, and how it is treated?

5. **Written assignment:** Describe **endotracheal intubation.**

   Discussion assignment: State the primary difference between endotracheal intubation and bronchoscopy.

Optional Internet Activity

*The goal of this activity is to help you learn more about medical terminology while improving your Internet skills. Select **one** of these two options and follow the instructions.*

1. **Internet Search:** Search for information about **SIDS.** Write a brief (one- or two-paragraph) report on something new you learned here and include the address of the web site where you found this information.

2. **Web Site:** To learn more about **asthma,** go to this web address: **http://lungusa.org/**. Under Diseases A to Z, search under A for asthma. Write a brief (one- or two-paragraph) report on something new you learned here.

The Human Touch: Critical Thinking Exercise

The following story and questions are designed to stimulate critical thinking through class discussion or as a brief essay response. There are no right or wrong answers to these questions.

Sylvia Gaylord works as a legal aide on the twelfth floor of an 18-story glass-and-steel monument to modern architectural technology in the center of the city. On clear days, the views are spectacular. From her cubicle, Sylvia's eye catches the edge of a beautiful blue and white skyscape as she reaches for her Medihaler. This is the third attack since she returned from lunch four hours ago—her asthma is really bad today. But if she leaves work early again, her boss will write her up. Sylvia concentrates on breathing normally.

Her roommate, Kelly, is a respiratory therapist at the county hospital. Kelly says Sylvia's asthma attacks are probably triggered by the city's high level of air pollution. That can't be true. They both run in the park every morning before work, and Sylvia rarely needs to use her inhaler. The problems start when she gets to work. The wheezing and coughing were so bad today that by the time she got up the elevator and into her cubicle, she could hardly breathe.

Last night, the cable news ran a story on the unhealthy air found in some buildings. They called it "sick building syndrome" and reported that certain employees developed allergic reactions just by breathing the air. "Hmmm," she thought, "it seems like more and more people are getting sick in our office. John has had the flu twice. Sid's bronchitis turned into bronchopneumonia, and Nging complains of sinusitis. Could this building have an air-quality problem?"

Suggested Discussion Topics

1. Discuss which environmental factors might cause an asthma attack.

2. Discuss what Sylvia might do to find out if her building has an air-quality problem.

3. Use proper medical terminology to describe what happens to Sylvia's airways during an asthma attack and how medications affect the symptoms.

4. Asthmatic medications, similar to Sylvia's inhaler, are easily available in drugstores without a prescription. Discuss the pros and cons of this practice.

5. If Sylvia's inhaler does not control her attack and her condition worsens, what steps should be taken promptly? Why?

Student Workbook and Student Activity CD-ROM

1. Go to your **Student Workbook** and complete the Learning Exercises for this chapter.

2. Go to the **Student Activity CD-ROM** and have fun with the exercises and games for this chapter.

8 The Digestive System

Structures, Word Parts, and Functions of the Digestive System

MAJOR STRUCTURES	RELATED WORD ROOTS	PRIMARY FUNCTIONS
Mouth	or/o	Begins preparation of food for digestion.
Pharynx	pharyng/o	Transports food from the mouth to the esophagus.
Esophagus	esophag/o	Transports food from the pharynx to the stomach.
Stomach	gastr/o	Breaks down food and mixes it with digestive juices.
Small intestines	enter/o	Completes digestion and absorption of most nutrients.
Large intestines	col/o	Absorbs excess water and prepares solid waste for elimination.
Rectum and Anus	an/o, proct/o, rect/o	Controls the excretion of solid waste.
Liver	hepat/o	Secretes bile and enzymes to aid in the digestion of fats.
Gallbladder	cholecyst/o	Stores bile and releases it to the small intestine as needed.
Pancreas	pancreat/o	Secretes digestive juices and enzymes into small intestine as needed.

Vocabulary Related to the Digestive System

Terms marked with the ❖ symbol are pronounced on the Student Activity CD-ROM that accompanies this text.

KEY WORD PARTS

- ☐ an/o
- ☐ cec/o
- ☐ chol/e
- ☐ cholecyst/o
- ☐ col/o, colon/o
- ☐ enter/o
- ☐ esophag/o
- ☐ gastr/o
- ☐ hepat/o_
- ☐ -lithiasis
- ☐ pancreat/o
- ☐ -pepsia
- ☐ proct/o
- ☐ rect/o
- ☐ sigmoid/o

KEY MEDICAL TERMS

- ☐ achlorhydria (ah-klor-HIGH-dree-ah) ❖
- ☐ aerophagia (ay-er-oh-FAY-jee-ah)
- ☐ amebic dysentery
  (ah-MEE-bik DIS-en-ter-ee) ❖
- ☐ anastomosis (ah-nas-toh-MOH-sis) ❖
- ☐ anoplasty (AY-noh-plas-tee)
- ☐ anorexia (an-oh-RECK-see-ah) ❖
- ☐ anoscopy (ah-NOS-koh-pee) ❖
- ☐ aphthous ulcers (AF-thus UL-serz) ❖
- ☐ bilirubin (bill-ih-ROO-bin) ❖
- ☐ borborygmus (bor-boh-RIG-mus) ❖
- ☐ botulism (BOT-you-lizm) ❖
- ☐ bruxism (BRUCK-sizm) ❖
- ☐ bulimia (byou LIM ee-ah or boo-LEE-mee-ah) ❖
- ☐ cholecystalgia (koh-lee-sis-TAL-jee-ah) ❖
- ☐ cholecystectomy (koh-lee-sis-TECK-toh-mee) ❖
- ☐ cholecystitis (koh-lee-sis-TYE-tis) ❖
- ☐ choledocholithotomy
  (koh-led-oh-koh-lih-THOT-oh-mee) ❖
- ☐ cholelithiasis (koh-lee-lih-THIGH-ah-sis) ❖
- ☐ cholera (KOL-er-ah) ❖
- ☐ cirrhosis (sih-ROH-sis) ❖
- ☐ colitis (koh-LYE-tis) ❖
- ☐ colonoscopy (koh-lun-OSS-koh-pee) ❖
- ☐ colostomy (koh-LAHS-toh-mee) ❖
- ☐ diverticulectomy
  (dye-ver-tick-you-LECK-toh-mee) ❖
- ☐ diverticulitis (dye-ver-tick-you-LYE-tis) ❖
- ☐ duodenal ulcers (dew-oh-DEE-nal or
  dew-ODD-eh-nal UL-serz) ❖
- ☐ dyspepsia (dis-PEP-see-ah) ❖
- ☐ dysphagia (dis-FAY-jee-ah)
- ☐ emesis (EM-eh-sis) ❖

- ☐ emetic (eh-MET-ick) ❖
- ☐ enteritis (en-ter-EYE-tis)
- ☐ eructation (eh-ruk-TAY-shun) ❖
- ☐ esophageal reflux
  (eh-sof-ah-JEE-al REE-flucks) ❖
- ☐ esophageal varices
  (eh-sof-ah-JEE-al VAYR-ih-seez) ❖
- ☐ esophagoplasty (eh-SOF-ah-go-plas-tee)
- ☐ gastroduodenostomy
  (gas-troh-dew-oh-deh-NOS-toh-mee) ❖
- ☐ gastroenteritis (gas-troh-en-ter-EYE-tis) ❖
- ☐ gastrorrhagia (gas-troh-RAY-jee-ah) ❖
- ☐ gastrorrhea (gas-troh-REE-ah) ❖
- ☐ gastrorrhexis (gas-troh-RECK-sis) ❖
- ☐ gastrostomy (gas-TROS-toh-mee) ❖
- ☐ gingivectomy (jin-jih-VECK-toh-mee)
- ☐ gingivitis (jin-jih-VYE-tis)
- ☐ hematemesis (hee-mah-TEM-eh-sis or
  hem-ah-TEM-eh-sis) ❖
- ☐ hemoccult (HEE-moh-kult) ❖
- ☐ hemorrhoidectomy
  (hem-oh-roid-ECK-toh-mee) ❖
- ☐ hepatitis (hep-ah-TYE-tis) ❖
- ☐ hepatomegaly (hep-ah-toh-MEG-ah-lee) ❖
- ☐ hepatorrhaphy (hep-ah-TOR-ah-fee) ❖
- ☐ hepatorrhexis (hep-ah-toh-RECK-sis) ❖
- ☐ hepatotomy (hep-ah-TOT-oh-mee)
- ☐ herpes labialis (HER-peez lay-bee-AL-iss)
- ☐ hiatal hernia (high-AY-tal HER-nee-ah) ❖
- ☐ hyperemesis (high-per-EM-eh-sis) ❖
- ☐ ileectomy (ill-ee-ECK-toh-mee) ❖
- ☐ ileitis (ill-ee-EYE-tis)
- ☐ ileocecal (ill-ee-oh-SEE-kull)
- ☐ ileostomy (ill-ee-OS-toh-mee) ❖
- ☐ ileus (ILL-ee-us) ❖
- ☐ inguinal hernia (ING-gwih-nal HER-nee-ah) ❖
- ☐ intussusception (in-tus-sus-SEP-shun) ❖
- ☐ jaundice (JAWN-dis) ❖
- ☐ maxillofacial (mack-sill-oh-FAY-shul)
- ☐ melena (meh-LEE-nah or MEL-eh-nah) ❖
- ☐ nasogastric intubation
  (nay-zoh-GAS-trick in-too-BAY-shun)
- ☐ orthodontist (or-thoh-DON-tist) ❖
- ☐ periodontitis (pehr-ee-oh-don-TYE-tis) ❖
- ☐ peristalsis (pehr-ih-STAL-sis)
- ☐ pica (PYE-kah) ❖
- ☐ proctoplasty (PROCK-toh-plas-tee) ❖
- ☐ pyrosis (pye-ROH-sis) ❖
- ☐ regurgitation (ree-gur-jih-TAY-shun) ❖
- ☐ salmonella (sal-moh-NEL-ah) ❖
- ☐ sigmoidoscopy (sig-moi-DOS-koh-pee) ❖
- ☐ volvulus (VOL-view-lus) ❖

Upon completion of this chapter, you should be able to:

1. Identify and describe the major structures and functions of the digestive system.
2. Describe the processes of digestion, absorption, and metabolism.
3. Recognize, define, spell, and pronounce terms related to the pathology and diagnostic and treatment procedures of the digestive system.

FUNCTIONS OF THE DIGESTIVE SYSTEM

The digestive system is also known as the **alimentary canal** (**al**-ih-**MEN**-tar-ee) (**aliment** means to nourish and **-ary** means pertaining to). This system is responsible for

- The intake and digestion of food
- The absorption of nutrients from digested food
- The elimination of solid waste products

STRUCTURES OF THE DIGESTIVE SYSTEM

The major structures of the digestive system include the **oral cavity** (mouth), **pharynx** (throat), **esophagus, stomach, small intestine, large intestine, rectum,** and **anus.**

Accessory organs related to the digestive system include the **liver, gallbladder,** and **pancreas** (Figure 8.1).

THE GASTROINTESTINAL TRACT

The structures of the digestive system are also described as the **gastrointestinal** (**gas**-troh-in-**TESS**-tih-nal) or **GI tract** (**gastr/o** means stomach, **intestin** means intestine, and **-al** means pertaining to).

- The **upper GI tract** consists of the mouth, esophagus, and stomach.
- The **lower GI tract** is made up of the small intestine, large intestines, rectum, and anus. The intestines are sometimes referred to as the **bowels.**
- When these terms are used to describe diagnostic procedures, the small intestine is usually included with the upper GI tract.

THE ORAL CAVITY

The major structures of the oral cavity, also known as the **mouth,** are the lips, hard and soft palates, salivary glands, tongue, teeth, and the periodontium (Figure 8.2).

The Lips

The **lips,** also known as **labia** (**LAY**-bee-ah), form the opening to the oral cavity (singular, **labium**). (The labia are also part of the female genitalia.) Another word part relating to the lips of the mouth is **cheil/o.**

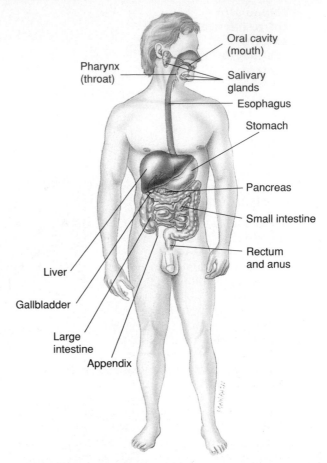

Oral cavity (mouth)
Pharynx (throat)
Salivary glands
Esophagus
Stomach
Pancreas
Small intestine
Rectum and anus
Liver
Gallbladder
Large intestine
Appendix

FIGURE 8.1 Major structures and accessory organs of the digestive system.

The Palate

The **palate** (**PAL**-at), which forms the roof of the mouth, consists of two parts: the hard and soft palates.

- The **hard palate** forms the bony anterior portion of the palate that is covered with specialized mucous membrane.
- **Rugae** (**ROO**-gay), which are irregular ridges or folds in the mucous membrane, cover the anterior portion of the hard palate. Rugae are also found in the stomach (singular, **ruga**).
- The **soft palate** forms the flexible posterior portion of the palate. It has the important role of closing off the nasal passage during swallowing so food does not move upward into the nasal cavity.

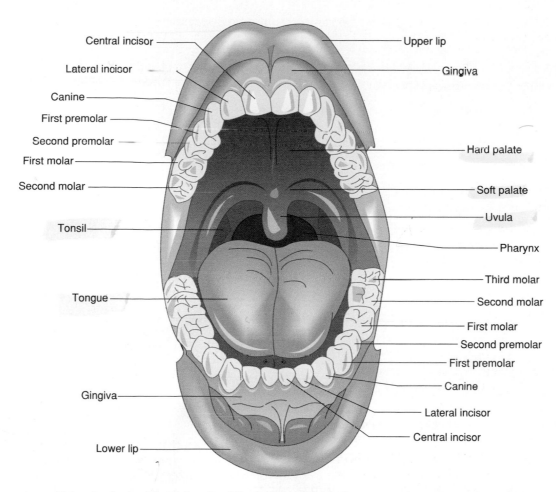

Central incisor — Upper lip

Lateral incisor — Gingiva

Canine —

First premolar —

Second premolar —

First molar — Hard palate

Second molar — Soft palate

— Uvula

Tonsil — Pharynx

— Third molar

— Second molar

Tongue — First molar

— Second premolar

— First premolar

Gingiva — Canine

— Lateral incisor

— Central incisor

Lower lip —

FIGURE 8.2 Major structures of the oral cavity. (The maxillary third molars are missing in this adult dentition.)

● The **uvula** (**YOU**-view-lah), which hangs from the free edge of the soft palate, helps in producing sounds and speech.

The Tongue

The **tongue,** which is very strong and flexible, aids in speech and moves food during chewing and swallowing.

● The upper surface of the tongue has a tough protective covering and contains the **papillae,** which are also known as the **taste buds.**

● The underside of the tongue is highly vascular and covered with delicate tissue. (*Highly vascular* means containing many blood vessels.) It is this structure that makes it possible for medications placed under the tongue to be quickly absorbed into the bloodstream.

Terms Related to the Teeth

● The term **dentition** (den-**TISH**-un) refers to the natural teeth arranged in the **maxillary** (upper) and **mandibular** (lower) arches.

● **Edentulous** (ee-**DEN**-too-lus) means without teeth. This term is used after the natural teeth have been lost.

● Human dentition includes four types of teeth: **incisors** and **canines** (also known as **cuspids**) that are used for biting and tearing; plus **premolars** (also known as **bicuspids**) and **molars** that are used for chewing and grinding.

● The **primary dentition,** also known as the **deciduous dentition** (dee-**SID**-you-us) or **baby teeth,** consists of 20 teeth (eight incisors, four canines, eight molars, and no premolars). The primary teeth are lost normally and replaced by the permanent teeth.

● The **permanent dentition** consists of 32 teeth (eight incisors, four canines, eight premolars, and twelve molars). These teeth are designed to last a lifetime.

● As used in dentistry, **occlusion** (ah-**KLOO**-zhun) is any contact between the chewing surfaces of the maxillary (upper) and mandibular (lower) teeth. **Malocclusion** (**mal**-oh-**KLOO**-zhun) is any deviation from a normal occlusion.

Structures and Tissues of the Teeth

● The **crown** of the tooth is the portion that is visible in the mouth. It is covered with **enamel,** the strongest tissue in the body (Figure 8.3).

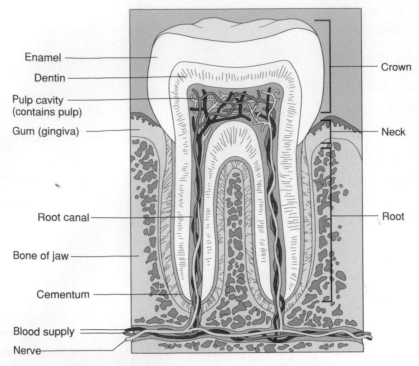

Enamel

Dentin

Pulp cavity
(contains pulp)

Gum (gingiva)

Root canal

Bone of jaw

Cementum

Blood supply

Nerve

Crown

Neck

Root

FIGURE 8.3   Structures and tissues of the tooth.

- The **root** of the tooth holds the tooth securely in place within the dental arch. The root is protected by **cementum.** The crown and root meet at the **neck** of the tooth.
- **Dentin** makes up the bulk of the tooth and is protected by the enamel and cementum.
- The **pulp chamber** is the inner area of the crown of the tooth that runs downward to form the **root canals.** The **pulp** is made up of a rich supply of blood vessels and nerves.

The Periodontium

The **periodontium** (**pehr**-ee-oh-**DON**-shee-um) consists of the bone and soft tissues that surround and support the teeth (**peri-** means surrounding, **odonti** means the teeth, and **-um** is the noun ending).

- The **gingiva** (**JIN**-jih-vah), also known as the **gums,** is the specialized mucous membrane that surrounds the teeth, covers the bone of the dental arches, and continues to form the lining of the cheeks.

The Salivary Glands

The **salivary glands** (**SAL**-ih-ver-ee) secrete **saliva** that moistens food, begins the digestive process, and cleanses the mouth (see Figure 8.1).

- There are three pairs of salivary glands: **parotid glands** (pah-**ROT**-id) located on the face in front of and slightly lower than each ear, **sublingual glands** located on the underside of the tongue, and **submandibular glands** located on the floor of the mouth.

THE PHARYNX

The **pharynx** (**FAR**-inks), also known as the **throat,** is the common passageway for both respiration and digestion (see Chapter 7).

- During swallowing, food is prevented from moving from the pharynx into the lungs by the **epiglottis** (**ep**-ih-**GLOT**-is), which closes off the entrance to the trachea (windpipe). This closing allows food to move safely into the esophagus.

THE ESOPHAGUS

The **esophagus** (eh-**SOF**-ah-gus), also known as the **gullet,** is a collapsible tube that leads from the pharynx to the stomach (see Figure 8.1).

- The **lower esophageal sphincter** (**SFINK**-ter), also known as the **cardiac sphincter,** is a ringlike muscle that controls the flow between the esophagus and the stomach. When this functions normally, stomach contents do not flow back into the esophagus.

THE STOMACH

The stomach is a saclike organ composed of the **fundus** (upper, rounded part), **body** (main portion), and **antrum** (lower part) (Figure 8.4).

- **Rugae** are the folds in the mucosa lining the stomach. Glands located within these folds produce the gastric juices that aid in digestion and mucus that forms the protective coating of the lining of the stomach.

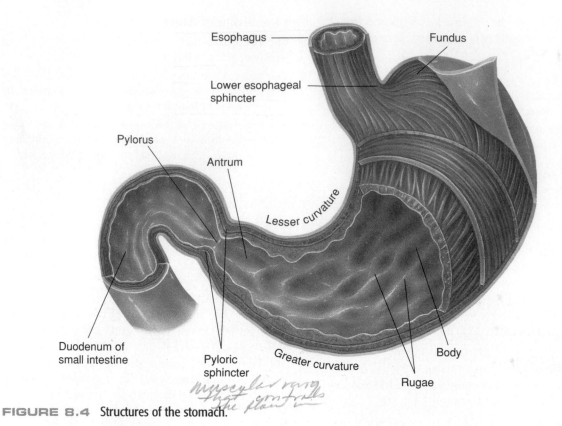

FIGURE 8.4 Structures of the stomach.

- The **pylorus** (pye-**LOR**-us) is the narrow passage connecting the stomach with the small intestine.

- The **pyloric sphincter** is the muscle ring that controls the flow from the stomach to the duodenum of the small intestine.

THE SMALL INTESTINE

The **small intestine** extends from the pyloric sphincter to the first part of the large intestine. It is here that the nutrients from food are absorbed into the bloodstream. The small intestine is a coiled organ up to 20 feet in length. However, it is known as the small intestine because it is smaller in diameter than the large intestine (see Figure 8.1).

Parts of the Small Intestine

The small intestine consists of these three parts: the duodenum, jejunum, and ileum.

- The **duodenum** (**dew**-oh-**DEE**-num *or* dew-**ODD**-eh-num), the first portion of the small intestine, extends from the pylorus to the jejunum.

- The **jejunum** (jeh-**JOO**-num), the middle portion of the small intestine, extends from the duodenum to the ileum.

- The **ileum** (**ILL**-ee-um), the last portion of the small intestine, extends from the jejunum to the cecum of the large intestine.

- The **ileocecal sphincter** (**ill**-ee-oh-**SEE**-kull) controls the flow from the ileum of the small intestine into the cecum of the large intestine.

THE LARGE INTESTINE

The large intestine extends from the end of the small intestine to the anus. The waste products of digestion are processed in the large intestine and then excreted through the anus (Figure 8.5).

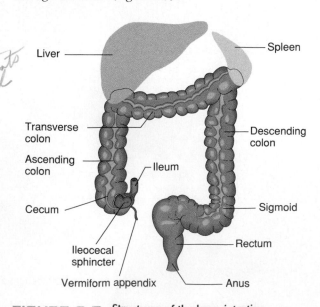

FIGURE 8.5 Structures of the large intestine.

- The major parts of the large intestine are the **cecum, colon, rectum,** and **anus.**

The Cecum

The **cecum** (**SEE**-kum) is a pouch that lies on the right side of the abdomen. It extends from the end of the ileum to the beginning of the colon.

- The **vermiform appendix,** commonly called the **appendix,** hangs from the lower portion of the cecum. (The name *vermiform* refers to its wormlike shape.) The appendix, which consists of lymphatic tissue, serves no known function in the digestive system.

The Colon

The colon is subdivided into four parts:

- The **ascending colon** travels upward from the cecum to the undersurface of the liver.
- The **transverse colon** passes horizontally from right to left toward the spleen.
- The **descending colon** travels down the left side of the abdominal cavity to the sigmoid colon.
- The **sigmoid colon** (**SIG**-moid) is an S-shaped structure that continues from the descending colon above and joins with the rectum below.

The Rectum and Anus

- The **rectum,** which is the last division of the large intestine, ends at the anus.
- The **anus** is the lower opening of the digestive tract. The flow of waste through the anus is controlled by the two **anal sphincter muscles.**
- The term **anorectal** (**ah**-noh-**RECK**-tal) refers to the anus and rectum as a single unit (**an/o** means anus, **rect** means rectum, and **-al** means pertaining to).

ACCESSORY DIGESTIVE ORGANS

The following organs are referred to as accessory organs because they play a key role in the digestive process but are not part of the gastrointestinal tract (Figure 8.6).

The Liver

The liver is located in the right upper quadrant of the abdomen and has several important functions. The term **hepatic** (heh-**PAT**-ick) means pertaining to the liver (**hepat** means liver and **ic** means pertaining to).

- The liver removes excess **glucose** (**GLOO**-kohs), also known as **blood sugar,** from the bloodstream and stores it as **glycogen** (**GLYE**-koh-jen) (a form of starch). When the blood sugar level is low, the liver converts glycogen back into glucose and releases it for use by the body.

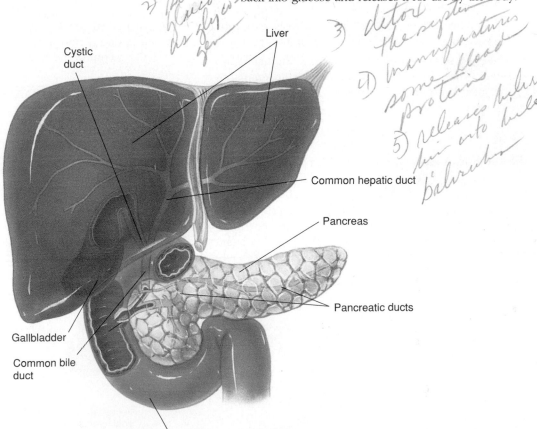

FIGURE 8.6 Accessory digestive organs: the liver, gallbladder, and pancreas.

- The liver destroys old erythrocytes (red blood cells), removes poisons from the blood, and manufactures some blood proteins.

- **Bilirubin** (bill-ih-**ROO**-bin), a pigment produced from the destruction of hemoglobin, is released by the liver in bile. Excess bilirubin in the blood is associated with jaundice.

- The liver secretes **bile,** which is a digestive juice containing enzymes that break down fat. The term *biliary* (**BILL**-ee-air-ee), as in the biliary system, means pertaining to bile.

- Bile travels down the **common hepatic duct** to the **cystic duct** that leads to the gallbladder where the bile is stored.

The Gallbladder

The **gallbladder** is a pear-shaped sac located under the liver. It stores and concentrates the bile for later use.

- The term **cholecystic** (**koh**-lee-**SIS**-tick) means pertaining to the gallbladder (**cholecyst** means gallbladder and **-ic** means pertaining to).

- When bile is needed, the gallbladder contracts, forcing the bile out through the **cystic duct** and into the **common bile duct** that carries it into the duodenum of the small intestine.

The Pancreas

The **pancreas** (**PAN**-kree-as) is a feather-shaped organ located posterior to (behind) the stomach. It has important roles in both the digestive and endocrine systems.

The endocrine functions plus the pathology and procedures related to the pancreas are discussed further in Chapter 13.

- The pancreas synthesizes and secretes **pancreatic juices.** These juices are made up of sodium bicarbonate (to help neutralize stomach acids) and digestive enzymes (to process the protein, carbohydrates, and fats in food).

- The pancreatic juices leave the pancreas through the **pancreatic ducts** that join the **common bile duct** just before the entrance to the duodenum.

DIGESTION

Digestion is the process by which complex foods are broken down into nutrients in a form the body can use. The flow of food through the digestive system is shown in Figure 8.7.

- **Enzymes** (**EN**-zimes) are responsible for the chemical changes that break foods down into simpler forms of nutrients for use by the body.

- A **nutrient** is a substance, usually from food, that is necessary for normal functioning of the body.

METABOLISM

- **Metabolism** (meh-**TAB**-oh-lizm) is the sum of anabolism and catabolism. That is, this term includes *all* of the processes involved in the body's use of these nutrients (**metabol** means change and **-ism** means condition).

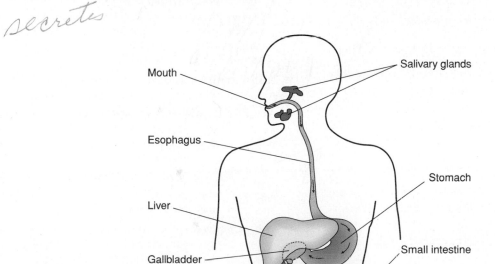

FIGURE 8.7 A schematic diagram showing the pathway of food through the digestive system.

- **Anabolism** (an-**NAB**-oh-lizm) is the building up of body cells and substances from nutrients.
- **Catabolism** (kah-**TAB**-oh-lizm), which is the opposite of anabolism, is the breaking down of body cells or substances, releasing energy and carbon dioxide.

ABSORPTION

Absorption (ab-**SORP**-shun) is the process by which completely digested nutrients are taken into the circulatory system by passing through the capillaries located in the walls of the small intestine.

- Fats and fat-soluble vitamins are absorbed into the lymphatic system through **villi** (**VILL**-eye), the tiny hairlike projections that line the walls of the small intestine (singular, **villus**).

THE ROLE OF THE MOUTH, SALIVARY GLANDS, AND ESOPHAGUS

- **Mastication** (**mass**-tih-**KAY**-shun), also known as **chewing,** breaks food down into smaller pieces and mixes it with saliva. Saliva contains an enzyme that begins the chemical breakdown to convert starches into sugar.
- During swallowing, food travels from the mouth into the pharynx and on into the **esophagus.**
- In the esophagus, food moves downward through the action of gravity and peristalsis. **Peristalsis** (**pehr**-ih-**STAL**-sis) is a series of wavelike contractions of the smooth muscles in a single direction.

THE ROLE OF THE STOMACH

- The **gastric juices** of the stomach contain **hydrochloric acid** and digestive enzymes.
- Few nutrients enter the bloodstream through the walls of the stomach. Instead, the churning action of the stomach works with the gastric juices to convert the food to chyme.
- **Chyme** (**KYM**) is the semifluid mass of partly digested food that passes from the stomach, through the pyloric sphincter, and into the small intestine.

THE ROLE OF THE SMALL INTESTINE

Food is moved through the intestines by peristaltic action and digestion is completed in the duodenum after the chyme has been mixed with bile and pancreatic juice.

- Bile breaks apart large fat globules into smaller particles so enzymes in the pancreatic juices can digest the fats. This action is called **emulsification** and must be completed before the nutrients can be absorbed into the body.

THE ROLE OF THE LARGE INTESTINE

The role of the entire large intestine is to receive the solid waste products of digestion and store them until they are eliminated from the body.

- Excess water is absorbed from the food waste through the walls of the large intestine and solid feces are formed. **Feces** (**FEE**-seez), also known as **stools,** are solid body wastes expelled through the rectum and anus.
- **Defecation** (**def**-eh-**KAY**-shun), also known as a **bowel movement,** is the evacuation or emptying of the large intestines.
- Gas is frequently produced by the normal, friendly bacteria in the colon, which helps to further break down food. The gas that is passed out of the body through the rectum is known as **flatulence** or **flatus.**
- **Borborygmus** (**bor**-boh-**RIG**-mus) is the rumbling noise caused by the movement of gas in the intestine.

MEDICAL SPECIALTIES RELATED TO THE DIGESTIVE SYSTEM

- A **dentist** holds a Doctor of Dental Surgery (DDS) or Doctor of Medical Dentistry (DMD) degree and specializes in diagnosing and treating diseases and disorders of teeth and tissues of the oral cavity.
- A **gastroenterologist** (**gas**-troh-**en**-ter-**OL**-oh-jist) specializes in diagnosing and treating diseases and disorders of the stomach and intestines (**gastr/o** means stomach, **enter** means small intestine, and **-ologist** means specialist).
- An **internist** specializes in diagnosing and treating diseases and disorders of the internal organs.
- An **orthodontist** (**or**-thoh-**DON**-tist) is a dental specialist in the prevention or correction of abnormalities in the positioning of the teeth and related facial structures.
- A **periodontist** (**pehr**-ee-oh-**DON**-tist) is a dental specialist who prevents or treats disorders of the tissues surrounding the teeth.
- A **proctologist** (prock-**TOL**-oh-jist) specializes in disorders of the colon, rectum, and anus (**proct** means anus and rectum and **-ologist** means specialist).

PATHOLOGY OF THE DIGESTIVE SYSTEM

TISSUES OF THE ORAL CAVITY

- **Aphthous ulcers** (**AF**-thus), also known as **canker sores,** are recurrent blisterlike sores that break and form lesions on the soft tissues lining the mouth.

Although the exact cause is unknown, the appearance of these sores is associated with stress, certain foods, or fever.

- **Herpes labialis** (**HER** peez **lay** bee-**AL**-iss), also known as **cold sores** or **fever blisters,** are blister-like sores caused by the herpes simplex virus that occur on the lips and adjacent tissue.

- A **cleft lip,** also known as a **harelip,** is a congenital defect resulting in a deep fissure of the lip running upward to the nose. (As used here, a **fissure** is a deep groove or opening.)

- A **cleft palate** is a congenital fissure of the palate that involves the upper lip, hard palate, and/or soft palate. If not corrected, this opening between the nose and mouth makes it difficult for the child to eat and speak.

DENTAL DISEASES

- **Bruxism** (**BRUCK**-sizm) is involuntary grinding or clenching of the teeth that usually occurs during sleep and is associated with tension or stress. Bruxism wears away tooth structure, damages periodontal tissues, and injures the temporomandibular joint.

- **Dental calculus** (**KAL**-kyou-luhs) is hardened dental plaque on the teeth that irritates the surrounding tissues. The term *calculus* also describes hard deposits, commonly known as **stones,** formed in any part of the body.

- **Dental caries** (**KAYR**-eez), also known as **tooth decay** or a **cavity,** is an infectious disease that destroys the enamel and dentin of the tooth. If the decay process is not arrested, the pulp can be exposed and become infected.

- **Dental plaque** (**PLACK**) is a soft deposit consisting of bacteria and bacterial by-products that builds up on the teeth and is a major cause of dental caries and periodontal disease. (*Plaque* also means a patch or small differentiated area on a body surface or the buildup of deposits of cholesterol in blood vessels.)

- **Periodontal disease,** also known as **periodontitis** (**pehr**-ee-oh-don-**TYE**-tis), is an inflammation of the tissues that surround and support the teeth (**peri-** means surrounding, **odont** means tooth or teeth, and **-itis** means inflammation). This progressive disease is classified according to the degree of tissue involvement.

- **Gingivitis** (**jin**-jih-**VYE**-tis), an inflammation of the gums, is the earliest stage of periodontal disease (**gingiv** means gums and **-itis** means inflammation).

- **Halitosis** (hal-ih-**TOH**-sis), also known as **bad breath,** may be caused by dental diseases or respiratory or gastric disorders (**halit** means breath and **-osis** means condition of).

- **Temporomandibular disorders** (**tem**-poh-roh-man-**DIB**-you-lar) (**TMD**), also known as **myofas-**cial pain dysfunction (MPD),** are a group of complex symptoms including pain, headache, or difficulty in chewing that are related to the functioning of the temporomandibular joint.

ESOPHAGUS

- **Dysphagia** (dis-**FAY**-jee-ah) is difficulty in swallowing (**dys-** means difficult and **-phagia** means swallowing).

- **Esophageal reflux** (eh-**sof**-ah-**JEE**-al **REE**-flucks), also known as **gastroesophageal reflux disease** or **GERD,** is the upward flow of stomach acid into the esophagus. (*Reflux* means a backward or return flow.)

- **Esophageal varices** (eh-**sof**-ah-**JEE**-al **VAYR**-ih-seez) are enlarged and swollen veins at the lower end of the esophagus. Severe bleeding occurs if one of these veins ruptures.

- A **hiatal hernia** (high-**AY**-tal **HER**-nee-ah) is a protrusion of part of the stomach through the esophageal sphincter in the diaphragm (**hiat** means opening and **-al** means pertaining to). This condition may cause esophageal reflux and pyrosis (Figure 8.8).

- **Pyrosis** (pye-**ROH**-sis), also known as **heartburn,** is the burning sensation caused by the return of acidic stomach contents into the esophagus (**pyr** means fever or fire and **-osis** means abnormal condition).

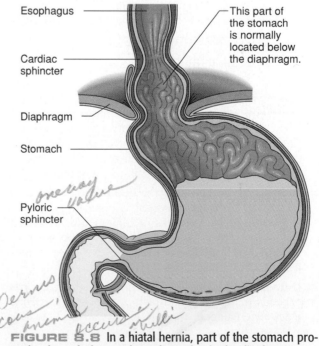

Esophagus

This part of the stomach is normally located below the diaphragm.

Cardiac sphincter

Diaphragm

Stomach

Pyloric sphincter

FIGURE 8.8 In a hiatal hernia, part of the stomach protrudes through the esophageal opening in the diaphragm.

STOMACH

- **Gastritis** (gas-**TRY**-tis) is an inflammation of the stomach (**gastr** means stomach and **-itis** means inflammation).
- **Gastroenteritis** (gas-troh-en-ter-**EYE**-tis) is an inflammation of the stomach and intestines, especially the small intestine (**gastr/o** means stomach, **enter** means small intestine, and **-itis** means inflammation).
- **Gastrorrhagia** (gas-troh-**RAY**-jee-ah) is bleeding from the stomach (**gastro** means stomach and **rrhagia** means bleeding).
- **Gastrorrhea** (gas-troh-**REE**-ah) is the excessive flow of gastric secretions (**gastr/o** is stomach and **-rrhea** means abnormal flow).
- **Gastrorrhexis** (gas-troh-**RECK**-sis) is a rupture of the stomach (**gastr/o** means stomach and **-rrhexis** means rupture).

Peptic Ulcers

A **peptic ulcer (PU)** is a lesion of the mucous membranes of the digestive system (**pept** means digestion, and **-ic** means pertaining to). These ulcers, which are frequently caused by the bacterium *Helicobacter pylori,* may occur in the lower end of the esophagus, the stomach, or in the duodenum.

- **Gastric ulcers** are peptic ulcers that occur in the stomach.
- **Duodenal ulcers** (dew-oh-**DEE**-nal *or* dew-**ODD**-eh-nal **UL**-serz) are peptic ulcers that occur in the upper part of the small intestine and are the most common form of peptic ulcer.
- A **perforating ulcer** involves erosion through the entire thickness of the organ wall.

EATING DISORDERS

- **Anorexia** (an-oh-**RECK**-see-ah) is the lack or loss of appetite for food.
- **Anorexia nervosa** is an eating disorder characterized by a refusal to maintain a minimally normal body weight and an intense fear of gaining weight. Compulsive dieting and excessive exercising often cause the patient to become emaciated. (*Emaciated* [ee-**MAY**-shee-ayt-ed] means abnormally thin.)
- **Bulimia** (byou-**LIM**-ee-ah *or* boo-**LEE**-mee-ah), also known as **bulimia nervosa**, is an eating disorder characterized by episodes of binge eating followed by inappropriate compensatory behavior such as self-induced vomiting or misuse of laxatives, diuretics, or other medications.
- **Dehydration** is a condition in which fluid loss exceeds fluid intake and disrupts the body's normal electrolyte balance.

- **Malnutrition** is a lack of proper food or nutrients in the body, either due to a shortage of food or the improper absorption or distribution of nutrients.
- **Obesity** (oh-**BEE**-sih-tee) is an excessive accumulation of fat in the body. The term *obese* is usually used to refer to individuals who are 20 percent to 30 percent over the established standards for height, age, sex, and weight.
- **Pica** (**PYE**-kah) is an eating disorder in which there is persistent eating of nonnutritional substances such as clay. These abnormal cravings are sometimes associated with pregnancy.

DIGESTION AND VOMITING

- **Achlorhydria** (ah-klor-**HIGH**-dree-ah) is the absence of hydrochloric acid from gastric secretions.
- **Aerophagia** (ay-er-oh-**FAY**-jee-ah) is the spasmodic swallowing of air followed by eructations (**aer/o** means air and **-phagia** means swallowing).
- **Eructation** (eh-ruk-**TAY**-shun) is the act of belching or raising gas orally from the stomach.
- **Dyspepsia** (dis-**PEP**-see-ah), also known as **indigestion,** is an impairment of digestion (**dys-** means painful and **-pepsia** means digestion).
- **Emesis** (**EM**-eh-sis), also known as **vomiting,** means to expel the contents of the stomach through the esophagus and out of the mouth.
- **Hematemesis** (hee-mah-**TEM**-eh-sis *or* hem-ah-**TEM**-eh-sis) is vomiting blood (**hemat** means blood and **-emesis** means vomiting).
- **Hyperemesis** (high-per-**EM**-eh-sis) means excessive vomiting (**hyper-** means excessive and **-emesis** means vomiting).
- **Nausea** (**NAW**-see-ah) is the sensation that leads to the urge to vomit.
- **Regurgitation** (ree-gur-jih-**TAY**-shun) is the return of swallowed food into the mouth.

INTESTINAL DISORDERS

- **Colorectal cancer** is a common form of cancer that often first manifests itself in polyps in the colon.
- **Diverticulitis** (dye-ver-tick-you-**LYE**-tis) is inflammation of one or more diverticulum (**diverticul** means diverticulum and **-itis** means inflammation). A **diverticulum** (dye-ver-**TICK**-you-lum) is a pouch or sac occurring in the lining or wall of a tubular organ including the intestines (plural, **diverticula**).

Inflammatory Bowel Diseases

Chronic inflammatory diseases of the gastrointestinal tract are known as **inflammatory bowel diseases (IBDs).**

- **Colitis** (koh-**LYE**-tis) is an inflammation of the colon (**col** means colon and **-itis** means inflammation).

- **Crohn's disease** is a chronic autoimmune disorder involving any part of the gastrointestinal tract but most commonly resulting in scarring and thickening of the walls of ileum, colon, or both.

- **Enteritis** (**en**-ter-**EYE**-tis) is an inflammation of the small intestines (**enter** means small intestine and **-itis** means inflammation).

- **Ileitis** (**ill**-ee-**EYE**-tis) is an inflammation of the ileum (**ile** means the ileum and **-itis** means inflammation).

- **Spastic colon,** also known as **irritable bowel syndrome (IBS),** is a disorder of the motility (ability to move spontaneously) of the entire GI tract. It is characterized by abdominal pain, nausea, gas, constipation, and/or diarrhea.

Intestinal Obstructions

- **Ileus** (**ILL**-ee-us) is a temporary stoppage of intestinal peristalsis that may be accompanied by severe pain, abdominal distention, vomiting, absence of passage of stools, fever, and dehydration. Ileus may be present for 24 to 72 hours after abdominal surgery.

- **Intestinal adhesions** (ad-**HEE**-zhunz) abnormally hold together parts of the intestine where they normally should be separate. This condition, which is caused by inflammation or trauma, can lead to intestinal obstruction.

- **Intestinal obstruction** is a complete stoppage or serious impairment to the passage of the intestinal contents. A mechanical obstruction may result from a blockage that can be due to many causes, including the presence of a tumor.

- In a **strangulating obstruction,** the blood flow to a segment of the intestine is cut off. This may lead to gangrene (tissue death) and perforation.

- **Volvulus** (**VOL**-view-lus) is twisting of the intestine (bowel) on itself that causes an obstruction (Figure 8. 9).

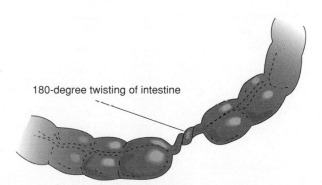

180-degree twisting of intestine

FIGURE 8.9 Volvulus is the twisting of the bowel on itself.

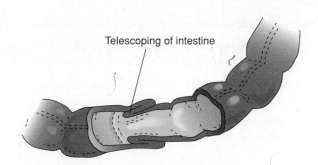

Telescoping of intestine

FIGURE 8.10 Intussusception is the telescoping of the bowel on itself.

- **Intussusception** (**in**-tus-sus-**SEP**-shun) is the telescoping of one part of the intestine into the opening of an immediately adjacent part. This is typically a condition found in infants and young children (Figure 8.10).

- An **inguinal hernia** (**ING**-gwih-nal **HER**-nee-ah) is the protrusion of a small loop of bowel through a weak place in the lower abdominal wall or groin.

Infectious Diseases of the Intestines

Infectious diseases of the intestines may be transmitted through contaminated food and water or through poor sanitation practices. The more common of these diseases are discussed in Table 8.1.

ANORECTAL DISORDERS

- **Bowel incontinence** (in-**KON**-tih-nents) is the inability to control the excretion of feces. (Urinary incontinence refers to the inability to control urination and is discussed further in Chapter 9.)

- **Constipation** is a decrease in frequency in the passage of stools, or difficulty in passing hard, dry stools.

- **Diarrhea** (**dye**-ah-**REE**-ah) is an abnormal frequency of loose or watery stools that may lead to dehydration (**dia** means through and **-rrhea** means abnormal flow).

- **Hemorrhoids** (**HEM**-oh-roids), also known as **piles,** are enlarged veins in or near the anus that may cause pain and bleeding.

- **Melena** (meh-**LEE**-nah or **MEL**-eh-nah) is the passage of black stools containing digested blood.

LIVER

- **Cirrhosis** (sih-**ROH**-sis) is a progressive degenerative disease of the liver characterized by the disturbance of the structure and function of the liver. It frequently results in jaundice and ultimately hepatic failure (Figure 8.11).

Table 8.1

INFECTIOUS DISEASES OF THE INTESTINES

Disease	Causative Agent	Symptoms
Amebic dysentery (ah-**MEE**-bik **DIS**-en-**ter**-ee)	Entamoeba histolytica amoeba	Frequent, watery stools often with blood and mucus accompanied by pain, fever, and dehydration
Botulism (**BOT**-you-lizm)	Clostridium botulinum	Food poisoning that is characterized by paralysis and is often fatal
Cholera (**KOL**-er-ah)	Vibrio cholerae	Severe diarrhea, vomiting, and dehydration that can be fatal if not treated
E. coli	Escherichia coli	Watery diarrhea that becomes bloody but is not usually accompanied by fever.
Salmonella (**sal**-moh-**NEL**-ah), nontyphoidal	Salmonella	Severe diarrhea, nausea, and vomiting accompanied by a high fever
Typhoid fever (also known as **enteric fever**)	Salmonella typhi	Headache, delirium, cough, watery diarrhea, rash, and a high fever

- **Hepatomegaly** (**hep**-ah-toh-**MEG**-ah-lee) is the enlargement of the liver (**hepat/o** means liver and **-megaly** means enlargement).
- **Hepatorrhexis** (**hep**-ah-toh-**RECK**-sis) means rupture of the liver (**hepat/o** means liver and **-rrhexis** means rupture).
- **Jaundice** (**JAWN**-dis), also known as **icterus** (**ICK**-ter-us), is a yellow discoloration of the skin and other tissues caused by greater than normal amounts of bilirubin in the blood.

Hepatitis

Hepatitis (**hep**-ah-**TYE**-tis) is an inflammation of the liver that is usually caused by a virus but may also be caused by toxic substances (**hepat** means liver and **-itis** means inflammation). The five varieties of hepatitis viruses are shown in Table 8.2.

GALLBLADDER

- **Cholecystalgia** (**koh**-lee-sis-**TAL**-jee-ah) is pain in the gallbladder (**cholecyst** means gallbladder and **-algia** means pain).
- **Cholecystitis** (**koh**-lee-sis-**TYE**-tis) is inflammation of the gallbladder (**cholecyst** means gallbladder and **-itis** means inflammation).
- A **gallstone,** also known as **biliary calculus,** is a hard deposit that forms in the gallbladder and bile ducts (plural, **calculi**). The formation of stones is discussed further in Chapter 9.
- **Cholelithiasis** (**koh**-lee-lih-**THIGH**-ah-sis) is the presence of gallstones in the gallbladder or bile ducts

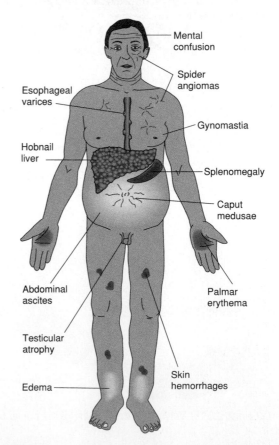

FIGURE 8.11 Clinical features of cirrhosis of the liver in the male.

Table 8.2

HEPATITIS FROM A TO E

A **Hepatitis virus A (HVA),** also known as **infectious hepatitis,** is transmitted by contaminated food and water.

B **Hepatitis virus B (HVB),** also known as **serum hepatitis,** is bloodborne and can be prevented through vaccination. (Bloodborne means transmitted through direct contact with blood or body fluids contaminated with the virus.) Blood transfusions, sexual contact, and IV drug abuse are possible sources of contact with contaminated blood.

C **Hepatitis virus C (HVC),** is bloodborne, and there is no vaccine to prevent this disease. HVC is a described as a silent epidemic because it can be present in the body for years and destroy the liver before any symptoms appear. This outcome is most likely to occur among individuals who received blood transfusions before 1992, when testing began to detect this virus.

D **Hepatitis virus D (HVD)** is bloodborne, and there is no vaccine to prevent this disease.

E **Hepatitis virus E (HVE)** is transmitted through contaminated food and water.

(**chole** means bile or gall and **-lithiasis** means presence of stones).

DIAGNOSTIC PROCEDURES OF THE DIGESTIVE SYSTEM

- **Abdominal CT,** or **CT scan,** is a radiographic procedure that produces a detailed cross section of the tissue structure within the abdomen, showing, for example, the presence of a tumor or obstruction. CT stands for **computed tomography** (**tom/o** means slice or cut and **-graphy** means the process of recording).

- An **abdominal ultrasound** is a noninvasive test used to visualize internal organs by using very high frequency sound waves.

- **Anoscopy** (ah-NOS-koh-pee) is the visual examination of the anal canal and lower rectum using a short speculum called an **anoscope** (AY-no-skope). A **speculum** (SPECK-you-lum) is an instrument used to enlarge the opening of any body cavity to facilitate inspection of its interior.

- An **upper GI series,** or **barium swallow,** and **lower GI series,** or **barium enema (BE),** are radiographic studies to examine the digestive system.

Barium is used as a contrast medium to make these structures visible.

- The term **enema** also describes a solution placed into the rectum and colon to empty the lower intestine through bowel activity. One purpose of an enema is to clear the bowels in preparation for an endoscopic examination.

- **Hemoccult** (HEE-moh-kult), also known as the **fecal occult blood test** or **FOBT,** is a laboratory test for hidden blood in the stools (**hem** means blood and **-occult** means hidden or difficult to see). A test kit may be used at home and the specimens are delivered to a laboratory or physician's office for evaluation.

- **Stool samples** are specimens of feces that are examined for content and characteristics. For example, fatty stools might indicate the presence of pancreatic problems. Cultures of the stool sample can be examined in the laboratory for the presence of bacteria or **O & P,** which are **ova** (parasite eggs) and **parasites.**

ENDOSCOPIC PROCEDURES

An **endoscope** is an instrument used for visual examination of internal structures (**endo-** means within and **-scope** means an instrument for visual examination). Endoscopes are also used for obtaining biopsy samples, controlling bleeding, removing foreign objects, as well as for other surgical and treatment procedures.

- **Colonoscopy** (koh-lun-OSS-koh-pee) is the direct visual examination of the inner surface of the colon, from the rectum to the cecum (**colon/o** means colon and **-scopy** means visual examination).

- **Gastrointestinal endoscopy** is the endoscopic examination of the interior of the esophagus, stomach, and duodenum.

- **Proctoscopy** is the endoscopic examination of the rectum and anus (**proct/o** means anus and rectum and **-scopy** is the visual examination).

- **Sigmoidoscopy** (sig-moi-DOS-koh-pee) is the use of an endoscope for the direct visual examination of the interior of the entire rectum, sigmoid colon, and possibly a portion of the descending colon.

TREATMENT PROCEDURES OF THE DIGESTIVE SYSTEM
MEDICATIONS

- **Acid blockers,** which are taken before eating, block the effects of histamine that signals the stomach to produce acid.

- An **antiemetic** (an-tih-ee-MET-ick) prevents or relieves nausea and vomiting.

- An **emetic** (eh-MET-ick) produces vomiting.

- **Laxatives** are medications or foods given to stimulate bowel movements.

- **Oral rehydration therapy (ORT)** is a treatment in which a solution of electrolytes is administered orally to counteract the dehydration that may accompany severe diarrhea.

ORAL CAVITY AND ESOPHAGUS

- **Esophagoplasty** (eh-**SOF**-ah-go-**plas**-tee) is the surgical repair of the esophagus (**esophag/o** means esophagus and **-plasty** means surgical repair).

- An **extraction,** as the term is used in dentistry, is the surgical removal of a tooth.

- A **gingivectomy** (**jin**-jih-**VECK**-toh-mee) is the surgical removal of diseased gingival tissue (**gingiv** means gingival tissue and **-ectomy** means surgical removal).

- **Maxillofacial surgery** (mack-**sill**-oh-**FAY**-shul) is specialized surgery of the face and jaws to correct deformities, treat diseases, and repair injuries.

- **Palatoplasty** (**PAL**-ah-toh-**plas**-tee) is surgical repair of a cleft palate (**palat/o** means palate and **-plasty** means surgical repair).

STOMACH

- A **gastrectomy** (gas-**TRECK**-toh-mee) is the surgical removal of all or a part of the stomach (**gastr** means stomach and **-ectomy** means surgical removal).

- A **gastrotomy** (gas-**TROT**-oh-mee) is a surgical incision into the stomach (**gastr** means stomach and **-otomy** means a surgical incision into).

- **Nasogastric intubation** (**nay**-zoh-**GAS**-trick **in**-too-**BAY**-shun) is the placement of a tube through the nose and into the stomach.

INTESTINES

- **Anoplasty** (**AY**-noh-**plas**-tee) is the surgical repair of the anus (**an/o** means anus and **-plasty** means surgical repair).

- A **colectomy** (koh-**LECK**-toh-mee) is the surgical removal of all or part of the colon (**col** means colon and **-ectomy** means surgical removal).

- A **colotomy** (koh-**LOT**-oh-mee) is a surgical incision into the colon (**col** means colon and **-otomy** means a surgical incision into).

- A **diverticulectomy** (**dye**-ver-**tick**-you-**LECK**-toh-mee) is the surgical removal of a diverticulum (**diverticul** means diverticulum and **-ectomy** means surgical removal).

- A **gastroduodenostomy** (**gas**-troh-**dew**-oh-deh-**NOS**-toh-mee) is the removal of the pylorus of the stomach and the establishment of an anastomosis between the upper portion of the stomach and the duodenum (Figure 8.12). An **anastomosis** (ah-**nas**-toh-**MOH**-sis) is a surgical connection between two hollow or tubular structures (plural, **anastomoses**).

- A **hemorrhoidectomy** (hem-oh-roid-**ECK**-toh-mee) is the surgical removal of hemorrhoids (**hemorrhoid** means piles and **-ectomy** means surgical removal).

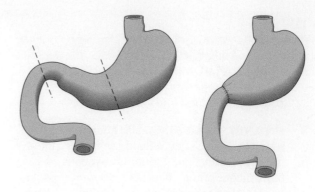

FIGURE 8.12 In a gastroduodenostomy, an anastomosis is formed where the stomach and duodenum are surgically joined.

- An **ileectomy** (ill-ee-**ECK**-toh-mee) is the surgical removal of the ileum (**ile** means the ileum, and **-ectomy** means surgical removal. Notice that this is term is spelled with a double *e.*)

Ostomies

An **ostomy** (**OSS**-toh-mee) is a surgical procedure to create an artificial opening between an organ and the body surface. This opening is called a **stoma** (**STOH**-mah). *Ostomy* can be used alone as a noun to describe a procedure or as a suffix with the word part that describes the organ involved.

- A **gastrostomy** (gas-**TROS**-toh-mee) is the surgical creation of an artificial opening into the stomach (**gastr** means stomach and **-ostomy** means surgically creating an opening). This procedure is frequently performed for the placement of a permanent feeding tube.

- An **ileostomy** (ill-ee-**OS**-toh-mee) is the surgical creation of an opening between the ileum, at the end of the small intestine, and the abdominal wall (**ile** means small intestine and **-ostomy** means surgically creating an opening).

- A **colostomy** (koh-**LAHS**-toh-mee) is the surgical creation of an opening between the colon and the body surface (**col** means colon and **-ostomy** means surgically creating an opening). The entire segment of the intestine below the ostomy is usually removed and an effluent (moved discharge) flows from the stoma. A colostomy *may* be temporary, to divert feces from an area that needs to heal. Colostomies are named for the part of the colon where the stoma, or exit point, is located (Figure 8.13).

THE RECTUM AND ANUS

- A **proctectomy** (prock-**TECK**-toh-mee) is the surgical removal of the rectum (**proct** means rectum and **-ectomy** means surgical removal).

- **Proctopexy** (**PROCK**-toh-**peck**-see) is the surgical fixation of the rectum to an adjacent tissue or organ (**proct/o** means rectum and **-pexy** means surgical fixation).

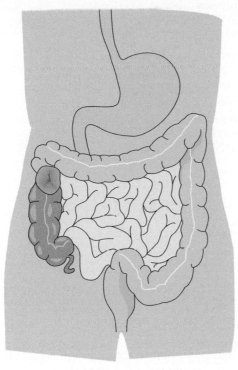

Ascending colostomy

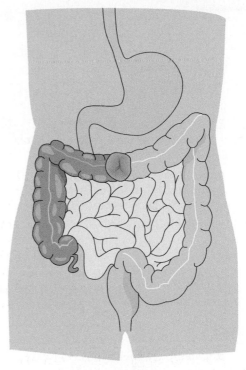

Transverse colostomy

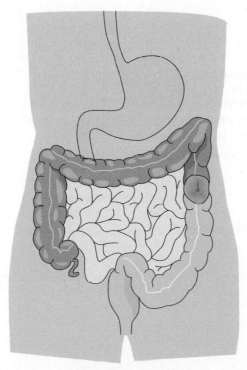

Descending colostomy

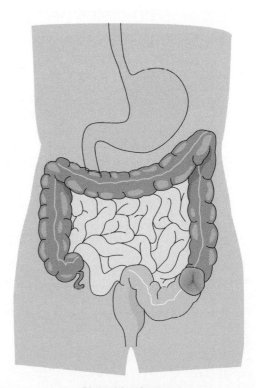

Sigmoid colostomy

FIGURE 8.13 Colostomy sites vary depending on the part of the bowel removed. The stoma, or new opening, is located at the end of the remaining intestine (shown in brown). The portion that has been removed is shown in blue.

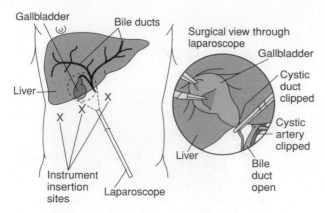

Surgical view through laparoscope

FIGURE 8.14 A lap choley is the surgical removal of the gallbladder using a laparoscope and other instruments.

- **Proctoplasty** (**PROCK**-toh-**plas**-tee) is the surgical repair of the rectum (**proct/o** means rectum and **-plasty** means surgical repair).

LIVER

- A **hepatectomy** (hep-ah-**TECK**-toh-mee) is the surgical removal of all or part of the liver (**hepat** means liver and **-ectomy** means surgical removal).

- **Hepatotomy** (hep-ah-**TOT**-oh-mee) is a surgical incision into the liver (**hepat** means liver and **-otomy** means surgical incision).

- **Hepatorrhaphy** (hep-ah-**TOR**-ah-fee) means to suture the liver (**hepat/o** means liver and **-rrhaphy** means to suture).

- A **liver transplant** is an option for a patient whose liver has failed for a reason other than liver cancer. Because liver tissue regenerates, a partial transplant, in which only part of a liver is donated, may be adequate.

GALLBLADDER

- A **choledocholithotomy** (koh-**led**-oh-koh-lih-**THOT**-oh-mee) is an incision in the common bile duct for the removal of gallstones (**choledoch/o** means the common bile duct, **lith** means stone, and **-otomy** means surgical incision).

- **Laparoscopic cholecystectomy** (koh-lee-sis-**TECK**-toh-mee), also known as a **lap choley,** is the surgical removal of the gallbladder using a laparoscope and other instruments while working through very small openings in the abdominal wall (Figure 8.14).

Career Opportunities

In addition to the medical specialties already discussed, some of the health occupations involving the treatment of the digestive system include

- **Dental hygienist:** works under the supervision of a dentist, is licensed to remove stains and deposits from the teeth, take and develop x-rays, and assist the patient in developing and maintaining good dental health

- **Dental assistant:** works under the supervision of a dentist, preparing patient for examinations, passing instruments during procedures, taking and developing x-rays (depending upon certification), sterilizing instruments, and/or performing receptionist and practice management duties

- **Dental laboratory technician:** makes and repairs dental appliances such as crowns, bridges, and orthodontic appliances, according to the specifications of dentists

- **Registered Dietitian (RD):** licensed to assess

patients' dietary needs, manage food service systems, and supervise and train personnel. Some specialties include

Pediatric dietitian
Total parenteral nutrition (TPN) needs dietitian
Renal (kidney) dietitian
Diabetic patient care dietitian
Weight management dietitian

- **Dietetic technician, registered (DTR):** works under a dietitian to plan menus, prepare food, and provide basic dietary instruction

- **Dietetic assistant** or **food service worker:** assists in menu selection, food preparation and service, and cleanup

- **Sanitarian:** performs environmental health inspections, and encourages compliance with public standards for food safety, water purity, waste disposal, and air quality

Health Occupation Profile: CERTIFIED DENTAL ASSISTANT

Debbie Robinson, 26, is a certified dental assistant (CDA). "The first time I thought about a career in dentistry was when I was 12 years old. I had such a great experience as a child going to the dentist. Everyone in the office was kind and helpful and made my visits a lot of fun. I searched out information on different professions in dentistry and found that becoming a dental assistant was a great track for me. I received my classroom and clinical training in a one-year program in which I earned a certificate of completion. I took the National Board Exam and passed, so now my title is Certified Dental Assistant. Because of my great experiences as a child, I decided to pursue a job in a pediatric dental office. This type of practice allows me to assist in treating children and individuals with special needs. Being a dental assistant provides me with the real satisfaction that I had hoped to find in my job."

STUDY BREAK

You may remember that an *eponym* is a word that derives from someone's name. Many people believe that a common slang word associated with *defecation,* or the elimination of solid waste products, comes from the name of the inventor of the toilet, Thomas Crapper.

This is only partially true. There was indeed a Thomas Crapper, an English inventor and plumber of the nineteenth century who set about to improve the water closet (WC) already in common use at the time. Ironically, although he did hold nine patents of his own, he bought the patent for a device allowing a toilet to flush more effectively from its actual inventor, Albert Giblin. But the name of Crapper's company, T. Crapper—Chelsea, was emblazoned on new, improved toilets throughout England.

When American soldiers passed through England during World War I, they picked up the habit of using *crapper* as a slang term for the WC. Thomas Crapper thus achieved a dubious place in our language through an eponym that is frowned upon, but still in use, today.

Review Time

Write the answers to the following questions on a separate piece of paper or in your notebook. In addition, be prepared to take part in the classroom discussion.

1. **Written assignment:** Using your own words, describe **peptic ulcers** and state one possible cause of this condition.

   Discussion assignment: Describe the difference between **gastric** and **duodenal ulcers.**

2. **Written assignment:** Using terms a patient would understand, describe how **hepatitis A** and **hepatitis B** are transmitted.

   Discussion assignment: Why is being immunized against hepatitis B of particular importance to healthcare workers?

3. **Written assignment:** Using terms a physician would understand, describe the differences between an **ileostomy** and a **colostomy.**

   Discussion assignment: Mr. Hernandez has a colostomy but has never mentioned it to his friends or to his employer. As a healthcare worker, what is your ethical responsibility in maintaining confidentiality concerning his condition?

4. **Written assignment:** Using terms the family would understand, describe the differences between a **cleft lip** and a **cleft palate.**

   Discussion assignment: What are some of the emotions that parents feel when their child is born with this type of defect?

5. **Written assignment:** Describe the differences between **GERD** and **pyrosis.**

   Discussion assignment: Do you think taking the well-advertised over-the-counter products should replace getting medical advice on these problems?

Optional Internet Activity

The goal of this activity is to help you learn more about medical terminology while improving your Internet skills. Select one of these two options and follow the instructions.

1. **Internet Search:** Search for the **Bad Bug Book** to learn more about foodborne diseases. Write a brief (one- or two-paragraph) report on something new you learned here and include the address of the web site where you found this information.

2. **Web Site:** To learn more about the many types of **hepatitis,** go to this web address: **http://www. hepnet.com/.** Write a brief (one- or two-paragraph) report on something new you learned about any one type of hepatitis.

The Human Touch: Critical Thinking Exercise

The following story and questions are designed to stimulate critical thinking through class discussion or as a brief essay response. There are no right or wrong answers to these questions.

"Stick the landing and our team walks away with the gold!" Coach Schaefer meant to be supportive as she squeezed Claire's shoulder. "What you mean is beat Leia's score for the Riverview team and we'll win," Claire thought sarcastically. She watched as Leia's numbers were shown from her last vault. A 6.8 out of a possible 7. "Great, just great! She chooses a less difficult vault, but with that toothpick body she gets more height than I ever will!" She wondered if Leia was naturally that thin, or did she use the secret method—you can't gain weight if the food doesn't stay in your stomach.

All season it had been that way. Everyone seemed to be watching the rivalry between West High's Claire and Riverview's "tiny-mighty" Leia. Claire was pretty sure that her 10-pound weight loss had improved both her floor routine and her tricky dismount off the beam. "I'm less than a half point behind, so coach should be happy," she thought. But just last week Coach Schaefer had a long talk with her when she got dizzy and fell off the balance beam. She asked Claire the one question she swore she'd never answer: "Just what have you been doing to lose the weight?"

Claire felt her hands sweat. "Just stick the landing," she told herself, but her body had a different agenda. Starved for fuel, her muscles failed, and the gold slipped out of reach.

Suggested Discussion Topics

1. Who do you think sets the standards for how a person thinks he or she should look?

2. List several eating disorders. What personality traits do you think cause a person to develop eating disorders?

3. Discuss why anorexia and bulimia usually occur in young women between the ages of 12 and 28.

4. Athletes sometime abuse their bodies through dieting or drugs to achieve peak performances. What should the groups that oversee competitive athletics do about this practice?

5. Imagine you have a daughter. How would you know if she had an eating disorder? What kind of treatment might help her?

Student Workbook and Student Activity CD-ROM

1. Go to your **Student Workbook** and complete the Learning Exercises for this chapter.

2. Go to the **Student Activity CD-ROM** and have fun with the exercises and games for this chapter.

CHAPTER

9

The Urinary System

Overview of Structures, Word Parts, and Functions of the Urinary System

MAJOR STRUCTURES	RELATED WORD PARTS	PRIMARY FUNCTIONS
Kidneys	nephr/o, ren/o	Filter the blood to remove waste products, maintain electrolyte concentrations, and remove excess water to maintain the fluid volume within the body.
Renal pelvis	pyel/o	Collects urine produced by the kidneys.
Urine	-uria, urin/o	Liquid waste products to be excreted.
Ureters	ureter/o	Transport urine from the kidneys to the bladder.
Urinary bladder	cyst/o, vesic/o	Stores urine until it is excreted.
Urethra	urethr/o	Transports urine from the bladder through the urethral meatus, where it is excreted from the body.

Vocabulary Related to the Urinary System

Terms marked with the ❖ symbol are pronounced on the Student Activity CD-ROM that accompanies this text.

KEY WORD PARTS

- [ ] dia-
- [ ] -cele
- [ ] cyst/o
- [ ] -ectasis
- [ ] glomerul/o
- [ ] lith/o
- [ ] -lysis
- [ ] nephr/o
- [ ] -pexy
- [ ] pyel/o
- [ ] ren/o
- [ ] -tripsy
- [ ] ureter/o
- [ ] urethr/o
- [ ] -uria

KEY MEDICAL TERMS

- [ ] anuria (ah-NEW-ree-ah) ❖
- [ ] catheterization (kath-eh-ter-eye-ZAY-shun) ❖
- [ ] cystalgia (sis-TAL-jee-ah) ❖
- [ ] cystectomy (sis-TECK-toh-mee) ❖
- [ ] cystitis (sis-TYE-tis) ❖
- [ ] cystocele (SIS-toh-seel) ❖
- [ ] cystography (sis-TOG-rah-fee) ❖
- [ ] cystolith (SIS-toh-lith) ❖
- [ ] cystopexy (sis-toh-peck-see) ❖
- [ ] cystorrhagia (sis-toh-RAY-jee-ah) ❖
- [ ] cystorrhaphy (sis-TOR-ah-fee) ❖
- [ ] cystoscopy (sis-TOS-koh-pee) ❖
- [ ] diuresis (dye-you-REE-sis) ❖
- [ ] diuretics (dye-you-RET-icks)
- [ ] dysuria (dis-YOU-ree-ah) ❖
- [ ] enuresis (en-you-REE-sis) ❖
- [ ] epispadias (ep-ih-SPAY-dee-as) ❖
- [ ] glomerulonephritis
  (gloh-mer-you-loh-neh-FRY-tis) ❖
- [ ] glomerulus (gloh-MER-you-lus)
- [ ] hemodialysis (hee-moh-dye-AL-ih-sis) ❖
- [ ] homeostasis (hoh-mee-oh-STAY-sis)
- [ ] hydronephrosis (high-droh-neh-FROH-sis) ❖
- [ ] hydroureter (high-droh-you-REE-ter)
- [ ] hypospadias (high-poh-SPAY-dee-as) ❖
- [ ] incontinence (in-KON-tih-nents)
- [ ] interstitial cystitis (in-ter-STISH-al sis-TYE-tis)
- [ ] lithotomy (lih-THOT-oh-mee)
- [ ] lithotripsy (LITH-oh-trip-see) ❖
- [ ] meatotomy (mee-ah-TOT-oh-mee) ❖

- [ ] micturition (mick-too-RISH-un)
- [ ] nephrectasis (neh-FRECK-tah-sis) ❖
- [ ] nephritis (neh-FRY-tis)
- [ ] nephrolith (NEF-roh-lith) ❖
- [ ] nephrolithiasis (nef-roh-lih-THIGH-ah-sis) ❖
- [ ] nephrolithotomy (nef-roh-lih-THOT-oh-mee) ❖
- [ ] nephrologist (neh-FROL-oh-jist)
- [ ] nephrolysis (neh-FROL-ih-sis) ❖
- [ ] nephropathy (neh-FROP-ah-thee)
- [ ] nephropexy (NEF-roh-peck-see) ❖
- [ ] nephroptosis (nef-rop-TOH-sis) ❖
- [ ] nephropyosis (nef-roh-pye-OH-sis) ❖
- [ ] nephrosis (neh-FROH-sis) ❖
- [ ] nephrostomy (neh-FROS-toh-me)
- [ ] nephrotic syndrome (neh-FROT-ick) ❖
- [ ] nocturia (nock-TOO-ree-ah) ❖
- [ ] oliguria (ol-ih-GOO-ree-ah) ❖
- [ ] paraspadias (par-ah-SPAY-dee-as) ❖
- [ ] peritoneal dialysis
  (pehr-ih-toh-NEE-al dye-AL-ih-sis) ❖
- [ ] polyuria (pol-ee-YOU-ree-ah) ❖
- [ ] pyelitis (pye-eh-LYE-tis) ❖
- [ ] pyelogram (PYE-eh-loh-gram) ❖
- [ ] pyelonephritis (pye-eh-loh-neh-FRY-tis) ❖
- [ ] pyeloplasty (PYE-eh-loh-plas-tee) ❖
- [ ] pyelotomy (pye-eh-LOT-oh-mee) ❖
- [ ] suprapubic (soo-prah-PYOU-bick)
- [ ] uremia (you-REE-mee-ah) ❖
- [ ] ureterectasis (you-ree-ter-ECK-tah-sis) ❖
- [ ] ureterectomy (you-ree-ter-ECK-toh-mee) ❖
- [ ] ureterolith (you-REE-ter-oh-lith) ❖
- [ ] ureteroplasty (you-REE-ter-oh-plas-tee) ❖
- [ ] ureterorrhagia (you-ree-ter-oh-RAY-jee-ah) ❖
- [ ] ureterorrhaphy (you-ree-ter-OR-ah-fee)
- [ ] ureterostenosis
  (you-ree-ter-oh-steh-NOH-sis) ❖
- [ ] urethralgia (you-ree-THRAL-jee-ah) ❖
- [ ] urethritis (you-reh-THRIGH-tis) ❖
- [ ] urethropexy (you-REE-throh-peck-see) ❖
- [ ] urethroplasty (you-REE-throh-plas-tee) ❖
- [ ] urethrorrhagia (you-ree-throh-RAY-jee-ah) ❖
- [ ] urethrorrhaphy (you-reh-THROR-ah-fee) ❖
- [ ] urethrorrhea (you-ree-throh-REE-ah) ❖
- [ ] urethrostenosis (you-ree-throh-steh-NOH-sis) ❖
- [ ] urethrostomy (you-reh-THROS-toh-mee) ❖
- [ ] urethrotomy (you-reh-THROT-oh-mee) ❖
- [ ] urography (you-ROG-rah-fee) ❖
- [ ] vesicovaginal fissure (ves-ih-koh-VAG-ih-nahl)

Upon completion of this chapter, you should be able to:

1. Describe the major functions of the urinary system.
2. Name and describe the structures of the urinary system.
3. Recognize, define, spell, and pronounce terms related to the pathology and diagnostic and treatment procedures of the urinary system.

FUNCTIONS OF THE URINARY SYSTEM

The urinary system performs many functions that are important in maintaining **homeostasis** (**hoh**-mee-oh-**STAY**-sis), a state of equilibrium that produces a constant internal environment throughout the body (**home/o** means sameness and **-stasis** means control). To achieve this, the urinary system

● Maintains the proper balance of water, salts, and acids in the body fluids by removing excess fluids from the body or reabsorbing water as needed.

● Constantly filters the blood to remove urea and other waste materials from the bloodstream. **Urea** (you-**REE**-ah) is the major waste product of protein metabolism.

● Converts these waste products and excess fluids into **urine** in the kidneys and excretes them from the body via the urinary bladder.

STRUCTURES OF THE URINARY SYSTEM

The urinary system consists of two kidneys, two ureters, one bladder, and a urethra (Figure 9.1). The adrenal glands, which are part of the endocrine system, are located on the top of the kidneys.

THE KIDNEYS

The kidneys constantly filter the blood to remove waste products and excess water. These are excreted as urine, which is 95 percent water and 5 percent other wastes.

● The two kidneys are located retroperitoneally with one on each side of the vertebral column below the diaphragm. *Retroperitoneally* means located behind the peritoneum, which is the membrane that lines the abdominal cavity.

● Each kidney consists of two layers that surround the **renal pelvis** (Figure 9.2A). *Renal* (**REE**-nal) means pertaining to the kidneys.

● The **renal cortex** (**KOR**-tecks) is the outer layer of the kidney. It contains over one million microscopic units called **nephrons.**

● The **medulla** (meh-**DULL**-ah) is the inner layer, and it contains most of the urine-collecting tubules. (A *tubule* is a small tube.)

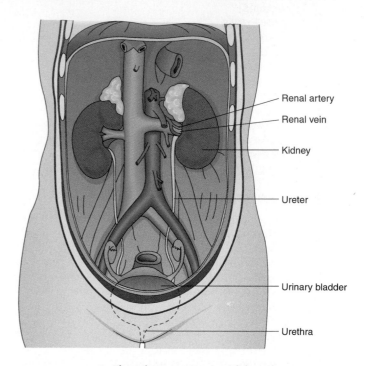

- Renal artery
- Renal vein
- Kidney
- Ureter
- Urinary bladder
- Urethra

FIGURE 9.1 The primary structures of the urinary system: the kidneys, ureters, urinary bladder, and urethra.

The Nephrons

Nephrons (**NEF**-rons) are the functional units of the kidneys. They form urine by the processes of filtration, reabsorption, and secretion (Figure 9.2B).

● Each nephron contains a **glomerulus** (gloh-**MER**-you-lus), which is a cluster of capillaries surrounded by a membrane called the Bowman's capsule (plural, **glomeruli**).

● Blood flows into the kidney through the renal artery. It is filtered in the capillaries of the glomerulus and leaves the kidney through the renal vein.

● Waste products pass through a series of urine-collecting tubules and are transported to the **renal pelvis** before entering the ureters.

● **Urochrome** (**YOU**-roh-krome) is the pigment that gives urine its normal yellow-amber or straw color (**ur/o** means urine and **-chrome** means color). The color of urine can be influenced by normal factors such as the amount of liquid consumed or by diseases and medications.

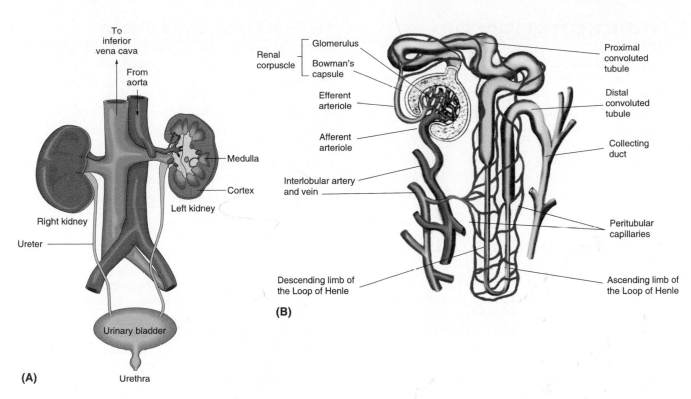

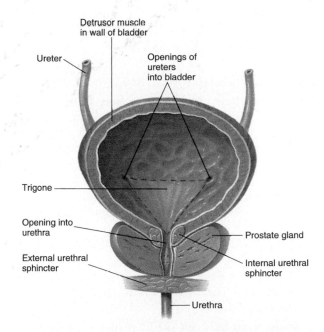

FIGURE 9.2 Structures and blood flow of the kidneys. (A) The kidneys, ureters, and bladder. (B) A nephron unit and its associated structures. The small arrows indicate the flow of blood through the nephron.

THE URETERS

The **ureters** (you-**REE**-ters) are narrow tubes, each about 10 to 12 inches long. Each ureter carries urine from a kidney to the urinary bladder.

THE URINARY BLADDER

The **urinary bladder** (Figure 9.3) is a hollow muscular organ that is a reservoir for urine. It is located in the anterior portion of the pelvic cavity behind the pubic symphysis and stores about one pint of urine. In a pregnant woman the uterus rests on the bladder and this pressure may decrease its capacity.

THE URETHRA

The **urethra** (you-**REE**-thrah) is the tube extending from the bladder to the outside of the body. (*Caution:* The spellings of *ureter* and *urethra* are very similar!)

● Two **urinary sphincters,** one located at either end of the urethra, control the flow of urine from the bladder into the urethra and out of the urethra through the urethral meatus. (A *sphincter* is a ringlike muscle that closes a passageway.)

● The **urethral meatus** (you-**REE**-thrahl mee-**AY**-tus), also known as the **urinary meatus,** is the external opening of the urethra.

● The **female urethra** is approximately 1.5 inches long. The urethral meatus is located between the clitoris and the opening of the vagina. In the female, the urethra conveys only urine (see Figure 9.3).

FIGURE 9.3 The anatomy of the urinary bladder in the male.

● The **male urethra** is approximately eight inches long, and the urethral meatus is located at the tip of the penis. In the male, the urethra conveys both urine and semen. The neck of the urethra is surrounded by the prostate gland (see Figure 9.3), which is part of the reproductive system and is discussed further in Chapter 14.

THE EXCRETION OF URINE

As the bladder fills up, pressure is placed on the base of the urethra, resulting in the urge to **urinate** or **micturate.**

- **Urination,** also known as **micturition** (**mick**-too-**RISH**-un) or **voiding,** is the normal process of excreting urine.
- Urination requires the coordinated contraction of the bladder muscles and relaxation of the sphincters. This action forces the urine through the urethra and out through the urinary meatus.

MEDICAL SPECIALTIES RELATED TO THE URINARY SYSTEM

- A **nephrologist** (neh-**FROL**-oh-jist) specializes in diagnosing and treating diseases and disorders of the kidneys (**nephr** means kidney and **-ologist** means specialist).
- A **urologist** (you-**ROL**-oh-jist) specializes in diagnosing and treating diseases and disorders of the urinary system of females and the genitourinary system of males (**ur** means urine and **-ologist** means specialist).

PATHOLOGY OF THE URINARY SYSTEM

RENAL FAILURE

Renal failure, also known as **kidney failure,** is the inability of the kidney or kidneys to perform their functions. The body cannot replace damaged nephrons. When too many nephrons have been destroyed, the result is kidney failure.

- **Anuria** (ah-**NEW**-ree-ah), also known as **anuresis** (**an**-you-**REE**-sis), is the complete suppression (stopping) of urine formation by the kidneys (**an-** means without and **-uria** means urination).
- **Uremia** (you-**REE**-mee-ah), also known as **uremic poisoning,** is a toxic condition caused by excessive amount of urea and other waste products in the bloodstream (**ur** means urine and **-emia** means blood condition).
- **Acute renal failure (ARF)** has sudden onset and is characterized by uremia. ARF may be caused by many factors, including a drop in blood volume or blood pressure due to injury or surgery.
- **Chronic renal failure (CRF)** is a progressive disease that may be caused by a variety of conditions. When kidney function is insufficient, dialysis or transplantation is required.
- **End-stage renal disease (ESRD)** refers to the late stages of chronic renal failure.

NEPHROTIC SYNDROME

Nephrotic syndrome (neh-**FROT**-ick) **(NS)** is a general group of kidney diseases (**nephr/o** means kidney and **-tic** means pertaining to). The following are characteristics of kidney malfunction diseases:

- **Edema** (excessive fluid in the body tissue)
- **Hyperproteinuria** (abnormally *high* concentrations of protein [albumin] in the urine)
- **Hypoproteinemia** (abnormally *low* concentrations of protein [albumin] in the blood)
- **Hyperlipidemia** (abnormally *large* amount of lipids in the blood)

Nephrosis

- **Nephrosis** (neh-**FROH**-sis) and **nephropathy** (neh-**FROP**-ah-thee) both mean diseases of the kidney, and these terms are used interchangeably with nephrotic syndrome (**nephr** means kidney and **-osis** means abnormal condition).
- **Diabetic nephropathy** is a result of the damage to the kidney's capillary blood vessels that is caused by long-term diabetes mellitus (**nephr/o** means kidney and **-pathy** means disease).

THE KIDNEYS

- **Glomerulonephritis** (gloh-**mer**-you-loh-neh-**FRY**-tis) is an inflammation of the kidney involving primarily the glomeruli (**glomerul/o** means glomeruli, **nephr** means kidney, and **-itis** means inflammation). In acute glomerulonephritis, the urine is dark brown or black. This condition is often related to an autoimmune problem.
- **Hydronephrosis** (**high**-droh-neh-**FROH**-sis) is the dilation (enlargement) of the renal pelvis of one or both kidneys (**hydr/o** means water, **nephr** means kidney, and **-osis** means abnormal condition). This is the result of an obstruction of the flow of urine (Figure 9.4).
- **Nephrectasis** (neh-**FRECK**-tah-sis) is the distention of a kidney (**nephr** means kidney and **-ectasis** means enlargement or stretching. *Distention* means the state of being enlarged).
- **Nephritis** (neh-**FRY**-tis) is an inflammation of the kidney (**nephr** means kidney and **-itis** means inflammation).
- **Nephroptosis** (**nef**-rop-**TOH**-sis), also known as a **floating kidney,** is the downward displacement of the kidney (**nephr/o** means kidney and **-ptosis** means or dropping down).
- **Nephropyosis** (**nef**-roh-pye-**OH**-sis) is suppuration of the kidney (**nephr/o** means kidney, **py** means pus, and **-osis** means condition). *Suppuration* means the formation or discharge of pus.
- **Pyelitis** (pye-eh-**LYE**-tis) is an inflammation of the renal pelvis (**pyel** means renal pelvis and **-itis** means inflammation).

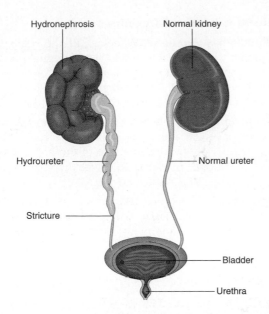

FIGURE 9.4 Hydroureter and hydronephrosis resulting from a urethral stricture.

- **Pyelonephritis** (**pye**-eh-loh-neh-**FRY**-tis) is an inflammation of the renal pelvis and of the kidney (**pyel/o** means renal pelvis, **nephr** means kidney, and **-itis** means inflammation).

- **Renal colic** (**REE**-nal **KOLL**-ick) is an acute pain in the kidney area that is caused by blockage during the passage of a kidney stone.

STONES

A **stone,** also known as **calculus** (**KAL**-kyou-luhs), is an abnormal mineral deposit (plural, **calculi**). These stones vary in size from small sandlike granules to the size of marbles and are named for the organ or tissue where they are located. See Figure 9.5 and Table 9.1.

- **Nephrolithiasis** (nef-roh-lih-**THIGH**-ah-sis) is a disorder characterized by the presence of stones in the kidney (**nephr/o** means kidney and **-lithiasis** means the presence of stones).

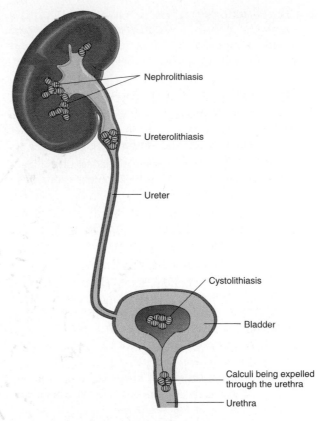

FIGURE 9.5 Calculi of the urinary system.

THE URETERS

- **Hydroureter** (**high**-droh-you-**REE**-ter) is the distention (stretching out) of the ureter with urine that cannot flow because the ureter is blocked (**hydr/o** means water and **-ureter** means ureter). See Figure 9.4.

- **Ureterectasis** (you-**ree**-ter-**ECK**-tah-sis) is the distention of a ureter (**ureter** means ureter and **-ectasis** means enlargement).

- **Ureterorrhagia** (you-**ree**-ter-oh-**RAY**-jee-ah) is the discharge of blood from the ureter (**ureter/o** means ureter and **-rrhagia** means bleeding).

Table 9.1

TYPES AND LOCATIONS OF URINARY STONES

Type of Stone	Word Parts	Location
Cystolith (**SIS**-toh-lith)	**cyst/o** means bladder and **-lith** means stone	Urinary bladder
Nephrolith (**NEF**-roh-lith), also known as **renal calculus** or a **kidney stone**	**nephr/o** means kidney and **-lith** means stone	Kidney
Ureterolith (you-**REE**-ter-oh-**lith**)	**ureter/o** means ureter and **-lith** means stone	Ureter

- **Ureterostenosis** (you-**ree**-ter-oh-steh-**NOH**-sis) is a stricture of the ureter (**ureter/o** means ureter, and **-stenosis** means abnormal narrowing). A *stricture* is an abnormal band of tissue narrowing a body passage.

THE URINARY BLADDER

- **Cystalgia** (sis-**TAL**-jee-ah) and **cystodynia** (**sis**-toh-**DIN**-ee-ah) both mean pain in the urinary bladder (**cyst** means bladder and **-algia** means pain).

- **Cystitis** (sis-**TYE**-tis) is an inflammation of the bladder (**cyst** mean bladder and **-itis** means inflammation).

- **Interstitial cystitis** (**in**-ter-**STISH**-al sis-**TYE**-tis) is an inflammation within the wall of the bladder. This is a chronic condition with symptoms similar to those of cystitis.

- A **cystocele** (**SIS**-toh-seel) is a hernia of the bladder through the vaginal wall (**cyst/o** means bladder and **-cele** means hernia).

- **Cystorrhagia** (sis-toh-**RAY**-jee-ah) is bleeding from the bladder (**cyst/o** means bladder and **-rrhagia** means bleeding).

- **Urinary tract infections (UTIs)** usually begin in the bladder. These infections occur more frequently in women because of the shortness of the urethra and the proximity of its opening to the vagina and rectum.

- A **vesicovaginal fissure** (ves-ih-koh-**VAG**-ih-nahl) is an abnormal opening between the bladder and vagina (**vesic/o** means bladder, **vagin** means vagina, and **-al** means pertaining to).

THE URETHRA

- Blockage of the urethra can cause urine to back up into the ureters. This condition, which is called **reflux,** can eventually result in damage to the kidneys.

- **Urethralgia** (you-ree-**THRAL**-jee-ah) is pain in the urethra (**urethr** means urethra and **-algia** means pain).

- **Urethritis** (you-reh-**THRIGH**-tis) is an inflammation of the urethra (**urethr** means urethra and **-itis** means inflammation).

- **Urethrorrhagia** (you-ree-throh-**RAY**-jee-ah) is bleeding from the urethra (**urethr/o** means urethra and **-rrhagia** means bleeding).

- **Urethrorrhea** (you-**ree**-throh-**REE**-ah) is an abnormal discharge from the urethra (**urethr/o** means urethra and **-rrhea** means abnormal flow).

- **Urethrostenosis** (you-**ree**-throh-steh-**NOH**-sis) is the stricture or stenosis of the urethra (**urethr/o** means urethra and **-stenosis** means tightening or narrowing).

Abnormal Urethral Openings

- **Epispadias** (ep-ih-**SPAY**-dee-as) in the male is a congenital abnormality in which the urethral opening is located on the dorsal (upper surface) of the penis (**epi-** means over). In the female with epispadias, the urethral opening is in the region of the clitoris.

- **Hypospadias** (**high**-poh-**SPAY**-dee-as) in the male is a congenital abnormality in which the urethral opening is on the undersurface of the penis (**hypo-** means below). In the female with hypospadias the urethral opening is into the vagina.

- **Paraspadias** (par-ah-**SPAY**-dee-as) is a congenital abnormality in males in which the urethral opening is on one side of the penis (**para-** means beside).

URINATION

- **Diuresis** (dye-you-**REE**-sis) is the increased excretion of urine (**diur** means increasing the output of urine and **-esis** means an abnormal condition).

- **Dysuria** (dis-**YOU**-ree-ah) is difficult or painful urination (**dys-** means painful and **-uria** means urination). This condition is frequently associated with UTIs.

- **Enuresis** (en-you-**REE**-sis) is the involuntary discharge of urine. **Nocturnal enuresis,** which occurs during sleep, is also known as **bed-wetting.** (*Nocturnal* means night.)

- **Nocturia** (nock-**TOO**-ree-ah) is excessive urination during the night (**noct** means night and **-uria** means urination).

- **Oliguria** (ol-ih-**GOO**-ree-ah) means scanty urination (**olig** means scanty and **-uria** means urination).

- **Polyuria** (pol-ee-**YOU**-ree-ah) means excessive urination (**poly-** means many and **-uria** means urination).

- **Urinary retention** is the inability to void or empty the bladder.

Incontinence

- **Incontinence** (in-**KON**-tih-nents) means the inability to control excretory functions.

- **Urinary incontinence** is the inability to control the voiding of urine.

- **Urinary stress incontinence** is the inability to control the voiding of urine under physical stress such as running, sneezing, laughing, or coughing.

- **Urge incontinence** is when urination occurs involuntarily as soon as an urgent desire to urinate is felt. This urge may be triggered by a physical movement rather than by a full bladder.

DIAGNOSTIC PROCEDURES OF THE URINARY SYSTEM

- **Catheterization** (**kath**-eh-ter-eye-**ZAY**-shun) is the insertion of a sterile catheter through the urethra and into the urinary bladder. This is most commonly performed to withdraw urine, relieve urinary retention pressures, or prevent incontinence during surgical procedures. A catheter may also be used to place fluid, such as a chemotherapy solution, into the bladder.

- **Cystoscopy** (sis-**TOS**-koh-pee), which is also known as **cysto,** is the visual examination of the urinary bladder using a cystoscope (**cyst/o** means bladder and **-scopy** means visual examination). A **cystoscope** (**SIS**-toh-**skope**) also is used for treatment procedures such as the removal of tumors (Figure 9.6).

- An **intravenous pyelogram** (**PYE**-eh-loh-**gram**) (**IVP**) is a radiographic (x-ray) study of the kidneys and ureters in which iodine is injected into a vein as a contrast medium to define these structures more clearly (**pyel/o** means renal pelvis and **-gram** means record).

- A **KUB** (kidneys, ureters, bladder) is a radiographic study of these structures without the use of a contrast medium. This study is also referred to as a **flat-plate of the abdomen.**

- **Intravenous urography** (you-**ROG**-rah-fee) is the radiographic visualization of the urinary tract with the use of a contrast medium (Figure 9.7). The resulting record is called a **urogram** (**ur/o** means urine and **-gram** means record).

- **Excretory urography** is so named because it traces the action of the kidney as it processes and excretes dye injected into the bloodstream.

- **Retrograde urography** is a radiograph of the urinary system taken after dye has been placed in the urethra through a sterile catheter and caused to flow upward (backward) through the urinary tract.

- **Cystography** (sis-**TOG**-rah-fee) is a radiographic examination of the bladder after instillation of a contrast medium via a urethral catheter. The resulting film is called a **cystogram** (**cyst/o** means bladder, and **-gram** means record).

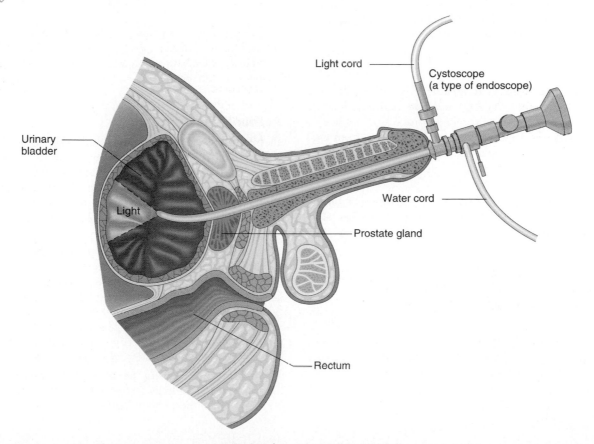

FIGURE 9.6 Use of a cystoscope to examine the interior of the bladder in a male.

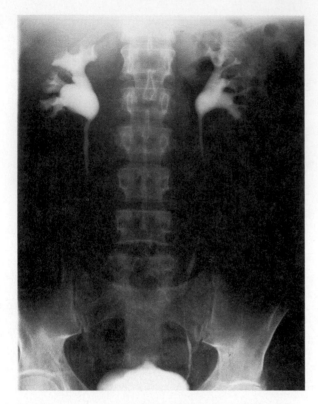

FIGURE 9.7 An intravenous urogram showing the internal structures of the kidneys and ureters.

- **Voiding cystourethrography** (**sis**-toh-you-ree-**THROG**-rah-fee) (**VCUG**) may be performed after cystography. In this diagnostic procedure, a fluoroscope is used to examine the flow of urine from the bladder and through the urethra (**cyst/o** means bladder, **urethr/o** means urethra, and **-graphy** means process of recording).

- **Urinalysis** (**you**-rih-**NAL**-ih-sis) is the examination of urine to determine the presence of abnormal elements. These tests are discussed further in Chapter 15.

TREATMENT PROCEDURES OF THE URINARY SYSTEM

MEDICATIONS

Diuretics (**dye**-you-**RET**-icks) are medications administered to increase urine secretion to rid the body of excess sodium and water.

DIALYSIS

Dialysis (dye-**AL**-ih-sis) is a procedure to remove waste products from the blood of patients whose kidneys no longer function (**dia-** means complete or through and **-lysis** means separation). The two types of dialysis in common use are hemodialysis and peritoneal dialysis.

Hemodialysis

Hemodialysis (**hee**-moh-dye-**AL**-ih-sis) (**HD**) filters waste products from the patient's blood. A shunt implanted in the patient's arm is connected to the artifical kidney machine, and arterial blood flows through the filters. The filters contain **dialysate,** a solution made up of water and electrolytes, which removes excess fluids and waste from the blood. After these are removed, the blood is returned to the body through a vein (Figure 9.8).

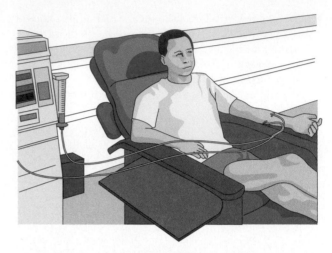

FIGURE 9.8 Hemodialysis filters waste from the patient's blood. A shunt implanted in the patient's arm allows blood to leave the body via an artery, be filtered by the dialysis machine, and returned via a vein.

Peritoneal Dialysis

In **peritoneal dialysis** (**pehr**-ih-toh-**NEE**-al dye-**AL**-ih-sis), the lining of the peritoneal cavity acts as the filter to remove waste from the blood. Dialysate solution is run into the peritoneal cavity, and the fluid is exchanged through a catheter implanted in the abdominal wall. This type of dialysis is used for renal failure and certain types of poisoning (Figure 9.9).

- **Continuous ambulatory peritoneal dialysis** (**CAPD**) provides ongoing dialysis as the patient goes about his daily activities. In this procedure, a dialysate solution is instilled from a plastic container worn under the patient's clothing. Every six to eight hours, the used solution is drained back into this bag and the bag is discarded. A new bag is then attached, the solution is instilled, and the process continues.

- **Continuous cycling peritoneal dialysis (CCPD)** uses a machine to cycle the dialysate fluid during the night while the patient sleeps.

KIDNEYS

- A **renal transplantation,** also known as a **kidney transplant,** is the grafting of a donor kidney into the body to replace the recipient's failed kidneys (see Figure 9.10 on page 170).

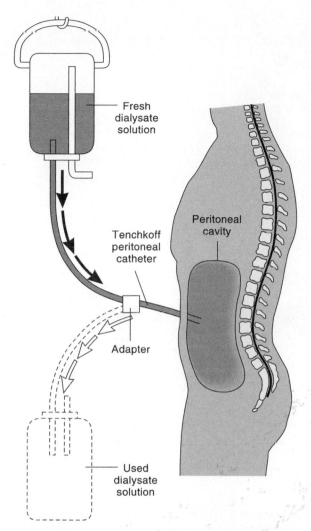

FIGURE 9.9 Peritoneal dialysis removes waste through a fluid exchange in the peritoneal cavity.

- **Nephrolysis** (neh-**FROL**-ih-sis) is the freeing of a kidney from adhesions (**nephr/o** means kidney and **-lysis** means setting free). An **adhesion** (ad-**HEE**-zhun) is a band of fibers that holds structures together abnormally.

  Note: The suffix **-lysis** means setting free; however, it also means destruction. Therefore, the term *nephrolysis* can also describe a pathologic condition in which there is the destruction of kidney substance.

- **Nephropexy** (**NEF**-roh-**peck**-see) is the surgical fixation of a floating kidney (**nephr/o** means kidney and **-pexy** means surgical fixation).

- A **nephrostomy** (neh-**FROS**-toh-mee) is the establishment of an opening between the pelvis of the kidney through its cortex to the exterior of the body (**nephr** means kidney and **-ostomy** means creating an opening).

- **Pyeloplasty** (**PYE** eh-loh-**plas**-tee) is the surgical repair of the renal pelvis (**pyel/o** means the renal pelvis and **-plasty** means surgical repair).

- A **pyelotomy** (pye-eh-**LOT**-oh-mee) is a surgical incision into the renal pelvis (**pyel** means the renal pelvis and **-otomy** means surgical incision).

Removal of Kidney Stones

- **Lithotripsy** (**LITH**-oh-**trip**-see), also known as **extracorporeal shockwave lithotripsy** or **ESWL,** is the destruction of a kidney stone with the use of ultrasonic waves traveling through water (**lith/o** means stone and **-tripsy** means to crush). *Extracorporeal* means situated or occurring outside the body.

- A **nephrolithotomy** (nef-roh-lih-**THOT**-oh-mee) is the surgical removal of a kidney stone through an incision in the kidney (**nephr/o** means kidney, **lith** means stone, and **-otomy** means surgical incision).

THE URETERS

- A **ureterectomy** (**you**-ree-ter-**ECK**-toh-mee) is the surgical removal of a ureter (**ureter** means ureter and **-ectomy** means surgical removal).

- **Ureteroplasty** (you-**REE**-ter-oh-**plas**-tee) is the surgical repair of a ureter (**ureter/o** means ureter and **-plasty** means surgical repair).

- **Ureterorrhaphy** (**you**-ree-ter-**OR**-ah-fee) is the suturing of a ureter (**ureter/o** means ureter and **-rrhaphy** means to suture).

THE URINARY BLADDER

- A **cystectomy** (sis-**TECK**-toh-mee) is the surgical removal of all or part of the urinary bladder (**cyst** means bladder and **-ectomy** means surgical removal).

- **Cystopexy** (**sis**-toh-**peck**-see) is the surgical fixation of the bladder to the abdominal wall (**cyst/o** means bladder and **-pexy** means surgical fixation).

- **Cystorrhaphy** (sis-**TOR**-ah-fee) means suturing of the bladder (**cyst/o** means bladder and **-rrhaphy** means to suture).

- A **lithotomy** (lih-**THOT**-oh-mee) is a surgical incision for the removal of a stone, usually from the bladder (**lith** means stone and **-otomy** means surgical incision). This term also is used to describe a physical examination position, as discussed further in Chapter 15.

- A **suprapubic catheter** (soo-prah-**PYOU**-bick) is an indwelling catheter placed into the bladder through a small incision made through the abdominal wall just *above* (**supra-** means above) the pubic bone. (*Indwelling* means something that remains inside the body for a prolonged time.) See Figure 9.11.

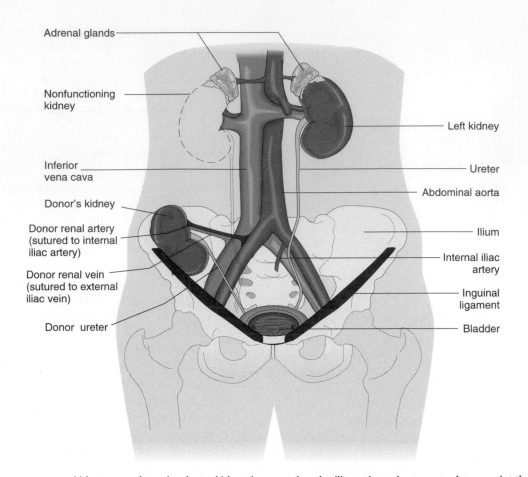

Adrenal glands

Nonfunctioning kidney

Inferior vena cava

Donor's kidney

Donor renal artery (sutured to internal iliac artery)

Donor renal vein (sutured to external iliac vein)

Donor ureter

Left kidney

Ureter

Abdominal aorta

Ilium

Internal iliac artery

Inguinal ligament

Bladder

FIGURE 9.10 In a kidney transplant, the donor kidney is sutured to the iliac vein and artery at a lower point than the nonfunctioning kidney, which is not removed.

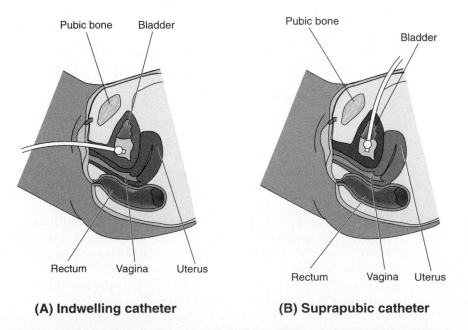

Pubic bone   Bladder

Rectum   Vagina   Uterus

(A) Indwelling catheter

Pubic bone

Bladder

Rectum   Vagina   Uterus

(B) Suprapubic catheter

FIGURE 9.11 Types of urinary catheterization. (A) An indwelling catheter. (B) A suprapubic catheter.

THE URETHRA

- A **meatotomy** (**mee**-ah-**TOT**-oh-mee) is an incision of the urinary meatus to enlarge the opening (**meat** means meatus and **-otomy** means surgical incision).

- **Urethropexy** (you-**REE**-throh-**peck**-see) is the surgical fixation of the urethra usually for the correction of urinary stress incontinence (**urethr/o** means urethra and **-pexy** means surgical fixation).

- **Urethroplasty** (you-**REE**-throh-**plas**-tee) is the surgical repair of the urethra (**urethr/o** means urethra and **-plasty** means surgical repair).

- A **urethrostomy** (**you**-reh-**THROS**-toh-mee) is the surgical creation of a permanent opening between the urethra and the skin (**urethr** means urethra and **-ostomy** means creating an opening).

- A **urethrotomy** (**you**-reh-**THROT**-oh-mee) is a surgical incision into the urethra for relief of a stricture (**urethr** means urethra and **-otomy** means surgical incision).

Career Opportunities

In addition to the medical specialties already discussed, some of the health occupations involving the treatment of the urinary system include

- **Dialysis technician:** operates the hemodialysis machine; also provides emotional support and nutritional counseling for dialysis patients

- **Urology/nephrology (or renal) licensed practical nurse** or **certified nursing assistant:** provides care and information to patients with urinary and kidney problems

STUDY BREAK

Most human infants are potty trained at around age two or three. Until that time, babies are clothed in diapers to absorb their *urinary output* and other excretions. The average baby will go through 5,000 to 6,000 diaper changes! The majority of parents today use disposable diapers, so we tend to forget that these are a somewhat recent invention.

Over the course of time, many different methods of diapering a baby have been used:

- Native Americans packed the soft insides of milkweed around their babies' bottoms before strapping them into papoose boards.

- Eskimos gathered moss during the summer and placed it inside the animal skins in which the mothers carried their babies.

- Cotton diapers, still in use today, are what our term *diaper* (meaning a diamond-patterned fabric) comes from.

Health Occupation Profile: UROLOGIST

Dr. Arthur Sonneland, MD, is a urologist specializing in diseases of the urogenital system. "About half of my work time is spent performing surgery on the prostate, bladder, or kidneys. I also do surgical repairs to help control female incontinence. The other half of my practice is consulting with patients in the office."

"My father was also a urologist, so it was probably natural for me to follow in his footsteps. Urology may not be the most popular field for medical students looking for a possible career. But I've found it to be a fascinating surgical specialty, with a wide variety of diseases to treat and yet a 'sane' lifestyle (most of the time), with very little nighttime emergency duty."

Review Time

Write the answers to the following questions on a separate piece of paper or in your notebook. In addition, be prepared to take part in the classroom discussion.

1. **Written assignment:** Using terms a physician would understand, describe the difference between **hemodialysis** and **peritoneal dialysis.**

   Discussion assignment: How would being on dialysis affect the quality of life of the patient?

2. **Written assignment:** Using terms a patient would understand, describe the difference between a **nephrolithotomy** and **ESWL** for the removal of a kidney stone.

   Discussion assignment: Mr. Morrison has a kidney stone and is in a lot of pain. Which type of treatment do you think Mr. Morrison would prefer for the removal of this stone?

3. **Written assignment:** Describe the difference between **epispadias** and **hypospadias** in the male.

   Discussion assignment: How do these two conditions affect the female?

4. **Written assignment:** Describe the difference between **acute renal failure** and **chronic renal failure.**

   Discussion assignment: What are some of the causes of these two conditions?

5. **Written assignment:** Describe the difference between a **cystocele** and a **vesicovaginal fissure.**

   Discussion assignment: What are some of the possible complications that might result from either of these conditions if it has not been repaired?

Optional Internet Activity

*The goal of this activity is to help you learn more about medical terminology while improving your Internet skills. Select **one** of these two options and follow the instructions.*

1. **Internet Search:** Search for information about a **kidney transplant.** Write a brief (one- or two-paragraph) report on something new you learned here and include the address of the web site where you found this information.

2. **Web Site:** To learn more about **bladder diseases,** go to this web address: **http://www.bladderdiseases.com/.** Write a brief (one- or two-paragraph) report on something new you learned here.

The Human Touch: Critical Thinking Exercise

The following story and questions are designed to stimulate critical thinking through class discussion or as a brief essay response. There are no right or wrong answers to these questions.

"Guess what—my baby sister is getting married, and she wants me to give her away!" Cody Gantry let out a whoop as he read the e-mail out loud to his wife. He could imagine his sister's smiling face as she sat at her computer on the other side of the Atlantic. Cody and Billie Jean were only two years apart, and she had followed in her big brother's footsteps and joined the Army when she graduated from high school. Stationed in Germany, she worked on sensitive computerized targeting systems. Now he knew why she so often mentioned a fellow officer named Jon Vorheese.

Cody's mind drifted back to his own military career in South Korea. It had been cut short when a nephrolith led to hydronephrosis. Severe nephropyosis developed, and the Army doctors were forced to perform a nephrectomy. He had received a medical discharge and been sent stateside just three days shy of his twenty-fifth birthday.

Back at home, Cody married his high school sweetheart and went to work in the local garage. Now, Cody was almost 30 and needed dialysis weekly as the result of kidney failure. He was on a waiting list for a kidney transplant, but there was a chronic shortage of donor organs.

Cody certainly felt well enough to make a short trip to Germany for Billie Jean's wedding. But what if a donor kidney finally became available right before he was scheduled to leave or while he was away? Would his urologist approve of his leaving the country while on dialysis? He was certain there were hospitals in Berlin with dialysis facilities, but he'd heard that in some countries, a shortage of dialysis equipment meant that the procedure was available only to residents. He'd do almost anything for the chance to walk his sister down the aisle on her big day.

Suggested Discussion Topics

1. Explain the two types of dialysis procedures in terms that your mother or father would understand.
2. Discuss what could happen to Cody if he skipped one or more of his dialysis treatments.
3. Dialysis is not as common in many countries as it is in the United States. Discuss the possible reasons.
4. Cody is a veteran with a medical discharge. Is his health care covered as a veteran's benefit or by a private insurance company? Would a private insurance company pay for his treatment while overseas?
5. Cody needs a kidney transplant. Discuss your views on ethical ways in which recipients should be selected. What could be done to improve the supply of donor organs?

Student Workbook and Student Activity CD-ROM

1. Go to your **Student Workbook** and complete the Learning Exercises for this chapter.
2. Go to the **Student Activity CD-ROM** and have fun with the exercises and games for this chapter.

10 The Nervous System

Overview of Structures, Word Parts, and Functions of the Nervous System

MAJOR STRUCTURES	RELATED WORD PARTS	PRIMARY FUNCTIONS
Brain	encephal/o	Coordinates all activities of the body and receives and transmits messages throughout the body.
Spinal cord	myel/o	Transmits nerve impulses between the brain, limbs, and lower part of the body.
Nerves	neur/i, neur/o	Receive and transmit messages to and from all parts of the body.
Sensory Organs: 　Ears (hearing) 　Eyes (sight) 　Nose (smell) 　Skin (touch) 　Tongue (taste)		Receive external stimulation and transmit it to the sensory neurons. The eyes and ears are discussed further in Chapter 11.

Vocabulary Related to the Nervous System

Terms marked with the ❖ symbol are pronounced on the Student Activity CD-ROM that accompanies this text.

KEY WORD PARTS

- [ ] ambul/o
- [ ] cephal/o
- [ ] concuss/o
- [ ] contus/o
- [ ] ech/o
- [ ] encephal/o
- [ ] -esthesia
- [ ] klept/o
- [ ] mening/o
- [ ] myel/o
- [ ] narc/o
- [ ] neur/i, neur/o
- [ ] -phobia
- [ ] psych/o
- [ ] somn/o

KEY MEDICAL TERMS

- [ ] **acrophobia** (ack-roh-**FOH**-bee-ah) ❖
- [ ] **Alzheimer's disease** (**ALTZ**-high-merz) ❖
- [ ] **amnesia** (am-**NEE**-zee-ah) ❖
- [ ] **amobarbital** (am-oh-**BAR**-bih-tal) ❖
- [ ] **amyotrophic lateral sclerosis** (ah-my-oh-**TROH**-fick) ❖
- [ ] **analgesic** (an-al-**JEE**-zick) ❖
- [ ] **anesthesia** (an-es-**THEE**-zee-ah) ❖
- [ ] **anesthesiologist** (an-es-thee-zee-**OL**-oh-jist) ❖
- [ ] **anesthetic** (an-es-**THET**-ick) ❖
- [ ] **anesthetist** (ah-**NES**-thch-tist) ❖
- [ ] **anxiety state**
- [ ] **aphasia** (ah-**FAY**-zee-ah)
- [ ] **autistic** (aw-**TISS**-tick)
- [ ] **barbiturate** (bar-**BIT**-you-rayt)
- [ ] **Bell's palsy**
- [ ] **catatonic** (kat-ah-**TON**-ick)
- [ ] **cerebral** (**SER**-eh-bral *or* seh-**REE**-bral) ❖
- [ ] **cerebral palsy** (**SER**-eh-bral *or* seh-**REE**-bral **PAWL**-zee) ❖
- [ ] **cerebrovascular accident** (ser-eh-broh-**VAS**-kyou-lar) ❖
- [ ] **claustrophobia** (klaws-troh-**FOH**-bee-ah) ❖
- [ ] **cognition** (kog-**NISH**-un) ❖
- [ ] **comatose** (**KOH**-mah-tohs)
- [ ] **concussion** (kon-**KUSH**-un) ❖
- [ ] **contusion** (kon-**TOO**-zhun) ❖
- [ ] **cranial hematoma** (hee-mah-**TOH**-mah) ❖
- [ ] **craniocele** (**KRAY**-nee-oh-seel) ❖
- [ ] **delirium** (dee-**LIR**-ee-um) ❖
- [ ] **delirium tremens** (dee-**LIR**-ee-um **TREE**-mens)
- [ ] **delusion** (dee-**LOO**-zhun) ❖
- [ ] **dementia** (dee-**MEN**-shee-ah) ❖

- [ ] **dyslexia** (dis-**LECK**-see-ah) ❖
- [ ] **echoencephalography** (eck-oh-en-**sef**-ah-**LOG**-rah-fee) ❖
- [ ] **electroconvulsive therapy** (ee-leck-troh-kon-**VUL**-siv) ❖
- [ ] **electroencephalography** (ee-leck-troh-en-**sef**-ah-**LOG**-rah-fee) ❖
- [ ] **empathy** (**EM**-pah-thee) ❖
- [ ] **encephalitis** (en-sef-ah-**LYE**-tis) ❖
- [ ] **encephalography** (en-sef-ah-**LOG**-rah-fee) ❖
- [ ] **epidural anesthesia** (ep-ih-**DOO**-ral an-es-**THEE**-zee-ah) ❖
- [ ] **grand mal epilepsy** (**GRAN MAHL EP**-ih-**lep**-see) ❖
- [ ] **Guillain-Barré syndrome** (gee-**YAHN**-bah-**RAY**) ❖
- [ ] **hallucination** (hah-**loo**-sih-**NAY**-shun) ❖
- [ ] **hemorrhagic** (hem-oh-**RAJ**-ick) ❖
- [ ] **hydrocephalus** (high-droh-**SEF**-ah-lus) ❖
- [ ] **hyperesthesia** (**high**-per-es-**THEE**-zee-ah)
- [ ] **hypochondriasis** (**high**-poh-kon-**DRY**-ah-sis) ❖
- [ ] **kleptomania** (klep-toh-**MAY**-nee-ah) ❖
- [ ] **malingering** (mah-**LING**-ger-ing)
- [ ] **meningitis** (men-in-**JIGH**-tis) ❖
- [ ] **meningocele** (meh-**NING**-goh-**seel**) ❖
- [ ] **migraine headache** (**MY**-grayn) ❖
- [ ] **multiple sclerosis** (skleh-**ROH**-sis) ❖
- [ ] **Munchausen syndrome** (**MUHN**-chow-zen) ❖
- [ ] **myelitis** (my-eh-**LYE**-tis) ❖
- [ ] **myelography** (my-eh-**LOG**-rah-fee) ❖
- [ ] **myelosis** (my-eh-**LOH**-sis) ❖
- [ ] **narcissistic** (nahr-sih-**SIS**-tick) ❖
- [ ] **narcolepsy** (**NAR**-koh-lep-see) ❖
- [ ] **neurologist** (new-**ROL**-oh-jist) ❖
- [ ] **paresthesia** (par-es-**THEE**-zee-ah) ❖
- [ ] **Parkinson's disease**
- [ ] **peripheral neuropathy** (new-**ROP**-ah-thee) ❖
- [ ] **petit mal epilepsy** (peh-**TEE MAHL EP**-ih-**lep**-see) ❖
- [ ] **poliomyelitis** (poh-lee-oh-**my**-eh-**LYE**-tis) ❖
- [ ] **posttraumatic stress disorder**
- [ ] **psychiatrist** (sigh-**KYE**-ah-trist) ❖
- [ ] **psychologist** (sigh-**KOL**-oh-jist) ❖
- [ ] **pyromania** (pye-roh-**MAY**-nee-ah) ❖
- [ ] **schizophrenia** (skit-soh-**FREE**-nee-ah) ❖
- [ ] **sciatica** (sigh-**AT**-ih-kah) ❖
- [ ] **seizure** (**SEE**-zhur)
- [ ] **syncope** (**SIN**-koh-pee) ❖
- [ ] **tetanus** (**TET**-ah-nus)
- [ ] **thalamotomy** (thal-ah-**MOT**-oh-mee) ❖
- [ ] **tic douloureux** (**TICK** doo-loo-**ROO**) ❖
- [ ] **transient ischemic attack** (iss-**KEE**-mick) ❖

Upon completion of this chapter, you should be able to:

1. Describe the functions and structures of the nervous system.
2. Identify the major divisions of the nervous system and describe the structures of each by location and function.
3. Identify the medical specialists who treat disorders of the nervous system.
4. Recognize, define, spell, and pronounce terms related to the pathology and diagnostic and treatment procedures of the nervous system.
5. Recognize, define, spell, and pronounce terms related to the pathology and diagnostic and treatment procedures of mental health disorders.

FUNCTIONS OF THE NERVOUS SYSTEM

The nervous system, with the brain as its center, coordinates and controls all bodily activities. When the brain ceases functioning, the body dies.

STRUCTURES OF THE NERVOUS SYSTEM

The major structures of the nervous system are the brain, spinal cord, nerves, and sensory organs. For descriptive purposes, the nervous system is divided into three parts: the central, peripheral, and autonomic nervous systems (Figure 10.1).

- The **central nervous system (CNS)** includes the brain and spinal cord.
- The **peripheral nervous system (PNS)** includes the 12 pairs of cranial nerves extending from the brain and the 31 pairs of spinal nerves extending from the spinal cord.
- The **autonomic nervous system (ANS)** includes the peripheral nerves and ganglia on either side of the spinal cord. (*Note:* Some textbooks include the ANS as a division of the peripheral nervous system. Both ways are correct.)

THE NERVES

A **nerve** is one or more bundles of neuron cells (impulse carrying fibers) that connect the brain and the spinal cord with other parts of the body.

- A **tract** is a bundle or group of nerve fibers located within the brain or spinal cord. **Ascending tracts** carry nerve impulses *toward* the brain. **Descending tracts** carry nerve impulses *away from* the brain.
- A **ganglion** (**GANG**-glee-on) is a knotlike mass or group of nerve cell bodies located outside the central nervous system (plural, **ganglia** or **ganglions**).

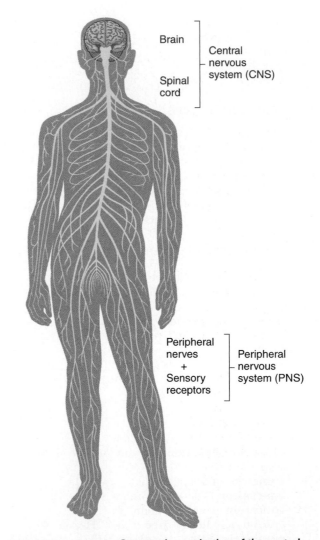

FIGURE 10.1 Structural organization of the central and peripheral nervous systems.

- A **plexus** (**PLECK**-sus) is a network of intersecting nerves and blood or lymphatic vessels (see Figure 10.10).

- **Innervation** (**in**-err-**VAY**-shun) is the supply of nerves to a body part. It also means the stimulation of a body part through the action of nerves.
- **Receptors** are sites in the sensory organs (eyes, ears, skin, nose, and taste buds) that receive external stimulation. The receptors send the stimulus through the sensory neurons to the brain for interpretation. Eyes and ears are discussed further in Chapter 11.
- A **stimulus** is anything that excites or activates a nerve and causes an impulse (plural, **stimuli**).
- An **impulse** is a wave of excitation transmitted through nerve fibers and neurons.

THE REFLEXES

A **reflex** (**REE**-flecks) is an automatic, involuntary response to some change, either inside or outside the body. Deep tendon reflexes are discussed in Chapter 4.

- Maintenance of the heart rate, breathing rate, and blood pressure are reflex actions.
- Coughing, sneezing, and reactions to painful stimuli are also reflex actions.

THE NEURONS

A **neuron** (**NEW**-ron) is the basic cell of the nervous system. The three types of neurons are described according to their function. These are summarized in Table 10.1.

- The mnemonic **ACE** can help you remember the types of neurons and their roles: **A**fferent (sending), **C**onnecting (associative), **E**fferent (motor). (A *mnemonic* is a device intended to aid memory.)

Table 10.1

TYPES OF NEURONS

Afferent neurons (**AF**-er-ent)
Also known as **sensory neurons,** they emerge from the skin or sense organs and carry impulses toward the brain and spinal cord.

Connecting neurons   Also known as **associative neurons,** they carry impulses from one neuron to another.

Efferent neurons (**EF**-er-ent)
Also known as **motor neurons,** they carry impulses away from the brain and spinal cord and toward the muscles and glands.

Neuron Parts

- Each neuron consists of a cell body, several dendrites, a single axon, and terminal end fibers (Figure 10.2).

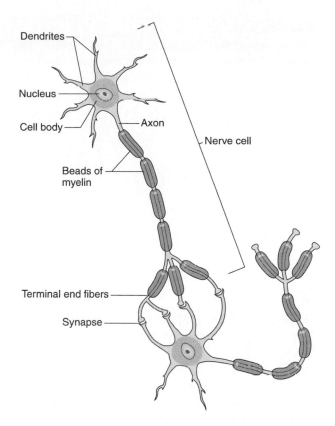

FIGURE 10.2 The structures of a neuron.

- The **dendrites** (**DEN**-drytes) are rootlike structures that receive impulses and conduct them to the cell body.
- The **axon** (**ACK**-son) extends away from the cell body and conducts impulses away from the nerve cell. Some axons, but not all, are protected by a white fatty tissue covering called **myelin** (**MY**-eh-lin).
- **Terminal end fibers** are the branching fibers of the neuron that lead the nervous impulse away from the axon and toward the synapse.

SYNAPSES

A **synapse** (**SIN**-apps) is the space between two neurons or between a neuron and a receptor organ.

NEUROTRANSMITTERS

A **neurotransmitter** (**new**-roh-trans-**MIT**-er) is a chemical messenger that transmits messages between nerve cells by making it possible for the nerve impulse to jump across the synapse from one neuron to another.

- At least 30 neurotransmitters have been identified. Each neurotransmitter is located within a specific group of neurons and has specific functions. Examples are shown in Table 10.2.

Table 10.2

EXAMPLES OF NEUROTRANSMITTERS AND THEIR FUNCTIONS	
Acetylcholine (**ass**-eh-til-**KOH**-leen)	Released at some synapses in the spinal cord and at neuromuscular junctions; influences muscle action.
Dopamine (**DOH**-pah-meen)	Released within the brain; is thought to cause some forms of psychosis and abnormal movement disorders such as Parkinson's disease.
Endorphins (en-**DOR**-fins)	Released within the spinal cord in the pain condition pathway; inhibit the conduction of pain impulses and act as natural pain relievers.
Serotonin (**sehr**-oh-**TOH**-nin or **seer**-oh-**TOH**-nin)	Released in the brain; has roles in sleep and pleasure recognition.

NEUROGLIA

The **neuroglia** (new-**ROG**-lee-ah), also known as **glial cells,** are the supportive and connective cells of the nervous system. *Glial* means pertaining to glue, and neuroglia is sometimes referred to as *nerve glue.*

MYELIN SHEATH

A **myelin sheath** is the white protective covering over some nerve cells including parts of the spinal cord, white matter of the brain, and most peripheral nerves (Figure 10.3).

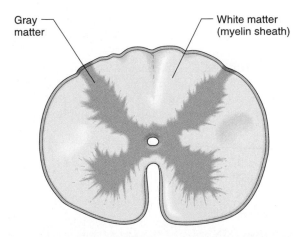

Gray matter

White matter (myelin sheath)

FIGURE 10.3 A cross section of the spinal cord showing the white matter (myelin sheath) that protects the gray matter (nerve tissue).

- **White matter.** The myelin sheath gives nerve fibers a white color, and the myelinated axons of nerves are referred to as *white matter.* The term **myelinated** (**MY**-eh-lih-**nayt**-ed) means having a myelin sheath.
- **Gray matter.** Those portions of nerves that *do not* have a myelin sheath are gray and make up the *gray matter* of the brain and spinal cord.

THE CENTRAL NERVOUS SYSTEM

The **central nervous system (CNS)** is made up of the brain and spinal cord. These structures are protected externally by the bones of the cranium and spinal column (see Chapter 3). Within these bony structures, the brain and spinal cord are protected by the meninges and cerebrospinal fluid.

The brain parts are shown in Figure 10.4. The body functions controlled by these brain parts are summarized in Table 10.3. Notice that the functions vital to life support are located in the most protected portion of the brain.

THE MENINGES

The **meninges** (meh-**NIN**-jeez) are three layers of connective tissue membrane that enclose the brain and spinal cord (singular, **meninx**). These are the dura mater, arachnoid membrane, and pia mater (Figure 10.5).

The Dura Mater

The **dura mater** (**DOO**-rah **MAY**-ter) is the thick, tough, outermost membrane of the meninges.

- The **epidural space** (**ep**-ih-**DOO**-ral) is located *above* the dura mater and within the surrounding bone walls (**epi-** means above and **-dural** means pertaining to dura mater). It contains fat and supportive connective tissues to cushion the dura mater.
- The **subdural space** (sub-**DOO**-ral) is located *below* the dura membrane and above the arachnoid membrane (**sub-** means below and **-dural** means pertaining to dura mater).

The Arachnoid Membrane

The **arachnoid membrane** (ah-**RACK**-noid), which resembles a spider web, is the second layer surrounding the brain and spinal cord.

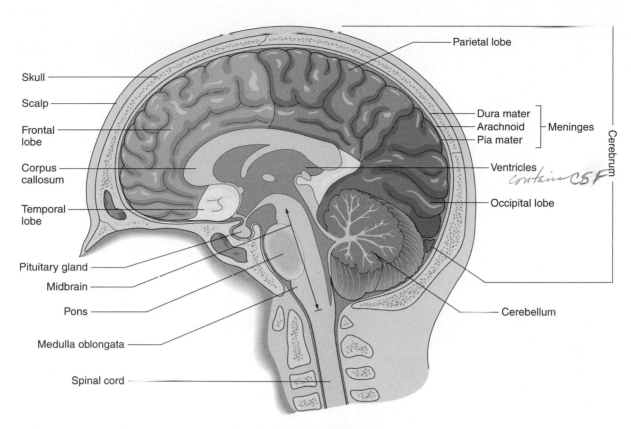

FIGURE 10.4 A cross section showing the major parts of the brain.

Table 10. 3

BRAIN PARTS AND WHAT THEY CONTROL	
Brain Part	**Controls**
Cerebrum—uppermost and least protected layer of the brain	Is responsible for the highest level of thought including judgment, memory, association, and critical thinking.
Thalamus—located below the cerebrum	Monitors sensory stimuli by suppressing some and magnifying others.
Hypothalamus—located below the thalamus.	Controls vital bodily functions (see Table 10.4).
Cerebellum—located in the lower back of the cranium below the cerebrum	Coordinates muscular activity for smooth and steady movements.
Pons—located in the brainstem at the base of the brain	Nerves cross over so that one side of the brain controls the opposite side of the body.
Medulla oblongata—most protected part of the brain	Controls the basic vital functions of life.

● The arachnoid membrane is loosely attached to the other meninges to allow space for fluid between the layers.

● The **subarachnoid space,** located below the arachnoid membrane and above the pia mater, contains cerebrospinal fluid.

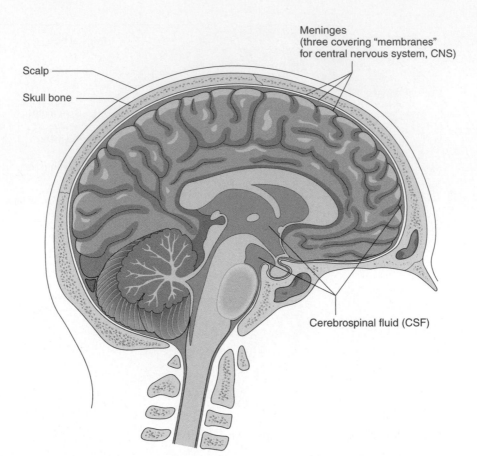

Scalp

Skull bone

Meninges
(three covering "membranes"
for central nervous system, CNS)

Cerebrospinal fluid (CSF)

FIGURE 10.5 A cross section of the brain showing the protective coverings. The cerebrospinal fluid is shown in pink.

The Pia Mater

The **pia mater,** the third layer of the meninges, is located nearest to the brain and spinal cord. It consists of delicate connective tissue with a rich supply of blood vessels.

CEREBROSPINAL FLUID

Cerebrospinal fluid (CSF) is a clear, colorless, watery fluid produced by special capillaries within the ventricles of the brain.

- The CFS flows throughout the brain and around the spinal cord, and its functions are to nourish, cool, and cushion these organs from shock or injury.

THE CEREBRUM

The **cerebrum** (seh-**REE**-brum) is the largest and uppermost portion of the brain. It is responsible for all thought, judgment, memory, association, and discrimination.

- The term **cerebral** (**SER**-eh-bral *or* seh-**REE**-bral) means pertaining to the cerebrum or brain.

- The **cerebral cortex,** made up of gray matter, is the outer layer of the cerebrum and is arranged in folds.

The Cerebral Hemispheres

The cerebrum is divided into the **left hemisphere** and the **right hemisphere** (Figure 10.6). These are also referred to as the left brain and right brain.

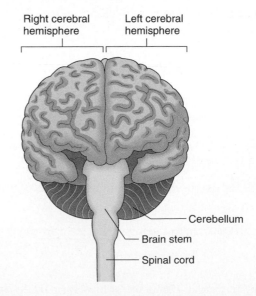

Right cerebral
hemisphere

Left cerebral
hemisphere

Cerebellum

Brain stem

Spinal cord

FIGURE 10.6 An anterior view showing the brain divided into right and left hemispheres.

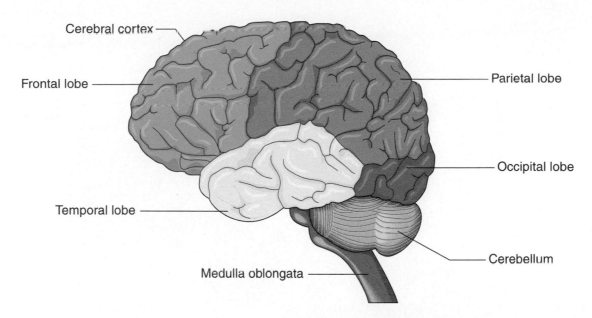

FIGURE 10.7 A left lateral view of the exterior of the brain with the lobes shown in color.

- The two cerebral hemispheres are connected at the lower midpoint by the **corpus callosum** (**KOR**-pus kah-**LOH**-sum). See Figures 10.4 and 10.8.

The Lobes of the Brain

Each hemisphere of the cerebrum is divided into four **lobes,** and each lobe is named for the bone of the cranium covering it (Figure 10.7).

- The **frontal lobe** controls motor functions.
- The **parietal lobe** receives and interprets nerve impulses from the sensory receptors.
- The **occipital lobe** controls eyesight.
- The **temporal lobe** controls the senses of hearing and smell.

The Ventricles

The four **ventricles** located within the middle region of the cerebrum contain CFS. (A *ventricle* is a small cavity, such as the ventricles of the brain and of the heart.)

THE THALAMUS

The **thalamus** (**THAL**-ah-mus), which is located below the cerebrum, produces sensations by relaying impulses to and from the cerebral cortex and the sense organs of the body (Figure 10.8).

The Hypothalamus

The **hypothalamus** (**high**-poh-**THAL**-ah-mus), located below the thalamus, has seven major regulatory functions. These are summarized in Table 10.4.

- The hypothalamus communicates with other parts of the body by secreting neurohormones. (A *neurohormone* is a hormone secreted by, or acting on, a part of the nervous system.)

Table 10.4

REGULATORY FUNCTIONS OF THE HYPOTHALAMUS

1. Regulates and integrates the autonomic nervous system, thereby controlling heart rate, blood pressure, respiratory rate, and digestive tract activity.

2. Regulates emotional responses and behavior.

3. Regulates body temperature.

4. Regulates food intake by controlling hunger sensations.

5. Regulates water balance and thirst.

6. Regulates sleep-wakefulness cycles.

7. Regulates endocrine system activity.

THE CEREBELLUM

The **cerebellum** (**ser**-eh-**BELL**-um) is the second largest part of the brain. It is located at the back of the head below the posterior part of the cerebrum.

- The cerebellum receives incoming messages regarding movement within joints, muscle tone, and positions of the body. From here, messages are relayed to the different parts of the brain that control skeletal muscles.

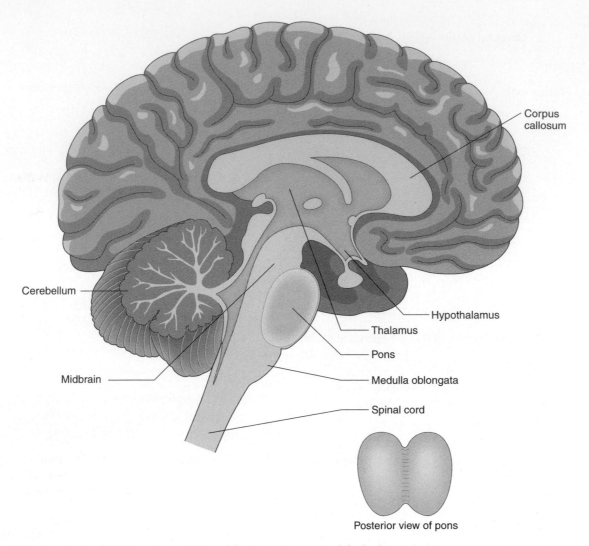

Corpus callosum

Cerebellum

Hypothalamus

Thalamus

Pons

Midbrain

Medulla oblongata

Spinal cord

Posterior view of pons

FIGURE 10.8 A schematic representation of the inner structures of the brain.

THE BRAINSTEM

The **brainstem** is the stalklike portion of the brain that connects the cerebral hemispheres with the spinal cord. It is made up of the midbrain, pons, and medulla oblongata.

The Midbrain

The **midbrain** extends from the lower surface of the cerebrum to the pons. It is a short narrow segment that provides conduction pathways to and from higher and lower centers.

The Pons

The **pons** (**PONZ**), which means bridge, is situated at the base of the brain. It is here that nerve cells cross from one side of the brain to control the opposite side of the body.

- The nerves that control the left side of the body are found in the right side of the brain. Because the nerves cross at the pons, an injury to the right side of the brain affects the left side of the body.

- The nerves that control the right side of the body are found in the left side of the brain. Because the nerves cross at the pons, an injury to the left side of the brain affects the right side of the body.

The Medulla Oblongata

The **medulla oblongata** (meh-**DULL**-ah **ob**-long-**GAH**-tah) is located at the lowest part of the brainstem. It controls basic life functions including the muscles of respiration, heart rate, and blood pressure.

THE SPINAL CORD

The **spinal cord (SC)** is the pathway for impulses going to and from the brain.

- The spinal cord contains all the nerves that affect the limbs and lower part of the body.

- The spinal cord is protected by CFS and is surrounded by the three meninges.

- The gray matter in the spinal cord, which is not protected by a myelin sheath, is located in the internal section. The myelinated white matter composes the outer portion of the spinal cord (see Figure 10.3).

THE PERIPHERAL NERVOUS SYSTEM

The **peripheral nervous system (PNS)** consists of the cranial nerves (extending from the brain) and the spinal nerves (extending from the spinal cord).

THE CRANIAL NERVES

The 12 pairs of **cranial nerves** originate from the undersurface of the brain. Each nerve of a pair serves half of the body, and the two nerves are identical in function and structure.

● The cranial nerves are identified by Roman numerals and are named for the area or function they serve (Figure 10.9).

THE SPINAL NERVES

The 31 pairs of **spinal nerves** are usually named for the artery they accompany or the body part they innervate (Figure 10.10).

● For example, the femoral nerve innervates muscles associated with the femur (the bone of the upper leg).

THE AUTONOMIC NERVOUS SYSTEM

The **autonomic nervous system (ANS)** controls the involuntary actions of the body (Figure 10.11).

● The ANS is subdivided into two divisions: the **sympathetic** and **parasympathetic nervous systems.**

● As shown in Table 10.5, one division balances the activity of the other to maintain homeostasis. **Homeostasis (hoh-**mee-oh-**STAY**-sis) is the process of maintaining the constant internal environment of the body.

MEDICAL SPECIALTIES RELATED TO THE NERVOUS SYSTEM

● An **anesthesiologist** (**an-**es-**thee**-zee-**OL**-oh-jist) is a physician who specializes in administering anesthetic agents before and during surgery (**an-** means without, **esthesi** means feeling, and **-ologist** means specialist).

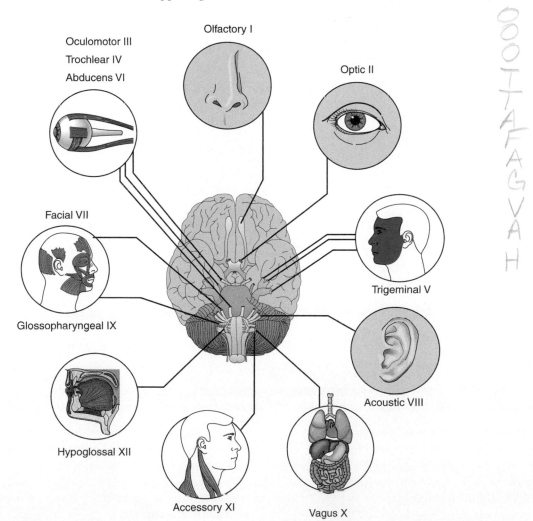

FIGURE 10.9 Cranial nerves are identified with Roman numerals and are named for the area or function they serve.

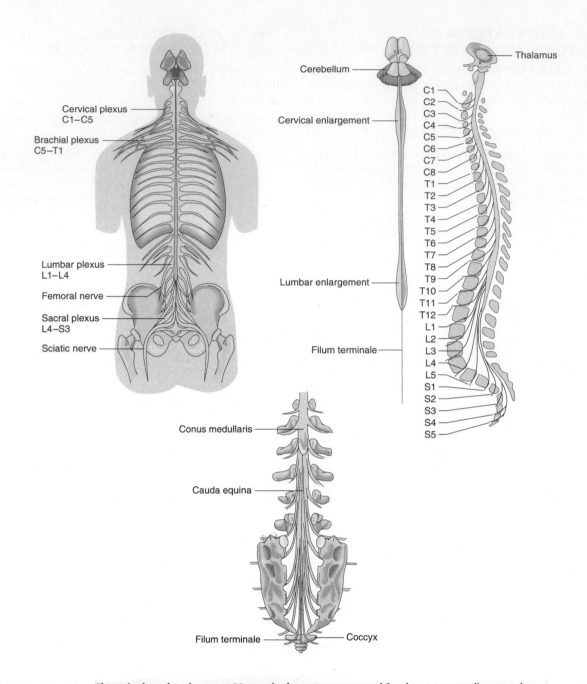

FIGURE 10.10 The spinal cord and nerves. Most spinal nerves are named for the corresponding vertebrae.

Table 10.5

DIVISIONS OF THE AUTONOMIC NERVOUS SYSTEM AND THEIR CONTRASTING ACTIONS

Sympathetic Nervous System	Parasympathetic Nervous System
Prepares the body for emergency and stressful situations by increasing the breathing rate, heart rate, and blood flow to muscles.	Returns the body to normal after a stressful response. It also maintains normal body functions during ordinary circumstances that are not emotionally or physically stressful.

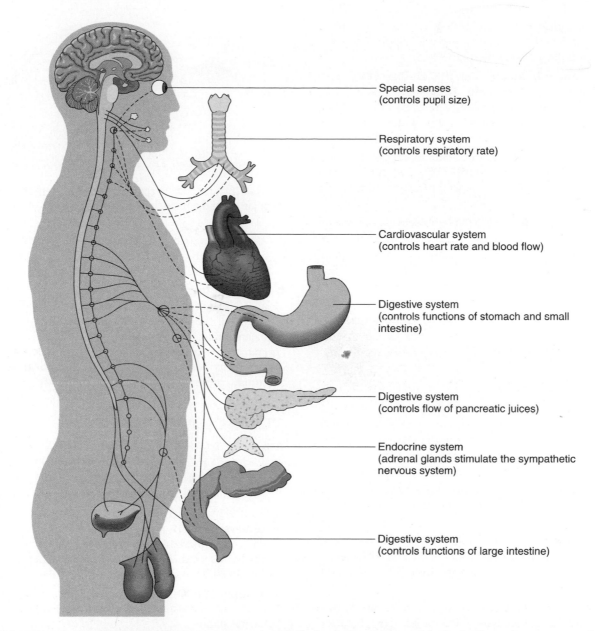

Special senses
(controls pupil size)

Respiratory system
(controls respiratory rate)

Cardiovascular system
(controls heart rate and blood flow)

Digestive system
(controls functions of stomach and small intestine)

Digestive system
(controls flow of pancreatic juices)

Endocrine system
(adrenal glands stimulate the sympathetic nervous system)

Digestive system
(controls functions of large intestine)

FIGURE 10.11 The autonomic nervous system controls the involuntary actions of the body. Shown here are examples of this interaction with the major body systems.

- An **anesthetist** (ah-**NES**-theh-tist) is a person trained in administering anesthesia but who is not necessarily a physician, for example, a nurse anesthetist (**an-** means without, **esthet** means feeling, and **-ist** means specialist).

- A **neurologist** (new-**ROL**-oh-jist) specializes in diagnosing and treating diseases and disorders of the nervous system (**neur** means nerve and **-ologist** means specialist).

- A **neurosurgeon** is a physician who specializes in surgery of the nervous system.

- A **psychiatrist** (sigh-**KYE**-ah-trist) holds a Medical Doctor (MD) degree and specializes in diagnosing and treating chemical dependencies, emotional problems, and mental illness (**psych** means mind and **-iatrist** means specialist).

- A **psychologist** (sigh-**KOL**-oh-jist) holds an advanced degree, other than a medical degree, and specializes in evaluating and treating emotional problems (**psych** means mind and **-ologist** means specialist).

PATHOLOGY OF THE NERVOUS SYSTEM

HEAD AND MENINGES

- **Cephalalgia** (**sef**-ah-**LAL**-jee-ah), also known as a **headache,** is pain in the head (**cephal** means head and **-algia** means pain). It is also known as **cephalodynia** (**sef**-ah-loh-**DIN**-ee-ah).

- A **migraine headache** (**MY**-grayn) is a syndrome characterized by sudden, severe, sharp headache usually present on only one side.

- An **encephalocele** (en-**SEF**-ah-loh-**seel**), also known as a **craniocele** (**KRAY**-nee-oh-**seel**), is a congenital gap in the skull with herniation of brain substance (**encephal/o** means brain and **-cele** means hernia). Compare this with a meningocele.

- **Hydrocephalus** (high-droh-**SEF**-ah-lus) is an abnormally increased amount of CFS within the brain (**hydr/o** means water, **cephal** means head, and **-us** is a singular noun ending).

- A **meningocele** (meh-**NING**-goh-**seel**) is the protrusion of the membranes of the brain or spinal cord through a defect in the skull or spinal column (**mening/o** means meninges and **-cele** means hernia). Compare this with an encephalocele.

- **Meningitis** (men-in-**JIGH**-tis) is an inflammation of the meninges of the brain or spinal cord (**mening** means meninges and **-itis** means inflammation) (plural, **meningitides**). Compare with *encephalitis*.

DISORDERS OF THE BRAIN

- **Alzheimer's disease** (**ALTZ**-high-merz) (**AD**) is a group of disorders associated with degenerative changes in the brain structure that lead to characteristic symptoms including progressive memory loss, impaired cognition, and personality changes.

- **Cognition** (kog-**NISH**-un) describes the mental activities associated with thinking, learning, and memory.

- **Encephalitis** (en-sef-ah-**LYE**-tis) is an inflammation of the brain (**encelphal** means brain and **-itis** means inflammation) (plural, **encephalitides**). Compare with *meningitis*.

- **Parkinson's disease** (**PD**) is a chronic, slowly progressive, degenerative CNS disorder. It is characterized by fine muscle tremors, a masklike facial expression, and a shuffling gait. (*Gait* means manner of walking.)

- **Tetanus** (**TET**-ah-nus), also known as **lockjaw,** is an acute and potentially fatal bacterial infection of the CNS caused by the tetanus bacillus. Tetanus can be prevented through immunization.

BRAIN INJURIES

- **Amnesia** (am-**NEE**-zee-ah) is a disturbance in the memory marked by a total or partial inability to recall past experiences. The cause may be a brain injury, illness, or psychological disturbance.

- A **concussion** (kon-**KUSH**-un), also called a **cerebral concussion,** is a violent shaking up or jarring of the brain (**concuss** means shaken together and **-ion** means condition) (Figure 10.12).

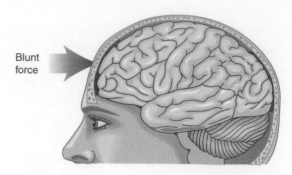

FIGURE 10.12   A concussion is the violent shaking up or jarring of the brain.

- A **cerebral contusion** (kon-**TOO**-zhun) is the bruising of brain tissue as a result of a head injury (**contus** means bruise and **-ion** means condition).

- A **cranial hematoma** (hee-mah-**TOH**-mah *or* hemah-**TOH**-mah) is a collection of blood trapped in the tissues of the brain (**hemat** means blood and **-oma** means tumor). Named for their location, the types of cranial hematomas include **epidural hematoma, subdural hematoma,** and **intracerebral hematoma** (Figure 10.13).

LEVELS OF CONSCIOUSNESS *LOC*

- **Conscious,** also known as **alert,** means being awake, aware, and responding appropriately.

- **Syncope** (**SIN**-koh-pee), also known as **fainting,** is the brief loss of consciousness caused by a brief lack of oxygen in the brain.

- **Lethargy** (**LETH**-ar-jee) is a lowered level of consciousness marked by listlessness, drowsiness, and apathy. As used here, *apathy* means indifference and a reduced level of activity.

- A **stupor** (**STOO**-per) is a state of impaired consciousness marked by a lack of responsiveness to environmental stimuli.

- A **coma** (**KOH**-mah) is a profound (deep) state of unconsciousness marked by the absence of spontaneous eye movements, no response to painful stimuli, and no vocalization (speech). **Comatose** (**KOH**-mahtohs) refers to a person who is in a coma.

Delirium and Dementia

- **Delirium** (dee-**LIR**-ee-um) is a potentially reversible condition often associated with a high fever that comes on suddenly. A *delirious* patient is confused, disoriented, and unable to think clearly.

- **Dementia** (dee-**MEN**-shee-ah) is a slowly progressive decline in mental abilities including memory, thinking, judgment, and the ability to pay attention.

BRAIN TUMORS

A **brain tumor** is an abnormal growth within the brain that may be either benign (not life threatening) or malig-

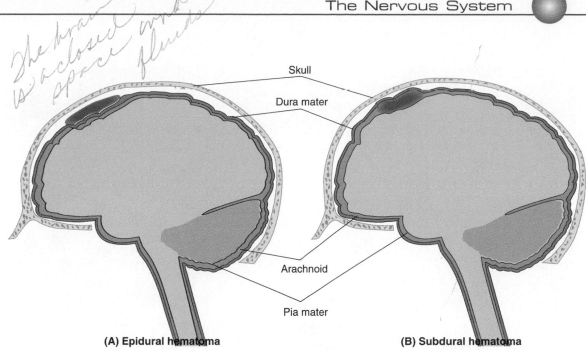

The brain is a closed space and fluids (handwritten annotation)

Skull

Dura mater

Arachnoid

Pia mater

(A) Epidural hematoma   **(B) Subdural hematoma**

FIGURE 10.13 Cranial hematomas. (Left) Epidural hematoma. (Right) Subdural hematoma.

nant (life threatening). A malignant brain tumor may originate in the brain as the primary site, or it may spread from a secondary site in another part of the body.

● Any abnormal growth in the brain can cause damage in two ways. First, if the tumor is invasive, it destroys brain tissue. Second, because the skull is hard, the tumor can damage the brain by causing pressure on it (Figure 10.14).

STROKES

A **stroke,** also known as a **cerebrovascular accident** (**ser**-eh-broh-**VAS**-kyou-lar) **(CVA)**, is damage to the brain that occurs when the blood flow to the brain is disrupted because a blood vessel supplying it either is blocked or has ruptured (Figure 10.15).

Ischemic Attacks

● A **transient ischemic attack** (iss-**KEE**-mick) **(TIA)** is the temporary interruption in the blood supply to the brain. Symptoms include weakness, dizziness, or loss of balance. These pass within a few minutes. However, a TIA may be a warning of an impending stroke.

● The most common type of stroke in older people is an **ischemic stroke** in which the flow of blood in the brain is blocked. This may be caused by a narrowing of the carotid artery or by a **cerebral thrombosis** in which a thrombus (clot) blocks the artery. This disruption of blood flow usually affects the cerebrum and damages the controls of movement, language, and senses.

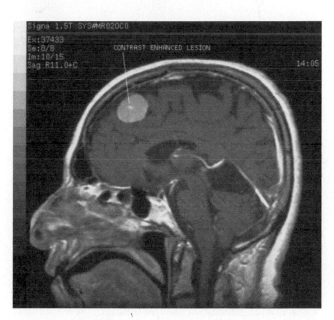

FIGURE 10.14 A brain tumor visualized by magnetic resonance imaging (MRI).

● **Aphasia** (ah-**FAY**-zee-ah) is the loss of the ability to speak, write, or comprehend the written or spoken word (**a-** means without and **-phasia** means speech). Aphasia is often due to brain damage associated with a stroke.

● A carotid endarterectomy, described in Chapter 5, may be performed to prevent an ischemic stroke by opening a blocked artery before a stroke occurs.

Hemorrhagic Stroke

In a **hemorrhagic stroke** (**hem**-oh-**RAJ**-ick), also known as a **bleed,** a blood vessel in the brain leaks or ruptures.

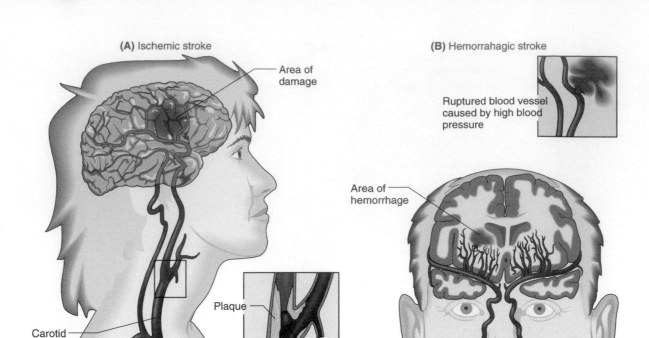

(A) Ischemic stroke

Area of damage

Carotid artery

Plaque

Thrombotic blood clot

(B) Hemorrahagic stroke

Ruptured blood vessel caused by high blood pressure

Area of hemorrhage

FIGURE 10.15   Stroke damage reflects the affected area of the brain. (A) Ischemic stroke. (B) Hemorrhagic stroke. *(By permission of Mayo Foundation; from June 1995 "Medical Essay,"* Supplement to Mayo Clinic Health Letter.)

This type of stroke is less common than ischemic strokes, but is more deadly. A hemorrhagic stroke affects the area of the brain damaged by the leaking blood (Figure 10.16).

SLEEP DISORDERS

- **Insomnia** is the prolonged or abnormal inability to sleep. This condition is usually a symptom of another problem such as depression, pain, or excessive caffeine.

- **Narcolepsy** (**NAR**-koh-**lep**-see) is a syndrome characterized by recurrent uncontrollable seizures of drowsiness and sleep (**narc/o** means stupor and **-lepsy** means seizure).

- **Somnambulism** (som-**NAM**-byou-lizm), also known as **noctambulism** or **sleepwalking,** is the condition of walking without awakening (**somn** means sleep, **ambul** means to walk, and **-ism** means condition of).

- **Somnolence** (**SOM**-noh-lens) is a condition of unnatural sleepiness or semiconsciousness approaching coma. A *somnolent* person usually can be aroused by verbal stimuli.

THE SPINAL CORD

- **Myelitis** (**my**-eh-**LYE**-tis) is an inflammation of the spinal cord (**myel** means spinal cord [and bone marrow] and **-itis** means inflammation). Myelitis also means inflammation of bone marrow.

- A **myelosis** (my-eh-**LOH**-sis) is a tumor of the spinal cord (**myel** means spinal cord [and bone marrow] and **-osis** means abnormal condition). Myelosis also

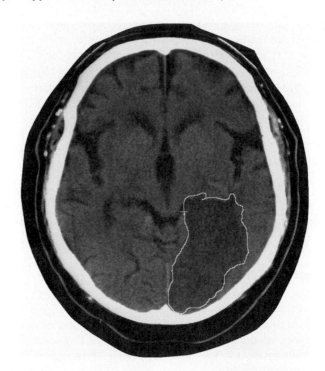

FIGURE 10.16   MRI of a brain, with the area of a bleed visible in the lower right.

means an abnormal proliferation of bone marrow tissue.

- **Multiple sclerosis** (skleh-**ROH**-sis) **(MS)** is a progressive autoimmune disorder characterized by scattered patches of demyelination of nerve fibers of the brain and spinal cord. Demyelination, which is the loss of this protective myelin covering, disrupts the transmission of nerve impulses and causes symptoms including tremors, paralysis, and speech disturbances.

- **Poliomyelitis** (**poh**-lee-oh-**my**-eh-**LYE**-tis), also known as **polio**, is a viral infection of the gray matter of the spinal cord that may result in paralysis. This can be prevented through immunization (**poli/o** means gray, **myel** means spinal cord, and **-itis** means inflammation).

- **Postpolio syndrome** is the recurrence later in life of some polio symptoms in individuals who have had poliomyelitis and have recovered from it.

- **Radiculitis** (rah-**dick**-you-**LYE**-tis), also known as a **pinched nerve**, is an inflammation of the root of a spinal nerve (**radicul** means root or nerve root and **-itis** means inflammation). This term usually applies to that portion of the root that lies between the spinal cord and the intervertebral canal of the spinal column.

- **Spinal cord injuries (SCIs)** are discussed in Chapter 4 under Paralysis.

NERVES

- **Amyotrophic lateral sclerosis** (ah-**my**-oh-**TROH**-fick) **(ALS)**, also known as **Lou Gehrig's disease,** is a degenerative disease of the motor neurons in which patients become progressively weaker until they are completely paralyzed. Intellect, eye motion, bladder function, and sensations are spared.

- **Bell's palsy** is paralysis of the facial (seventh cranial) nerve that causes drooping only on the affected side of the face. Compare with *tic douloureux*.

- **Guillain-Barré syndrome** (gee-**YAHN**-bah-**RAY**) **(GBS)**, also known as **acute ascending polyneuritis,** is characterized by rapidly worsening muscle weakness that may lead to temporary paralysis. GBS is presumed to be an autoimmune reaction that may occur after a mild infection, surgery, or an immunization.

- **Peripheral neuropathy** (new-**ROP**-ah-thee), also known as **peripheral neuritis** (new-**RYE**-tis), is a painful condition of the nerves of the hands and feet due to peripheral nerve damage that may be caused by disease such as diabetes, alcoholism, autoimmune diseases, and exposure to toxic substances.

- **Tic douloureux** (**TICK** doo-loo-**ROO**), also known as **trigeminal neuralgia,** is inflammation of the trigeminal (fifth cranial) nerve. It is characterized by sudden, intense, sharp pain on one side of the face. Compare with *Bell's palsy*.

- **Sciatica** (sigh-**AT**-ih-kah) is inflammation of the sciatic nerve that results in pain along the course of the nerve through the thigh and leg.

ABNORMAL SENSATIONS

- **Causalgia** (kaw-**ZAL**-jee-ah) is an intense burning pain after an injury to a sensory nerve (**caus** means burning and **-algia** means pain).

- **Hyperesthesia** (**high**-per-es-**THEE**-zee-ah) means a condition of excessive sensitivity to stimuli (**hyper-** means excessive and **-esthesia** means sensation or feeling).

- **Paresthesia** (**par**-es-**THEE**-zee-ah) is an abnormal sensation, such as burning, tingling, or numbness, for no apparent reason (**par-** means abnormal and **-esthesia** means sensation or feeling).

CEREBRAL PALSY

Cerebral palsy (**SER**-eh-bral *or* seh-**REE**-bral **PAWL**-zee) **(CP)** is a condition characterized by poor muscle control, spasticity, and other neurologic deficiencies caused by an injury to the part of the brain that controls muscle movements. This injury occurs during pregnancy, birth, or soon after birth. CP occurs most often in premature or low-birthweight infants.

CONVULSIONS AND SEIZURES

The terms **convulsion** and **seizure** (**SEE**-zhur) are used interchangeably to describe a sudden, violent, involuntary contraction of a group of muscles caused by a disturbance in brain function. Convulsions have many causes including brain injury, lesions, or extreme high fever.

- A **generalized seizure,** also known as a **generalized tonic-clonic seizure,** is characterized by a loss of consciousness with tonic convulsions followed by clonic convulsions. (These are sometimes described as tonic and clonic phases of a generalized seizure.)

- A **tonic convulsion** is a state of continuous muscular contraction that results in rigidity and violent spasms.

- A **clonic convulsion** is a state marked by the alternate contraction and relaxation of muscles, resulting in jerking movements of the face, trunk, or extremities.

- A **partial seizure,** also known as a **localized seizure,** begins with specific motor, sensory, or psychomotor phenomena without loss of consciousness.

EPILEPSY

Epilepsy (**EP**-ih-**lep**-see) is a group of neurologic disorders characterized by recurrent episodes of seizures.

- **Grand mal epilepsy** (**GRAN MAHL EP**-ih-**lep**-see), which is the more severe form, is characterized by generalized tonic-clonic seizures.

- **Petit mal epilepsy** (peh-**TEE MAHL EP**-ih-**lep**-see), also known as **absence epilepsy,** is the milder form in which there is a sudden, temporary loss of consciousness, lasting only a few seconds. Seizures are very mild, do not include convulsive movements, and may not be noticed.

- An **epileptic aura** is a manifestation, such as a particular smell or light, which may be experienced just before a seizure.

MENTAL HEALTH

Although described as mental disorders, the following conditions are often caused by physical changes, substance abuse, medications, or any combination of those factors.

DEVELOPMENTAL DISORDERS

- **Mental retardation** is significantly below average general intellectual functioning that is accompanied by a significant limitation in adaptive functioning.

- An **autistic disorder** (aw-**TISS**-tick), also known as **autism** (**AW**-tizm), is a disorder in which a young child cannot develop normal social relationships, behaves in compulsive and ritualistic ways, and frequently has poor communication skills.

- **Attention deficit disorder (ADD)** is a short attention span and impulsiveness that is inappropriate for the child's developmental age.

- An **attention deficit/hyperactivity disorder (ADHD)** is a pattern of inattention and hyperactivity that is inappropriate for the child's developmental age. This condition may persist into adulthood.

- **Dyslexia** (dis-**LECK**-see-ah), also known as a **reading disorder,** is a learning disability characterized by reading achievement that falls substantially below that expected given the individual's chronological age, measured intelligence, and age-appropriate education.

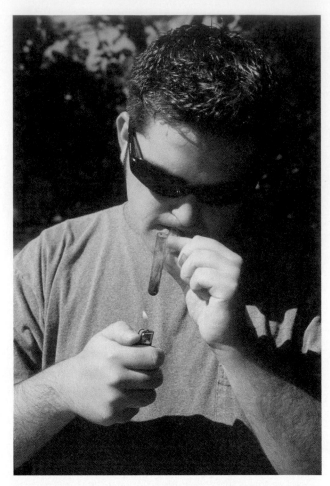

FIGURE 10.17 Substance abuse includes the use of illegal drugs.

SUBSTANCE-RELATED DISORDERS

An **addiction** is the compulsive and overwhelming involvement with a specific activity despite the fact that it causes significant health hazards plus recurrent legal and social problems. The addiction may be to actions such as gambling or smoking. Abused substances include alcohol, medications, and illegal drugs (Figure 10.17).

- For example, **alcoholism** (**AL**-koh-hol-izm) is chronic alcohol dependence or abuse with specific signs and symptoms of withdrawal. *Withdrawal* is a psychological or physical syndrome (or both) caused by the abrupt cessation (stopping) of the use of a drug in a habituated individual.

- **Delirium tremens** (dee-**LIR**-ee-um **TREE**-mens) **(DTs)** is a form of acute organic brain syndrome due to alcohol withdrawal and is characterized by sweating, tremor, restlessness, anxiety, mental confusion, and hallucinations.

SCHIZOPHRENIA AND OTHER PSYCHOTIC DISORDERS

- A **psychotic disorder** (sigh-**KOT**-ick) is characterized by the derangement of personality, loss of contact with reality, and deterioration of normal social functioning.

- **Schizophrenia** (**skit**-soh-**FREE**-nee-ah) is a psychotic disorder characterized by delusions, hallucinations, disorganized speech that is often incoherent, and disruptive or catatonic behavior.

- A **delusion** (dee-**LOO**-zhun) is a false personal belief that is maintained despite obvious proof or evidence to the contrary.

- A **hallucination** (hah-**loo**-sih-**NAY**-shun) is a sense perception (sight, touch, sound, smell, or taste) that has no basis in external stimulation.

- **Catatonic behavior** (**kat**-ah-**TON**-ick) is marked by a lack of responsiveness, stupor, and a tendency to remain in a fixed posture.

MOOD DISORDERS

- A **manic episode** is a distinct period during which there is an abnormally, and persistently elevated, expansive and irritable mood.

- A **major depressive episode** is a prolonged period during which there is either a depressed mood or the loss of interest or pleasure in nearly all activities.

- A **bipolar disorder,** also known as a **manic-depressive episode,** is a clinical course characterized by the occurrence of manic episodes alternating with depressive episodes.

PANIC DISORDERS

- **Panic disorders** are characterized by the sudden, unanticipated recurrence of a group of symptoms known as a panic attack. Once a person has experienced a panic attack, he or she will go to great lengths to avoid having it happen again.

- A **panic attack** includes intense feelings of apprehension, fearfulness, terror, and impending doom. Physical symptoms include shortness of breath, profuse sweating, heart palpitations, chest pain, and choking sensations.

ANXIETY DISORDERS

- An **anxiety state** is a feeling of apprehension, tension, or uneasiness that stems from the anticipation of danger, the source of which is largely unknown or unrecognized.

- An **obsessive-compulsive disorder** is a pattern of specific behaviors such as repeated hand washing. *Obsessions* are persistent ideas, thoughts, or images that cause the individual anxiety or distress. *Compulsions* are repetitive behaviors the goal of which is to prevent or reduce anxiety or stress.

- **Posttraumatic stress disorder (PTSD)** is the development of characteristic symptoms after a psychologically traumatic event such as witnessing a shooting, surviving a natural disaster, or being held as a hostage. Symptoms include numbed responsiveness to external stimuli, anxiety, sleep disorders, restlessness, difficulty concentrating, and depression.

PHOBIAS

- A **phobia** (**FOH**-bee-ah) is a persistent irrational fear of a specific thing or situation. This fear is strong enough to cause avoidance of that thing or situation.

- **Acrophobia** (**ack**-roh-**FOH**-bee-ah) is an excessive fear of being in high places (**acr/o** means top and **-phobia** means abnormal fear).

- **Agoraphobia** (**ag**-oh-rah-**FOH**-bee-ah) is an overwhelming and irrational fear of leaving the familiar setting of home or venturing into the open (**agor/a** means market place and **-phobia** means abnormal fear).

- **Claustrophobia** (**klaws**-troh-**FOH**-bee-ah) is an abnormal fear of being in narrow or enclosed spaces (**claustr/o** means barrier and **-phobia** means abnormal fear).

SOMATOFORM DISORDERS

- **Somatoform** (soh-**MAT**-oh-**form**) is the term used to describe the presence of physical symptoms that suggest general medical conditions not explained by the patient's actual medical condition.

- A **conversion disorder,** such as paralysis of an arm or disturbance of vision, is characterized by a change in function that suggests a physical disorder but has no physical cause. Apparently these symptoms are an expression of the patient's psychological problems that he has converted into physical symptoms.

- **Hypochondriasis** (**high**-poh-kon-**DRY**-ah-sis) is characterized by a preoccupation with fears of having, or the idea that one does have, a serious disease based on misinterpretation of one or more bodily signs or symptoms.

IMPULSE-CONTROL DISORDERS

- **Kleptomania** (**klep**-toh-**MAY**-nee-ah) is a disorder characterized by a recurrent failure to resist impulses to steal objects not for immediate use or their monetary value (**klept/o** means to steal and **-mania** means madness).

- **Pyromania** (**pye**-roh-**MAY**-nee-ah) is a disorder characterized by a recurrent failure to resist impulses to set fires (**pyr/o** means fire and **-mania** means madness).

PERSONALITY DISORDERS

- A **personality disorder** is an enduring pattern of inner experience and behavior that deviates markedly from the expectations of the individual's culture. This pattern is pervasive and inflexible, has an onset in adolescence or early adulthood, is stable over time, and leads to distress or impairment.

- An **antisocial personality disorder** is a pattern of disregard for, and violation of, the rights of others. This pattern brings the individual into continuous conflict with society.

- A **narcissistic personality disorder** (**nahr**-sih-**SIS**-tick) is a pattern of an exaggerated need for admiration and complete lack of empathy. *Empathy* (**EM**-pah-thee) is the ability to understand another person's mental and emotional state without becoming personally involved.

OTHER CONDITIONS

- **Malingering** (mah-**LING**-ger-ing) is characterized by the intentional creation of false or grossly exaggerated physical or psychological symptoms, motivated by external incentives such as avoiding work.

- **Munchausen syndrome** (**MUHN**-chow-zen), named for a German nobleman in the 1700s, is a condition in which the "patient" repeatedly makes up clinically convincing simulations of disease for the purpose of gaining medical attention.

- **Munchausen syndrome by proxy** is a form of child abuse. Although seeming very concerned about the child's well-being, the abusive parent will falsify an illness in a child by making up or creating symptoms and then seeking medical treatment for the child.

DIAGNOSTIC PROCEDURES OF THE NERVOUS SYSTEM

- **Computed tomography,** also known as a **CT scan,** and **magnetic resonance imaging (MRI)** are important diagnostic tools of the nervous system because they can image the soft tissue structures of the brain and spinal cord (see Figures 10.14 and 10.16). These diagnostic techniques are discussed further in Chapter 15.

- **Echoencephalography** (eck-oh-en-**sef**-ah-**LOG**-rah-fee) is the use of ultrasound imaging to diagnose a shift in the midline structures of the brain (**ech/o** means sound, **encephal/o** means brain, and **-graphy** means the process of recording).

- **Electroencephalography** (ee-**leck**-troh-en-**sef**-ah-**LOG**-rah-fee) (**EEG**) is the process of recording the electrical activity of the brain through the use of electrodes attached to the scalp (**electr/o** means electric, **encephal/o** means brain, and **-graphy** means the process of recording). The resulting record is called an **electroencephalogram.** This electrical activity may also be displayed on a monitor as brain waves.

- **Encephalography** (en-**sef**-ah-**LOG**-rah-fee) is a radiographic study demonstrating the intracranial fluid-containing spaces of the brain (**encephal/o** means brain and **-graphy** means the process of recording). The resulting record is called an **encephalogram.**

- **Myelography** (**my**-eh-**LOG**-rah-fee) is a radiographic study of the spinal cord after the injection of a contrast medium (**myel/o** means spinal cord and **-graphy** means the process of recording). The resulting record is called a **myelogram.**

- Determining the patient's **level of consciousness (LOC)** is an important part of a neurologic evaluation. The LOC is established by observing the patient and evaluating his or her reactions to stimuli.

TREATMENT PROCEDURES OF THE NERVOUS SYSTEM

MEDICATIONS TO TREAT MENTAL DISORDERS

- **Tranquilizers,** also known as **antianxiety drugs,** suppress anxiety and relax muscles.

- An **antidepressant** prevents or relieves depression.

- An **antipsychotic** (**an**-tih-sigh-**KOT**-ick) is used to treat symptoms of severe psychiatric disorders.

- **Psychotropic drugs** (**sigh**-koh-**TROP**-pick) are capable of affecting the mind, emotions, and behavior and are used in the treatment of mental illnesses.

PAIN CONTROL

- **Transcutaneous electronic nerve stimulation (TENS)** is a method of pain control by the application of electronic impulses to the nerve endings through the skin.

- An **analgesic** (**an**-al-**JEE**-zick) is a drug that relieves pain without affecting consciousness.

- **Nonnarcotic analgesics** such as aspirin are used for mild to moderate pain.

- **Narcotic analgesics** such as morphine, Demerol, and codeine are used to relieve severe pain. However, they may cause physical dependence or addiction.

SEDATIVE AND HYPNOTIC MEDICATIONS

- A **sedative** depresses the CNS to produce calm and diminished responsiveness without producing sleep. **Sedation** is the effect produced by a sedative.

- A **hypnotic** depresses the CNS and usually produces sleep.

- A **barbiturate** (bar-**BIT**-you-rayt) is a class of drugs whose major action is a calming or depressed effect on the CNS.

- **Amobarbital** (**am**-oh-**BAR**-bih-tal) is a barbiturate used as a sedative and hypnotic.

- **Phenobarbital** (**fee**-noh-**BAR**-bih-tal) is a barbiturate used as a sedative and as an anticonvulsant.

- An **anticonvulsant** (**an**-tih-kon-**VUL**-sant) prevents seizures and convulsions.

ANESTHESIA

Anesthesia (**an**-es-**THEE**-zee-ah) is the absence of normal sensation, especially sensitivity to pain (**an-** means without and **-esthesia** means feeling).

- An **anesthetic** (**an**-es-**THET**-ick) is the medication used to induce anesthesia. The anesthetic may be topical, local, regional, or general.

- **Topical anesthesia** numbs only the tissue surface and is applied as a liquid, ointment, or spray.

- **Local anesthesia** is the loss of sensation in a limited area and is produced by injecting an anesthetic solution near that area.

- **Regional anesthesia,** the temporary interruption of nerve conduction, is produced by injecting an anesthetic solution near the nerves to be blocked.

- **Epidural anesthesia** (**ep**-ih-**DOO**-ral **an**-es-**THEE**-zee-ah) is regional anesthesia produced by injecting a local anesthetic into the epidural space of the lumbar or sacral region of the spine.

- **Spinal anesthesia** is produced by injecting an anesthetic into the subarachnoid space that is located below the arachnoid membrane and above the pia mater that surrounds the spinal cord.

- **General anesthesia** involves the total loss of body sensation and consciousness as induced by various anesthetic agents, given primarily by inhalation or intravenous injection.

BRAIN AND HEAD

- **Electroshock therapy,** also known as **electroconvulsive therapy** (ee-**leck**-troh-kon-**VUL**-siv) **(ECT),** is a controlled convulsion produced by the passage of an electric current through the brain. ECT is used primarily in the treatment of depression and mental disorders that do not respond to other forms of therapy.

- A **lobectomy** (loh-**BECK**-toh-mee) is surgical removal of a portion of the brain to treat brain cancer or seizure disorders that cannot be controlled with medication.

- A **thalamotomy** (**thal**-ah-**MOT**-oh-mee) is a surgical incision into the thalamus (**thalam** means thalamus and **-otomy** means surgical incision). This procedure, which destroys brain cells, is performed to quiet the tremors of Parkinson's disease, to treat some psychotic disorders, or to stop intractable pain.

NERVES

- A **neurectomy** (new-**RECK**-toh-mee) is the surgical removal of a nerve (**neur** means nerve and **-ectomy** means surgical removal).

- **Neuroplasty** (**NEW**-roh-**plas**-tee) is the surgical repair of a nerve or nerves (**neur/o** means nerve and **-plasty** means surgical repair).

- **Neurorrhaphy** (new-**ROR**-ah-fee) is suturing together of the ends of a severed nerve (**neur/o** means nerve and **-rrhaphy** means to suture).

- A **neurotomy** (new-**ROT**-oh-mee) is a surgical incision or the dissection of a nerve (**neur** means nerve and **-otomy** means a surgical incision).

Career Opportunities

In addition to the medical specialties already discussed, some of the health occupations involving the treatment of the nervous system include

- **Electroencephalographic (EEG) technologist:** operates an electroencephalograph, recording the electrical activity of the brain for diagnosis and evaluation

- **Electroneurodiagnostic technologist:** in addition to performing EEGs, performs nerve conduction tests, measures sensory and physical responses to specific stimuli, and conducts sleep studies and ambulatory monitoring

- **Polysomnographic technologist:** administers sleep disorder evaluations

- **Social worker:** trained to help people make adjustments in their lives or to refer them to community resources for assistance; also called case managers, counselors, or sociologists. Some specialties include

Child welfare and family counseling	Health care social work
Correctional (prison) counseling	Occupational social work
Geriatrics and hospice work	Psychiatric social work

- **Social services assistant:** aids social workers by maintaining records and performing other administrative tasks, often for a government agency

- **Psychiatric** or **mental health technician, assistant,** and **aide:** work under the supervision of a psychiatrist or psychologist to help patients with care and rehabilitation. They may also observe and report behavior.

- **Art, music,** and **dance therapists:** use creative arts for nonverbal expression of feelings, for communication, and for social integration. They may work with patients suffering from mental disorders, emotional trauma, or other social, psychological, or physical problems.

- **Recreational therapist:** uses creative arts and other activities such as sports and field trips to improve the patient's physical, emotional, and mental well-being.

Health Occupation Profile: MENTAL HEALTH WORKER

Shawn Goldwyn, 28, is a mental health worker in a psychiatric hospital. "In my job, I help people who are experiencing some form of mental crisis. Some of my patients have hallucinations or hear voices telling them to hurt themselves or others. Others have experienced severe trauma in their lives, have chemical imbalances that make them extremely aggressive or uninhibited, or are so profoundly depressed that suicide feels like the only option. My job is to make sure they are in a safe and supportive environment. Sometimes, I help run groups to teach different coping skills and ways to manage anger, anxiety, or depression. Most of the time, I sit and listen to them talk."

"I have always been a good listener. In high school, friends would seek me out to tell me their problems. This job is perfect for someone with lots of patience and understanding. It also helps to be flexible. Some days are very chaotic, and I never know what will happen next; other days are quieter and more predictable. Every day is different, and I like that."

STUDY BREAK

We all know that hitting your funny bone is not really funny.

The sudden, sharp pain we associate with the "funny bone" comes from the *ulnar nerve*. Why does it hurt so much when it is hit? The ulnar nerve is a long one running from the spinal cord to the fingertips. In most places along the way, it is protected by muscle or fat. But when it runs past the elbow joint, it is close to the skin. When you accidentally hit your elbow (which is easy to do, because it sticks out), you hit the ulnar nerve against the bone, causing a sharp pain or tingling sensation.

The ankle also has a nerve that runs close to the surface and can cause similar pain. But, because the ankle doesn't move about as widely as the elbow, it is less likely to be bumped sharply.

And why do we call the bone that carries the ulnar nerve to the elbow a funny bone? Because its scientific name, the *humerus*, sounds a lot like the word *humorous*.

Review Time

Write the answers to the following questions on a separate piece of paper or in your notebook. In addition, be prepared to take part in the classroom discussion.

1. **Written assignment:** Using terms a physician would understand, describe the difference between an **encephalocele** and a **meningocele**.

   Discussion assignment: Discuss how the word parts tell you what these terms mean.

2. **Written assignment:** Describe the difference between a **concussion** and a **contusion**.

   Discussion assignment: How could each type of injury occur?

3. **Written assignment:** Using terms a patient would understand, describe the difference between a **panic attack** and an **anxiety state**.

   Discussion assignment: How would each condition affect the quality of life for the patient?

4. **Written assignment:** Research and report on the full name and dates of the person for whom **Alzheimer's disease** is named.

   Discussion assignment: Mr. Greene has just been diagnosed with Alzheimer's disease. What should his family be prepared to face in the months and years ahead?

5. Written assignment: Describe the difference between an **ischemic stroke** and a **hemorrhagic stroke.**

Discussion assignment: Why is receiving treatment quickly so important for a stroke patient?

Optional Internet Activity

The goal of this activity is to help you learn more about medical terminology while improving your Internet skills. Select **one** of these two options and follow the instructions.

1. Internet Search: Search for information about **Alzheimer's disease.** Write a brief (one- or two-paragraph) report on something new you learned here and include the address of the web site where you found this information.

2. Web Site: To learn more about **brain injuries** go to this web address: **http://www.braincenter. org/.** Explore the site and then write a brief (one- or two-paragraph) report on something new you learned here.

The Human Touch: Critical Thinking Exercise

The following story and questions are designed to stimulate critical thinking through class discussion or as a brief essay response. There are no right or wrong answers to these questions.

Calle Washington read the information Dr. Thakker gave her with numb disbelief. "Multiple sclerosis is a neurological disorder characterized by demyelination of nerve fibers in the brain and spinal column. This disease may be progressively debilitating with symptoms that could include numbness, paralysis, ataxia, pain, and blindness. Some patients do experience life-threatening complications. This disease attacks young adults. It affects more women than men."

"Well, I sure fit the profile," thought Calle bitterly. She took a deep breath, trying to quiet the fluttering in her stomach. How could this happen now? Everything was so perfect. Her wedding gown was getting its last alterations, and the tickets for her honeymoon in Jamaica were in the desk drawer. Gabe was putting the final touches on the house where they planned on raising their family. Suddenly, her fairy tale life was turning into a nightmare.

She couldn't expect Gabe to waste his future caring for someone in a wheelchair, could she? And what would happen once her fellow teachers at the day care center noticed that her balance was sometimes off? She couldn't risk hurting one of the children, but if she lost her job she'd lose her health insurance. Dr. Thakker had said there were new drugs for MS, but he'd mentioned that they were very expensive. And what about the children that she and Gabe both wanted? Could she still have a baby and take care of it?

"Maybe I should take out an ad that says 'Twenty-five year old female seeks cure for deadly disease before marrying Prince Charming,'" she thought, trying to laugh through her tears.

Suggested Discussion Topics

1. Discuss whether Calle and Gabe should go ahead with the wedding.

2. How might Calle's condition affect her job? Should she be asked to resign?

3. If Calle loses her job at the day care center and tries to find work elsewhere, should she disclose the fact that she has MS?

4. Insurance companies want the people they insure to have a physical examination and provide information about previous illnesses and diseases. Discuss whether you think this is an ethical practice. If you think it is not ethical, why do you think the insurance companies do it?

5. What federal legislation is designed to help disabled individuals? Do you think this law would apply to Calle's situation?

Student Workbook and Student Activity CD-ROM

1. Go to your **Student Workbook** and complete the Learning Exercises for this chapter.
2. Go to the **Student Activity CD-ROM** and have fun with the exercises and games for this chapter.

11

Special Senses: The Eyes and Ears

● Overview of Structures, Word Parts, and Functions of the Eyes and Ears

MAJOR STRUCTURES	RELATED WORD PARTS	PRIMARY FUNCTIONS
Eyes	**opt/i, opt/o, optic/o, ophthalm/o**	Receptor organs for the sense of sight.
Adnexa of the eye		Accessory structures that provide external protection and movement for the eyes.
Lacrimal apparatus	**lacrim/o, dacry/o**	Produces, stores, and removes tears.
Iris	**ir/i, ir/o, irid/o, irit/o**	Controls the amount of light entering the eye.
Lens	**phac/o**	Focuses rays of light on the retina.
Retina	**retin/o**	Converts light images into electrical impulses and transmits them to the brain.
Ears	**acous/o, acout/o, audi/o, audit/o, ot/o**	Receptor organs for the sense of hearing; also help to maintain balance.
Outer ear	**pinn/i**	Transmits sound waves to the middle ear.
Middle ear	**myring/o, tympan/o**	Transmits sound waves to the inner ear.
Inner ear	**labyrinth/o**	Receives sound vibrations and transmits them to the brain.

Vocabulary Related to the Special Senses

Terms marked with the ❖ symbol are pronounced on the Student Activity CD-ROM that accompanies this text.

KEY WORD PARTS

- [ ] blephar/o
- [ ] -cusis
- [ ] dacryocyst/o
- [ ] irid/o
- [ ] kerat/o
- [ ] -metry
- [ ] ophthalm/o
- [ ] -opia
- [ ] ot/o
- [ ] presby/o
- [ ] pseud/o
- [ ] retin/o
- [ ] scler/o
- [ ] trop/o
- [ ] tympan/o

KEY MEDICAL TERMS

- [ ] accommodation (ah-kom-oh-DAY-shun) ❖
- [ ] adnexa (ad-NECK-sah) ❖
- [ ] amblyopia (am-blee-OH-pee-ah) ❖
- [ ] ametropia (am-eh-TROH-pee-ah) ❖
- [ ] anisocoria (an-ih-so-KOH-ree-ah) ❖
- [ ] astigmatism (ah-STIG-mah-tizm) ❖
- [ ] audiologist (aw-dee-OL-oh-jist)
- [ ] blepharoptosis (blef-ah-roh-TOH-sis or blef-ah-rop-TOH-sis) ❖
- [ ] cataract (KAT-ah-rakt) ❖
- [ ] chalazion (kah-LAY-zee-on) ❖
- [ ] conjunctivitis (kon-junk-tih-VYE-tis) ❖
- [ ] conjunctivoplasty (kon-junk-TYE-voh-plas-tee)
- [ ] convergence (kon-VER-jens)
- [ ] dacryocystitis (dack-ree-oh-sis-TYE-tis) ❖
- [ ] diplopia (dih-PLOH-pee-ah) ❖
- [ ] ectropion (eck-TROH-pee-on) ❖
- [ ] emmetropia (em-eh-TROH-pee-ah) ❖
- [ ] entropion (en-TROH-pee-on) ❖
- [ ] esotropia (es-oh-TROH-pee-ah) ❖
- [ ] eustachitis (you-stay-KYE-tis) ❖
- [ ] exotropia (eck-soh-TROH-pee-ah) ❖
- [ ] fenestration (fen-es-TRAY-shun) ❖
- [ ] glaucoma (glaw-KOH-mah) ❖
- [ ] hemianopia (hem-ee-ah-NOH-pee-ah) ❖
- [ ] hordeolum (hor-DEE-oh-lum) ❖
- [ ] hyperopia (high-per-OH-pee-ah) ❖
- [ ] intravenous fluorescein angiography (flew-oh-RES-ee-in) ❖
- [ ] iridectomy (ir-ih-DECK-toh-mee) ❖
- [ ] iritis (eye-RYE-tis) ❖
- [ ] keratitis (ker-ah-TYE-tis) ❖

- [ ] keratotomy (ker-ah-TOT-oh-mee) ❖
- [ ] labyrinthectomy (lab-ih-rin-THECK-toh-mee) ❖
- [ ] labyrinthitis (lab-ih-rin-THIGH-tis) ❖
- [ ] mastoidectomy (mas-toy-DECK-toh-mee)
- [ ] mastoiditis (mas-toy-DYE-tis)
- [ ] Ménière's syndrome (men-ee-AYRZ or men-YEHRS) ❖
- [ ] monochromatism (mon-oh-KROH-mah-tizm) ❖
- [ ] myopia (my-OH-pee-ah) ❖
- [ ] myringectomy (mir-in-JECK-toh-mee) ❖
- [ ] myringitis (mir-in-JIGH-tis) ❖
- [ ] myringotomy (mir-in-GOT-oh-mee) ❖
- [ ] nyctalopia (nick-tah-LOH-pee-ah) ❖
- [ ] nystagmus (nis-TAG-mus) ❖
- [ ] ophthalmologist (ahf-thal-MOL-oh-jist) ❖
- [ ] optometrist (op-TOM-eh-trist) ❖
- [ ] otitis media (oh-TYE-tis MEE-dee-ah) ❖
- [ ] otomycosis (oh-toh-my-KOH-sis) ❖
- [ ] otoplasty (OH-toh-plas-tee) ❖
- [ ] otopyorrhea (oh-toh-pye-oh-REE-ah) ❖
- [ ] otorrhagia (oh-toh-RAY-jee-ah) ❖
- [ ] otosclerosis (oh-toh-skleh-ROH-sis)
- [ ] papilledema (pap-ill-eh-DEE-mah) ❖
- [ ] patulous (PAT-you-lus)
- [ ] phacoemulsification (fay-koh-ee-mul-sih-fih-KAY-shun or fack-koh-ee-mul-sih-fih-KAY-shun) ❖
- [ ] presbycusis (pres-beh-KOO-sis) ❖
- [ ] presbyopia (pres-bee-OH-pee-ah) ❖
- [ ] purulent otitis media (PYOU-roo-lent oh-TYE-tis MEE-dee-ah)
- [ ] retinopexy (RET-ih-noh-peck-see)
- [ ] scleritis (skleh-RYE-tis)
- [ ] scotoma (skoh-TOH-mah) ❖
- [ ] stapedectomy (stay-peh-DECK-toh-mee)
- [ ] strabismus (strah-BIZ-mus) ❖
- [ ] synechia (sigh-NECK-ee-ah) ❖
- [ ] tarsectomy (tahr-SECK-toh-mee) ❖
- [ ] tarsorrhaphy (tahr-SOR-ah-fee) ❖
- [ ] tinnitus (tih-NIGH-tus) ❖
- [ ] tonometry (toh-NOM-eh-tree) ❖
- [ ] trabeculoplasty (trah-BECK-you-loh-plas-tee) ❖
- [ ] tympanectomy (tim-pah-NECK-toh-mee) ❖
- [ ] tympanocentesis (tim-pah-noh-sen-TEE-sis)
- [ ] tympanometry (tim-pah-NOM-eh-tree) ❖
- [ ] tympanoplasty (tim-pah-noh-PLAS-tee)
- [ ] tympanostomy tubes (tim-pan-OSS-toh-mee)
- [ ] vertigo (VER-tih-go)
- [ ] xerophthalmia (zeer-ahf-THAL-mee-ah) ❖

Upon completion of this chapter, you should be able to:

1. Describe the functions and structures of the eyes and adnexa.

2. Recognize, define, spell, and pronounce terms related to the pathology and diagnostic and treatment procedures of eye disorders.

3. Describe the functions and structures of the ears.

4. Recognize, define, spell, and pronounce terms related to the pathology and diagnostic and treatment procedures of ear disorders.

MEDICAL SPECIALTIES RELATED TO THE EYES AND EARS

- An **audiologist** (aw-dee-**OL**-oh-jist) specializes in the measurement of hearing function and the rehabilitation of persons with hearing impairments (**audi** means hearing and **-ologist** means specialist).

- An **ophthalmologist** (ahf-thal-**MOL**-oh-jist) specializes in diagnosing and treating diseases and disorders of the eye (**ophthalm** means eye and **-ologist** means specialist).

- An **optometrist** (op-**TOM**-eh-trist) holds a Doctor of Optometry (OD) degree and specializes in measuring the accuracy of vision to determine whether corrective lenses or eyeglasses are needed (**opt/o** means vision and **-metrist** means one who measures).

- An **otolaryngologist** (oh-toh-**lar**-in-**GOL**-oh-jist) is a physician who specializes in the care of the ears, nose, and throat (**ot/o** means ear, **laryng** means larynx, and **-ologist** means specialist).

FUNCTIONS OF THE EYES AND EARS

The eyes and ears are sensory receptor organs. Abbreviations used to describe these sensory organs are listed in Table 11.1.

FUNCTIONS OF THE EYES

The functions of the eyes are to receive images and transmit them to the brain.

- The term **optic** means pertaining to the eye or sight (**opt** means sight and **-ic** means pertaining to).

- **Ocular** (**OCK**-you-lar) means pertaining to the eye (**ocul** means eye and **-ar** means pertaining to).

- **Extraocular** (**eck**-strah-**OCK**-you-lar) means outside the eyeball (**extra-** means on the outside, **ocul** means eye, and **-ar** means pertaining to).

- **Intraocular** (**in**-trah-**OCK**-you-lar) means within the eyeball (**intra-** means within, **ocul** means eye, and **-ar** means pertaining to).

FUNCTIONS OF THE EARS

The functions of the ears are to receive sound impulses and transmit them to the brain. The inner ear also helps to maintain balance.

- The term **auditory** (**AW**-dih-**tor**-ee) means pertaining to the sense of hearing (**audit** means hearing or sense of hearing and **-ory** means pertaining to).

- **Acoustic** (ah-**KOOS**-tick) means relating to sound or hearing (**acous** means hearing or sound and **-tic** means pertaining to).

Table 11.1

COMPARISON OF ABBREVIATIONS RELATING TO THE EYES AND EARS			
Eyes		**Ears**	
OD	Right eye	AD	Right ear
OS	Left eye	AS	Left ear
OU	Each eye or both eyes	AU	Each ear or both ears

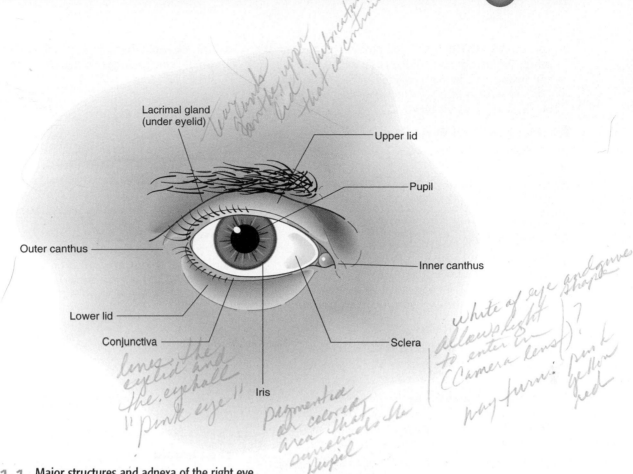

Handwritten annotations (partially legible):
tear ducts upper and lower lid; lubrication that is continuous
lines the eyelid and the eyeball "pink eye"
pigmented or colored area that surrounds the pupil
white of eye and gives shape; allows light to enter in (Camera lens)? may turn pink yellow red

FIGURE 11.1 Major structures and adnexa of the right eye.

STRUCTURES OF THE EYES

ADNEXA OF THE EYES

The **adnexa** (ad-**NECK**-sah) of the eyes, also known as **adnexa oculi,** include the orbit, eye muscles, eyelids, eyelashes, conjunctiva, and lacrimal apparatus (Figure 11.1). *Adnexa* means the appendages or accessory structures of an organ.

The Orbit

The **orbit,** also known as the **eye socket,** is the bony cavity of the skull that contains and protects the eyeball and its associated muscles, blood vessels, and nerves.

The Eye Muscles

The six major muscles attached to each eye make possible a wide range of movement (Figure 11.2).

● The muscles of both eyes work together in coordinated movements that enable normal binocular vision. *Binocular* refers to the use of both eyes working together.

The Eyelids

The **upper** and **lower eyelids** of each eye protect the eyeball from foreign matter, excessive light, and impact.

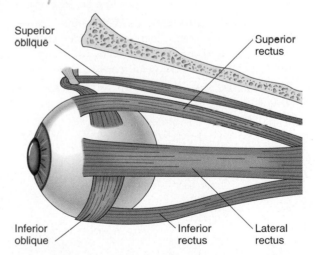

FIGURE 11.2 Six muscles, arranged in three pairs, make major eye movement possible. These are the superior and inferior rectus, superior and inferior oblique, and lateral and medial rectus (not visible here).

● The **canthus** (**KAN**-thus) is the angle where the upper and lower eyelids meet (plural, **canthi**).

● The **inner canthus** is where the eyelids meet nearest the nose. The **epicanthus** (**ep**-ih-**KAN**-thus) is a vertical fold of skin on either side of the nose. In some people, this covers the inner canthus.

- The **tarsus** (**TAHR**-suhs), also known as the **tarsal plate,** is the platelike framework within the upper and lower eyelids that provides stiffness and shape. *Caution: Tarsus* also refers to the seven tarsal bones of the instep (plural, **tarsi**).

The Eyebrows and Eyelashes

The **eyebrows** and **eyelashes** prevent foreign matter from reaching the eyes.

- The edges of the eyelids contain **cilia** (**SIL**-ee-ah), also known as **eyelashes,** and oil-producing sebaceous glands.

The Conjunctiva

The **conjunctiva** (**kon**-junk-**TYE**-vah) is the mucous membrane that lines the underside of each eyelid and continues to form a protective covering over the exposed surface of the eyeball (plural, **conjunctivae**).

The Lacrimal Apparatus

The **lacrimal apparatus** (**LACK**-rih-mal), also known as the **tear apparatus,** consists of the structures that produce, store, and remove tears.

- The **lacrimal glands** are located above the outer corner of each eye. These glands secrete **lacrimal fluid,** also known as **tears,** that maintains moisture on the anterior surface of the eyeball.

- **Lacrimation** (**lack**-rih-**MAY**-shun) is the normal continuous secretion of tears by the lacrimal glands.

- The **lacrimal canaliculi** (**LACK**-rih-mal **kan**-ah-**LICK**-you-lye) are the ducts at the inner corner of each eye. These ducts collect tears and drain them into the lacrimal sac (singular, **canaliculus**).

- The **lacrimal sac,** also known as the **dacryocyst** (**DACK**-ree-oh-sist) or **tear sac,** is an enlargement of the upper portion of the lacrimal duct.

- The **lacrimal duct,** also known as the **nasolacrimal duct,** is the passageway that drains lacrimal fluid into the nose.

THE EYEBALL

The eyeball, also known as the **globe,** is a one-inch sphere with walls made up of three layers: the sclera, choroid, and retina (Figure 11.3). The interior of the eye is divided into anterior and posterior segments.

THE SCLERA AND CORNEA

The **sclera** (**SKLEHR**-ah), also known as the **white of the eye,** is the fibrous tissue outer layer of the eye. It maintains the shape of the eye and protects the delicate inner layers of tissue. *Caution:* **scler/o** means the white of the eye, and it also means hard.

- The **cornea** (**KOR**-nee-ah) is the transparent anterior portion of the sclera. It is the cornea that provides most of the optical power of the eye.

THE UVEAL TRACT

The **uveal tract** (**YOU**-vee-ahl), also known as the **uvea** (**YOU**-vee-ah), is the vascular layer of the eye. It includes the choroid, iris, and ciliary body (Figure 11.4).

The Choroid

The **choroid** (**KOH**-roid), also known as the **choroid layer** or **choroid coat,** is the opaque middle layer of the eyeball. *Opaque* (oh-**PAYK**) means that light cannot pass through this substance.

- The choroid contains many blood vessels and provides the blood supply for the entire eye.

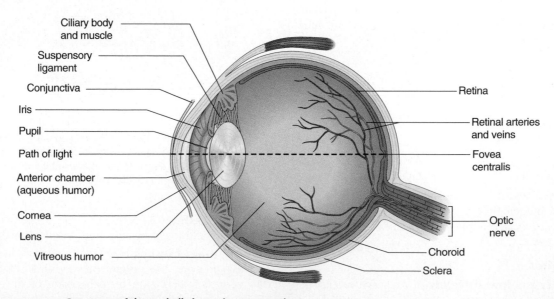

FIGURE 11.3 Structures of the eyeball shown in cross section.

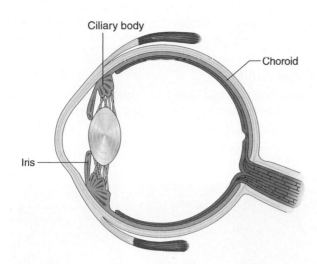

FIGURE 11.4 The uveal tract includes the choroid, iris, and ciliary body.

The Iris, Pupil, and Lens

- The **iris** is the pigmented (colored) muscular layer that surrounds the pupil.
- The **pupil** is the black circular opening in the center of the iris that permits light to enter the eye.
- Muscles within the iris control the amount of light that is allowed to enter. To *decrease* the amount of light, these circular muscles contract and make the opening smaller. To *increase* the amount of light, the muscles dilate (relax) and make the opening larger.
- The **lens,** also known as the **crystalline lens,** is the clear, flexible, curved structure that focuses images on the retina. It is held in place by the suspensory ligaments from the ciliary body. It is contained within a clear capsule and is located behind the iris and pupil.

The Ciliary Body

The **ciliary body** (**SIL**-ee-ehr-ee), which is located within the choroid, is a set of muscles and suspensory ligaments that adjust the lens to refine the focus of light rays on the retina (see Figure 11.4).

- To focus on nearby objects, these muscles adjust the lens to make it *thicker.*
- To focus on distant objects, these muscles stretch the lens so it is *thinner.*

THE RETINA

The **retina** (**RET**-ih-nah) is the sensitive inner nerve layer of the eye located between the posterior chamber and the choroid layer at the back of the eye.

- The retina contains specialized light-sensitive cells called **rods** (black and white receptors) and **cones** (color receptors).
- These rods and cones receive images and convert them into nerve impulses.

The Macula Lutea and Fovea Centralis

- The **macula lutea** (**MACK**-you-lah **LOO**-tee-ah) is a clearly defined yellow area in the center of the retina (**macula** means spot and **lutea** means yellow). This is the area of sharpest central vision.
- The **fovea centralis** (**FOH**-vee-ah sen-**TRAH**-lis) is a pit in the middle of the macula lutea. Color vision is best in this area because it contains a high concentration of cones.

The Optic Disk and Nerve

- The **optic disk,** also known as the **blind spot,** is the region in the eye where the nerve endings of the retina gather to form the optic nerve. It is called the blind spot because it does not contain any rods or cones.
- The **optic nerve,** also known as the **second cranial nerve (CN II),** transmits the nerve impulses from the retina to the brain.

SEGMENTS OF THE EYE

The eye is divided into anterior and posterior segments.

Anterior Segment of the Eye

The front one-third of the eyeball, known as the **anterior segment,** is divided into anterior and posterior chambers (Figure 11.5).

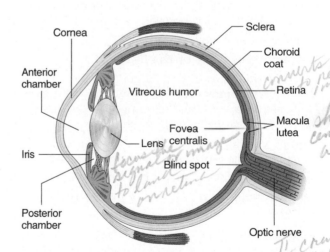

FIGURE 11.5 The anterior portion of the eye (in front of the lens) contains aqueous humor. The posterior portion (behind the lens capsule) is filled with vitreous humor.

- The **anterior chamber** is located behind the inner surface of the cornea and in front of the iris. The **posterior chamber** is located between the back of the iris and the front of the lens.
- These chambers are filled with **aqueous fluid,** also known as **aqueous humor.** A *humor* is any clear body liquid or semifluid substance.

● This fluid nourishes the intraocular structures and is constantly filtered and drained through the **trabecular meshwork** and the **canal of Schlemm** (Figure 11.6).

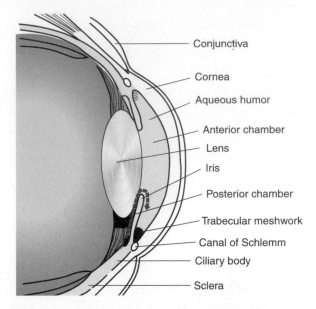

Conjunctiva

Cornea

Aqueous humor

Anterior chamber

Lens

Iris

Posterior chamber

Trabecular meshwork

Canal of Schlemm

Ciliary body

Sclera

FIGURE 11.6 The flow of aqueous humor.

● This constant drainage regulates **intraocular pressure (IOP),** which normally is between 12 and 21 mm Hg (see Diagnostic Procedures of the Eye).

Posterior Segment of the Eye

● The **posterior** two-thirds of the eyeball is filled with **vitreous humor** (**VIT**-ree-us), which is also known as **vitreous gel.** This soft, clear, jellylike mass aids the eye in maintaining its shape.

● The posterior portion of the eye is lined with the retina and its related structures.

NORMAL ACTION OF THE EYES

● **Accommodation** (ah-**kom**-oh-**DAY**-shun) is the process whereby the eyes make adjustments for seeing objects at various distances. These adjustments include constriction (narrowing) and dilation (widening) of the pupil, movement of the eyes, and changes in the shape of the lens.

● **Convergence** (kon-**VER**-jens) is the simultaneous inward movement of the two eyes (toward each other), usually in an effort to maintain single binocular vision as an object comes nearer.

● **Emmetropia** (em-eh-**TROH**-pee-ah) **(EM)** is the normal relationship between the refractive power of the eye and the shape of the eye that enables light rays to focus correctly on the retina (**emmetr** means in proper measure and **-opia** means vision condition). Compare this with *hyperopia* and *myopia.*

● **Refraction** is the ability of the lens to bend the light rays to help them focus on the retina (see Figure 11.11A)

Visual Acuity

Visual acuity is the ability to distinguish object details and shape at a distance. Normal vision is stated as 20/20.

● A **Snellen chart** is used to measure visual acuity. The results are recorded as two numbers in fraction form (Figure 11.7).

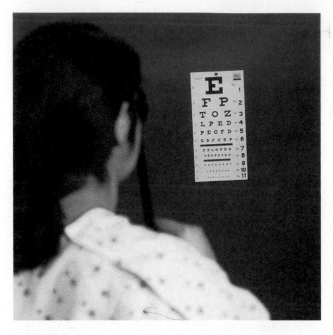

FIGURE 11.7 A Snellen chart is used to measure visual acuity.

● The **first number** indicates the distance from the chart, which is standardized at 20 feet. The **second number** indicates the deviation from the norm based on the ability to read lines of letters on the chart.

● For example, a person with 20/40 vision can read at 20 feet what someone with normal vision could read at 40 feet.

PATHOLOGY OF THE EYES

EYELIDS

● **Blepharoptosis** (**blef**-ah-roh-**TOH**-sis *or* **blef**-ah-rop-**TOH**-sis) is drooping of the upper eyelid (**blephar/o** means eyelid and **-ptosis** means drooping or sagging), see Figure 11.8A.

● **Ectropion** (eck-**TROH**-pee-on) is the eversion (turning outward) of the edge of the eyelid (**ec-** mean out, **trop** means turn, and **-ion** means condition), see Figure 11.8B.

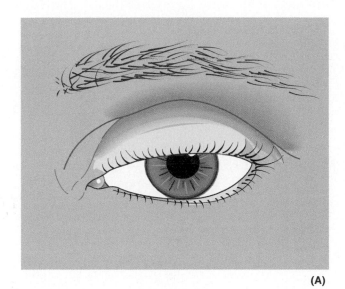

(A)

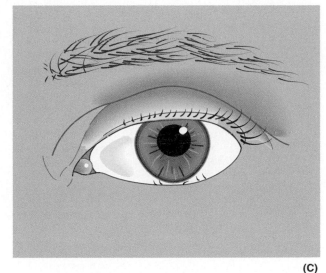

(C)

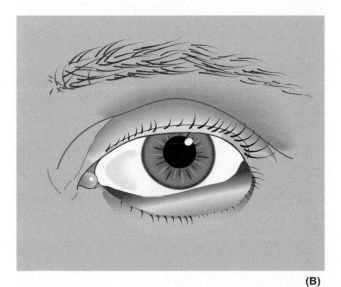

(B)

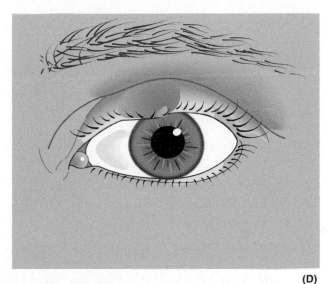

(D)

FIGURE 11.8 Disorders of the eyelid. (A) Blepharoptosis. (B) Ectropion. (C) Entropion. (D) Hordeolum.

- **Entropion** (en-**TROH**-pee-on) is the inversion (turning inward) of the edge of the eyelid (**en-** means in, **trop** means turn, and **-ion** means condition), see Figure 11.8C.

- A **hordeolum** (hor-**DEE**-oh-lum), also known as a **stye,** is an infection of one or more glands at the border of the eyelid, see Figure 11.8D.

- A **chalazion** (kah-**LAY**-zee-on), also known as an **internal hordeolum,** is a localized swelling of the eyelid resulting from obstruction of one of the sebaceous (oil-producing) glands of the eyelid.

ADDITIONAL ADNEXA PATHOLOGY

- **Dacryocystitis** (**dack**-ree-oh-sis-**TYE**-tis) is an inflammation of the lacrimal sac and is associated with faulty tear drainage (**dacryocyst** means tear sac and **-itis** means inflammation).

- **Conjunctivitis** (kon-**junk**-tih-**VYE**-tis), also known as **pinkeye,** is an inflammation of the conjunctiva (**conjunctiv** means conjunctiva and **-itis** means inflammation).

- **Xerophthalmia** (**zeer**-ahf-**THAL**-mee-ah), also known as **dry eye,** is drying of eye surfaces characterized by the loss of luster of the conjunctiva and cornea (**xer-** means dry, **ophthalm** means eye, and **-ia** means abnormal condition).

SCLERA, CORNEA, AND IRIS

- **Scleritis** (skleh-**RYE**-tis) is an inflammation of the sclera (**scler** means white of eye and **-itis** means inflammation). *Note:* **scler/o** also means hard.

- **Keratitis** (**ker**-ah-**TYE**-tis) is an inflammation of the cornea (**kerat** means cornea and **-itis** means inflammation). *Note:* **kerat/o** also means hard.

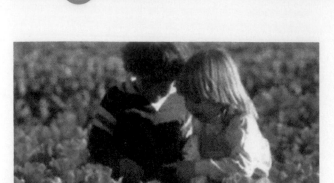

normal vision

(A)

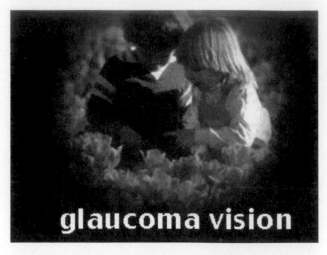

glaucoma vision

(C)

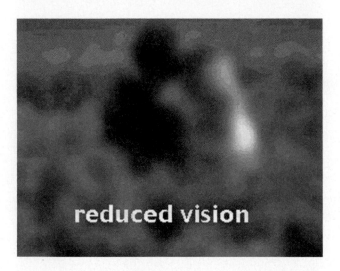

reduced vision

(B)

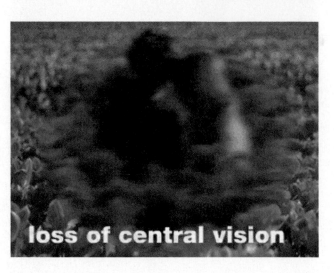

loss of central vision

(D)

FIGURE 11.9 Normal vision and pathologic vision changes. (A) Normal vision. (B) Vision reduced by cataracts. (C) The loss of peripheral vision caused by untreated glaucoma. (D) The loss of central vision due to macular degeneration.

- A **corneal abrasion** is an injury, such as a scratch or irritation, to the outer layers of the cornea.

- A **corneal ulcer** is a pitting of the cornea caused by an infection or injury. Although these ulcers heal with treatment, they may leave a cloudy scar that impairs vision.

- **Iritis** (eye-**RYE**-tis) is an inflammation of the iris (**irit** means iris, and **-itis** means inflammation).

- **Synechia** (sigh-**NECK**-ee-ah) is an adhesion that binds the iris to any adjacent structure (plural, **synechiae**). An *adhesion* (ad-**HE**-zhun) holds structures together abnormally.

THE EYE

- **Anisocoria** (**an**-ih-so-**KOH**-ree-ah) is a condition in which the pupils are unequal in size (**anis/o** means

unequal, **cor** means pupil, and **-ia** means abnormal condition). This may be congenital (present at birth) or caused by a head injury, aneurysm, or pathology of the central nervous system.

- A **cataract** (**KAT**-ah-rakt) is the loss of transparency of the lens. This may be congenital (present at birth) or caused by trauma (injury) or disease. However, the formation of most cataracts is associated with aging (see Figure 11.9B).

- **Choked disk,** also known as **papilledema** (**pap**-ill-eh-**DEE**-mah), is swelling and inflammation of the optic nerve at the point of entrance through the optic disk. This swelling is caused by increased intracranial pressure and may be due to a tumor pressing on the optic nerve.

- **Floaters,** also known as **vitreous floaters,** are particles that float in the vitreous fluid and cast shadows on the retina. Floaters occur normally with aging or in association with vitreous detachments, retinal tears, or intraocular inflammations.

- **Nystagmus** (nis-**TAG**-mus) is an involuntary, constant, rhythmic movement of the eyeball.

- In a **retinal detachment,** also known as a **detached retina,** the retina is pulled away from its normal position of being attached to the choroid in the back of the eye. A **retinal tear** occurs when the retina tears (develops a hole) as it is pulled away from its normal position.

- **Uveitis** (**you**-vee-**EYE**-tis) is an inflammation anywhere in the uveal tract (**uve** means uveal tract and **-itis** means inflammation). It may affect the choroid, iris, or ciliary body and has many possible causes, including diseases elsewhere in the body. Uveitis can rapidly damage the eye and produce complications including cataracts, detached retina, and glaucoma.

Glaucoma

Glaucoma (glaw-**KOH**-mah) is a group of diseases characterized by increased intraocular pressure (IOP), resulting in damage to the optic nerve and retinal nerve fibers. If left untreated, this pressure damages the optic nerve and causes the loss of peripheral vision and eventually blindness (see Figure 11.9C).

- In **open-angle glaucoma,** which is the most common form of glaucoma, the trabecular meshwork becomes blocked.

- In **closed-angle glaucoma,** the opening between the cornea and iris narrows so that fluid cannot reach the trabecular meshwork. This narrowing may cause a sudden increase in pressure and produce severe pain, nausea, redness of the eye, and blurred vision. Without immediate treatment, blindness may occur in as little as two days.

- Glaucoma does not produce symptoms noticed by the patient until the optic nerve has been damaged. However, it can be detected before damage occurs through regular eye examinations including tonometry and visual field testing (see Diagnostic Procedures of the Eyes).

Macular Degeneration

Macular degeneration (**MACK**-you-lar) is a gradually progressive condition that results in the loss of central vision but not in total blindness (Figure 11.9D). This condition, which most frequently affects older people, is also known as **age-related macular degeneration (AMD).**

- **Dry type macular degeneration,** which accounts for 90 percent of cases, is caused by the atrophy (deterioration) of the macula.

- **Wet type macular degeneration** is associated with the formation of new blood vessels that produce small hemorrhages.

FUNCTIONAL DEFECTS

- **Diplopia** (dih-**PLOH**-pee-ah), also known as **double vision,** is the perception of two images of a single object (**dipl** means double and **-opia** means vision condition).

- **Hemianopia** (**hem**-ee-ah-**NOH**-pee-ah) is blindness in one half of the visual field.

- **Monochromatism** (**mon**-oh-**KROH**-mah-tizm), also known as **color blindness,** is the lack of the ability to distinguish colors (**mon/o** means one, **chromat** means color, and **-ism** means condition).

- **Nyctalopia** (**nick**-tah-**LOH**-pee-ah), also known as **night blindness,** is a condition in which the individual has difficulty seeing at night (**nyctal** means night and **-opia** means vision condition).

- **Presbyopia** (**pres**-bee-**OH**-pee-ah) describes the changes in the eyes that occur with aging (**presby** means old age and **-opia** means vision condition). With aging, the lens becomes less flexible, and the muscles of the ciliary body become weaker. The result is that the eyes are no longer able to focus the image properly on the retina.

Strabismus

- **Strabismus** (strah-**BIZ**-mus), also known as a **squint,** is a disorder in which the eyes cannot be directed in a parallel manner toward the same object (Figure 11.10).

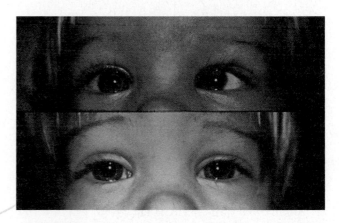

FIGURE 11.10 A child with strabismus before and after corrective treatment. (Courtesy of the National Eye Institute.)

- **Esotropia** (**es**-oh-**TROH**-pee-ah), also known as **cross-eyes,** is strabismus characterized by an inward deviation of one eye in relation to the other (**eso-** means inward, **trop** means turn, and **-ia** means abnormal condition).

- **Exotropia** (**eck**-soh-**TROH**-pee-ah), also known as **walleye,** is strabismus characterized by the outward deviation of one eye relative to the other (**exo-** means outward, **trop** means turn, and **-ia** means abnormal condition).

REFRACTIVE DISORDERS

A **refractive disorder** is a condition in which the lens and cornea do not bend light so that it focuses properly on the retina. (Normal refraction is shown in Figure 11.11A.)

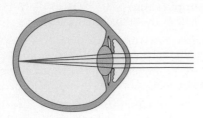

(A) Normal eye
Light rays focus on the retina

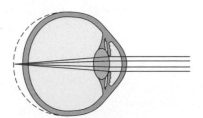

(B) Hyperopia (farsightedness)
Light rays focus beyond
the retina

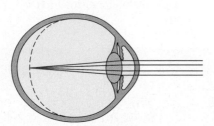

(C) Myopia (nearsightedness)
Light rays focus in front
of the retina

FIGURE 11.11 Refraction. (A) Normal eye. (B) Hyperopia (farsightedness). (C) Myopia (nearsightedness).

- **Ametropia** (**am**-eh-**TROH**-pee-ah) is any error of refraction in which images do not focus properly on the retina (**ametr** means out of proportion and **-opia** means vision condition). Astigmatism, hyperopia, and myopia are all froms of ametropia.
- **Astigmatism** (ah-**STIG**-mah-tizm) is a condition in which the eye does not focus properly because of uneven curvatures of the cornea.
- **Hyperopia** (**high**-per-**OH**-pee-ah), also known as **farsightedness,** is a defect in which light rays focus beyond the retina (**hyper-** means excessive and **-opia** means vision condition). This condition occurs most commonly after age 40 (see Figure 11.11B).
- **Myopia** (my-**OH**-pee-ah), also known as **nearsightedness,** is a defect in which light rays focus in front

of the retina. This condition occurs most commonly in school-aged children (see Figure 11.11C).

BLINDNESS

- **Amblyopia** (**am**-blee-**OH**-pee-ah) is a dimness of vision or the partial loss of sight without detectable disease of the eye (**ambly** means dim or dull and **-opia** means vision condition).
- **Blindness** is the inability to see. Although some sight remains, **legal blindness** is the point at which, under law, an individual is considered to be blind. A commonly used standard is that a person is legally blind when his or her best-corrected vision is reduced to 20/200 or less (see Normal Action of the Eyes).
- **Scotoma** (skoh-**TOH**-mah), also known as a **blind spot,** is an abnormal area of absent or depressed vision surrounded by an area of normal vision.

DIAGNOSTIC PROCEDURES OF THE EYES

- **Visual acuity measurement** (ah-**KYOU**-ih-tee) is an evaluation of the eye's ability to distinguish object details and shape (see Normal Action of the Eyes.)
- **Refraction** is an examination procedure to determine an eye's refractive error and the best corrective lenses to be prescribed. A **diopter** (dye-**AHP**-tur) is a unit of measurement of lens refractive power.
- **Tonometry** (toh-**NOM**-eh-tree) measures **intraocular pressure (IOP).** Abnormally high pressure may be an indication of glaucoma.
- In preparation for an examination of the interior of the eye, it is necessary to **dilate** (**DYE**-layt) the pupils. Dilation is accomplished by administering **mydriatic drops** (**mid**-ree-**AT**-ick) that produce temporary paralysis, which forces the pupils to remain wide open even in the presence of bright light. (*Dilation* is the artificial enlargement of an opening.)

SPECIALIZED DIAGNOSTIC PROCEDURES

- **Fluorescein staining** (**flew**-oh-**RES**-ee-in) is used to visualize a corneal abrasion (injury). When the stain is applied, corneal abrasions are stained bright green.
- In **intravenous fluorescein angiography** (**flew**-oh-**RES**-ee-in **an**-jee-**OG**-rah-fee) **(IVFA),** a dye is injected into a vein in the arm, and pictures are taken as the dye passes through the blood vessels in the retina. This test allows the examiner to detect leaking blood vessels within the eye.
- A **visual field test** is used to determine losses in peripheral vision. Such a loss is characteristic of glaucoma.

TREATMENT PROCEDURES OF THE EYES

THE ORBIT AND EYELIDS

- **Orbitotomy** (**or**-bih-**TOT**-oh-mee) is a surgical incision into the orbit for biopsy, abscess drainage, or the removal of a tumor mass or foreign object (**orbit** means bony socket and **-otomy** means surgical incision).

- A **tarsectomy** (tahr-**SECK**-toh-mee) is the surgical removal of a segment of the tarsal plate of the upper or lower eyelid (**tars** means eyelid and **-ectomy** means surgical removal).

- **Tarsorrhaphy** (tahr-**SOR**-ah-fee) is the partial or complete suturing together of the upper and lower eyelids (**tars/o** means eyelid and **-rrhaphy** means to suture). This procedure is performed to provide protection to the eye when the lids are paralyzed and unable to close normally.

- Cosmetic procedures relating to the eyelids are discussed further in Chapter 12.

CONJUNCTIVA, CORNEA, AND IRIS

- **Conjunctivoplasty** (**kon**-junk-**TYE**-voh-**plas**-tee) is the surgical repair of the conjunctiva (**conjunctiv** means conjunctiva and **-plasty** means surgical repair).

- A **corneal transplant**, also known as **keratoplasty** (**KER**-ah-toh-**plas**-tee), is the surgical replacement of scarred or diseased cornea with clear corneal tissue from a donor (**kerat/o** means cornea and **-plasty** means surgical repair).

- An **iridectomy** (**ir**-ih-**DECK**-toh-mee) is the surgical removal of a portion of the iris tissue (**irid** means iris and **-ectomy** means surgical removal).

- **Radial keratotomy** (ker-ah-**TOT**-oh-mee) **(RK)** is used to correct myopia (**kerat** means cornea, and **-otomy** means surgical incision). During the surgery, incisions made partially through the cornea cause it to flatten.

CATARACT SURGERY

- **Lensectomy** (len-**SECK**-toh-mee) is the general term used to describe the surgical removal of a cataract-clouded lens.

- **Extracapsular cataract extraction (ECCE)** is the removal of a cloudy lens that leaves the posterior lens capsule intact (Figure 11.12).

- **Intracapsular cataract extraction (ICCE)** is the removal of a cloudy lens including the surrounding capsule.

- **Phacoemulsification** (**fay**-koh-ee-**mul**-sih-fih-**KAY**-shun *or* **fack**-koh-ee-**mul**-sih-fih-**KAY**-shun) is the use

Lens Implant Surgery for Cataracts

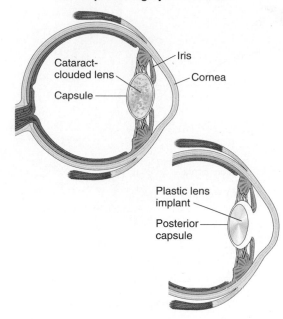

FIGURE 11.12 In an extracapsular extraction, the lens is removed, the posterior lens capsule is left intact, and an intraocular lens (IOL) is placed.

of ultrasonic vibration to shatter and break up a cataract making it easier to remove.

- An **intraocular lens (IOL)** is a plastic lens that is surgically implanted to replace the natural lens.

- **Aphakia** (ah-**FAY**-kee-ah) is the absence of the lens of an eye after cataract extraction (**a-** means without, **phak** means lens, and **-ia** means abnormal condition).

- **Pseudophakia** (**soo**-doh-**FAY**-kee-ah) is an eye in which the natural lens is replaced with an IOL (**pseudo/o** means false, **phak** means lens, and **-ia** means abnormal condition).

LASER TREATMENTS

Lasers have a wide range of applications in the treatment of eye disorders. (For more details on how lasers work, see Chapter 12.) In the treatment of eye disorders, lasers are used for the following reasons:

- To treat **open-angle glaucoma** by creating an opening that allows fluid to drain properly to prevent pressure buildup within the eye. This procedure is known as **laser trabeculoplasty** (trah-**BECK**-you-loh-**plas**-tee).

- To treat **closed-angle glaucoma** by creating an opening in the iris to allow proper drainage. This procedure is known as **laser iridotomy** (ir-ih-**DOT**-oh-mee).

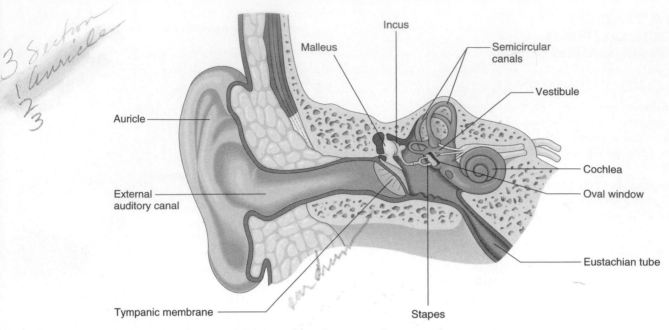

FIGURE 11.13 Structures of the ear shown in cross section.

- To treat some forms of **macular degeneration** by sealing leaking or damaged blood vessels.
- To treat **retinal tears** by sealing the torn portion.
- To reattach a **detached retina.** This procedure is also known as **retinopexy** (**RET**-ih-noh-**peck**-see).
- To correct **refraction disorders** by reshaping of the top layer of the cornea. This procedure is known as **photo refractive keratectomy** (**ker**-ah-**TECK**-toh-mee) or **PRK.**
- To remove **clouded tissue** that may form in the posterior portion of the lens capsule after cataract extraction.

STRUCTURES OF THE EARS

The ear is divided into three separate regions: the outer ear, middle ear, and inner ear (Figure 11.13).

THE OUTER EAR

- The **pinna** (**PIN**-nah), also known as the **auricle,** is the external portion of the ear. This structure catches sound waves and transmits them into the external auditory canal.
- The **external auditory canal** transmits sound waves from the pinna to the middle ear.
- **Cerumen** (seh-**ROO**-men), also known as **earwax,** is secreted by ceruminous glands that line the auditory canal. This sticky yellow-brown substance has protective functions as it traps small insects, dust, debris, and certain bacteria to prevent them from entering the middle ear.

THE MIDDLE EAR

- The **tympanic membrane** (tim-**PAN**-ick) **(TM),** also known as the **eardrum,** is located between the outer and middle ear (Figure 11.14). (The word parts **myring/o** and **tympan/o** both mean tympanic membrane.)

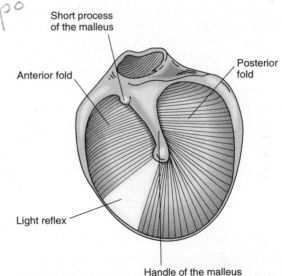

FIGURE 11.14 Schematic of the normal tympanic membrane as viewed from the auditory canal.

- When sound waves reach it, this membrane transmits the sound by vibrating.
- The middle ear is surrounded by the **mastoid cells,** which are hollow air spaces located in the mastoid process of the temporal bone. An infection in the middle ear can rapidly spread to these cells.

The Auditory Ossicles

The **auditory ossicles** (**OSS**-ih-kulz) are three small bones found in the middle ear. These bones transmit the sound waves from the eardrum to the inner ear by vibration. These bones, which are named for their shapes, are the

- **Malleus** (**MAL**-ee-us), also known as the **hammer**
- **Incus** (**ING**-kus), also known as the **anvil**
- **Stapes** (**STAY**-peez), also known as the **stirrup**

The Eustachian Tubes

The **eustachian tubes** (you-**STAY**-shun *or* you-**STAY**-kee-an) are also known as the **auditory tubes.** These narrow tubes, which lead from the middle ear to the nasopharynx, equalize the air pressure in the middle ear with that of the outside atmosphere.

THE INNER EAR

The **inner ear,** also known as the **labyrinth** (**LAB**-ih-rinth), contains the sensory receptors for hearing and balance.

- The **oval window,** located under the base of the stapes, is the membrane that separates the middle ear from the inner ear.
- The **cochlea** (**KOCK**-lee-ah) is the spiral passage that leads from the oval window.
- The **cochlear duct,** located within the cochlea, is filled with fluid that vibrates when the sound waves strike it.
- The **organ of Corti,** also located within the cochlea, is the receptor site that receives these vibrations and relays them to the **auditory nerve fibers,** which transmit them to the auditory center of the cerebral cortex, where they are interpreted and heard.
- The three **semicircular canals,** also located within the inner ear, contain **endolymph** (a liquid) and sensitive hairlike cells. The bending of these hairlike cells in response to the movements of the head sets up impulses in nerve fibers to help maintain equilibrium. *Equilibrium* is the state of balance.
- The **acoustic nerves** (cranial nerve VIII) transmit this information to the brain, and the brain sends messages to muscles in all parts of the body to ensure that equilibrium is maintained.

NORMAL ACTION OF THE EARS

- Sound waves enter the ear through the pinna, travel down the auditory canal, and strike the tympanic membrane between the outer and middle ear. This process is called **air conduction.**
- As the eardrum vibrates, it moves the auditory ossicles, and these conduct sound waves through the middle ear. This process is called **bone conduction.**

- Sound vibrations reach the inner ear via the oval window. The structures of the inner ear receive the sound waves and relay them to the brain. This process is called **sensorineural conduction.**

PATHOLOGY OF THE EARS

THE OUTER EAR

- **Impacted cerumen** is an accumulation of cerumen that forms a solid mass adhering to the walls of the external auditory canal. *Impacted* means lodged or wedged firmly in place.
- **Otalgia** (oh-**TAL**-gee-ah), also known as an **ear-ache,** is pain in the ear (**ot** means ear and **-algia** means pain).
- **Otitis** (oh-**TYE**-tis) means any inflammation of the ear (**ot** means ear and **-itis** means inflammation). The second term gives the location of the inflammation.
- **Otitis externa** is an inflammation of the outer ear.
- **Otomycosis** (oh-toh-my-**KOH**-sis), also known as **swimmer's ear,** is a fungal infection of the external auditory canal (**ot/o** means ear, **myc** means fungus, and **-osis** means abnormal condition).
- **Otopyorrhea** (oh-toh-pye-oh-**REE**-ah) is the flow of pus from the ear (**ot/o** means ear, **py/o** means pus, and **-rrhea** means abnormal flow).
- **Otorrhagia** (oh-toh-**RAY**-jee-ah) is bleeding from the ear (**ot/o** means ear and **-rrhagia** means bleeding).

THE MIDDLE EAR

- **Eustachitis** (you-stay-**KYE**-tis) is an inflammation of the eustachian tube (**eustach** means eustachian tube and **-Itis** means inflammation).
- **Mastoiditis** (mas-toy-**DYE**-tis) is an inflammation of any part of the mastoid process (**mastoid** means mastoid process and **-itis** means inflammation).
- **Myringitis** (mir-in-**JIGH**-tis) is an inflammation of the tympanic membrane (**myring** means eardrum and **-itis** means inflammation).
- **Otosclerosis** (oh-toh-skleh-**ROH**-sis) is ankylosis of the bones of the middle ear resulting in a conductive hearing loss (**ot/o** means ear, and **-sclerosis** means abnormal hardening). *Ankylosis* (ang-kih-**LOH**-sis) means fused together.
- **Patulous eustachian tube** (**PAT**-you-lus) is distention of the eustachian tube. *Patulous* means extended, spread wide open.

Otitis Media

- **Acute otitis media** (oh-**TYE**-tis **MEE**-dee-ah) **(AOM)** is an inflammation of the middle ear usually associated with an upper respiratory infection that is most commonly seen in young children.

(A) Serous otitis media

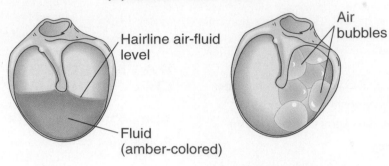

Hairline air-fluid level

Air bubbles

Fluid (amber-colored)

(B) Acute purulent otitis media

Early

Late

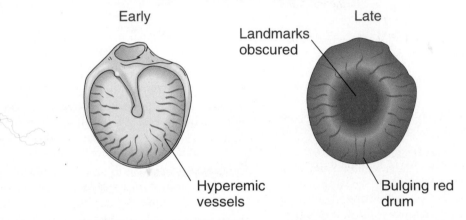

Landmarks obscured

Hyperemic vessels

Bulging red drum

FIGURE 11.15 The tympanic membrane in the presence of otitis media. (A) Serious otitis media. (B) Acute purulent otitis media. *Hyperemic* means increased blood within these vessels.

- **Serous otitis media** (**SEER**-us oh-**TYE**-tis **MEE**-dee-ah) (**SOM**) is a fluid buildup in the middle ear that may follow acute otitis media or be caused by an obstruction of the eustachian tube (Figure 11.15A).

- SOM is also known as **otitis media with effusion**. *Effusion* (eh-**FEW**-zhun) is the escape of fluid from blood or lymphatic vessels into the tissues or a cavity.

- **Purulent otitis media** (**PYOU**-roo-lent oh-**TYE**-tis **MEE**-dee-ah) is a buildup of pus within the middle ear (Figure 11.15B).

THE INNER EAR

- **Labyrinthitis** (**lab**-ih-rin-**THIGH**-tis) is an inflammation of the labyrinth that may result in vertigo and deafness.

- **Vertigo** (**VER**-tih-goh), which is a symptom of several conditions, is described as a sense of whirling, dizziness, and the loss of balance.

- **Ménière's syndrome** (**men**-ee-**AYRZ** *or* men-**YEHRS**) is a chronic disease of the inner ear characterized by three main symptoms: attacks of vertigo, a fluctuating hearing loss (usually in one ear), and tinnitus.

- **Tinnitus** (tih-**NIGH**-tus) is a ringing, buzzing, or roaring sound in the ears.

HEARING LOSS

- **Deafness** is the complete or partial loss of the ability to hear. It may range from the inability to hear sounds of a certain pitch or intensity to a complete loss of hearing.

- A **conductive hearing loss** is one in which the outer or middle ear does not conduct sound vibrations to the inner ear normally.

- A **noise-induced hearing loss** is the result of the loss of sensitive hairlike cells of the inner ear. This damage is most commonly caused by repeated exposure to very intense noise such as aircraft engines, noisy equipment, and loud music.

- A **sensorineural hearing loss,** also known as **nerve deafness,** is a symptom of problems affecting the inner ear.

- **Presbycusis** (**pres**-beh-**KOO**-sis) is a progressive hearing loss occurring in old age (**presby** means old age and **-cusis** means hearing).

DIAGNOSTIC PROCEDURES OF THE EARS

- **Audiometry** (aw-dee-**OM**-eh-tree) is the use of an audiometer to measure hearing (**audio** means hearing and **-metry** means to measure).

- An **audiometer** (aw-dee-**OM**-eh-ter) is an electronic device that produces acoustic stimuli of a known frequency and intensity (**audi/o** means hearing and **-meter** means to measure).

- **Speech audiometry** measures the threshold of speech reception (hearing speech sounds) and speech discrimination (understanding speech sounds).

- An **evoked potential audiometer** is an instrument that detects response to sound stimuli by changes in the electroencephalogram (record of brain wave activity).

- **Tympanometry** (tim-pah-**NOM**-eh-tree) is the indirect measurement of acoustical energy absorbed or reflected by the middle ear (**tympan/o** means eardrum and **-metry** means to measure). In a conductive hearing loss, the middle ear absorbs relatively less sound and reflects relatively more sound. This test is used to test for middle ear effusion (fluid buildup) or eustachian tube obstruction. The resulting record is a **tympanogram.**

- **Monaural** (mon-**AW**-rahl) testing involves one ear (**mon-** means one, **aur** means hearing, and **-al** means pertaining to).

- **Binaural** (bye-**NAW**-rul *or* bin-**AW**-rahl) testing involves both ears (**bi-** means two, **aur** means hearing, and **-al** means pertaining to).

TREATMENT PROCEDURES OF THE EARS

THE OUTER EAR

- **Otoplasty** (**OH**-toh-**plas**-tee) is the surgical repair of the pinna of the ear (**ot/o** means ear and **-plasty** means surgical repair).

THE MIDDLE EAR

- A **mastoidectomy** (**mas**-toy-**DECK**-toh-mee) is the surgical removal of mastoid cells (**mastoid** means mastoid process and **-ectomy** means surgical removal).

- A **myringectomy** (**mir**-in-**JECK**-toh-mee), also known as a **tympanectomy** (tim-pah-**NECK**-toh-me), is the surgical removal of all or part of the tympanic membrane (**myring** means eardrum and **-ectomy** means surgical removal).

- A **myringotomy** (**mir**-in-**GOT**-oh-mee) is the surgical incision of the eardrum to create an opening for the placement of tympanostomy tubes (**myring** means eardrum and **-otomy** means surgical incision).

- **Tympanostomy tubes** (tim-pan-**OSS**-toh-mee), also known as **pediatric ear tubes,** are tiny ventilating tubes placed through the eardrum to provide ongoing drainage for fluids and to relieve pressure that can build up after ear infections.

- **Tympanocentesis** (tim-pah-noh-sen-**TEE**-sis) is the surgical puncture of the tympanic membrane with a needle to remove fluid from the middle ear (**tympan/o** means eardrum and **-centesis** means a surgical puncture to remove fluid).

- **Tympanoplasty** (tim-pah-noh-**PLAS**-tee) is the surgical correction of a damaged middle ear (**tympan/o** means eardrum and **-plasty** means a surgical repair).

- A **stapedectomy** (stay-peh-**DECK**-toh-mee) is the surgical removal of the stapes.

The Inner Ear

- A **fenestration** (fen-es-**TRAY**-shun) is a surgical procedure in which a new opening is made in the labyrinth of the inner ear to restore hearing.

- A **labyrinthectomy** (**lab**-ih-rin-**THECK**-toh-mee) is the surgical removal of the labyrinth (**labyrinth** means labyrinth and **-ectomy** means surgical removal).

- A **labyrinthotomy** (**lab**-ih-rin-**THOT**-oh-mee) is a surgical incision into the labyrinth (**labyrinth** means labyrinth and **-otomy** means a surgical incision).

Career Opportunities

In addition to the medical specialties already discussed, some of the health occupations involving the treatment of the eyes and ears include

- **Ophthalmic dispenser** or **dispensing optician:** places orders for prescribed ophthalmic laboratory work, helps patients select frames, adjusts finished glasses, and may fit patients for contact lenses

- **Ocularist:** a dispensing optician who specializes in fitting artificial eyes

- **Ophthalmic laboratory technician:** grinds, finishes, polishes, and mounts lenses for eyeglasses and contact lenses

- **Optometric technician (OpT)** or **paraoptometric:** works under the supervision of an ophthalmologist (or optometrist) preparing patients for examinations, performing receptionist duties, helping patients with frame selection, and instructing patients in the care and use of their contact lenses. An OpT also administers basic vision tests and teaches eye exercises.

- **Optometric assistant:** performs the same duties as an OpT, with the exception of administering vision testing and teaching eye exercises

- **Orientation and mobility instructor:** teaches visually challenged individuals how to move about safely in a variety of environments

- **Audiologist:** provides care to individuals with hearing problems, testing, diagnosing, and prescribing treatment. Audiologists also conduct noise-level testing in workplaces and work to prevent hearing loss.

- **Speech/language therapist** or **pathologist:** identifies, evaluates, and treats patients with speech and language disorders; may work with elementary or preschool children or in the rehabilitation of stroke patients

Health Occupation Profile: AUDIOLOGIST

Perry C. Hanavan is an audiologist in Sioux Falls, South Dakota. "As an audiologist, I identify, diagnose, treat, and manage individuals with communication disorders resulting from hearing loss. From diagnosing hearing problems in newborns to providing audiologic services to elderly persons who suffer a hearing loss, this profession provides challenging and stimulating career experiences across the life span."

"Audiologists select, dispense, and fit hearing aids and assistive listening devices and are a part of the cochlear implant team. Increasingly, audiologists rely on a variety of technologies to fit programmable and digital hearing aids, to assess auditory brain activity, and to assess middle ear and inner ear function."

"I was in search of a profession that included psychology, science, and technology when I discovered the fascinating field of audiology while in college. I am now an assistant professor, teaching audiology courses and supervising students providing audiologic services."

STUDY BREAK

Images seen through the *rods* and *cones* of the eye's *retina* are converted into nerve impulses to be interpreted by the brain. Sometimes, the brain gets confused by the images it receives, as is the case of an optical illusion. Try this famous Floating Finger optical illusion:

- Hold your hands in front of you at eye level. Point your index fingers toward each other. Leave a little space (an inch or so) between your two index fingers. With your fingers at eye level, focus on a wall or an object a few feet away.

- You should see a finger with two ends floating in between your two index fingers. If you have trouble seeing it, try moving your fingers closer to your eyes (still at eye level).

- For a different illusion, try this with your two index fingers actually touching each other.

Optical illusions are part of our everyday vision. Newspaper illustrations and computer screens, for example, are made up of small colored dots that our brain merges into solid images. If the optic nerve could transmit only literal impulses to the brain, we would not be able to enjoy television, animation, and many other wonderful optical illusions.

Review Time

Write the answers to the following questions on a separate piece of paper or in your notebook. In addition, be prepared to take part in the classroom discussion.

1. **Written assignment:** Using terms a physician would understand, describe the differences between **open-angle glaucoma** and **closed-angle glaucoma.**

   Discussion assignment: What test is performed to detect glaucoma?

2. **Written assignment:** Describe the differences between a **conductive hearing loss** and a **noise-induced hearing loss.**

   Discussion assignment: What steps can be taken to prevent a noise-induced hearing loss, and at what age should one begin taking these precautions?

3. **Written assignment:** Using terms a patient would understand, describe the difference in the vision loss between a patient with **glaucoma** and one with **macular degeneration.**

   Discussion assignment: How would each of these vision losses affect the patient's quality of life?

4. **Written assignment:** Describe the difference between **tinnitus** and **vertigo.**

   Discussion assignment: How would each of these conditions affect the patient?

5. **Written assignment:** Describe the difference between **hyperopia** and **myopia.**

   Discussion assignment: How would you explain each of these conditions to a young patient and her family?

Optional Internet Activity

*The goal of this activity is to help you learn more about medical terminology while improving your Internet skills. Select **one** of these two options and follow the instructions.*

1. **Internet Search:** Search for information about **glaucoma.** Write a brief (one- or two-paragraph) report on something new you learned here and include the address of the web site where you found this information.

2. **Web Site:** To learn more about **tinnitus,** go to this web address: **http://www.ata.org/.** Explore the site and then write a brief (one- or two-paragraph) report on something new you learned here.

The Human Touch: Critical Thinking Exercise

The following story and questions are designed to stimulate critical thinking through class discussion or as a brief essay response. There are no right or wrong answers to these questions.

William Davis is 62 years old. He was employed as a postal worker until his declining eyesight forced him into early retirement a few months ago. His wife, Mildred, died last year of complications from diabetes after a prolonged and expensive hospitalization. Mr. Davis does not trust the medical community and, because of this distrust, he has not been to a doctor since his wife's death.

Mr. Davis is not considered legally blind, but his presbyopia and the advancing cataract in his right eye are starting to interfere with his ability to take care of himself. He still drives to the market once a week, but angry drivers honk and yell at him. He pays for his groceries with a credit card because he is afraid the checker will cheat him if he accidentally gives her the wrong bill. He complains that the cleaning lady hides things from him and deliberately leaves the furniture out of place. When she leaves, he can't find his slippers or an ashtray. Yesterday, he put his lit pipe down in a wooden bowl by accident.

His son insists on taking him to see the ophthalmologist who treated his wife's diabetic retinopathy. Dr. Hsing believes Mr. Davis's sight can be improved in the right eye by performing cataract surgery. Mr. Davis listens in fear as the doctor explains. "Without this procedure your sight will only get worse."

Mr. Davis thinks about all the medical procedures that were tried on Mildred, and she died anyway. He doesn't want to go into the hospital, and he doesn't want any operations. But his son is talking about taking away his car if he doesn't do something about his failing sight. "What more can be taken away from me?" he thinks bitterly. "First my wife, then my job, and now my independence."

Suggested Discussion Topics

1. Discuss how Mr. Davis's loss of sight is affecting the way he treats others and is treated by them.
2. Mr. Davis is a patient at the clinic where you work. Discuss the ways you would adjust your usual routine to accommodate his needs.
3. Close your eyes and keep them closed for 15 minutes while a classmate or friend leads you around. Discuss how you felt and what could have been done to make the experience less stressful.
4. Discuss why cataract surgery would be scary to Mr. Davis and what Dr. Hsing and his staff could do to ease his apprehension.
5. If Mr. Davis does not go ahead with the surgery, available support groups can help him cope with his vision loss. What groups might help him deal with his grief and depression?

Student Workbook and Student Activity CD-ROM

1. Go to your **Student Workbook** and complete the Learning Exercises for this chapter.
2. Go to the **Student Activity CD-ROM** and have fun with the exercises and games for this chapter.

12

Skin: The Integumentary System

Overview of Structures, Word Parts, and Functions of the Integumentary System

Major Structures	Related Word Parts	Primary Functions
Skin	**cutane/o, dermat/o, derm/o**	Intact skin is the first line of defense for the immune system. Skin also waterproofs the body and is the major receptor for the sense of touch.
Sebaceous glands	**seb/o**	Secrete sebum (oil) to lubricate the skin and discourage the growth of bacteria on the skin.
Sweat glands	**hidr/o**	Secrete sweat to regulate body temperature and water content and excrete some metabolic waste.
Hair	**pil/i, pil/o**	Aids in controlling the loss of body heat.
Nails	**onych/o, ungu/o**	Protect the dorsal surface of the last bone of each finger and toe.

Vocabulary Related to the Skin

Terms marked with the ❖ symbol are pronounced on the Student Activity CD-ROM that accompanies this text.

KEY WORD PARTS

- [ ] **albin/o**
- [ ] **bi/o**
- [ ] **derm/o, dermat/o**
- [ ] **erythr/o**
- [ ] **hidr/o**
- [ ] **kerat/o**
- [ ] **lip/o**
- [ ] **melan/o**
- [ ] **myc/o**
- [ ] **onych/o**
- [ ] **pedicul/o**
- [ ] **pil/o**
- [ ] **rhytid/o**
- [ ] **seb/o**
- [ ] **xer/o**

KEY MEDICAL TERMS

- [ ] **abrasion** (ah-**BRAY**-zhun)
- [ ] **actinic keratosis** (ack-**TIN**-ick **kerr**-ah-**TOH**-sis) ❖
- [ ] **albinism** (**AL**-bih-niz-um) ❖
- [ ] **alopecia** (**al**-oh-**PEE**-shee-ah) ❖
- [ ] **anhidrosis** (an-high-**DROH**-sis) ❖
- [ ] **blepharoplasty** (**BLEF**-ah-roh-**plas**-tee) ❖
- [ ] **bulla** (**BULL**-ah)
- [ ] **carbuncle** (**KAR**-bung-kul) ❖
- [ ] **cauterization** (**kaw**-ter-eye-**ZAY**-shun) ❖
- [ ] **cellulitis** (**sell**-you-**LYE**-tis) ❖
- [ ] **chloasma** (kloh-**AZ**-mah) ❖
- [ ] **cicatrix** (sick-**AY**-tricks) ❖
- [ ] **comedo** (**KOM**-eh-doh) ❖
- [ ] **contusion** (kon-**TOO**-zhun)
- [ ] **debridement** (day-breed-**MON**) ❖
- [ ] **decubitus ulcer** (dee-**KYOU**-bih-tus) ❖
- [ ] **dermabrasion** (der-mah-**BRAY**-zhun) ❖
- [ ] **dermatitis** (der-mah-**TYE**-tis) ❖
- [ ] **dermatomycosis** (der-mah-toh-my-**KOH**-sis) ❖
- [ ] **dermatoplasty** (**DER**-mah-toh-**plas**-tee)
- [ ] **diaphoresis** (**dye**-ah-foh-**REE**-sis)
- [ ] **dyschromia** (dis-**KROH**-mee-ah) ❖
- [ ] **dysplastic nevi** (dis-**PLAS**-tick **NEE** vye) ❖
- [ ] **ecchymosis** (eck-ih-**MOH**-sis) ❖
- [ ] **eczema** (**ECK**-zeh-mah) ❖
- [ ] **epithelioma** (ep-ih-thee-lee-**OH**-mah) ❖
- [ ] **erythema** (er-ih-**THEE**-mah) ❖
- [ ] **exfoliative cytology** (ecks-**FOH**-lee-**ay**-tiv sigh-**TOL**-oh-jee) ❖
- [ ] **furuncle** (**FYOU**-rung-kul) ❖
- [ ] **gangrene** (**GANG**-green) ❖

- [ ] **granuloma** (**gran**-you-**LOH**-mah) ❖
- [ ] **hemangioma** (hee-**man**-jee-**OH**-mah *or* heh-**man**-jee-**OH**-mah) ❖
- [ ] **hirsutism** (**HER**-soot-izm) ❖
- [ ] **hyperhidrosis** (**high**-per-high-**DROH**-sis) ❖
- [ ] **impetigo** (**im**-peh-**TYE**-go) ❖
- [ ] **keloid** (**KEE**-loid) ❖
- [ ] **keratosis** (**kerr**-ah-**TOH**-sis)
- [ ] **koilonychia** (**koy**-loh-**NICK**-ee-ah) ❖
- [ ] **lipectomy** (lih-**PECK**-toh-mee)
- [ ] **lipedema** (lip-eh-**DEE**-mah)
- [ ] **lipocytes** (**LIP**-oh-sights)
- [ ] **lipoma** (lih-**POH**-mah)
- [ ] **liposuction** (**LIP**-oh-**suck**-shun *or* **LYE**-poh-**suck**-shun) ❖
- [ ] **lupus erythematosus** (**LOO**-pus er-ih-**thee**-mah-**TOH**-sus) ❖
- [ ] **macule** (**MACK**-youl) ❖
- [ ] **melanoma** (mel-ah-**NOH**-mah) ❖
- [ ] **miliaria** (**mill**-ee-**AYR**-ee-ah)
- [ ] **onychia** (oh-**NICK**-ee-ah) ❖
- [ ] **onychocryptosis** (**on**-ih-koh-krip-**TOH**-sis) ❖
- [ ] **onychomycosis** (**on**-ih-koh-my-**KOH**-sis) ❖
- [ ] **papilloma** (pap-ih-**LOH**-mah)
- [ ] **papule** (**PAP**-youl)
- [ ] **paronychia** (**par**-oh-**NICK**-ee-ah) ❖
- [ ] **pediculosis** (pee-**dick**-you-**LOH**-sis) ❖
- [ ] **petechiae** (pee-**TEE**-kee-ee) ❖
- [ ] **pruritus** (proo-**RYE**-tus) ❖
- [ ] **psoriasis** (soh-**RYE**-uh-sis) ❖
- [ ] **purpura** (**PUR**-pew-rah) ❖
- [ ] **purulent** (**PYOU**-roo-lent) ❖
- [ ] **putrefaction** (**pyou**-treh-**FACK**-shun) ❖
- [ ] **rhinophyma** (rye-noh-**FIGH**-muh) ❖
- [ ] **rhytidectomy** (rit-ih-**DECK**-toh-mee) ❖
- [ ] **rosacea** (roh-**ZAY**-shee-ah) ❖
- [ ] **scabies** (**SKAY**-beez) ❖
- [ ] **scleroderma** (**sklehr**-oh-**DER**-mah *or* **skleer**-oh-**DER**-mah) ❖
- [ ] **seborrhea** (seb-oh-**REE**-ah) ❖
- [ ] **seborrheic keratosis** (seb-oh-**REE**-ick **kerr**-ah-**TOH**-sis) ❖
- [ ] **subungual hematoma** (sub-**UNG**-gwal **hee**-mah-**TOH**-mah)
- [ ] **tinea** (**TIN**-ee-ah) ❖
- [ ] **urticaria** (**ur**-tih-**KAR**-ree-ah) ❖
- [ ] **verrucae** (veh-**ROO**-see) ❖
- [ ] **vesicle** (**VES**-ih-kul) ❖
- [ ] **vitiligo** (**vit**-ih-**LYE**-goh) ❖
- [ ] **wheal** (**WHEEL**) ❖
- [ ] **xeroderma** (zee-roh-**DER**-mah) ❖

FUNCTIONS OF THE INTEGUMENTARY SYSTEM

The **integumentary system** (in-**teg**-you-**MEN**-tah-ree), which makes up the outer covering of the body, serves many important functions beyond appearance.

FUNCTIONS OF THE SKIN

- The skin waterproofs the body and prevents fluid loss.
- Intact (unbroken) skin plays important roles in the immune system (see Chapter 6).
- Skin is the major receptor for the sense of touch.
- Skin helps the body synthesize (manufacture) vitamin D from the sun's ultraviolet light, while screening out harmful ultraviolet radiation.

FUNCTIONS OF RELATED STRUCTURES

- **Sebaceous glands** (seh-**BAY**-shus), also known as **oil glands,** secrete **sebum** (oil), which lubricates the skin and discourages the growth of bacteria on the skin.
- **Sweat glands** help regulate body temperature and water content by secreting sweat. Also, a small amount of metabolic waste is excreted through the sweat glands.
- **Hair** helps control the loss of body heat.
- **Nails** protect the dorsal surface of the last bone of each toe and finger.

STRUCTURES OF THE INTEGUMENTARY SYSTEM

The integumentary system consists of the skin and its related structures: sebaceous glands, sweat glands, hair, and nails (Figure 12.1).

THE SKIN

Skin covers the external surfaces of the body. The terms **derma** and **cutaneous** (kyou-**TAY**-nee-us) are both used to describe the skin (**cutane** means skin and **-ous** means pertaining to).

The skin is a complex system of specialized tissues and is made up of three strata (layers) of tissue (Figure 12.2):

- Epidermis
- Dermis
- Subcutaneous layer

THE EPIDERMIS

Epithelial tissues (ep-ih-**THEE**-lee-al) form a protective covering for *all* of the internal and external surfaces of the body. The **epidermis** (ep-ih-**DER**-mis), which is the outermost layer of the skin, is made up of several specialized epithelial tissues.

- **Squamous epithelial tissue** (**SKWAY**-mus), which forms the upper layer, consists of flat, scaly cells that are continuously sloughed off (shed). *Squamous* means scalelike.
- The epidermis does not contain any blood vessels or connective tissue and is dependent on lower layers for nourishment.
- Cells are produced in the lower **basal layer** and pushed upward. When these cells reach the surface, they die and become filled with keratin.
- **Keratin** (**KER**-ah-tin) is a fibrous, water-repellent protein. Soft keratin is a primary component of the epidermis. Hard keratin is found in the hair and nails.
- The basal cell layer also contains special cells called **melanocytes** (**MEL**-ah-noh-sights *or* meh-**LAN**-oh-sights). These cells produce and contain a dark brown to black pigment called **melanin** (**MEL**-ah-nin). The type and amount of melanin pigment determine the color of the skin.
- Melanin also protects the skin against some of the harmful ultraviolet rays of the sun. **Ultraviolet (UV)** refers to light that is beyond the visible spectrum at the violet end. Some UV rays help the skin produce vitamin D, but others can cause damage.

THE DERMIS

The **dermis** (**DER**-mis), also known as the **corium,** is the thick layer of living tissue directly below the epidermis. It contains connective tissue, blood and lymph vessels, nerve fibers, plus hair follicles and sebaceous and sweat glands.

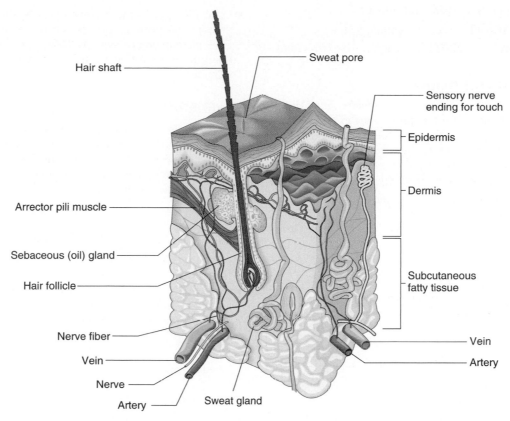

FIGURE 12.1 Structures of the skin.

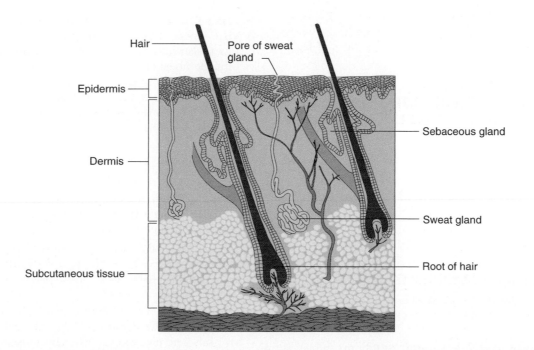

FIGURE 12.2 Layers of the skin.

Sensitive nerve endings in the dermis receive impulses that enable the body to recognize sensory stimuli such as touch, temperature, pain, and pressure.

- **Tactile** (**TACK**-til) means pertaining to touch.
- **Perception** is the ability to recognize sensory stimulus.

Tissues within the Dermis

- **Collagen** (**KOL**-ah-jen), which means glue, is a tough, yet flexible, fibrous protein material. In addition to being found in the skin, collagen is also found in bone, cartilage, tendons, and ligaments. Some cosmetics contain artificially produced collagen protein, which is claimed to minimize wrinkles.
- **Mast cells**, which are found in the connective tissue of the dermis, respond to injury or infection by producing and releasing substances including heparin and histamine.
- **Heparin** (**HEP**-ah-rin), which is released in response to injury, is an anticoagulant.
- **Histamine** (**HISS**-tah-meen), which is released in response to allergens, causes itching and increased mucus secretion.

THE SUBCUTANEOUS LAYER

The **subcutaneous layer,** located just below the skin, connects the skin to the surface muscles.

- This layer is made up of loose connective tissue and fatty **adipose tissue** (**AD**-ih-pohs). *Adipose* means fat.
- **Cellulite** is a nontechnical term for the subcutaneous deposit of fat, especially in the thighs and buttocks.
- **Lipocytes** (**LIP**-oh-sights), also known as **fat cells,** are predominant in the subcutaneous layer, where they manufacture and store large quantities of fat.

ASSOCIATED STRUCTURES OF THE INTEGUMENTARY SYSTEM

The structures associated with the integumentary system (Figure 12.3) are the

- Sebaceous glands
- Sweat glands
- Hair
- Nails

THE SEBACEOUS GLANDS

Sebaceous glands (seh-**BAY**-shus) are located in the dermis layer of the skin and are closely associated with hair follicles.

- These glands secrete **sebum** (**SEE**-bum), which is released through ducts opening into the hair follicles. From here, the sebum moves onto the surface and

lubricates the skin. Because sebum is slightly acidic, it also discourages the growth of bacteria on the skin.

- The milk-producing **mammary glands,** which are modified sebaceous glands, are often classified with the integumentary system. However, they also are part of the reproductive system and are discussed in Chapter 14.

THE SWEAT GLANDS

Sweat glands are tiny, coiled glands found on almost all body surfaces. They are most numerous in the palms of the hands, the soles of the feet, the forehead, and the armpits. Ducts from sweat glands open on the surface of the skin through **pores.**

- **Sweat,** also known as **perspiration,** is secreted by sweat glands and is made up of 99 percent water plus some salt and metabolic waste products.
- **Perspiring,** or secreting sweat, is a means of excreting excess water. It also cools the body as the sweat evaporates into the air. Body odor associated with sweat comes from the interaction of the perspiration with bacteria on the skin's surface.
- **Hidrosis** (high-**DROH**-sis) means the production and excretion of sweat (**hidr** means sweat and **-osis** means condition).

THE HAIR

Hair fibers are rodlike structures composed of tightly fused, dead protein cells filled with hard keratin. The darkness of the hair is determined by the amount of melanin produced by the melanocytes that surround the core of the hair shaft.

- **Hair follicles** are the sacs that hold the **root** of the hair fibers. The **arrector pili** (ah-**RECK**-tor **PYE**-lye), also known as the **erector muscles,** are tiny muscle fibers attached to the hair follicles that cause the hair to stand erect. In response to cold or fright, these muscles contract, causing raised areas of skin known as goose bumps. This action reduces heat loss through the skin.

THE NAILS

A nail, also known as an **unguis** (**UNG**-gwis), is the keratin plate covering the dorsal surface of the last bone of each toe and finger (plural, **ungues**). Each nail consists of these parts (Figure 12.4):

- The **nail body,** which is translucent, is closely molded to the surface of the underlying tissues. It is made up of hard, keratinized plates of epidermal cells.
- The **nail bed,** which joins the nail body to the underlying connective tissue, nourishes the nail. The blood vessels here give the nail its characteristic pink color.
- The **free edge,** which is the portion of the nail not attached to the nail bed, extends beyond the tip of the finger or toe.

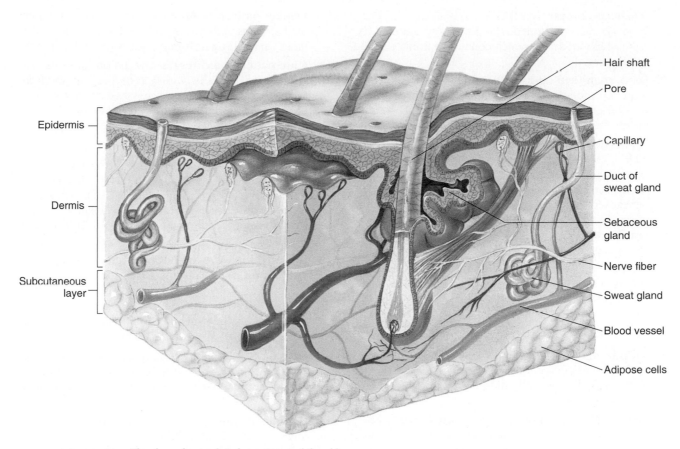

FIGURE 12.3 Glands and associated structures of the skin.

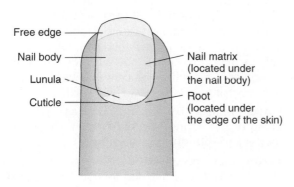

FIGURE 12.4 Structures of the fingernails and toe-nails.

- The **cuticle** is a narrow band of epidermis attached to the surface of the nail just in front of the root. (*Cuticle* means little skin.)

- The **lunula** (**LOO**-new-lah) is a pale half-moon-shaped region at the nail root and is generally found in the thumbnail and in varying degrees in other nails (plural, **lunulae**). *Lunula* means little moon.

- The **root** fastens the nail to the finger or toe by fitting into a groove in the skin.

MEDICAL SPECIALTIES RELATED TO THE INTEGUMENTARY SYSTEM

- A **dermatologist** (**der**-mah-**TOL**-oh-jist) specializes in diagnosing and treating disorders of the skin (**dermat** means skin and **-ologist** means specialist).

- A **cosmetic surgeon**, also known as a **plastic surgeon,** specializes in the surgical restoration and reconstruction of body structures. *Plastic* in this title refers to **–plasty,** the suffix meaning surgical repair.

PATHOLOGY OF THE INTEGUMENTARY SYSTEM

SEBACEOUS GLANDS

- **Acne vulgaris** (**ACK**-nee vul-**GAY**-ris) is a chronic inflammatory disease that is characterized by pustular eruptions of the skin in or near the sebaceous glands. Although common during puberty and adolescence, it also occurs in adults.

- A **comedo** (**KOM**-eh-doh) is a lesion formed by the buildup of sebum and keratin in a hair follicle (plural, **comedones**). Comedones are associated with acne vulgaris; when the sebum plug is exposed to air it oxidizes and becomes a **blackhead.**

- A **sebaceous cyst** (seh-**BAY**-shus) is a cyst of a sebaceous gland that contains yellow, fatty material. A *cyst* is a closed sac or pouch containing fluid or semisolid material.

- **Seborrhea** (seb-oh-**REE**-ah) is any of several common skin conditions in which there is an overproduction of sebum (**seb/o** means sebum and **-rrhea** means flow).

- **Seborrheic dermatitis** (seb-oh-**REE**-ick **der**-mah-**TYE**-tis) is an inflammation of the upper layers of the skin, caused by seborrhea. This results in the scaling of the scalp known as **dandruff.** Mild dandruff may be caused only by overactive oil glands. In newborns, this condition results in a scalp rash known as **cradle cap.**

- A **seborrheic keratosis** (seb-oh-**REE**-ick **kerr**-ah-**TOH**-sis) is a benign flesh-colored, brown, or black skin tumor. These growths tend to occur most often in the elderly.

SWEAT GLANDS

- **Anhidrosis** (an-high-**DROH**-sis) is the condition of lacking or being without sweat (**an-** means without, **hidr** means sweat, and **-osis** means abnormal condition).

- **Hyperhidrosis** (high-per-high-**DROH**-sis) is a condition of excessive sweating (**hyper-** means excessive, **hidr** means sweat, and **-osis** means abnormal condition).

- **Diaphoresis** (dye-ah-foh-**REE**-sis) means profuse, but not necessarily excessive, sweating.

- **Miliaria** (**mill**-ee-**AYR**-ee-ah), also known as **heat rash** and **prickly heat,** is an inflammation caused by trapped sweat. This produces a skin rash and itching. (Do not confuse this with *malaria,* an infectious disease.)

HAIR

Excessive Hairiness

- **Hirsutism** (**HER**-soot-izm) means abnormal hairiness (**hirsut** means hairy and **-ism** means condition). This term usually refers to the appearance of male body or facial hair patterns in the female.

Abnormal Hair Loss

- **Alopecia** (al-oh-**PEE**-shee-ah), also known as **baldness,** is the partial or complete loss of hair (**alopec** means baldness and **-ia** means condition).

- **Alopecia areata** is an autoimmune disorder in which there are well-defined bald areas, usually on the scalp and face.

- **Alopecia capitis totalis** is an uncommon condition characterized by the loss of all the hair on the scalp.

- **Alopecia universalis** is the total loss of hair on all parts of the body.

- **Female pattern baldness** is a condition in which the hair thins in the front and on the sides and sometimes on the crown. It rarely leads to total hair loss.

- **Male pattern baldness** is a common hair loss pattern in men, with the hairline receding from the front to the back until only a horseshoe-shaped area of hair remains in the back and on the temples.

NAILS

- **Clubbing** is abnormal curving of the nails that is often accompanied by enlargement of the fingertips. This condition can be hereditary or can be caused by changes associated with oxygen deficiencies related to coronary or pulmonary disease, which usually occurs in adults.

- **Koilonychia** (koy-loh-**NICK**-ee-ah), also known as **spoon nail,** is a malformation of the nails in which the outer surface is concave or scooped out (**koil** means hollow or concave, **onych** means fingernail or toenail, and **-ia** means condition). Koilonychia is often indicative of iron-deficiency anemia.

- **Onychia** (oh-**NICK**-ee-ah), also known as **onychitis** (on-ih-**KYE**-tis), is an inflammation of the matrix of the nail (**onych** means fingernail or toenail and **-ia** means condition).

- **Onychocryptosis** (on-ih-koh-krip-**TOH**-sis) means ingrown toenail (**onych/o** means fingernail or toenail, **crypt** means hidden, and **-osis** means abnormal condition).

- **Onychomycosis** (on-ih-koh-my-**KOH**-sis) is any fungal infection of the nail (**onych/o** means fingernail or toenail, **myc** means fungus, and **-osis** means abnormal condition). This condition, which is difficult to treat, may cause the nails to turn yellow, brown, or black and become thick or brittle, depending on what type of fungus is involved.

- **Onychophagia** (on-ih-koh-**FAY**-jee-ah) means nail biting or nail eating (**onych/o** means fingernail or toenail and **-phagia** means eating).

- **Paronychia** (par-oh-**NICK**-ee-ah) is an acute or chronic infection of the skin fold at the margin of a nail (**par-** means along side of, **onych** means fingernail or toenail, and **-ia** means condition).

- A **subungual hematoma** (sub-**UNG**-gwal **hee**-mah-**TOH**-mah), which is usually caused by an injury, is a collection of blood trapped in the tissues under a nail. Eventually, the body resorbs this blood.

PIGMENTATION

- **Albinism** (**AL**-bih-niz-um) is an inherited deficiency or absence of pigment in the skin, hair, and eyes due to an abnormality in production of melanin (**albin** means white and **-ism** means condition).

- **Chloasma** (kloh-**AZ**-mah), also known as **melasma** or the **mask of pregnancy,** is a pigmentation disorder characterized by brownish spots on the face. This may occur during pregnancy and usually disappears after delivery.

- **Dyschromia** (dis-**KROH**-mee-ah) is any disorder of the pigmentation of the skin or hair (**dys-** means bad, **chrom** means color, and **-ia** means condition).

- **Melanosis** (mel-ah-**NOH**-sis) is any condition of unusual deposits of black pigment in different parts of the body (**melan** means black and **-osis** means abnormal condition).

- **Vitiligo** (vit-ih-**LYE**-goh) is a condition in which a loss of melanocytes results in whitish areas of skin bordered by normally pigmented areas. The unpigmented skin is extremely sensitive to sunburn.

SURFACE LESIONS

A **lesion** (**LEE**-zhun) is a pathologic change of the tissues due to disease or injury. Lesions are described by their appearance, location, color, and size as measured in centimeters (cm) (Figure 12.5).

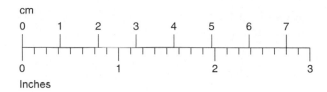

FIGURE 12.5 Lesions are described by length in centimeters. (*Note:* 2.5 centimeters equals 1 inch.)

- A **contusion** (kon-**TOO**-zhun) is an injury that does not break the skin and is characterized by swelling, discoloration, and pain.

- A **crust** is a collection of dried serum and cellular debris (Figure 12.6).

- An **ecchymosis** (eck-ih-**MOH**-sis), also known as a **bruise,** is a purplish area caused by hemorrhaging (bleeding) within the skin (plural, **ecchymoses**).

- A **macule** (**MACK**-youl) is a discolored, *flat* spot that is *less than* 1 cm in diameter. Freckles or flat moles are macules.

- **Nevi** (**NEE**-vye), also known as **moles,** are small dark skin growths that develop from melanocytes in the skin (plural, **nevus**). Normally, these growths are benign; however, **dysplastic nevi** (dis-**PLAS**-tick **NEE** vye) are atypical moles that may develop into skin cancer.

- A **nodule** (**NOD**-youl) is a small, *solid* bump. It may be felt within the skin or it may be raised as if it had formed below the surface of the skin and pushed upward. A cyst is a nodule.

- A **papule** (**PAP**-youl) is a small, solid, raised skin lesion that is *less than* 0.5 cm in diameter. Warts, insect bites, and skin tags are types of papules.

- **Petechiae** (pee-**TEE**-kee-ee), which are small pinpoint hemorrhages, are smaller versions of ecchymoses (bruises) (singular, **petechia**).

- A **plaque** (**PLACK**) is a solid, raised area of skin that is different from the area around it and *greater than* 0.5 cm in diameter. The lesions of psoriasis are plaques. (The term *plaque* also has several other meanings.)

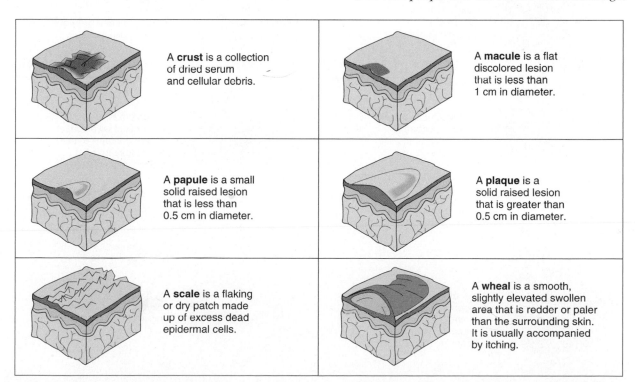

A **crust** is a collection of dried serum and cellular debris.

A **macule** is a flat discolored lesion that is less than 1 cm in diameter.

A **papule** is a small solid raised lesion that is less than 0.5 cm in diameter.

A **plaque** is a solid raised lesion that is greater than 0.5 cm in diameter.

A **scale** is a flaking or dry patch made up of excess dead epidermal cells.

A **wheal** is a smooth, slightly elevated swollen area that is redder or paler than the surrounding skin. It is usually accompanied by itching.

FIGURE 12.6 Surface lesions of the skin.

- A **scale** is a flaking or dry patch made up of excess dead epidermal cells. Some shedding of scales is normal. Excessive shedding of scales is associated with skin disorders such as psoriasis.

- **Verrucae** (veh-**ROO**-see), also known as **warts,** are skin lesions caused by the human papillomavirus (singular, **verruca**). **Plantar warts** develop on the sole of the foot.

- A **wheal** (**WHEEL**) is a smooth, *slightly elevated,* swollen area that is redder or paler than the surrounding skin and usually is accompanied by itching, for example, an insect bite or hives.

FLUID-FILLED LESIONS

- An **abscess** (**AB**-sess) is a localized collection of purulent exudate (pus) within a circumscribed area. *Purulent* (**PYOU**-roo-lent) means producing or containing pus. *Circumscribed* (**SER**-kum-skrybed) means contained within a limited area.

- A **bulla** (**BULL**-ah) is a large, circumscribed elevation of skin containing fluid that is *more than* 0.5 cm in diameter (Figure 12.7) (plural, **bullae**). A large blister is a bulla.

- A **cyst** is a closed sac or pouch containing fluid or semisolid material. The most common type of cyst is one filled with sebaceous (oily) secretions.

- A **pustule** (**PUS**-tyoul) is a small, circumscribed elevation of the skin containing pus. Pus-containing pimples, such as those associated with acne, are pustules.

- A **vesicle** (**VES**-ih-kul) is a circumscribed elevation of skin containing fluid that is *less than* 0.5 cm in diameter. A small blister is a vesicle.

LESIONS THROUGH THE SKIN

- An **abrasion** (ah-**BRAY**-zhun) is an injury in which superficial layers of skin are scraped or rubbed away. The term *abrasion* also describes treatment involving scraping or rubbing away skin.

- A **fissure** of the skin is a groove or cracklike sore (Figure 12.8). The term *fissure* also describes normal folds in the contours of the brain.

- A **laceration** (**lass**-er-**AY**-shun) is a torn or jagged wound or an accidental cut.

- A **puncture wound** is a deep hole made by a sharp object such as a nail. The risk for infection, especially tetanus, is greater with this type of wound.

- An **ulcer** (**UL**-ser) is an open sore or erosion of the skin or mucous membrane resulting in tissue loss and usually with inflammation. *Note:* Ulcers also occur inside the body. Those associated with the digestive system are discussed further in Chapter 8.

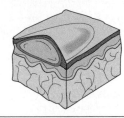
A **bulla** is a large vesicle that is more than 0.5 cm in diameter.

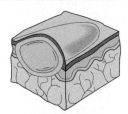
A **cyst** is a closed sac or pouch containing fluid or semisolid material.

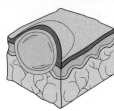
A **pustule** is a small circumscribed elevation of the skin containing pus.

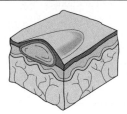
A **vesicle** is a circumscribed elevation of skin containing fluid that is less than 0.5 cm in diameter.

FIGURE 12.7 Fluid-filled lesions.

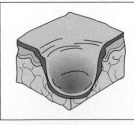
An **ulcer** is an open sore or erosion of the skin or mucous membrane resulting in tissue loss.

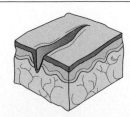
A **fissure** of the skin is a groove or cracklike sore.

FIGURE 12.8 Lesions through the skin.

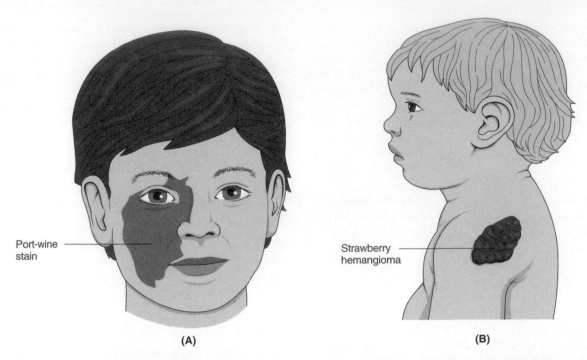

FIGURE 12.9 Types of birthmarks. (A) A port-wine stain is flat and is made up of pigmented cells. (B) A strawberry hemangioma is raised and is made up of blood vessels.

- A **decubitus ulcer** (dee-**KYOU**-bih-tus), also known as a **pressure ulcer** or **bedsore,** is an ulcerated area caused by prolonged pressure that cuts off circulation to a body part. *Decubitus* means lying down.

BIRTHMARKS

- A **port-wine stain** is a large, reddish purple discoloration of the face or neck. This discoloration will not resolve without treatment (Figure 12.9). See Laser Treatment of Skin Conditions.

- A **strawberry hemangioma** (hee-**man**-jee-**OH**-mah *or* heh-**man**-jee-**OH**-mah) is a soft, raised birthmark. This dark, reddish purple growth is a benign tumor made up of newly formed blood vessels. These usually resolve without treatment by about age seven years.

GENERAL SKIN CONDITIONS

- **Dermatitis** (der-mah-**TYE**-tis) is an inflammation of the upper layers of skin (**dermat** means skin and **-itis** means inflammation).

- **Contact dermatitis** is a localized allergic response caused by contact with an irritant or allergen. Symptoms include erythroderma (redness), itching, and rash (Figure 12.10).

- **Dermatosis** (der-mah-**TOH**-sis) is a general term used to denote any skin lesion or group of lesions or eruptions of any type that are *not* associated with inflammation (**dermat** means skin and **-osis** means abnormal condition) (plural, **dermatoses**).

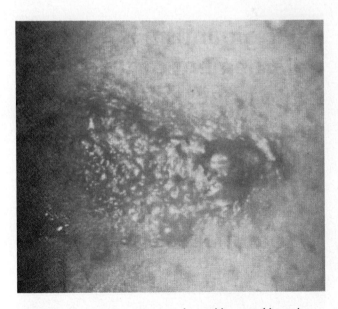

FIGURE 12.10 Contact dermatitis caused by poison oak. *(Courtesy of Timothy Berger, MD, Associate Clinical Professor, University of California, San Francisco.)*

- **Eczema** (**ECK**-zeh-mah) is an acute or chronic skin inflammation characterized by erythema, papules, vesicles, pustules, scales, crusts, scabs, and possibly itching. These symptoms may occur alone or in combination.

- **Erythema** (er-ih-**THEE**-mah) is any redness of the skin such as a nervous blush, inflammation, or mild sunburn (**erythem** means flushed and **-a** is a noun ending).

- **Lupus erythematosus** (**LOO**-pus er-ih-**thee**-mah-**TOH**-sus) (**LE**), also known as **systemic lupus erythematosus (SLE),** is an autoimmune disorder that is characterized by a red, scaly rash on the face and upper trunk. In addition to the skin, LE also involves other body systems.

- **Lipedema** (lip-eh-**DEE**-mah) is an abnormal swelling due to the collection of fat and fluid under the skin, usually between the calf and ankle (**lip** means fat and **-edema** means swelling). Compare with *lymphedema* in Chapter 6.

- **Pruritus** (proo-**RYE**-tus), also known as **itching,** is associated with most forms of dermatitis (**prurit** means itching and **-us** is a singular noun ending).

- **Psoriasis** (soh-**RYE**-uh-sis) is a chronic autoimmune disorder of the skin characterized by red papules covered with silvery scales that occur predominantly on the elbows, knees, scalp, back, and buttocks (Figure 12.11).

- **Purpura** (**PUR**-pew-rah) is a condition characterized by hemorrhage into the skin that causes spontaneous bruising (**purpur** means purple and **-a** is a noun ending).

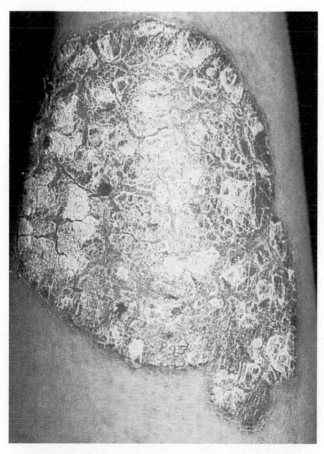

FIGURE 12.11 Psoriasis is characterized by silvery scales. (*Courtesy of Robert A. Silverman, MD, Clinical Associate Professor, Department of Pediatrics, Georgetown University.*)

- **Rosacea** (roh-**ZAY**-shee-ah) is a chronic condition of unknown cause that produces redness, tiny pimples, and broken blood vessels. It usually occurs on the central area of the face and appears most often in people with a fair complexion.

- **Scleroderma** (**sklehr**-oh-**DER**-mah *or* **skleer**-oh-**DER**-mah) is an autoimmune disorder that causes abnormal tissue thickening usually starting on the hands, feet, or face (**sclera/o** means hard and **-derma** means skin). Some forms of the disease spread to other body systems and can be fatal.

- **Urticaria** (**ur**-tih-**KAR**-ree-ah), also known as **hives,** is a skin condition characterized by localized areas of swelling accompanied by itching that is associated with an allergic reaction (**urtic** means rash and **-aria** means connected with).

- **Xeroderma** (zee-roh-**DER**-mah) is excessively dry skin (**xer/o** means dry and **-derma** means skin).

BACTERIAL SKIN INFECTIONS

- A **carbuncle** (**KAR**-bung-kul) is a cluster of furuncles (boils) that result in extensive sloughing of skin and scar formation.

- **Cellulitis** (**sell**-you-**LYE**-tis) is a diffuse infection of connective tissue with severe inflammation within the layers of the skin. *Diffuse* means widespread.

- **Furuncles** (**FYOU**-rung-kuls), also known as **boils,** are large tender, swollen, areas caused by staphylococcal infection around hair follicles.

- **Gangrene** (**GANG**-green) is tissue necrosis (death) that is usually associated with a loss of circulation. The tissue death is followed by bacterial invasion that causes putrefaction. **Putrefaction** (**pyou**-treh-**FACK**-shun) is decay that produces foul-smelling odors.

- **Impetigo** (im-peh-**TYE**-goh) is a highly contagious bacterial skin infection characterized by isolated pustules that become crusted and rupture.

- **Anthrax** (**AN**-thraks), which is caused by the bacterium *Bacillus anthracis,* is a contagious disease of warm-blooded animals including humans. In humans, it takes the form of **cutaneous anthrax,** which causes black sores on the skin, or **inhalation anthrax,** which causes severe respiratory symptoms.

FUNGAL SKIN INFECTIONS

- **Tinea** (**TIN**-ee-ah), also known as **ringworm,** is a fungal skin disease affecting different areas of the body. **Tinea capitis** is found on the scalps of children; **tinea pedis,** also known as **athlete's foot,** is found between the toes and on the feet; and **tinea cruris,** also known as **jock itch,** is found in the genital area.

- **Dermatomycosis** (**der**-mah-toh-my-**KOH**-sis), also known as **tinea versicolor,** is a fungal infection that

causes white to light brown areas on the skin (**dermat/o** means skin, **myc** means fungus, and **-osis** means abnormal condition).

PARASITIC SKIN INFESTATIONS

An **infestation** is the dwelling of a parasite on external surface tissue. Some parasites live temporarily on the skin; others lay eggs and reproduce there.

- **Scabies** (**SKAY**-beez) is a skin infection caused by an infestation with the itch mite.
- **Pediculosis** (pee-**dick**-you-**LOH**-sis) is an infestation with lice (**pedicul** means lice and **-osis** means abnormal condition). There are three types of lice, each attracted to a specific part of the body:
- **Pediculosis capitis** is an infestation with head lice.
- **Pediculosis corporis** is an infestation with body lice.
- **Pediculosis pubis** is an infestation with lice in the pubic hair and pubic region.

SKIN GROWTHS

- A **callus** (**KAL**-us) is a thickening of part of the skin on the hands or feet caused by repeated rubbing. (Compare with callus in Chapter 3.) A **clavus,** or **corn,** is a callus in the keratin layer of the skin covering the joints of the toes.
- A **cicatrix** (sick-**AY**-tricks) is a normal scar resulting from the healing of a wound (plural, **cicatrices**).
- **Granulation tissue** normally forms during the healing of a wound to create what will become scar tissue.
- **Granuloma** (gran-you-**LOH**-mah) is a general term used to describe small knotlike swellings of granulation tissue (**granul** meaning granular and **-oma** means tumor). Granulomas may result from inflammation, injury, or infection
- A **keloid** (**KEE**-loid) is an abnormally raised or thickened scar that is usually smooth and shiny (**kel** means growth or tumor and **-oid** means resembling).
- A **keratosis** (kerr-ah-**TOH**-sis) is any skin growth, such as a **wart** or a **callus,** in which there is overgrowth and thickening of the skin (**kerat** means hard or horny, and **-osis** means abnormal condition). *Note:* **kerat/o** also refers to the cornea of the eye (plural, **keratoses**).
- A **lipoma** (lih-**POH**-mah) is a benign fatty deposit under the skin that causes a bump (**lip** means fatty and **-oma** means tumor).
- A **papilloma** (pap-ih-**LOH**-mah) is a benign epithelial tumor that projects from the surrounding surface (**papill** means resembling a nipple and **-oma** means tumor.)

- **Polyp** (**POL**-ip) is a general term used most commonly to describe a mushroomlike growth from the surface of a mucous membrane, such as a polyp in the nose. These growths have many causes and are not necessarily malignant.
- **Rhinophyma** (rye-noh-**FIGH**-muh), also known as **bulbous nose,** is hyperplasia (overgrowth) of the tissues of the nose (**rhin/o** means nose and **-phyma** means growth). This condition is often associated with rosacea (see Figure 12.15).
- **Skin tags** are small flesh-colored or light brown growths that hang from the body by fine stalks. Skin tags are benign and tend to enlarge with age.

SKIN CANCER

Skin cancer is the most common form of cancer today, but fortunately most skin cancers are curable. Sun exposure is one of the main factors in predicting skin cancer.

- An **actinic keratosis** (ack-**TIN**-ick kerr-ah-**TOH**-sis) is a precancerous skin lesion caused by excessive exposure to the sun. Actinic keratoses are raised rough, dry, or scaly spots that are tan, brown, gray, or red.
- **Basal cell carcinoma** is a malignant tumor of the basal cell layer of the epidermis. Found mainly on the face, this is the most frequent and least harmful type of skin cancer. Basal cell carcinoma is slow growing and rarely spreads to other parts of the body. These lesions are smooth and raised and have a depression in the center. They are pink and tend to bleed easily (Figure 12.12).

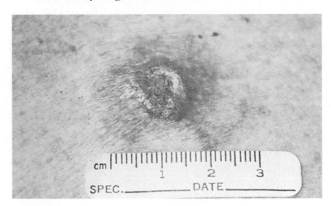

FIGURE 12.12 Basal cell carcinoma. (*Courtesy of Robert A. Silverman, MD, Clinical Associate Professor, Department of Pediatrics, Georgetown University.*)

- An **epithelioma** (ep-ih-thee-lee-**OH**-mah) is a benign or malignant tumor originating in the epidermis that may occur on the skin or mucous membranes (**epitheli** means epithelial tissue and **-oma** means tumor).
- **Malignant melanoma** (mel-ah-**NOH**-mah) (**MM**) is skin cancer derived from cells capable of forming melanin. This cancer can occur in the skin of any part of the body and may metastasize to the lungs, liver, and brain. These lesions are usually asymmetrical (not

evenly shaped), have irregular borders (ragged or blurred margins), have mixed colors (tan, brown, black, red, blue, and white), and are larger in diameter than a pencil eraser. Moles with these characteristics may be signs of malignant melanoma.

- **Squamous cell carcinoma** begins as a malignant tumor of the squamous cells of the epithelium, but it can quickly spread to other body systems. These cancers start as skin lesions that appear to be sores that will not heal or sores with a crusted, heaped-up look (Figure 12.13).

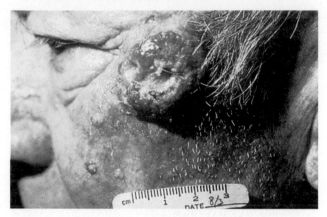

FIGURE 12.13 Squamous cell carcinoma. (*Courtesy of Robert A. Silverman, MD, Clinical Associate Professor, Department of Pediatrics, Georgetown University.*)

BURNS

A **burn** is an injury to body tissues caused by heat, flame, electricity, sun, chemicals, or radiation. The severity of a burn is described according to the percentage of the total body skin surface affected (more than 15 percent is considered serious). It is also described according to the depth or layers of skin involved (Table 12.1 and Figure 12.14).

DIAGNOSTIC PROCEDURES OF THE INTEGUMENTARY SYSTEM

A **biopsy** (**BYE**-op-see) is the removal of a small piece of living tissue for examination to confirm or establish a diagnosis (**bi-** means pertaining to life and **-opsy** means view of).

- In an **incisional biopsy** a piece, but not all, of the tumor or lesion is removed. *Incision* means to cut into.
- In an **excisional biopsy** the entire tumor or lesion and a margin of surrounding tissue are removed. *Excision* (eck-**SIH**-zhun) means the complete removal of a lesion or organ.
- In a **needle biopsy,** a hollow needle is used to remove a core of tissue for examination.
- **Exfoliative cytology** (ecks-**FOH**-lee-**ay**-tiv sigh-**TOL**-oh-jee) is a biopsy technique in which cells are scraped from the tissue and examined under a microscope.

TREATMENT PROCEDURES OF THE INTEGUMENTARY SYSTEM

TRANSDERMAL MEDICATIONS

The skin is able to absorb certain drugs and other chemical substances used to treat problems ranging from acne to angina attacks.

- A **topical** application is one that applies to a specific location. Topical medication is put on the skin to treat the area it is applied to.
- **Transdermal** refers to the application of medicine to unbroken skin so that it is absorbed continuously to produce a systemic effect (**trans-** means through or across, **derm** means skin, and **-al** means pertaining to). A transdermal patch may be used to convey medications such as nitroglycerin for angina pectoris, hormones for hormone replacement therapy, or scopolamine for motion sickness.

PREVENTIVE MEASURES

- **Sunscreen** that blocks out the harmful ultraviolet B (UVB) rays is sometimes measured in terms of the strength of the **sun protection factor (SPF)**. Some sunscreens also give protection against ultraviolet A (UVA).

Table 12.1

CLASSIFICATION OF BURN SEVERITY		
Type of Burn	**Also Known As**	**Layers of Skin Involved**
First-degree	**Superficial burns, sunburn**	No blisters, superficial damage to the epidermis
Second-degree	**Partial-thickness burns**	Blisters, superficial damage to the epidermis
Third-degree	**Full-thickness burns**	Damage to the epidermis, dermis, and subcutaneous layers

TISSUE REMOVAL

- **Cauterization** (**kaw**-ter-eye-**ZAY**-zhun) is the destruction of tissue by burning for therapeutic purposes. This technique is used in conjunction with **curettage** (**kyou**-reh-**TAHZH**) to remove and destroy basal cell tumors. *Curettage* is the removal of material from the surface by scraping.

- **Chemical peel,** also known as **chemabrasion** (keem-ah-**BRAY**-shun), is the use of chemicals to remove the outer layers of skin to treat acne scaring, fine wrinkling, and general keratoses.

- **Cryosurgery** is the destruction or elimination of abnormal tissue cells, such as warts or tumors, through the application of extreme cold, often by using liquid nitrogen.

- **Debridement** (day-breed-**MON**) is the removal of dirt, foreign objects, damaged tissue, and cellular debris from a wound to prevent infection and to promote healing.

- **Dermabrasion** (**der**-mah-**BRAY**-zhun) is a form of abrasion involving the use of revolving wire brushes or sandpaper.

- **Incision and drainage (I & D)** involves incision (cutting open) of a lesion, such as an abscess, and draining the contents.

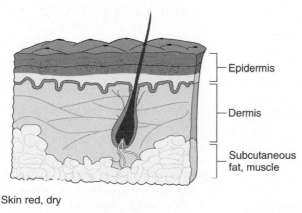

Skin red, dry

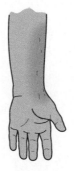

First degree, superficial

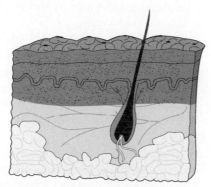

Blistered, skin moist, pink or red

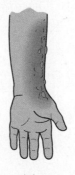

Second degree, partial thickness

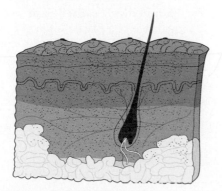

Charring, skin black, brown, red

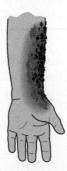

Third degree, full thickness

FIGURE 12.14 The degree of a burn is determined by the layers of skin involved.

- **Mohs' chemosurgery** is the use of a zinc chloride paste to remove recurrent tumors and scarlike basal cell carcinomas, with a minimum of normal tissue loss but complete removal of the tumor. As each layer is removed, it is examined microscopically, and the procedure continues until it is determined that the entire tumor has been removed. This technique is especially useful in treating basal cell epitheliomas.

LASER TREATMENT OF SKIN CONDITIONS

The term **laser** is an acronym for **l**ight **a**mplification by **s**timulated **e**mission of **r**adiation. An *acronym* (**ACK**-roh-nim) is a word formed from the initial letter or letters of the major parts of a compound term. Lasers are used to treat skin and many conditions affecting other body conditions.

Each type of laser derives its name from the substance (solid, liquid, or gas) within the laser tube. This substance is stimulated to emit light that is strengthened to a specific wavelength. The wavelength and power of the beam are the keys to the laser's effect on tissue. Some wavelengths are capable of destroying all skin tissue; others target tissue of a particular color.

- **Rhinophyma** is treated by using a carbon dioxide laser to reshape the nose by vaporizing the excess tissue (Figure 12.15).

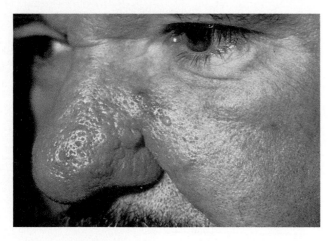

FIGURE 12.15 Rhinophyma before laser treatment. (*Courtesy of Robert A. Silverman, MD, Clinical Associate Professor, Department of Pediatrics, Georgetown University.*)

- **Port-wine stain** is treated using short pulses of laser light to remove the birthmark. Treatment may require many sessions because only a small section is treated at a time.
- **Tattoos** are removed by using lasers that target particular colors.

- Lasers are also used in the treatment of some skin cancers, precancer of the lip, and warts that recur around nails and on the soles of feet.

COSMETIC PROCEDURES

- **Blepharoplasty** (**BLEF**-ah-roh-**plas**-tee), also known as a **lid lift,** is the surgical reduction of the upper and lower eyelids (**blephar/o** means eyelid and **-plasty** means surgical repair).
- **Dermatoplasty** (**DER**-mah-toh-**plas**-tee), also known as a **skin graft,** is the replacement of damaged skin with tissue taken from a donor site on the patient's body (**dermat/o** means skin and **-plasty** means surgical repair).
- **Lipectomy** (lih-**PECK**-toh-mee) is the surgical removal of fat beneath the skin (**lip** means fat and **-ectomy** means surgical removal).
- **Liposuction** (**LIP**-oh-**suck**-shun *or* **LYE**-poh-**suck**-shun) is the surgical removal of fat beneath the skin with the aid of suction. It is also known as **suction-assisted lipectomy.**
- **Rhytidectomy** (**rit**-ih-**DECK**-toh-mee), also known as a **facelift,** is the surgical removal of excess skin for the elimination of wrinkles (**rhytid** means wrinkle and **-ectomy** means surgical removal).
- **Sclerotherapy** (**sklehr**-oh-**THER**-ah-pee), used in the treatment of spider veins (small veins that can be seen through the skin), involves injecting a sclerosing solution (saline solution) into the vein being treated. This solution irritates the tissue, causes swelling, and eventually closes off the vein.

Career Opportunities

In addition to the medical specialties already discussed, some of the health occupations involving the treatment of skin include:

- **Esthetician** (also spelled **aesthetician**): licensed to treat facial skin to maintain and improve its appearance through facials, massage, hair removal, and cosmetics
- **Paramedical esthetician:** works under the guidance of a plastic surgeon or dermatologist in pre- and postoperative skin care, including the use of corrective makeup to conceal scarring
- **Dermatology nurse certified (DNC):** an RN specially trained to provide care and information to dermatology patients
- **Burn care nurse:** an RN specializing in the treatment of burn patients

Health Occupation Profile: DERMATOLOGIST

Dr. Diane Thaler, MD, is a dermatologist and an assistant clinical professor in dermatology. "For me, medicine is a way of life. Not only do I see patients during the day, but I am also continuously reading and learning. The more one learns, the more one realizes how much more there is to know, and I'm always looking for new ideas to help my patients."

"It's a great feeling to help patients feel better when they leave my office than when they came in. Dermatology requires a trained eye and a passion for details and the 'trivia' of medicine, such as the Latin names of diseases; an understanding of infectious, inflammatory, and oncologic disease and of skin manifestations of internal disease as well as surgery and photobiology. I love the sleuthing involved in 'reading' these signs on the skin in order to help bring a patient to wellness."

STUDY BREAK

Despite the fact that about a million Americans develop skin cancer each year, many white Americans still consider a suntan to be a sign of good health and of having enough money for a beach vacation. Thousands of people die each year from *malignant melanoma,* yet we ignore the fact that skin cancer can often be directly linked to sun exposure or tanning salons.

In early times, a tan was considered a sign of outdoor labor, so it was a status symbol to be as white as possible. Yet, some of the ways of looking pale were as dangerous as getting a suntan:

- Greek and Roman women whitened their face with chalks and lead paints, a practice that sometimes caused a slow death by lead poisoning.

- In France both men and women wore fake beauty marks to emphasize the contrast with their light skin. Frequently these beauty marks were made of lead and eventually caused death by lead poisoning.

- In the 900s, some of the nobility bleached their skin with arsenic compounds. Unfortunately, this poison occasionally brought about a *truly* deadly pallor.

Review Time

Write the answers to the following questions on a separate piece of paper or in your notebook. In addition, be prepared to take part in the classroom discussion.

1. **Written assignment:** Using your own words, describe **acne vulgaris.**

   Discussion assignment: Tiffany's severe acne has never been treated. What psychological impact do you think having acne might have on her?

2. **Written assignment:** Describe the difference between **topical** and **transdermal** applications of medications.

   Discussion assignment: Give examples of medications that are administered using each mode of application.

3. **Written assignment:** Using terms a physician would understand, describe the difference between **eczema** and **psoriasis.**

   Discussion assignment: How would you describe each of these conditions in terms that the patient would understand?

4. **Written assignment:** Describe the difference between a **port-wine stain** and a **strawberry hemangioma.**

   Discussion assignment: Trisha Nelson was born with a small strawberry hemangioma on her face. How would you explain this condition and the prognosis to her parents?

5. **Written assignment:** Using terms a patient would understand, describe the difference between **blepharoplasty** and **rhytidectomy.**

   Discussion assignment: Be prepared to discuss in class some of the reasons why a patient might want to have either of these procedures performed.

Optional Internet Activity

*The goal of this activity is to help you learn more about medical terminology while improving your Internet skills. Select **one** of these two options and follow the instructions.*

1. **Internet Search:** Search for information about **skin cancer.** Write a brief (one- or two-paragraph) report on something new you learned here and include the address of the web site where you found this information.

2. **Web Site:** To learn more about **birthmarks,** go to this web address **http://www.birthmark.org**. Explore the site and then write a brief (one- or two-paragraph) report on something new you learned here.

The Human Touch: Critical Thinking Exercise

The following story and questions are designed to stimulate critical thinking through class discussion or as a brief essay response. There are no right or wrong answers to these questions.

"OK, guys, we're late again." Shaylene Boulay calls out to her two oldest sons, Nathan, Jr., 10, and Carl, 12. Grabbing the lunches Nate Sr. packed, she walks out the back door. "Come on Michel, school time!" Shaylene peers under the porch for her five-year-old. Their house is only a mile from the waterfront, and he loves to race cars between their dog Bubba's big paws in the cool sand underneath the porch. "Look at you!" As Shaylene dusts him off and heads to the truck, she notices that the rash of blisters on his leg is still bright red. "Must be ant bites," she thinks.

"Have a good day!" Shaylene hands Nathan and Carl their lunches as they hop out of the truck at the middle school. Next stop, Oak Creek Elementary. As Michel starts to get out, clutching his brown lunch bag tightly, his kindergarten teacher comes rushing over. "Michel, what are you doing here today? Didn't you give your mother the note from the nurse?"

"What note? Michel honey, did you forget to give Mama something from school?" Michel smiles sheepishly and reaches into his shorts pocket for a wadded up piece of paper. The note says: "We believe Michel has impetigo on his leg. This condition is very contagious. Please consult your doctor as soon as possible. We will need a note from him before we can allow Michel to reenter class."

"Oh no," Shaylene thinks. "I'm due for my shift at the diner in 15 minutes. Nobody's home to watch Michel. We don't have the money to see Dr. Gaines again already. And what if this rash on my arm is that thing Michel has?" She sits clutching the wheel of the old pickup, asking herself over and over, "What am I gonna do?"

Suggested Discussion Topics

1. Look up *impetigo* in a medical dictionary and read its description. Discuss how Shaylene could mistake the symptoms for something else.

2. You work in Dr. Gaines's office and the Boulays have an appointment today. What precautions would you take while seeing this family?

3. Shaylene is having difficulty understanding Dr. Gaines. She asks you to explain. Using information from a medical dictionary and terminology she can understand, describe the symptoms and treatment of impetigo.

4. Discuss Shaylene's responsibility to her children, her job, and the school. Provide her with a solution to her question, "What am I gonna do?"

5. What should Shaylene do to prevent her other children from getting impetigo?

Student Workbook and Student Activity CD-ROM

1. Go to your **Student Workbook** and complete the Learning Exercises for this chapter.

2. Go to the **Student Activity CD-ROM** and have fun with the exercises and games for this chapter.

13 The Endocrine System

● Overview of Structures, Word Parts, and Functions of the Endocrine System

MAJOR STRUCTURES	RELATED WORD ROOTS	PRIMARY FUNCTIONS
Adrenal glands (2)	adren/o	Regulate electrolyte levels, influence metabolism, and respond to stress.
Gonads 　Male testicles (2) 　Female ovaries (2)	gonad/o	Regulate development and maintenance of secondary sex characteristics.
Pancreatic islets	pancreat/o	Control blood sugar levels and glucose metabolism.
Parathyroid glands (4)	parathyroid/o	Regulate calcium levels throughout the body.
Pineal gland (1)	pineal/o	Influences the sleep-wakefulness cycle.
Pituitary gland (1)	pituit/o, pituitar/o	Controls the activity of the other endocrine glands.
Thymus (1)	thym/o	Plays a major role in the immune reaction.
Thyroid gland (1)	thyr/o, thyroid/o	Stimulates metabolism, growth, and activity of the nervous system.

Vocabulary Related to the Endocrine System

Terms marked with the ❖ symbol are pronounced on the Student Activity CD-ROM that accompanies this text.

KEY WORD PARTS

- ☐ acr/o
- ☐ adren/o
- ☐ crin/o
- ☐ -dipsia
- ☐ gonad/o
- ☐ -ism
- ☐ pancreat/o
- ☐ parathyroid/o
- ☐ pineal/o
- ☐ pituitar/o
- ☐ poly-
- ☐ somat/o
- ☐ thym/o
- ☐ thyr/o, thyroid/o
- ☐ -tropin

KEY MEDICAL TERMS

- ☐ **acromegaly** (ack-roh-**MEG**-ah-lee) ❖
- ☐ **Addison's disease** (**AD**-ih-sonz) ❖
- ☐ **adrenalitis** (ah-**dree**-nal-**EYE**-tis) ❖
- ☐ **aldosteronism** (al-**DOSS**-teh-roh-**niz**-em *or* al-doh-**STER**-ohn-izm) ❖
- ☐ **chemical thyroidectomy** (thigh-roi-**DECK**-toh-mee) ❖
- ☐ **cretinism** (**CREE**-tin-izm) ❖
- ☐ **Cushing's syndrome** (**KUSH**-ingz **SIN**-drohm) ❖
- ☐ **diabetes insipidus** (dye-ah-**BEE**-teez in-**SIP**-ih-dus) ❖
- ☐ **diabetes mellitus** (dye-ah-**BEE**-teez mel-**EYE**-tus *or* **MEL**-ih-tus) ❖
- ☐ **diabetic ketoacidosis** (kee-toh-**ass**-ih-**DOH**-sis) ❖
- ☐ **diabetic retinopathy** (ret-ih-**NOP**-ah-thee) ❖
- ☐ **electrolytes** (ee-**LECK**-troh-lytes) ❖
- ☐ **endocrinopathy** (en-doh-krih-**NOP**-ah-thee) ❖
- ☐ **epinephrine** (ep-ih-**NEF**-rin)
- ☐ **estrogen** (**ES**-troh-jen)
- ☐ **exophthalmos** (eck-sof-**THAL**-mos) ❖
- ☐ **fructosamine test** (fruck-**TOHS**-ah-meen) ❖
- ☐ **gestational diabetes mellitus** (jes-**TAY**-shun-al dye-ah-**BEE**-teez mel-**EYE**-tus *or* **MEL**-ih-tus) ❖
- ☐ **gigantism** (jigh-**GAN**-tiz-em *or* **JIGH**-en-tiz-em) ❖
- ☐ **glucagon** (**GLOO**-kah-gon)
- ☐ **glycohemoglobin** (glye-koh-**hee**-moh-**GLOH**-bin) ❖
- ☐ **goiter** (**GOI**-ter) ❖
- ☐ **gonadotropic hormone** (gon-ah-doh-**TROHP**-ick)
- ☐ **Graves' disease** (**GRAYVZ** dih-**ZEEZ**) ❖
- ☐ **growth hormone (GH)**
- ☐ **gynecomastia** (guy-neh-koh-**MAS**-tee-ah) ❖
- ☐ **Hashimoto's thyroiditis** (hah-shee-**MOH**-tohz thigh-roi-**DYE**-tis) ❖
- ☐ **hypercalcemia** (high-per-kal-**SEE**-mee-ah) ❖

- ☐ **hypercrinism** (high-per-**KRY**-nism) ❖
- ☐ **hyperglycemia** (high-per-glye-**SEE**-mee-ah) ❖
- ☐ **hypergonadism** (high-per-**GOH**-nad-izm) ❖
- ☐ **hyperinsulinism** (high-per-**IN**-suh-lin-izm) ❖
- ☐ **hyperparathyroidism** (high-per-**par**-ah-**THIGH**-roid-izm) ❖
- ☐ **hyperpituitarism** (high-per-pih-**TOO**-ih-tah-rizm) ❖
- ☐ **hyperthyroidism** (high-per-**THIGH**-roid-izm) ❖
- ☐ **hypocalcemia** (high-poh-kal-**SEE**-mee-ah) ❖
- ☐ **hypocrinism** (high-poh-**KRY**-nism) ❖
- ☐ **hypoglycemia** (high-poh-gly-**SEE**-mee-ah) ❖
- ☐ **hypogonadism** (high-poh-**GOH**-nad-izm) ❖
- ☐ **hypoparathyroidism** (high-poh-**par**-ah-**THIGH**-roid-izm) ❖
- ☐ **hypophysectomy** (high-**pof**-ih-**SECK**-toh-mee) ❖
- ☐ **hypopituitarism** (high-poh-pih-**TOO**-ih-tah-rizm) ❖
- ☐ **hypothyroidism** (high-poh-**THIGH**-roid-izm) ❖
- ☐ **insulin** (**IN**-suh-lin)
- ☐ **insulinoma** (in-suh-lin-**OH**-mah) ❖
- ☐ **laparoscopic adrenalectomy** (ah-**dree**-nal-**ECK**-toh-mee) ❖
- ☐ **lobectomy** (loh-**BECK**-toh-mee) ❖
- ☐ **metabolism** (meh-**TAB**-oh-**lizm**) ❖
- ☐ **myxedema** (**mick**-seh-**DEE**-mah) ❖
- ☐ **norepinephrine** (**nor**-ep-ih-**NEF**-rin)
- ☐ **oxytocin** (ock-sih-**TOH**-sin)
- ☐ **pancreatalgia** (**pan**-kree-ah-**TAL**-jee-ah) ❖
- ☐ **pancreatitis** (**pan**-kree-ah-**TYE**-tis) ❖
- ☐ **parathyroid hormone (PTH)**
- ☐ **parathyroidectomy** (**par**-ah-**thigh**-roi-**DECK**-toh-mee) ❖
- ☐ **pheochromocytoma** (fee-oh-**kroh**-moh-sigh-**TOH**-mah) ❖
- ☐ **pinealectomy** (**pin**-ee-al-**ECK**-toh-mee) ❖
- ☐ **pinealopathy** (**pin**-ee-ah-**LOP**-ah-thee) ❖
- ☐ **pituitarism** (pih-**TOO**-ih-tar-izm) ❖
- ☐ **pituitary adenoma** (pih-**TOO**-ih-**tair**-ee ad-eh-**NOH**-mah) ❖
- ☐ **polydipsia** (**pol**-ee-**DIP**-see-ah) ❖
- ☐ **polyuria** (**pol**-ee-**YOU**-ree-ah) ❖
- ☐ **progesterone** (proh-**JES**-ter-ohn)
- ☐ **prolactinoma** (proh-**lack**-tih-**NOH**-mah) ❖
- ☐ **steroid** (**STEHR**-oid)
- ☐ **testosterone** (tes-**TOS**-teh-rohn)
- ☐ **tetany** (**TET**-ah-nee) ❖
- ☐ **thymectomy** (thigh-**MECK**-toh-mee) ❖
- ☐ **thymitis** (thigh-**MY**-tis) ❖
- ☐ **thymoma** (thigh-**MOH**-mah) ❖
- ☐ **thymosin** (**THIGH**-moh-sin)
- ☐ **thyroid-stimulating hormone (TSH)**
- ☐ **thyromegaly** (thigh-roh-**MEG**-ah-lee) ❖
- ☐ **thyrotoxicosis** (**thy**-roh-**tock**-sih-**KOH**-sis) ❖
- ☐ **thyroxine** (thigh-**ROCK**-sin)

Objectives

Upon completion of this chapter, you should be able to:

1. Describe the role of the hypothalamus and endocrine glands in maintaining homeostasis.
2. Name and describe the functions of the primary hormones secreted by each of the endocrine glands.
3. Recognize, define, spell, and pronounce terms relating to the pathology and diagnostic and treatment procedures of the endocrine glands.

FUNCTIONS OF THE ENDOCRINE SYSTEM

The primary function of the endocrine system is to produce hormones. Because the hormones are secreted directly into the bloodstream, they are able to reach cells and organs throughout the body.

A **hormone** is a chemical messenger with a specialized function. The major hormones, their sources, and functions are described in Table 13.1.

STEROID HORMONES

Steroid hormones help control metabolism, inflammation, immune functions, salt and water balance, development of sexual characteristics, and the ability to withstand illness and injury.

- The term **steroid** (**STEHR**-oid) describes both hormones produced by the body and artificially produced hormones used in medications to duplicate the action of the naturally occurring steroids.

Table 13.1

HORMONES FROM A TO T

Hormone	Source	Functions
Aldosterone	Adrenal cortex	Aids in regulating the levels of salt and water in the body.
Androgens	Adrenal cortex and gonads	Influence sex-related characteristics.
Adrenocorticotropic hormone (ACTH)	Pituitary gland	Stimulates the growth and secretions of the adrenal cortex.
Antidiuretic hormone (ADH)	Pituitary gland	Helps control blood pressure by reducing the amount of water that is excreted.
Calcitonin	Thyroid gland	Works with the parathyroid hormone to regulate calcium levels in the blood and tissues.
Cortisol	Adrenal cortex	Regulates the metabolism of carbohydrates, fats and proteins in the body. Also has an anti-inflammatory action.
Epinephrine	Adrenal medulla	Stimulates the sympathetic nervous system.
Estrogen	Ovaries	Develops and maintains the female secondary sex characteristics and regulates the menstrual cycle.
Follicle-stimulating hormone (FSH)	Pituitary gland	In the female, stimulates the secretion of estrogen and the growth of ova (eggs). In the male, stimulates the production of sperm.

Table 13.1 – Continued

HORMONES FROM A TO T

Hormone	Source	Functions
Glucagon	Pancreatic islets	Increases the level of glucose in the bloodstream.
Growth hormone (GH)	Pituitary gland	Regulates the growth of bone, muscle, and other body tissues.
Human chorionic gonadotropin (HCG)	Placenta	Stimulates the secretion of the hormones required to maintain pregnancy.
Insulin (In)	Pancreatic islets	Regulates the transport of glucose to body cells and stimulates the conversion of excess glucose to glycogen for storage.
Lactogenic hormone (LTH)	Pituitary gland	Stimulates and maintains the secretion of breast milk.
Luteinizing hormone (LH)	Pituitary gland	In the female, stimulates ovulation. In the male, stimulates testosterone secretion.
Melatonin	Pineal gland	Influences the sleep-wakefulness cycle.
Norepinephrine	Adrenal medulla	Stimulates the sympathetic nervous system.
Oxytocin (OXT)	Pituitary gland	Stimulates uterine contractions during childbirth. Causes milk to flow from the mammary glands after childbirth.
Parathyroid hormone (PTH)	Parathyroid glands	Works with calcitonin to regulate calcium levels in the blood and tissues.
Progesterone	Ovaries	Completes preparation of the uterus for possible pregnancy.
Testosterone	Testicles	Stimulates the development of male secondary sex characteristics.
Thymosin	Thymus	Plays an important role in the immune system.
Thyroid hormones (T_4 and T_3)	Thyroid gland	Regulate the rate of metabolism.
Thyroid-stimulating hormone (TSH)	Pituitary gland	Stimulates the secretion of hormones by the thyroid gland.

Anabolic Steroids

Anabolic steroids (an-ah-**BOL**-ick), which are chemically related to the male sex hormone testosterone, have been used illegally by athletes to increase strength and muscle mass. This use usually can be detected through urine and blood testing.

- Serious side effects of anabolic steroid use include liver damage, altered body chemistry, testicular shrinkage and breast development in males, plus unpredictable mood swings and violence.

- Steroid use by teenagers also stops long bone development, resulting in shortened stature.

STRUCTURES OF THE ENDOCRINE SYSTEM

The major glands of the endocrine system are (Figure 13.1)

- One **pituitary gland** (divided into two lobes)
- One **thyroid gland**
- Four **parathyroid glands**

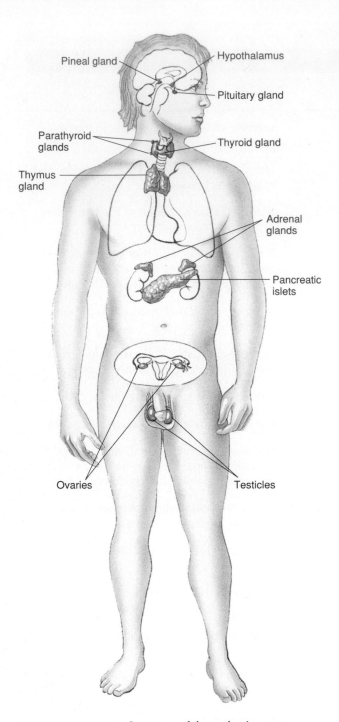

Pineal gland

Hypothalamus

Pituitary gland

Parathyroid glands

Thyroid gland

Thymus gland

Adrenal glands

Pancreatic islets

Ovaries

Testicles

FIGURE 13.1 Structures of the endocrine system.

- Two **adrenal glands**
- One **pancreas (pancreatic islets)**
- One **thymus**
- One **pineal gland**
- Two **gonads** (ovaries in females, testes in males)

MEDICAL SPECIALTIES RELATED TO THE ENDOCRINE SYSTEM

- An **endocrinologist** (**en**-doh-krih-**NOL**-oh-jist) specializes in diagnosing and treating diseases and malfunctions of the glands of internal secretion (**endo-** means within, **crin** means to secrete, and **-ologist** means specialist).

PATHOLOGY OF THE ENDOCRINE SYSTEM

- **Endocrinopathy** (**en**-doh-krih-**NOP**-ah-thee) is any disease due to a disorder of the endocrine system (**endo-** means within, **crin/o** means to secrete, and **-pathy** means disease).
- **Hypercrinism** (**high**-per-**KRY**-nism) is a condition caused by excessive secretion of any gland, especially an endocrine gland (**hyper-** means excessive, **crin** means to secrete, and **-ism** means condition).
- **Hypocrinism** (**high**-poh-**KRY**-nism) is a condition caused by deficient secretion of any gland, especially an endocrine gland (**hypo-** means deficient, **crin** means to secrete, and **-ism** means condition).

DIAGNOSTIC PROCEDURES RELATED TO THE ENDOCRINE SYSTEM

- Nuclear medicine and imaging techniques, which are described in Chapter 15, are used to diagnose and treat disorders affecting the endocrine system.
- Urine and blood testing are used to measure endocrine hormone levels and to detect the presence of anabolic steroids.

THE PITUITARY GLAND

The pea-sized **pituitary gland** (pih-**TOO**-ih-**tair**-ee) is located at the base of the brain just below the hypothalamus and is composed of anterior and posterior lobes.

FUNCTIONS OF THE PITUITARY GLAND

The primary function of the pituitary gland, also known as the **master gland,** is to control the activity of the other endocrine glands (Figure 13.2).

- The pituitary acts in response to stimuli from the hypothalamus of the brain. This system of checks and balances maintains an appropriate blood level of each hormone.

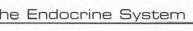

Thyroid feedback system

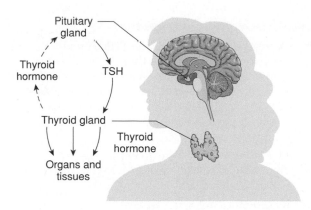

FIGURE 13.2 The pituitary gland secretes the thyroid-stimulating hormone, which signals the thyroid gland to produce thyroid hormones. These hormones travel through the bloodstream to organs and tissues throughout the body.

SECRETIONS OF THE PITUITARY GLAND: ANTERIOR LOBE

- The **adrenocorticotropic hormone (ACTH),** also known as **adrenotropin,** stimulates the growth and secretions of the adrenal cortex (**adren/o** means adrenal glands and **-tropin** means stimulating).

- The **follicle-stimulating hormone (FSH),** also known as **follitropin,** in the female stimulates the secretion of estrogen and the growth of ova (eggs) in the ovaries. In the male, it stimulates the production of sperm in the testicles.

- The **growth hormone (GH),** also known as **somatotropin (STH),** regulates the growth of bone, muscle and other body tissues (**somat/o** means body and **-tropin** means to stimulate).

- The **lactogenic hormone (LTH),** also known as **prolactin,** stimulates and maintains the secretion of breast milk after childbirth.

- The **luteinizing hormone (LH),** also known as **luteotropin,** stimulates ovulation in the female. In the male, it stimulates testosterone secretion.

- The **melanocyte-stimulating hormone (MSH),** also known as **melanotropin,** increases pigmentation of the skin (**melan/o** means black and **-tropin** means to stimulate or act on).

- The **thyroid-stimulating hormone (TSH),** also known as **thyrotropin,** stimulates the growth and secretions of the thyroid gland (**thyr/o** means thyroid and **-tropin** means to stimulate or act on).

SECRETIONS OF THE PITUITARY GLAND: POSTERIOR LOBE

- The **antidiuretic hormone (ADH)** maintains the water balance within the body by promoting the

reabsorption of water through the kidneys (see Chapter 9). When more ADH is secreted, less urine is produced. In contrast, when a **diuretic** (**dye**-you-**RET**-ick) is administered, urine secretion increases.

- **Oxytocin** (**ock**-sih-**TOH**-sin) **(OXT)** stimulates uterine contractions during childbirth. After childbirth, it stimulates the flow of milk from the mammary glands.

PATHOLOGY OF THE PITUITARY GLAND

- **Alcohol consumption** inhibits the secretion of ADH and results in increased urine output that can disrupt the body's fluid balance.

- **Acromegaly** (**ack**-roh-**MEG**-ah-lee) is enlargement of the extremities (hands and feet) caused by excessive secretion of growth hormone *after* puberty (**acr/o** means extremities and **-megaly** means abnormal enlargement). Compare with *gigantism*.

- **Gigantism** (jigh-**GAN**-tiz-em *or* **JIGH**-gen-tiz-em), which is also known as *giantism,* is abnormal overgrowth of the body caused by excessive secretion of growth hormone *before* puberty. Compare with *acromegaly.*

- **Hyperpituitarism** (**high**-per-pih-**TOO**-ih-tah-rizm) is pathology that results in the excessive secretion by the anterior lobe of the pituitary gland (**hyper-** means excessive, **pituitar** means pituitary, and **-ism** means condition).

- **Hypopituitarism** (**high**-poh-pih-**TOO**-ih-tah-rizm) is a condition of reduced secretion due to the partial or complete loss of the function of the anterior lobe of the pituitary gland (**hypo-** means deficient, **pituitar** means pituitary, and **-ism** means condition).

- A **pituitary adenoma** (**ad**-eh-**NOH**-mah) is a benign tumor of the pituitary gland that causes excess hormone secretion. An ACTH-secreting tumor stimulates the excess production of cortisol, which causes most cases of Cushing's syndrome (see Pathology of the Adrenal Glands).

- **Pituitarism** (pih-**TOO**-ih-tar-izm) is any disorder of pituitary function (**pituitar** means pituitary and **-ism** means condition).

- A **prolactin-producing adenoma,** also known as a **prolactinoma** (proh-**lack**-tih-**NOH**-mah), is a benign tumor of the pituitary gland that causes it to produce too much prolactin. In females, this overproduction causes infertility and changes in menstruation. In males, it causes impotence.

Diabetes Insipidus

Diabetes insipidus (**dye**-ah-**BEE**-teez in-**SIP**-ih-dus) is caused by insufficient production of the antidiuretic hormone (ADH) or by the inability of the kidneys to respond to ADH. Either cause allows too much fluid to be excreted, resulting in extreme polydipsia and polyuria.

- **Polydipsia** (pol-ee-**DIP**-see-ah) is excessive thirst (**poly-** means many and **-dipsia** means thirst).
- **Polyuria** (pol-ee-**YOU**-ree-ah) is excessive urination (**poly-** means many and **-uria** means urination).
- Diabetes insipidus is *not* similar to diabetes mellitus.

TREATMENT PROCEDURES OF THE PITUITARY GLAND

- A **hypophysectomy** (high-**pof**-ih-**SECK**-toh-mee) is use of radiation or surgery to remove all or part of the pituitary gland.
- **Human growth hormone therapy (GH),** also known as **recombinant GH,** is a synthetic version of naturally occurring growth hormone. It is administered to stimulate growth when the natural supply of growth hormone is insufficient for normal development.

THE THYROID GLAND

The butterfly-shaped **thyroid gland** lies on either side of the larynx, just below the thyroid cartilage (see Figure 13.1).

- The secretion of the thyroid hormones (T_4 and T_3) is controlled by the thyroid-stimulating hormone (TSH) secreted by the anterior lobe of the pituitary gland.
- The body's ability to secrete thyroid hormones depends on the uptake of iodine from food and water.

FUNCTIONS OF THE THYROID GLAND

The primary function of the thyroid gland is to regulate the body's metabolism.

- The term **metabolism** (meh-**TAB**-oh-**lizm**) includes *all* of the processes involved in the body's use of nutrients, including the rate at which they are utilized.
- The thyroid secretions also influence growth and the functioning of the nervous system.

SECRETIONS OF THE THYROID GLAND

- The primary thyroid hormones are **thyroxine (T_4)** (thigh-**ROCK**-sin) and **triiodothyronine (T_3)** (try-**eye**-oh-doh-**THIGH**-roh-neen).
- **Calcitonin** (**kal**-sih-**TOH**-nin), also known as **thyrocalcitonin,** works with the parathyroid hormone (PH) to regulate calcium levels in the blood and tissues. Calcitonin decreases blood levels by moving calcium into storage in the bones and teeth. Compare with PH under Secretions on the Parathyroid Glands.

PATHOLOGY OF THE THYROID GLAND

- **Thyroid cancer** is commonly first indicated by an enlargement of the thyroid gland. With early detection and treatment, the survival rate is high. Without

treatment, the cancer will spread to other parts of the body.

Insufficient Thyroid Secretion

- **Hypothyroidism** (**high**-poh-**THIGH**-roid-izm), also known as an **underactive thyroid,** is a deficiency of thyroid secretion (**hypo-** means deficient, **thyroid** means thyroid, and **-ism** means condition). Symptoms include fatigue, depression, sensitivity to cold, and a decreased metabolic rate.
- **Cretinism** (**CREE**-tin-izm) is a congenital lack of thyroid secretion. If treatment is not started soon after birth, cretinism causes arrested physical and mental development.
- **Myxedema** (**mick**-seh-**DEE**-mah) is a severe form of adult hypothyroidism. Symptoms include an enlarged tongue and puffiness of the hands and face.
- **Hashimoto's thyroiditis** (hah-shee-**MOH**-tohz **thigh**-roi-**DYE**-tis) is an autoimmune disorder in which the immune system mistakenly attacks thyroid tissue, setting up an inflammatory process that may progressively destroy the gland. This process may cause goiter or hypothyroidism.

Excessive Thyroid Secretion

- **Hyperthyroidism** (**high**-per-**THIGH**-roid-izm) is a condition of excessive thyroid hormones in the blood (**hyper-** means excessive, **thyroid** means thyroid, and **-ism** means condition). Symptoms include an increased metabolic rate, increased sweating, nervousness, and weight loss.
- **Graves' disease** (**GRAYVZ** dih-**ZEEZ**) is an autoimmune disorder characterized by hyperthyroidism, goiter, and exophthalmos.
- **Goiter** (**GOI**-ter), also known as **thyromegaly** (**thigh**-roh-**MEG**-ah-lee), is an abnormal enlargement of the thyroid gland that produces a swelling in the front part of the neck (**thyr/o** means thyroid and **-megaly** means abnormal enlargement).
- **Exophthalmos** (**eck**-sof-**THAL**-mos) is an abnormal protrusion of the eyes.
- **Thyrotoxicosis** (**thy**-roh-**tock**-sih-**KOH**-sis), also known as **thyroid storm,** is a life-threatening condition resulting from the release of excessive quantities of the thyroid hormones into the bloodstream (**thyr/o** means thyroid, **toxic** means poison, and **-osis** means abnormal condition).

DIAGNOSTIC AND TREATMENT PROCEDURES RELATED TO THE THYROID GLAND

- A **thyroid scan** is one means to measure thyroid function (see Chapter 15).
- An **antithyroid drug** is a medication administered to slow the ability of the thyroid gland to produce thyroid hormones.

- A **chemical thyroidectomy** (**thigh**-roi-**DECK**-toh-mee), also known as **radioactive iodine therapy,** is the administration of radioactive iodine to destroy thyroid cells. This is used to treat hyperthyroid disorders such as Graves' disease.

- A **lobectomy** (loh-**BECK**-toh-mee) is the removal of one lobe of the thyroid gland. This term is also used to describe the removal of a lobe of the liver, brain, or lung.

- A **thyroid-stimulating hormone assay** is a diagnostic test to measure circulating blood levels of TSH. This test is used to detect abnormal thyroid activity resulting from excessive pituitary stimulation.

THE PARATHYROID GLANDS

The four **parathyroid glands,** each of which is about the size of a grain of rice, are located within the thyroid gland (see Figure 13.1).

FUNCTIONS OF THE PARATHYROID GLANDS

The primary function of the parathyroid glands is to regulate calcium levels throughout the body. These calcium levels are important to the smooth functioning of the muscular and nervous systems.

SECRETIONS OF THE PARATHYROID GLANDS

Parathyroid hormone (PTH), also known as **parathormone,** works with calcitonin to regulate calcium levels in the blood and tissues. PTH increases calcium levels in the blood by mobilizing the release of calcium from storage in the bones and teeth. Compare with calcitonin under Secretions of the Thyroid Gland.

PATHOLOGY OF THE PARATHYROID GLANDS

Insufficient Parathyroid Secretion

- **Hypoparathyroidism** (**high**-poh-**par**-ah-**THIGH**-roid-izm) is a condition caused by an insufficient or

absent secretion of the parathyroid glands. This is usually accompanied by hypocalcemia and in severe cases leads to tetany. **Tetany** (**TET**-ah-nee) is an abnormal condition characterized by periodic painful muscle spasms (cramps) and tremors.

- **Hypocalcemia** (**high**-poh-kal-**SEE**-mee-ah) is characterized by abnormally low levels of calcium in the blood (**hypo-** means deficient, **calc** means calcium, and **-emia** means blood condition).

Excessive Parathyroid Secretion

- **Hyperparathyroidism** (**high**-per-**par**-ah-**THIGH**-roid-izm) (**HP**) is the overproduction of PTH. This causes hypercalcemia and may lead to weakened bones and the formation of kidney stones.

- **Hypercalcemia** (**high**-per-kal-**SEE**-mee-ah) is characterized by abnormally high concentrations of calcium circulating in the blood instead of being stored in the bones (**hyper-** means excessive, **calc** means calcium, and **-emia** means blood condition).

- **Primary HP** is caused by a diseased parathyroid gland. **Secondary HP** is caused by a problem elsewhere in the body. For example, kidney failure makes the body resistant to the action of PTH.

TREATMENT PROCEDURE OF THE PARATHYROID GLANDS

- A **parathyroidectomy** (**par**-ah-**thigh**-roi-**DECK**-toh-mee), which is the surgical removal of one or more of the parathyroid glands, is performed to control hyperparathyroidism.

THE ADRENAL GLANDS

The **adrenal glands,** also referred to as the **adrenals,** are located one on top of each kidney. Each adrenal gland consists of two parts: the **adrenal cortex,** which is the outer portion, and the **adrenal medulla,** which is the middle portion (Figure 13.3).

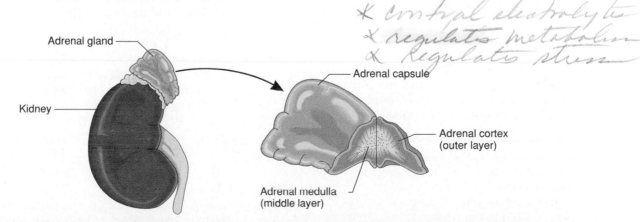

FIGURE 13.3 There is one adrenal gland on top of each kidney. Each adrenal gland is made up of two layers.

FUNCTIONS OF THE ADRENAL GLANDS

One of the primary functions of the adrenals is to control electrolyte levels within the body. **Electrolytes** (ee-**LECK**-troh-lytes) are mineral substances, such as sodium and potassium, found in the blood.

● Other important functions include helping to regulate metabolism and interacting with the sympathetic nervous system in response to stress.

SECRETIONS OF THE ADRENAL CORTEX

● **Corticosteroid** (**kor**-tih-koh-**STEHR**-oid) is the name given to any of the steroid hormones produced by the adrenal cortex or their synthetic equivalents. These are described in three groups: mineralocorticoids, glucocorticoids, and gonadocorticoids.

● **Mineralocorticoids** regulate the mineral salts in the body. The primary mineralocorticoid is **aldosterone** (al-**DOSS**-ter-ohn), which regulates the salt and water levels in the body by increasing sodium reabsorption in the kidneys. *Reabsorption* means returning a substance to the bloodstream instead of excreting it.

● **Glucocorticoids** regulate the metabolism of carbohydrates, fats, and proteins in the body. They also influence blood pressure and have an anti-inflammatory effect. The primary glucocorticoid is **cortisol** (**KOR**-tih-sol), which is also known as **hydrocortisone.**

● **Gonadocorticoids,** also known as **androgens** (**AN**-droh-jenz), are hormones that influence sex-related characteristics. Normally, in adults the production of androgens in the adrenal cortex is minimal; instead these hormones are produced in the male and female gonads.

SECRETIONS OF THE ADRENAL MEDULLA

● **Epinephrine** (**ep**-ih-**NEF**-rin), also called **adrenaline** (ah-**DREN**-uh-lin), and **norepinephrine** (nor-ep-ih-**NEF**-rin) stimulate the sympathetic nervous system. This stimulation causes an increase in the heart rate and increased blood pressure as well as the other symptoms associated with severe stress.

PATHOLOGY OF THE ADRENAL GLANDS

● **Adrenalitis** (ah-**dree**-nal-**EYE**-tis) is an inflammation of the adrenal glands (**adrenal** means adrenal glands and **-itis** means inflammation).

Insufficient Adrenal Secretions

● **Addison's disease** (**AD**-ih-sonz) is a progressive disease that occurs when adrenal glands do not produce enough cortisol. This underproduction may be due to a disorder of the adrenal glands or to inadequate secretion of ACTH by the pituitary gland. If untreated, it can produce a life-threatening addisonian crisis.

Excessive Adrenal Secretions

● **Aldosteronism** (al-**DOSS**-teh-roh-**niz**-em *or* al-doh-**STER**-ohn-izm) is an abnormality of electrolyte balance caused by excessive secretion of aldosterone.

● **Primary aldosteronism,** also known as **Conn's syndrome,** is aldosteronism due to disorders of the adrenal gland.

● **Secondary aldosteronism** is *not* caused by a disorder of the adrenal gland. It results from a disorder elsewhere in the body, such as a nephrotic syndrome (see Chapter 9).

● A **pheochromocytoma** (fee-oh-**kroh**-moh-sigh-**TOH**-mah) is a benign tumor of the adrenal medulla that causes the gland to produce excess epinephrine.

Cushing's Syndrome

● **Cushing's syndrome** (**KUSH**-ingz **SIN**-drohm) **(CS),** also known as **hypercortisolism,** is caused by prolonged exposure to high levels of cortisol. The symptoms include a rounded or "moon" face (Figure 13.4).

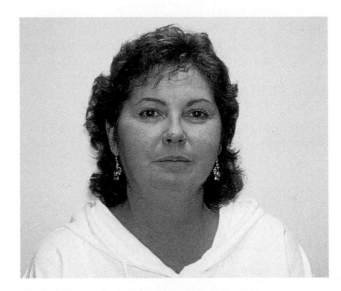

FIGURE 13.4 Cushing's syndrome causes a characteristic "moon" face. (*Courtesy of Matthew C. Leinung, MD, Albany Medical College, Albany, NY.*)

● CS may be caused by overproduction of cortisol by the body or by taking glucocorticoid hormone medications to treat inflammatory diseases such as asthma and rheumatoid arthritis.

TREATMENT PROCEDURES OF THE ADRENAL GLANDS

● A **laparoscopic adrenalectomy** (ah-**dree**-nal-**ECK**-toh-mee) is a minimally invasive surgical procedure to remove one or both adrenal glands (**adrenal** means adrenal gland and **-ectomy** means surgical removal).

- **Cortisone** (**KOR**-tih-sohn), also known as **hydrocortisone,** is the synthetic equivalent of corticosteroids produced by the body. Cortisone is administered to suppress inflammation, and in transplant recipients it is administered as an immunosuppressant to prevent organ rejection by the body.

- **Epinephrine** is a synthetic pharmaceutical used as a vasoconstrictor to treat conditions such as heart dysrhythmias and asthma attacks. A *vasoconstrictor* causes the blood vessels to contract.

THE PANCREATIC ISLETS

The **pancreas** (**PAN**-kree-as) is a feather-shaped organ located posterior to (behind) the stomach (see Figure 13.1). It primarily functions as part of the digestive system, and these functions are discussed in Chapter 8.

- The **pancreatic islets** (**pan**-kree-**AT**-ick **EYE**-lets), also known as the **islets of Langerhans** (**EYE**-lets of **LAHNG**-er-hahnz), are cells within the pancreas that have an endocrine function.

FUNCTIONS OF THE PANCREATIC ISLETS

The functions of the islets are to control blood sugar levels and glucose metabolism throughout the body.

SECRETIONS OF THE PANCREATIC ISLETS

- **Glucagon** (**GLOO**-kah-gon), which is produced by the **alpha cells** of the pancreatic islets, is secreted in response to low blood sugar. Glucagon increases the amount of glucose (sugar) in the bloodstream by stimulating the liver to convert glycogen into glucose.

- **Insulin** (**IN**-suh-lin) (**In**) is secreted by the **beta cells** of the pancreatic islets in response to high blood sugar. It functions in two ways. First, insulin allows glucose to enter the cells for use as energy. When additional glucose is *not* needed, insulin stimulates the liver to convert glucose into glycogen for storage (Figure 13.5).

PATHOLOGY OF THE PANCREAS

- **Hyperglycemia** (**high**-per-glye-**SEE**-mee-ah) is an abnormally high concentration of glucose in the blood (**hyper-** means excessive, **glyc** means sugar, and **-emia** means blood condition). Symptoms of hyperglycemia include polyuria and polydipsia.

- **Hyperinsulinism** (**high**-per-**IN**-suh-lin-izm) is a condition marked by excessive secretion of insulin that produces hypoglycemia (**hyper-** means excessive, **insulin** means insulin, and **-ism** means condition).

- **Hypoglycemia** (**high**-poh-glye-**SEE**-mee-ah) is an abnormally low concentration of glucose (sugar) in the blood (**hypo-** means deficient, **glyc** means sugar, and **-emia** means blood condition).

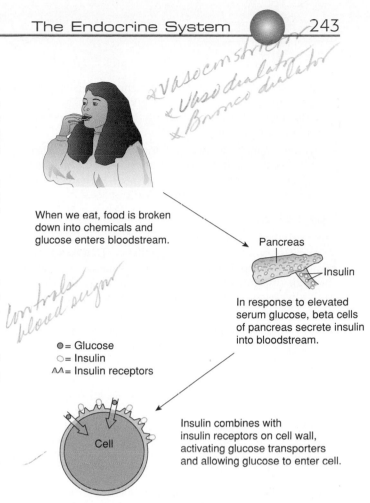

When we eat, food is broken down into chemicals and glucose enters bloodstream.

Pancreas

Insulin

In response to elevated serum glucose, beta cells of pancreas secrete insulin into bloodstream.

● = Glucose
○ = Insulin
⋀⋀ = Insulin receptors

Cell

Insulin combines with insulin receptors on cell wall, activating glucose transporters and allowing glucose to enter cell.

FIGURE 13.5   How insulin works.

- An **insulinoma** (**in**-suh-lin-**OH**-mah) is a benign tumor of the pancreas that causes hypoglycemia (**insulin** means insulin and **-oma** means tumor).

- **Pancreatalgia** (**pan**-kree-ah-**TAL**-jee-ah) means pain in the pancreas (**pancreat** means pancreas and **-algia** means pain).

- **Pancreatitis** (**pan**-kree-ah-**TYE**-tis) is an inflammation of the pancreas (**pancreat** means pancreas and **-itis** means inflammation).

DIABETES MELLITUS

- **Diabetes mellitus** (**dye**-ah-**BEE**-teez mel-**EYE**-tus or **MEL**-ih-tus) is a group of metabolic diseases characterized by hyperglycemia resulting from defects in insulin secretion, insulin action, or both.

- Although these are described as distinct types, many patients do not fit into a single category, and the treatment goals are to most effectively control the blood sugar levels and prevent diabetic complications.

Type 1 Diabetes

Type 1 diabetes, which was previously known as **insulin-dependent diabetes mellitus (IDDM)** or **juvenile diabetes,** is an autoimmune insulin deficiency disorder (*Note:* type 1 and type 2 diabetes are spelled with a small *t*).

- Because of the destruction of pancreatic islet beta cells, the body does not secrete enough insulin. Type 1 diabetes is treated with carefully regulated insulin replacement therapy.

- Symptoms include increased urination, constant thirst and hunger, weight loss, blurred vision, extreme fatigue, and slow healing. Only 1 in 10 individuals with diabetes has this form of the disease.

Type 2 Diabetes

Type 2 diabetes, which was previously known as **non-insulin-dependent diabetes mellitus (NIDDM)** or **adult-onset diabetes,** is an insulin resistance disorder. Although insulin is being produced, the body does not use it effectively. In an attempt to compensate, the body secretes more insulin.

- Type 2 diabetes may have no symptoms for years. When symptoms do occur, they include those of type 1 diabetes, plus recurring infections, irritability, and a tingling sensation in the hands or feet.

- Type 2 diabetes is treated with diet, exercise, and medications. Sulfonylureas are medications that lower blood sugar by causing the body to release more insulin. Other types of medications, such as Glucophage (metformin hydrochloride), work within the cells to help insulin let blood sugar in.

Gestational Diabetes Mellitus

Gestational diabetes mellitus (jes-**TAY**-shun-al **dye**-ah-**BEE**-teez mel-**EYE**-tus *or* **MEL**-ih-tus), also known as **GDM,** is the form of diabetes that occurs during some pregnancies. GDM usually disappears after delivery; however, many of these women later develop type 2 diabetes.

Diabetes Mellitus Diagnostic Procedures

- A **fasting blood sugar (FBS)** measures the glucose (blood sugar) levels after the patient has not eaten for 8 to 12 hours. This test is used to screen for and to monitor treatment of diabetes mellitus.

- A **glucose tolerance test** (**GLOO**-kohs) **(GTT)** is used to confirm diabetes mellitus and to aid in diagnosing hypoglycemia (low blood sugar).

- A **fingerstick blood sugar monitoring test** is performed at least once daily to determine how much insulin or other medications are required.

- **Hemoglobin A1c testing (HgA1c),** also known as the **HbA1c** or **glycohemoglobin testing (GHb),** uses blood tests that measure the average blood glucose level over the previous three to four months. These tests monitor how well blood sugar levels have been controlled during this time. **Glycohemoglobin** (glye-koh-**hee**-moh-**GLOH**-bin) **(GHb)** forms when glucose in the blood attaches to the hemoglobin.

- The **fructosamine test** (fruck-**TOHS**-ah-meen) measures average glucose levels over the past three weeks. The fructosamine test detects changes more rapidly than the HgA1c test.

Diabetic Emergencies

- **Hypoglycemia,** which is very low blood sugar, is caused by not eating at the proper time or by not adjusting medications properly. Treatment is to raise blood sugar rapidly with glucose tablets or another form of readily absorbed sugar.

- **Hyperglycemia,** which is very high blood sugar, is also known as **diabetic ketoacidosis** (kee-toh-**ass**-ih-**DOH**-sis) **(DKA).** This acute, life-threatening complication is caused by a severe insulin deficiency. If untreated, it may lead to a **diabetic coma** and possibly death.

Diabetic Complications

- Most diabetic complications result from the damage to blood vessels, particularly capillaries, caused by long-term high blood sugar. This damage affects the capillary beds in many organs such as the eyes and kidneys.

- **Heart disease** occurs because excess blood sugar makes the walls of the blood vessels sticky. This stickiness encourages atherosclerosis (plaque buildup) within these vessels that slows or blocks the normal flow of blood.

- **Kidney disease** may lead to renal failure due to blood vessel damage that reduces blood flow through the kidneys.

- **Peripheral neuropathy** (new-**ROP**-ah-thee) is damage to the nerves of the hands and feet. This can cause either extreme sensitivity or numbness.

- **Diabetic retinopathy (DR)** is a complication of diabetes that causes damage to the retina of the eye (**retin/o** means retina and **-pathy** means disease). *Retinopathy* (ret-ih-NOP-ah-thee) means any disease of the retina.

- One form of DR is **macular edema,** in which fluids from blood vessels leaking into the eye cause the macula to swell. Another form is **proliferative retinopathy.** Here fragile new blood vessels form and break, clouding vision and damaging the retina.

TREATMENT PROCEDURE OF THE PANCREAS

- A **pancreatectomy** (pan-kree-ah-**TECK**-toh-mee) is the surgical removal of the pancreas (**pancreat** means pancreas and **-ectomy** means surgical removal).

THE THYMUS

The **thymus** (**THIGH**-mus) is located near the midline in the anterior portion of the thoracic cavity. It is posterior to (behind) the sternum and slightly superior to (above) the heart. *Note:* The word part **thym/o** means thymus; however, it also means relationship to the soul or emotions.

FUNCTIONS OF THE THYMUS

The thymus plays an important role in the immune system, and these functions are discussed in Chapter 6.

SECRETIONS OF THE THYMUS

- **Thymosin** (**THIGH**-moh-sin) stimulates the maturation of lymphocytes into T cells of the immune system.

PATHOLOGY OF THE THYMUS

- **Thymitis** (thigh-**MY**-tis) is an inflammation of the thymus gland (**thym** means thymus, and **-itis** means inflammation).
- A **thymoma** (thigh-**MOH**-mah) is a usually benign tumor derived from the tissue of the thymus (**thym** means thymus and **-oma** means tumor).

TREATMENT PROCEDURE OF THE THYMUS

- A **thymectomy** (thigh-**MECK**-toh-mee) is the surgical removal of the thymus gland (**thym** means thymus and **-ectomy** means surgical removal).

THE PINEAL GLAND

The **pineal gland** (**PIN**-ee-al) is located in the central portion of the brain.

FUNCTIONS OF THE PINEAL GLAND

- The function of the pineal gland is not clearly understood. However, the pineal gland is known to influence the sleep-wakefulness cycle.

SECRETION OF THE PINEAL GLAND

- **Melatonin** (mel-ah-**TOH**-nin) influences the sleep and wakefulness portions of the circadian cycle. The term *circadian cycle* refers to the biological functions that occur within a 24-hour period.

PATHOLOGY OF THE PINEAL GLAND

- **Pinealopathy** (pin-ee-ah-**LOP**-ah-thee) is any disorder of the pineal gland (**pineal/o** means pineal gland and **-pathy** means disease).

TREATMENT PROCEDURES OF THE PINEAL GLAND

- A **pinealectomy** (pin-ee-al-**ECK**-toh-mee) is the surgical removal of the pineal body (**pineal** means pineal gland and **-ectomy** means surgical removal).

THE GONADS

The **gonads** (**GOH**-nadz), which are ovaries in females and testicles in males, are the gamete-producing glands. A **gamete** (**GAM**-eet) is a reproductive cell. This is the sperm in the male, and ova (eggs) in the female.

- A **gonadotropic hormone** (gon-ah-doh-**TROHP**-ick), also known as **gonadotropin,** is any hormone that stimulates the gonads.

FUNCTIONS OF THE GONADS

- The gonads secrete the hormones that are responsible for the development and maintenance of secondary sex characteristics.
- The additional functions of the glands are discussed in Chapter 14.

SECRETIONS OF THE TESTICLES

- **Testosterone** (tes-**TOS**-teh-rohn), which is secreted by the testicles, stimulates the development of male secondary sex characteristics (Figure 13.6).

SECRETIONS OF THE OVARIES

- **Estrogen** (**ES**-troh-jen) is important in the development and maintenance of the female secondary sex characteristics and in regulation of the menstrual cycle (Figure 13.7).
- **Progesterone** (proh-**JES**-ter-ohn) is the hormone released during the second half of the menstrual cycle by the corpus luteum in the ovary. Its function is to complete the preparations for pregnancy.
- If pregnancy occurs, the placenta takes over the production of progesterone.
- If pregnancy does not occur, secretion of the hormone stops and is followed by the menstrual period.

The Placenta

- The **placenta** is an organ formed during pregnancy that allows the exchange of nutrients, oxygen, and waste products between the mother and developing child during pregnancy. After the child is born, the placenta is expelled as the afterbirth.
- **Human chorionic gonadotropin** (kor-ee-**ON**-ick gon-ah-doh-**TROH**-pin) (**HCG**) is the hormone secreted by the placenta during pregnancy. HCG stimulates the corpus luteum to continue producing the hormones required to maintain the pregnancy.
- It also stimulates the hormones required to stimulate lactation after childbirth.

PATHOLOGY OF THE GONADS

- **Hypergonadism** (high-per-**GOH**-nad-izm) is the condition of excessive secretion of hormones by the sex glands (**hyper-** means excessive, **gonad** means sex gland, and **-ism** means condition).

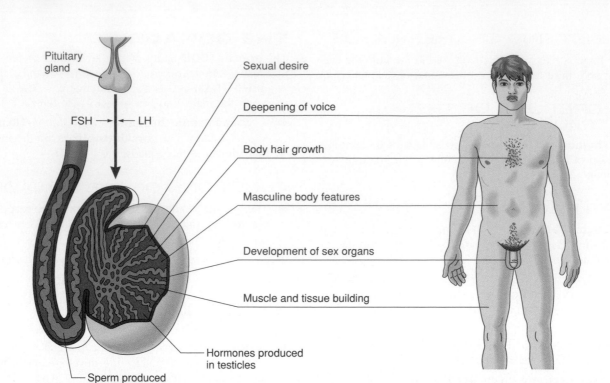

Pituitary gland

FSH → ← LH

Sexual desire

Deepening of voice

Body hair growth

Masculine body features

Development of sex organs

Muscle and tissue building

Hormones produced in testicles

Sperm produced in testicles

FIGURE 13.6 The secondary sex characteristics in the male produced by the secretion of testosterone.

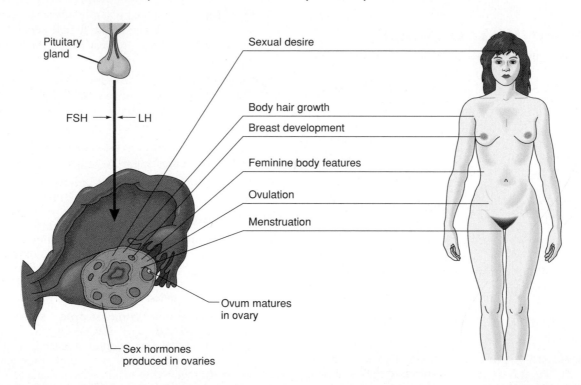

Pituitary gland

FSH → ← LH

Sexual desire

Body hair growth

Breast development

Feminine body features

Ovulation

Menstruation

Ovum matures in ovary

Sex hormones produced in ovaries

FIGURE 13.7 The secondary sex characteristics in the female produced by the secretion of estrogen.

● **Hypogonadism** (**high**-poh-**GOH**-nad-izm) is the condition of deficient secretion of hormones by the sex glands (**hypo-** means deficient, **gonad** means sex gland, and **-ism** means condition).

● **Gynecomastia** (**guy**-neh-koh-**MAS**-tee-ah) is the condition of excessive mammary development in the male (**gynec/o** means female, **mast** means breast, and **-ia** means abnormal condition).

TREATMENT PROCEDURES OF THE GONADS

Treatment procedures of the gonads are discussed in Chapter 14.

Review Time

Write the answers to the following questions on a separate piece of paper or in your notebook. In addition, be prepared to take part in the classroom discussion.

1. **Written assignment:** Using your own words, describe **acromegaly** and **gigantism.**

   Discussion assignment: What is the cause of each of these conditions?

2. **Written assignment:** Report on your research about the person for whom **Cushing's syndrome** was named. Include in your report his or her full name and dates.

   Discussion assignment: Use terms a physician could understand to describe the signs, symptoms, and causes of Cushing's syndrome.

3. **Written assignment:** Describe the primary difference between **type 1 diabetes** and **type 2 diabetes.**

   Discussion assignment: Lizzy, who is 79 years of age and overweight, has just been diagnosed with type 2 diabetes. How would you explain this condition to her?

4. **Written assignment:** Using terms a layperson would understand, explain the symptoms of **Graves' disease.**

Discussion assignment: What are the causes and treatment of Graves' disease?

5. **Written assignment:** Using your own words, describe **anabolic steroids.**

   Discussion assignment: What are the dangers of using anabolic steroids?

Optional Internet Activity

*The goal of this activity is to help you learn more about medical terminology while improving your Internet skills. Select **one** of these two options and follow the instructions.*

1. **Internet Search:** Search for information about **diabetes.** Write a brief (one- or two-paragraph) report on something new you learned here and include the address of the web site where you found this information.

2. **Web Site:** To learn more about **pituitary disorders,** go to this web address: **http://www.pituitary. org/.** Explore the site and then write a brief (one- or two-paragraph) report on something new you learned here.

The Human Touch: Critical Thinking Exercise

The following story and questions are designed to stimulate critical thinking through class discussion or as a brief essay response. There are no right or wrong answers to these questions.

By the time 14-year-old Jacob Tuls got home, he was sick enough for his mom to notice. He seemed shaky and confused and was sweaty even though the fall weather was cool. "Jake, let's get you a glass of juice right away," his mother said as calmly as she could. She was all too familiar with the symptoms of hypoglycemia brought on by Jake's type 1 diabetes. Ever since he was diagnosed at age six, she had carefully monitored his insulin, eating, and exercise. But now that he was in middle school, the ball was in his court, and it really worried her that he often seemed to mess up.

"Yeah, I know I shouldn't have gone so long without eating," Jake muttered once he was feeling better. "But you don't understand. I don't want to be different from the other kids." Before he could finish, his mom was on the telephone to the school nurse's office.

Jacob needed to inject himself with insulin three times a day. He knew what happened when his blood sugar got too high or if he didn't eat on schedule and it got too low. But when he was with his friends, he hated to go up to the chaperone on a field trip and say that he needed to eat something right away. And he hated it when some kid walked in while he was injecting. His mom had made arrangements with the school nurse for him to go to her office to get some privacy, but whenever he didn't show up between fourth and fifth periods, she'd come into the classroom to get him as if he was some kind of sick "dweeb."

He was tired of having this disease, sick of shots, and angry that he couldn't sleep late and skip meals like other kids. He made a face at his mother as she talked on the telephone to the nurse and slammed the back door on his way out to find his friend Joe.

Suggested Discussion Topics

1. What could Jacob's parents do to help him get through this rough time of his life?
2. Why is it more difficult for Jacob to maintain his injection routine in middle school than it was in elementary school?
3. Knowing that missing an insulin injection could cause a diabetic coma and death, why wouldn't Jacob be more conscientious?
4. Do you think Jacob's schoolmates talk about him, or does he just think they do? Discuss both possibilities.
5. People with juvenile diabetes can live close to a normal life span if they follow a healthy routine. Discuss stages in their lives at which they might have the most difficulties with this disease.

Student Workbook and Student Activity CD-ROM

1. Go to your **Student Workbook** and complete the Learning Exercises for this chapter.
2. Go to the **Student Activity CD-ROM** and have fun with the exercises and games for this chapter.

CHAPTER

14

The Reproductive Systems

● **Overview of Structures, Word Parts, and Functions of the Reproductive Systems**

MAJOR STRUCTURES	RELATED WORD PARTS	PRIMARY FUNCTIONS
Male		
Testicles, testes	**orch/o, orchid/o, test/i, test/o, testicul/o**	Produce sperm and the male hormone testosterone.
Female		
Ovaries	**oophor/o, ovari/o**	Produce ova (eggs) and female hormones.
Fallopian tubes	**salping/o**	Catch mature ova, provide the site for fertilization, transport ova to uterus.
Uterus	**hyster/o, metr/o, metri/o, uter/o**	Protects and supports the developing child.
Placenta	**placent/o**	Exchanges nutrients and waste between the mother and fetus during pregnancy.

Vocabulary Related to the Reproductive Systems

Terms marked with the ❖ symbol are pronounced on the Student Activity CD-ROM that accompanies this text.

KEY WORD PARTS

- ☐ cervic/o
- ☐ colp/o
- ☐ episi/o
- ☐ -gravida
- ☐ gynec/o
- ☐ mamm/o
- ☐ men/o
- ☐ metr/o
- ☐ nulli-
- ☐ oophor/o
- ☐ orchid/o
- ☐ ov/o
- ☐ -pexy
- ☐ prostat/o
- ☐ salping/o

KEY MEDICAL TERMS

- ☐ ablation (ab-**LAY**-shun) ❖
- ☐ abruptio placentae
  (ab-**RUP**-shee-oh plah-**SEN**-tee) ❖
- ☐ amenorrhea (ah-**men**-oh-**REE**-ah *or*
  ay-**men**-oh-**REE**-ah) ❖
- ☐ anorchism (an-**OR**-kizm) ❖
- ☐ azoospermia (ay-**zoh**-oh-**SPER**-mee-ah) ❖
- ☐ benign prostatic hypertrophy ❖
- ☐ cervical dysplasia (dis-**PLAY**-see-ah) ❖
- ☐ cervicitis (ser-vih-**SIGH**-tis)
- ☐ cesarean section (seh-**ZEHR**-ee-un **SECK**-shun)
- ☐ chlamydia (klah-**MID**-ee-ah)
- ☐ circumcision (ser-kum-**SIZH**-un)
- ☐ colposcopy (kol-**POS**-koh-pee)
- ☐ curettage (kyou-reh-**TAHZH**) ❖
- ☐ dilation (dye-**LAY**-shun) ❖
- ☐ dysmenorrhea (**dis**-men-oh-**REE**-ah) ❖
- ☐ eclampsia (eh-**KLAMP**-see-ah) ❖
- ☐ ectopic pregnancy (eck-**TOP**-ick) ❖
- ☐ endocervicitis (en-doh-ser-vih-**SIGH**-tis) ❖
- ☐ endometriosis (en-doh-mee-tree-**OH**-sis) ❖
- ☐ epididymitis (ep-ih-did-ih-**MY**-tis)
- ☐ episiorrhaphy (eh-**piz**-ee-**OR**-ah-fee) ❖
- ☐ episiotomy (eh-**piz**-ee-**OT**-oh-mee) ❖
- ☐ fibrocystic breast disease
  (**figh**-broh-**SIS**-tick) ❖
- ☐ gonorrhea (gon-oh-**REE**-ah) ❖
- ☐ gynecologist (**guy**-neh-**KOL**-oh-jist) ❖
- ☐ human papilloma virus (pap-ih-**LOH**-mah) ❖
- ☐ hypomenorrhea (**high**-poh-men-oh-**REE**-ah) ❖
- ☐ hysterectomy (hiss-teh-**RECK**-toh-mee) ❖
- ☐ hysteropexy (**HISS**-ter-oh-**peck**-see) ❖

- ☐ hysterosalpingography
  (**hiss**-ter-oh-**sal**-pin-**GOG**-rah-fee) ❖
- ☐ hysterosalpingo-oophorectomy (**hiss**-ter-oh-
  sal-**ping**-goh oh-**ahf**-oh-**RECK**-toh-mee) ❖
- ☐ hysteroscopy (**hiss**-ter-**OSS**-koh-pee) ❖
- ☐ leiomyoma (**lye**-oh-my-**OH**-mah) ❖
- ☐ leukorrhea (**loo**-koh-**REE**-ah) ❖
- ☐ mammography (mam-**OG**-rah-fee) ❖
- ☐ mammoplasty (**MAM**-oh-**plas**-tee) ❖
- ☐ menarche (meh-**NAR**-kee)
- ☐ menometrorrhagia
  (**men**-oh-**met**-roh-**RAY**-jee-ah) ❖
- ☐ menopause (**MEN**-oh-pawz)
- ☐ menstruation (**men**-stroo-**AY**-shun) ❖
- ☐ metrorrhea (**mee**-troh-**REE**-ah) ❖
- ☐ metrorrhexis (**mee**-troh-**RECK**-sis) ❖
- ☐ mittelschmerz (**MIT**-uhl-schmehrts) ❖
- ☐ multiparous (mul-**TIP**-ah-rus) ❖
- ☐ neonate (**NEE**-oh-nayt) ❖
- ☐ nulligravida (**null**-ih-**GRAV**-ih-dah) ❖
- ☐ nullipara (nuh-**LIP**-ah-rah) ❖
- ☐ obstetrician (**ob**-steh-**TRISH**-un) ❖
- ☐ oligomenorrhea (ol-ih-goh-**men**-oh-**REE**-ah) ❖
- ☐ oligospermia (ol-ih-goh-**SPER**-mee-ah) ❖
- ☐ oophorectomy (oh-ahf-oh-**RECK**-toh-mee) ❖
- ☐ oophoritis (oh-ahf-oh-**RYE**-tis) ❖
- ☐ orchidectomy (or-kih-**DECK**-toh-mee) ❖
- ☐ orchitis (or-**KYE**-tis) ❖
- ☐ ovariectomy (oh-vay-ree-**ECK**-toh-mee) ❖
- ☐ ovariorrhexis (oh-**vay**-ree-oh-**RECK**-sis) ❖
- ☐ Papanicolaou test (pap-ah-**nick**-oh-**LAY**-ooh) ❖
- ☐ perimenopause (pehr-ih-**MEN**-oh-pawz) ❖
- ☐ perineum (pehr-ih-**NEE**-um)
- ☐ placenta previa (plah-**SEN**-tah **PREE**-vee-ah) ❖
- ☐ preeclampsia (pree-ee-**KLAMP**-see-ah) ❖
- ☐ primigravida (prye-mih-**GRAV**-ih-dah)
- ☐ primipara (prye-**MIP**-ah-rah)
- ☐ prostatectomy (pros-tah-**TECK**-toh-mee)
- ☐ prostatitis (pros-tah-**TYE**-tis)
- ☐ pruritus vulvae (proo-**RYE**-tus **VUL**-vee)
- ☐ salpingo-oophorectomy
  (sal-**ping**-goh oh-**ahf**-oh-**RECK**-toh-mee) ❖
- ☐ syphilis (**SIF**-ih-lis)
- ☐ trichomonas (trick-oh-**MOH**-nas) ❖
- ☐ vaginal candidiasis (kan-dih-**DYE**-ah-sis) ❖
- ☐ vaginoplasty (vah-**JIGH**-noh-**plas**-tee) ❖
- ☐ varicocele (**VAR**-ih-koh-**seel**) ❖
- ☐ varicocelectomy
  (**var**-ih-koh-sih-**LECK**-toh-mee) ❖
- ☐ vasectomy (vah-**SECK**-toh-mee) ❖
- ☐ vasovasostomy (vas-oh-vah-**ZOS**-toh-mee *or*
  vay-zoh-vay-**ZOS**-toh-mee) ❖

Upon completion of this chapter, you should be able to:

1. Identify and describe the major functions and structures of the male reproductive system.
2. Recognize, define, spell, and pronounce the terms related to the pathology and diagnostic and treatment procedures of the male reproductive system.
3. Name at least six sexually transmitted diseases.
4. Identify and describe the major functions and structures of the female reproductive system.
5. Recognize, define, spell, and pronounce the terms related to the pathology and diagnostic and treatment procedures of the female reproductive system.
6. Recognize, define, spell, and pronounce the terms related to the pathology and diagnostic and treatment procedures of the female during pregnancy, childbirth, and the postpartum period.

FUNCTIONS OF THE MALE REPRODUCTIVE SYSTEM

The primary function of the male reproductive system is to produce millions of sperm and deliver them to unite with a single ovum (egg) to create a new life.

STRUCTURES OF THE MALE REPRODUCTIVE SYSTEM

Some of the structures of the male reproductive system also function as part of the urinary system. Urinary functions are discussed in Chapter 9.

THE EXTERNAL MALE GENITALIA

The term **genitalia** (**jen**-ih-**TAY**-lee-ah) means reproductive organs. The external genitalia are those reproductive organs located outside of the body cavity.

- Major external male organs include the penis, scrotum, and two testicles, each with an attached epididymis (Figure 14.1).

Scrotum

The **scrotum** (**SKROH**-tum) encloses, protects, and supports the testicles. It is suspended from the pubic arch behind the penis and lies between the thighs.

- In the male, the **perineum** (pehr-ih-**NEE**-um) is the region between the scrotum and the anus.

The Testicles

The **testicles,** also known as **testes,** are the two small egg-shaped glands that produce the spermatozoa (Figure 14.2) (singular, **testis**).

- The testicles develop within the abdomen of the male fetus and normally descend into the scrotum before birth or soon after birth.

- The **epididymis** (**ep**-ih-**DID**-ih-mis) is a tube at the upper part of each testicle. It runs down the length of the testicle then turns upward into the body, where it becomes a narrower tube called the vas deferens.

The Penis

The **penis** (**PEE**-nis) is the male sex organ that transports the sperm into the female vagina. The penis is composed of erectile tissue that, during sexual stimulation, fills with blood (under high pressure), causing an erection.

- The **glans penis** (glanz **PEE**-nis) is a soft sensitive region located at the tip of the penis.

- The **prepuce** (**PREE**-pyous), also known as the **foreskin,** covers and protects the glans penis.

INTERNAL MALE GENITALIA

The Vas Deferens

The **vas deferens** (vas **DEF**-er-enz) leads from the epididymis to the ejaculatory duct in the prostate.

The Seminal Vesicles

The **seminal vesicles** (**SEM**-ih-nal) are glands located at the base of the urinary bladder. These open into the vas deferens as it joins the urethra.

- These glands secrete a thick, yellow substance that nourishes the sperm cells and forms much of the volume of ejaculated semen.

- The **ejaculatory duct** is one of the two final portions of the seminal vesicles. This duct, which is formed by the union of the ductus deferens and the duct from the seminal vesicle, passes through the prostate gland and enters the urethra.

The Prostate Gland

The **prostate gland** (**PROS**-tayt) lies under the bladder and surrounds the upper end of the urethra in the region

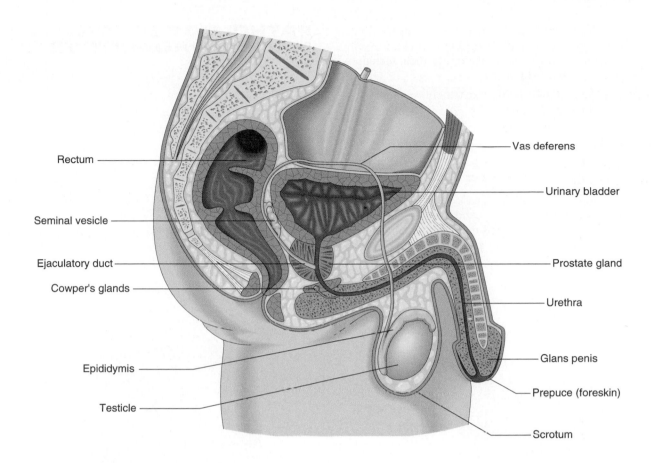

Rectum

Seminal vesicle

Ejaculatory duct

Cowper's glands

Epididymis

Testicle

Vas deferens

Urinary bladder

Prostate gland

Urethra

Glans penis

Prepuce (foreskin)

Scrotum

FIGURE 14.1 Cross section of the male reproductive organs.

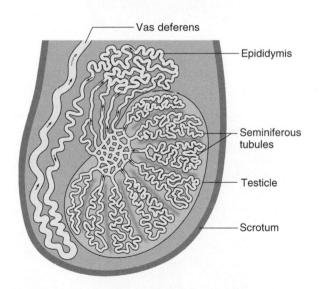

Vas deferens

Epididymis

Seminiferous tubules

Testicle

Scrotum

FIGURE 14.2 Cross section of structures contained within the scrotum. The arrows indicate the flow through these structures.

where the vas deferens enters the urethra (see Figure 9.3).

● The prostate gland secretes a thick fluid that, as part of the semen, aids the motility of the sperm.

The Cowper's Glands

Cowper's glands, also known as **bulbourethral glands** (**bul**-boh-you-**REE**-thral), are located on either side of the urethra just below the prostate gland, and their ducts open into the urethra.

● These glands secrete thick mucus that acts as a lubricant that tends to flow early during sexual excitement.

The Urethra

The **urethra** passes through the penis to the outside of the body. In the male, it serves both the reproductive and urinary systems.

THE SPERM AND SEMEN FORMATION

● The **sperm** are the male gametes. A **gamete** (**GAM**-eet) is a reproductive cell. Also known as **spermatozoa** (**sper**-mah-toh-**ZOH**-ah), sperm are formed in the seminiferous tubules of the testicles (singular, **spermatozoon**).

● After sperm are formed, they move into the epididymis, where they become motile and are temporarily stored. *Motile* means capable of spontaneous motion.

- From the epididymis, the sperm travel upward into the body and enter the vas deferens. There, the seminal vesicles and prostate gland add their secretions to form **semen** (**SEE**-men).

- At the peak of male sexual excitement, semen is ejaculated through the urethra.

MEDICAL SPECIALTIES RELATED TO THE MALE REPRODUCTIVE SYSTEM

- A **urologist** (you-**ROL**-oh-jist) specializes in diagnosing and treating diseases and disorders of the urinary system of females and the genitourinary system of males (**ur** means urine and **-ologist** means specialist).

THE PENIS

- **Balanitis** (**bal**-ah-**NIGH**-tis) is an inflammation of the glans penis and is often associated with phimosis (**balan** means glans penis and **-itis** means inflammation).

- **Phimosis** (figh-**MOH**-sis) is a narrowing of the opening of the foreskin so it cannot be retracted (pulled back) to expose the glans penis.

- **Impotence** (**IM**-poh-tens), also known as **erectile dysfunction,** is the inability of the male to achieve or maintain a penile erection.

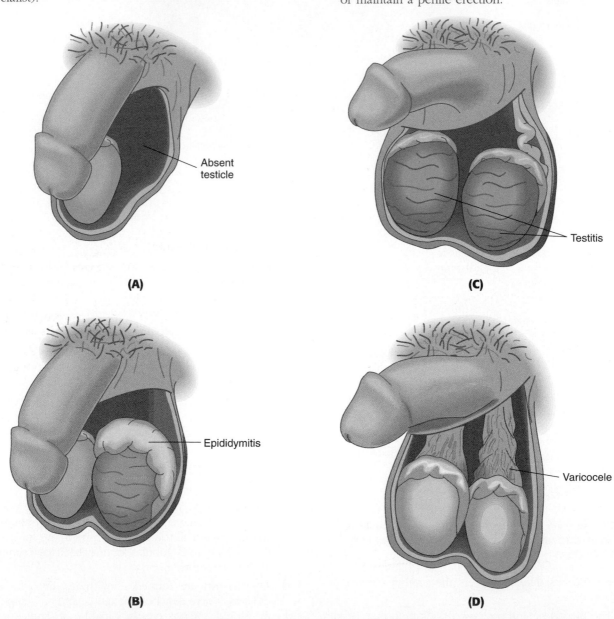

(A)

Absent testicle

(B)

Epididymitis

(C)

Testitis

(D)

Varicocele

FIGURE 14.3 Pathology of the testicles. (A) Anorchism in which one testicle is absent. (B) Epididymitis. (C) Testitus of both testicles. (D) Varicocele.

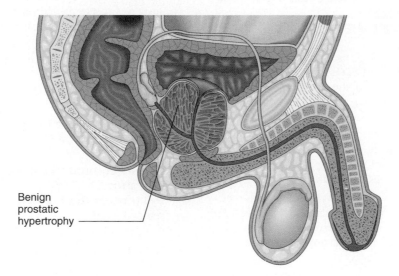

FIGURE 14.4 Benign prostatic hypertrophy. This enlarged prostate impinges on the bladder and slows the flow of urine through the urethra.

THE TESTICLES AND RELATED STRUCTURES

- **Anorchism** (an-**OR**-kizm) is the congenital absence of one or both testicles (**an-** means without, **orch** means testicle, and **-ism** means abnormal condition) (Figure 14.3A).

- **Cryptorchidism** (krip-**TOR**-kih-dizm), also known as an **undescended testis,** is a developmental defect in which one testicle fails to descend into the scrotum (**crypt/o** means hidden, **orchid** means testicle, and **-ism** means abnormal condition).

- **Epididymitis** (ep-ih-did-ih-**MY**-tis) is inflammation of the epididymis (**epididym** means epididymis and **-itis** means inflammation) (Figure 14.3B).

- A **hydrocele** (**HIGH**-droh-seel) is a hernia filled with fluid in the testicles or the tubes leading from the testicles (**hydro** means relating to water and **cele** means hernia).

- **Testitis** (tes-**TYE**-tis), also known as **orchitis** (or-**KYE**-tis), is inflammation of one or both testicles (**test** means testicle and **-itis** means inflammation) (Figure 14.3C).

- A **varicocele** (**VAR**-ih-koh-**seel**) is a varicose vein (abnormal enlargement of the vein) of the testicles that may cause male infertility (**varic/o** means varicose veins and **-cele** means swelling) (Figure 14.3D).

Sperm Count

- **Azoospermia** (ay-**zoh**-oh-**SPER**-mee-ah) is the absence of sperm in the semen (**a-** means without, **zoo** means life, **sperm** means sperm, and **-ia** means abnormal condition).

- **Oligospermia** (**ol**-ih-goh-**SPER**-mee-ah), also known as a **low sperm count,** is an abnormally low number of sperm in the ejaculate (**olig/o** means few, **sperm** means sperm, and **-ia** means abnormal condition).

THE PROSTATE GLAND

- **Benign prostatic hypertrophy (BPH),** also known as **prostatomegaly** (**pros**-tah-toh-**MEG**-ah-lee) or an **enlarged prostate,** is an abnormal enlargement of the prostate gland (Figure 14.4).

- **Prostate cancer** is one of the most common cancers among men. The disease may grow slowly with no symptoms, or it may grow aggressively and spread throughout the body.

- **Prostatitis** (**pros**-tah-**TYE**-tis) is an inflammation of the prostate gland (**prostat** means prostate gland and **-itis** means inflammation).

- **Prostatorrhea** (**pros**-tah-toh-**REE**-ah) is an abnormal flow of prostatic fluid discharged through the urethra (**prostat/o** means prostate gland and **-rrhea** means abnormal flow).

DIAGNOSTIC PROCEDURES OF THE MALE REPRODUCTIVE SYSTEM

- **Prostate-specific antigen (PSA)** is a blood test to screen for prostate cancer. Values greater than 10 are significant indicators for prostate cancer.

- **Sperm analysis (SA),** also known as **sperm count,** is the testing of freshly ejaculated semen to determine the volume plus the sperm count, shape, size, and motility (ability to move).

- **Testicular self-examination (TSE)** is an important self-help step in early detection of testicular cancer.

TREATMENT PROCEDURES OF THE MALE REPRODUCTIVE SYSTEM

GENERAL

- **Circumcision** (**ser**-kum-**SIZH**-un) is the surgical removal of the foreskin of the penis and is usually performed a few days after birth.

- An **orchidectomy** (**or**-kih-**DECK**-toh-mee) is the surgical removal of one or both testicles (**orchid** means testicle and **-ectomy** means surgical removal). This procedure is also known as an **orchectomy, orchiectomy** (**or**-kee-**ECK**-toh-mee), or **testectomy.**

- A **varicocelectomy** (**var**-ih-koh-sih-**LECK**-toh-mee) is the removal of a portion of an enlarged vein to relieve a varicocele (**varic/o** means varicose vein, **cele** means swelling, and **-ectomy** means surgical removal).

MALE STERILIZATION

Sterilization is any procedure rendering an individual (male or female) incapable of reproduction.

- **Castration** (kas-**TRAY**-shun), also known as **bilateral orchidectomy,** is the surgical removal or destruction of both testicles.

- A **vasectomy** (vah-**SECK**-toh-mee) is the male sterilization procedure in which a portion of the vas deferens is surgically removed (**vas** means vas deferens and **-ectomy** means surgical removal). This surgery prevents sperm from entering the ejaculate but does not change the volume of semen (Figure 14.5).

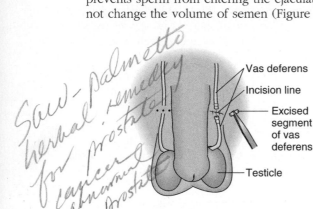

FIGURE 14.5 In a vasectomy, a portion of the vas deferens is removed to prevent sperm from becoming part of the semen.

- A **vasovasostomy** (vas-oh-vah-**ZOS**-toh-mee *or* vay-zoh-vay-**ZOS**-toh-mee) is a procedure to restore fertility to a vasectomized male.

PROSTATE CANCER TREATMENT

- The term **ablation** (ab-**LAY**-shun) means the removal or destruction of the function of a body part.

This technique, which is used to treat conditions such as prostate cancer, may involve surgery, chemical destruction, electrocautery, extreme cold, or radiation.

- A **prostatectomy** (**pros**-tah-**TECK**-toh-mee) is the surgical removal of all or part of the prostate gland (**prostat** means prostate and **-ectomy** means surgical removal).

- A **radical prostatectomy** is the surgical removal of the entire prostate gland, the seminal vesicles, and some surrounding tissue.

- A **transurethral prostatectomy** (**trans**-you-**REE**-thral **pros**-tah-**TECK**-toh-mee) **(TURP),** also known as a **transurethral resection of the prostate,** is the removal of all or part of the prostate through the urethra (Figure 14.6).

- **Radiation therapy (RT)** and **hormone therapy (HT)** are additional treatments used to control prostate cancer.

SEXUALLY TRANSMITTED DISEASES

Sexually transmitted diseases (STDs), also known as **venereal diseases (VDs),** are transmitted through sexual intercourse or other genital contact. **Venereal** (veh-**NEER**-ee-ahl) means pertaining to, relating to, or transmitted by sexual contact.

- **Bacterial vaginosis** (**vaj**-ih-**NOH**-sis) **(BV)** is a sexually transmitted bacterial infection of the vagina (**vagin** means vagina and **-osis** means abnormal condition). BV may cause complications during pregnancy and an increased risk of HIV infection.

- **Chlamydia** (klah-**MID**-ee-ah), which is caused by the bacterium *Chlamydia trachomatis,* is highly contagious. Unless there is early treatment with antibiotics, it may cause sterility in both males and females.

- **Genital herpes** (**HER**-peez) **(HSV-2)** is caused by the herpes simplex virus and is highly contagious. Symptoms include itching or burning before the appearance of lesions (sores). Antiviral drugs ease symptoms; however, currently there is no cure and lesions may recur at any time.

- **Gonorrhea** (**gon**-oh-**REE**-ah), which is caused by the bacterium *Neisseria gonorrhoeae,* is highly contagious. It is characterized by painful urination and an abnormal discharge and may affect other body structures, including the eyes. This disease may be transmitted to the child during birth. All newborns receive one drop of silver nitrate or penicillin in each eye immediately after birth to prevent gonorrhea infection of the eyes.

- **Human immunodeficiency virus (HIV),** which affects the immune system (see Chapter 6), is transmitted through exposure to infected body fluids, particularly through sexual intercourse with an infected partner.

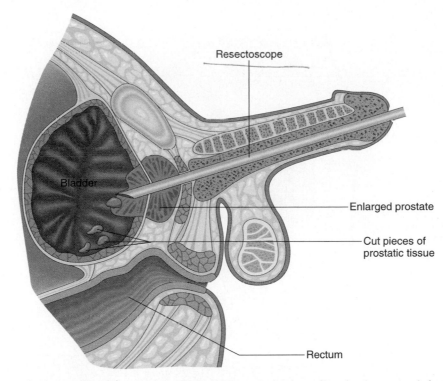

FIGURE 14.6 A transurethral resection of the prostate (TURP) being performed to relieve benign prostatic hypertrophy.

- The **human papilloma virus** (**pap**-ih-**LOH**-mah) **(HPV),** also known as **genital warts,** is caused by the *human papillomavirus.* It is highly contagious and increases the risk of genital and cervical cancer.

- **Syphilis** (**SIF**-ih-lis) is highly contagious and is caused by the spirochete *Treponema pallidum.* Before symptoms appear, syphilis can be detected through the VDRL (Venereal Disease Research Laboratory) blood test.

- **Trichomonas** (**trick**-oh-**MOH**-nas), also known as **trich,** is a vaginal inflammation caused by the protozoan parasite *Trichomonas vaginalis.* It may cause complications during pregnancy and increases the risk of HIV infection.

FUNCTIONS OF THE FEMALE REPRODUCTIVE SYSTEM

The primary functions of the female reproductive system are the creation and support of new life.

- The ovaries produce eggs to be fertilized by the sperm.

- The uterus provides the environment and support for the developing child.

- After birth, the breasts produce milk to feed the child.

STRUCTURES OF THE FEMALE REPRODUCTIVE SYSTEM

THE EXTERNAL FEMALE GENITALIA

- The external female genitalia are located below the mons pubis. The **mons pubis** (monz **PYOU**-bis) is a rounded fleshy prominence over the pubic symphysis (Figures 14.7 and 14.8).

- The female external genitalia are also known collectively as the **vulva** (**VUL**-vah) or the **pudendum** (pyou-**DEN**-dum) (plural, **pudenda**).

The Labia *the lips to protect external genitalia*

The **labia majora** and **labia minora** are the vaginal lips that protect the external genitalia and the urethral meatus. The **urethral meatus** is the external opening of the urethra (see Chapter 9).

The Clitoris

The **clitoris** (**KLIT**-oh-ris) is an organ of sensitive, erectile tissue located anterior to (in front of) the vaginal opening and the urethral meatus.

Bartholin's Glands

Bartholin's glands are two small, rounded glands on either side of the vaginal opening that produce a mucus secretion to lubricate the vagina.

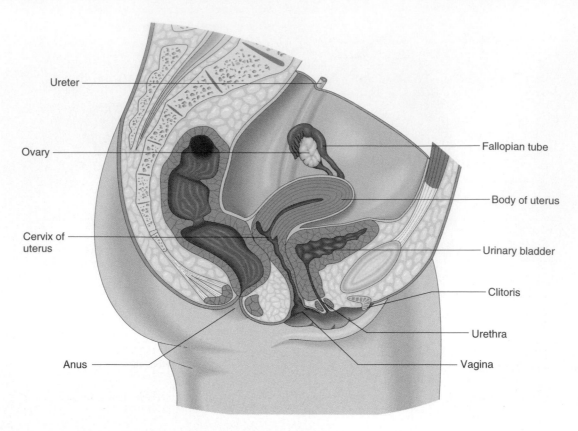

Ureter

Ovary

Cervix of
uterus

Anus

Fallopian tube

Body of uterus

Urinary bladder

Clitoris

Urethra

Vagina

FIGURE 14.7   Cross section of the female reproductive organs.

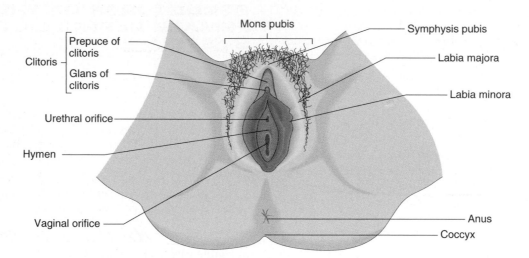

Mons pubis

Symphysis pubis

Prepuce of
clitoris

Clitoris

Glans of
clitoris

Urethral orifice

Hymen

Vaginal orifice

Labia majora

Labia minora

Anus

Coccyx

FIGURE 14.8   External genitalia of the female.

The Perineum

In the female, the **perineum** (pehr-ih-**NEE**-um) is the region between the vaginal orifice (opening) and the anus.

THE MAMMARY GLANDS

The **mammary glands,** also known as **breasts,** are milk-producing glands that develop during puberty (Figure 14.9). Each breast is fixed to the overlying skin and the underlying pectoral muscles by suspensory ligaments (see also Figure 6.12).

● The **areola** (ah-**REE**-oh-lah) is the dark-pigmented area that surrounds the **nipple.**

● The **mammary glands,** also known as **lactiferous glands** of the breast, produce milk after childbirth.

● The **lactiferous duct** (lack-**TIF**-er-us) carries milk from the mammary glands to the nipple.

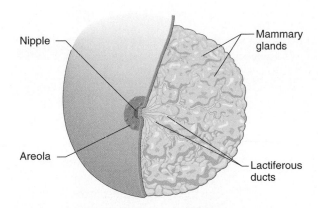

Nipple

Mammary glands

Areola

Lactiferous ducts

FIGURE 14.9 Structures of the breast.

INTERNAL FEMALE GENITALIA

The major female reproductive organs are located in the pelvic cavity and are protected by the bony pelvis (Figure 14.10). They include two ovaries, two fallopian tubes, one uterus, and the vagina.

The Ovaries

covered with small pockets called follicle

The **ovaries** (**OH**-vah-rees) are a pair of small almond-shaped organs located in the lower abdomen, one on either side of the uterus.

- A **follicle** (**FOL**-lick-kul) is a fluid-filled sac containing a single ovum (egg). There are thousands of these sacs on the surface of the ovaries.
- The **ova** (**OH**-vah), also known as eggs, are the female gametes (singular, **ovum**). Normally, each month one ovum matures and is released.

The Fallopian Tubes

carries the ovum from ovaries to uterus

The two **fallopian tubes,** also known as **uterine tubes,** carry the ovum downward from the ovary to the uterus. These tubes also carry sperm upward from the vagina and uterus.

- Each **fallopian tube** (fal-**LOH**-pee-an) extends from the upper end of the uterus to a point near but not attached to an ovary.
- The **infundibulum** (**in**-fun-**DIB**-you-lum) is the funnel-shaped opening into each fallopian tube. The **fimbriae** (**FIM**-bree-ee), which are the fringed fingerlike extensions of this opening, catch the ovum when it leaves the ovary (**fimbri** means fringe and **-ae** is a plural noun ending) (singular, **fimbria**).

The Uterus

vascular membrane lining

The **uterus** (**YOU**-ter-us) is a pear-shaped organ with muscular walls and a mucous membrane lining filled with a rich supply of blood vessels.

- The uterus is situated between the urinary bladder and the rectum and midway between the sacrum and the pubic bone.

The Parts of the Uterus

The uterus consists of three major anatomic areas.

- The **fundus** (**FUN**-dus) is the bulging rounded part above the entrance of the fallopian tubes (see Figure 14.10).
- The **corpus** (**KOR**-pus), also known as the **body,** is the middle portion.
- The **cervix** (**SER**-vicks), also known as the **cervix uteri,** is the lower narrow portion that extends into the vagina.

the lowest part of uterus that extend into vagina

The Tissues of the Uterus

The uterus is composed of three major layers of tissue.

- The **perimetrium** (pehr-ih-**MEE**-tree-um) is the tough membrane outer layer (**peri-** means surrounding, **metri** means uterus, and **-um** is a singular noun ending).

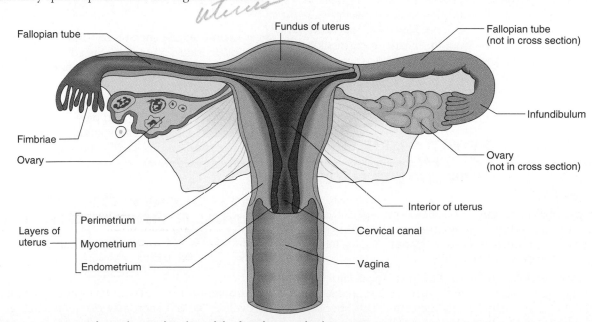

Fallopian tube

Fundus of uterus

Fallopian tube (not in cross section)

Fimbriae

Ovary

Infundibulum

Ovary (not in cross section)

Interior of uterus

Layers of uterus
- Perimetrium
- Myometrium
- Endometrium

Cervical canal

Vagina

FIGURE 14.10 Schematic anterior view of the female reproductive organs.

- The **myometrium** (my-oh-**MEE**-tree-um) is the muscular middle layer (**my/o** means muscle, **metri** means uterus, and **-um** is a singular noun ending).

- The **endometrium** (en-doh-**MEE**-tree-um) is the inner layer, which consists of specialized epithelial mucosa (**endo-** means within, **metri** means uterus, and **-um** is a singular noun ending).

The Vagina

The **vagina** (vah-**JIGH**-nah) is a muscular tube lined with mucosa that extends from the cervix to the outside of the body. (The word parts **colp/o** and **vagin/o** both mean vagina.)

- The **hymen** (**HIGH**-men) is a membranous fold of tissue that partly or completely covers the external vaginal orifice. An *orifice* is an entrance into, or an outlet from, a body cavity or canal.

MENSTRUATION

Menstruation (men-stroo-**AY**-shun), also known as **menses** (**MEN**-seez), is the normal periodic discharge of a bloody fluid from the nonpregnant uterus.

- **Menarche** (meh-**NAR**-kee) is the beginning of the menstrual function, which begins at puberty (**men** means menstruation and **-arche** means beginning).

- The average **menstrual cycle** consists of 28 days. These are grouped into four phases and are summarized in Table 14.1.

- **Menopause** (**MEN**-oh-pawz) is the normal stopping of the monthly menstrual periods (**men/o** means menstruation and **-pause** means stopping). Menopause, which officially begins 12 months after a woman's final menstrual period, occurs at the average age of 52.

- **Perimenopause** (pehr-ih-**MEN**-oh-pawz) is the term used to designate the transition phase between regular menstrual periods and no periods at all (**peri-** means surrounding, **men/o** means menstruation, and **-pause** means stopping). During this phase, which can last as long as 10 years, changes in hormone production may cause symptoms including hot flashes, mood swings, and disturbed sleep.

MEDICAL SPECIALTIES RELATED TO THE FEMALE REPRODUCTIVE SYSTEM

- A **gynecologist** (guy-neh-**KOL**-oh-jist) specializes in diagnosing and treating diseases and disorders of the female reproductive system (**gynec** means female and **-ologist** means specialist).

- An **obstetrician** (ob-steh-**TRISH**-un) specializes in providing medical care to women during pregnancy, childbirth, and immediately thereafter. This specialty is referred to as **obstetrics** (ob-**STET**-ricks).

Table 14.1

PHASES OF THE MENSTRUAL CYCLE

Days 1–5	**Menstrual Phase.** These are the days when the endometrial lining of the uterus is sloughed off and discharged through the vagina as the menstrual flow.
Days 6–12	**Postmenstrual Phase.** After the menstrual period, estrogen secreted by the ovary stimulates the lining of the uterus to prepare itself to receive a zygote (fertilized egg). The pituitary gland secretes follicle-stimulating hormone (FSH), causing an ovum to mature.
Days 13–14	**Ovulatory Phase.** On about the 13th or 14th day of the cycle, a mature ovum is released. When ovulation occurs, the egg leaves the ovary to travel slowly down the fallopian tube. During this time, the female is fertile and can become pregnant.
Days 15–28	**Premenstrual Phase.** If fertilization does not occur, hormone levels change to cause the breakdown of the uterine endometrium and the beginning of a new menstrual cycle.

- A **neonatologist** (nee-oh-nay-**TOL**-oh-jist) specializes in diagnosing and treating disorders of the newborn (**neo-** means new, **nat** means born, and **-ologist** means specialist).

- A **pediatrician** (pee-dee-ah-**TRISH**-un) specializes in diagnosing, treating, and preventing disorders and diseases of children. This specialty is known as **pediatrics** (**ped** means child, and **-iatrics** means the medical practice of).

PATHOLOGY OF THE FEMALE REPRODUCTIVE SYSTEM

THE OVARIES AND FALLOPIAN TUBES

- **Anovulation** (an-ov-you-**LAY**-shun) is the failure to ovulate. Menstruation may continue although ovulation does not occur.

- **Oophoritis** (**oh**-ahf-oh-**RYE**-tis) is an inflammation of an ovary (**oophor** means ovary and **-itis** means inflammation).

- **Ovarian cancer** is the third most common cancer of the female reproductive system; however, more women die of it than from other forms.

- **Ovariorrhexis** (oh-**vay**-ree-oh-**RECK**-sis) is the rupture of an ovary (**ovari/o** means ovary and **-rrhexis** means to rupture).

- **Pelvic inflammatory disease (PID)** is any inflammation of the female reproductive organs not associated with surgery or pregnancy. PID frequently occurs as a complication of STDs and can lead to infertility, tubal pregnancy, and other serious disorders.

- The **polycystic ovary syndrome (PCOS),** also known as **Stein-Leventhal syndrome,** is characterized by enlargement of the ovaries caused by the presence of many cysts. This condition, which is due to a hormonal imbalance, may cause infertility, menstrual abnormalities, and the development of secondary male characteristics such as hair growth.

- **Pyosalpinx** (**pye**-oh-**SAL**-pinks) is an accumulation of pus in the fallopian tube (**py/o** means pus and **-salpinx** means fallopian tube).

- **Salpingitis** (**sal**-pin-**JIGH**-tis) is an inflammation of a fallopian tube (**salping** means fallopian or eustachian tube and **-itis** means inflammation). *Caution:* This term also means inflammation of the eustachian tube of the middle ear.

THE UTERUS

- **Endometriosis** (en-doh-**mee**-tree-**OH**-sis) is a condition in which endometrial tissue escapes the uterus and grows outside the uterus on other structures in the pelvic cavity (**endo-** means within, **metri** means uterus, and **-osis** means abnormal condition).

- A **fibroid,** also known as a **leiomyoma** (lye-oh-my-**OH**-mah), is a benign tumor composed of muscle and fibrous tissue that occurs in the wall of the uterus.

- **Metrorrhea** (mee-troh-**REE**-ah) is an abnormal uterine discharge (**metr/o** means uterus and **-rrhea** means abnormal flow).

- **Metrorrhexis** (**mee**-troh-**RECK**-sis) means rupture of the uterus (**metr/o** means uterus and **-rrhexis** means to rupture).

- **Pyometritis** (pye-oh-meh-**TRY**-tis) is a purulent (pus-containing) inflammation of the uterus (**py/o** means pus, **metr** means uterus, and **-itis** means inflammation).

- **Uterine cancer** occurs most commonly after menopause, and one of the earliest symptoms is abnormal bleeding from the uterus.

Abnormal Uterine Positions

- **Anteflexion** (an-tee-**FLECK**-shun), as shown in Figure 14.7, is the normal position of the uterus. In this position, it is bent forward (**ante-** means forward, **flex** means bend, and **-ion** means condition).

- **Anteversion** (an-tee-**VER**-zhun), as shown in Figure 14.11, is abnormal tipping, tilting, or turning forward of the entire uterus, including the cervix (**ante-** means forward and **-version** means to turn).

- **Prolapse** (proh-**LAPS**) **of the uterus,** as shown in Figure 14.11, is a falling or sinking down of the uterus until it protrudes through the vaginal opening. *Prolapse* means downward placement.

- **Retroflexion** (ret-roh-**FLECK**-shun), as shown in Figure 14.11, is abnormal tipping with the body of the uterus bent, forming an angle with the cervix (**retro-** means backward, **flex** means to bend, and **-ion** means condition).

- **Retroversion** (ret-roh-**VER**-zhun), as shown in Figure 14.11, is abnormal tipping of the entire uterus backward, with the cervix pointing toward the pubic symphysis (**retro-** means backward and **-version** means to turn).

THE CERVIX

- **Cervical cancer** is the second most common cancer in women and usually affects women between the ages of 35 and 55. It can be detected early through routine Pap tests.

- **Cervical dysplasia** (**SER**-vih-kal dis-**PLAY**-see-ah), also known as **precancerous lesions,** is the abnormal growth of cells of the cervix that may be

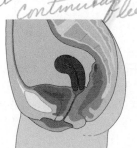 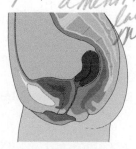 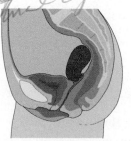 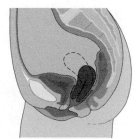

| Anteversion | Retroversion | Retroflexion | Prolapse |

FIGURE 14.11 Abnormal positions of the uterus.

PMS

detected on a Pap smear. If not treated, these cells may become malignant. *Dysplasia* is the abnormal growth of cells.

- **Cervicitis** (ser-vih-**SIGH**-tis) is an inflammation of the cervix (**cervic** means cervix and **-itis** means inflammation).

- **Endocervicitis** (en-doh-**ser**-vih-**SIGH**-tis) is an inflammation of the mucous membrane lining of the cervix (**endo-** means within, **cervic** means cervix, and **-itis** means inflammation).

THE VAGINA

- **Colporrhexis** (kol-poh-**RECK**-sis) means laceration (tearing) of the vagina (**colp/o** means vagina and **-rrhexis** means to rupture).

- **Leukorrhea** (loo-koh-**REE**-ah) is a profuse white mucus discharge from the uterus and vagina (**leuk/o** means white and **-rrhea** means abnormal flow).

- **Pruritus vulvae** (proo-**RYE**-tus **VUL**-vee) is a condition of severe itching of the external female genitalia. *Pruritus* means itching.

- **Vaginal candidiasis** (kan-dih-**DYE**-ah-sis), which is caused by the yeast *Candida albicans,* is the most commonly occurring vaginal yeast infection. Symptoms include itching, burning, and irritation.

- **Vaginitis** (vaj-ih-**NIGH**-tis), also known as **colpitis** (kol-**PYE**-tis), is an inflammation of the lining of the vagina (**vagin** means vagina and **-itis** means inflammation).

THE EXTERNAL GENITALIA

- **Vulvodynia** (vul-voh-**DIN**-ee-ah) is a nonspecific syndrome of unknown cause characterized by chronic burning, pain during sexual intercourse, itching, or stinging irritation of the vulva (**vulv/o** means vulva and **-dynia** means pain).

- **Vulvitis** (vul-**VYE**-tis) is an inflammation of the vulva (**vulv** means vulva and **-itis** means inflammation).

THE BREASTS

- **Breast cancer** and its treatment are discussed in Chapter 6.

- **Fibrocystic breast disease** (**figh**-broh-**SIS**-tick) is the presence of single or multiple cysts in the breasts. These cysts are usually benign but may become malignant.

- A **galactocele** (gah-**LACK**-toh-seel), also known as a **galactoma** (gal-ack-**TOH**-mah), is a cystic enlargement of the mammary gland containing milk (**galact/o** means milk and **-cele** means hernia).

- **Mastitis** (mas-**TYE**-tis) is an inflammation of the breast. It usually is associated with lactation but may occur for other reasons (**mast** means breast and **-itis** means inflammation).

MENSTRUAL DISORDERS

- **Amenorrhea** (ah-**men**-oh-**REE**-ah *or* ay-**men**-oh-**REE**-ah) is an absence of menstrual periods (**a-** means without, **men/o** means menstruation, and **-rrhea** means abnormal flow). This condition is normal only before puberty, during pregnancy, during breast-feeding, and after menopause.

- **Dysmenorrhea** (dis-men-oh-**REE**-ah) is abdominal pain caused by uterine cramps during a menstrual period (**dys-** means bad, **men/o** means menstruation, and **-rrhea** means abnormal flow).

- **Hypomenorrhea** (high-poh-men-oh-**REE**-ah) is a small amount of menstrual flow during a shortened regular menstrual period (**hypo-** means deficient, **men/o** means menstruation, and **-rrhea** means abnormal flow).

- **Menorrhagia** (men-oh-**RAY**-jee-ah) is an excessive amount of menstrual flow over a longer duration than of a normal period (**men/o** means menstruation and **-rrhagia** means abnormal bleeding).

- **Menometrorrhagia** (men-oh-**met**-roh-**RAY**-jee-ah) is excessive uterine bleeding occurring both during the menses and at irregular intervals (**men/o** means menstruation, **metr/o** means uterus, and **-rrhagia** means abnormal bleeding).

- **Mittelschmerz** (**MIT**-uhl-schmehrts) means pain between menstrual periods (from German, meaning "middle pain"). This usually occurs at the time of ovulation.

- **Oligomenorrhea** (ol-ih-goh-men-oh-**REE**-ah) means a markedly reduced menstrual flow and also abnormally infrequent menstruation or relative amenorrhea (**olig/o** means scanty, **men/o** means menstruation, and **-rrhea** means abnormal flow).

- **Polymenorrhea** (pol-ee-men-oh-**REE**-ah) means abnormally frequent menstruation (**poly-** means many, **men/o** means menstruation, and **-rrhea** means abnormal flow).

- **Premenstrual syndrome (PMS)** includes symptoms occurring within the two-week period before menstruation such as bloating, edema, headaches, mood swings, and breast discomfort.

PMS

DIAGNOSTIC PROCEDURES OF THE FEMALE REPRODUCTIVE SYSTEM

- **Breast self-examination (BSE)** is an important self-care procedure for the early detection of breast cancer.

- **Colposcopy** (kol-**POS**-koh-pee) is the direct visual examination of the tissues of the cervix and vagina using a **colposcope** (**colp/o** means vagina and **-scopy** means visual examination).

- **Endovaginal ultrasound** (**en**-doh-**VAJ**-ih-nal) is a diagnostic test to determine the cause of abnormal vaginal bleeding. In this procedure, an ultrasound transducer placed in the vagina uses sound waves to create images of the uterus and ovaries.

- **Hysterosalpingography** (**hiss**-ter-oh-**sal**-pin-**GOG**-rah-fee) is a radiographic examination of the uterus and fallopian tubes after the injection of radiopaque material (**hyster/o** means uterus, **salping/o** means tube, and **-graphy** means process of recording).

- **Hysteroscopy** (**hiss**-ter-**OSS**-koh-pee) is the direct visual examination of the interior of the uterus using the magnification of a **hysteroscope** (**HISS**-ter-oh-skope) (see Figure 2.9).

- **Mammography** (mam-**OG**-rah-fee) is a radiographic examination of the breast (Figures 14.12 and 14.13). The resulting record is called a **mammogram.**

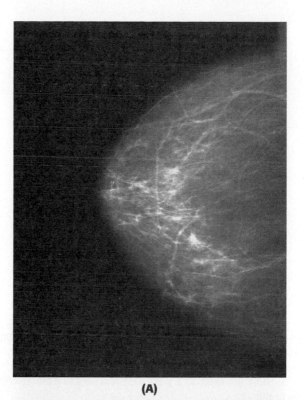

(A)

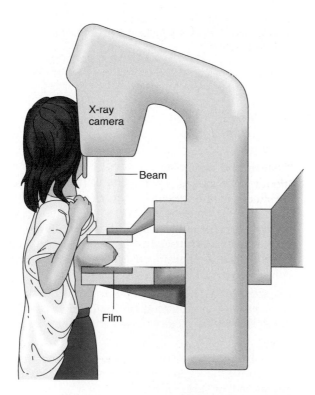

FIGURE 14.12 In mammography, the breast is gently flattened and then radiographed from above.

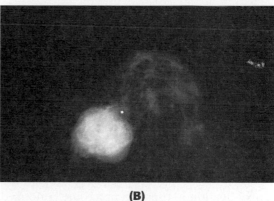

(B)

FIGURE 14.13 Mammograms. (A) A normal film. (B) A film in which a large mass is visible.

TREATMENT PROCEDURES OF THE FEMALE REPRODUCTIVE SYSTEM

MEDICATIONS

- **Birth control pills** are a form of hormones administered to prevent pregnancy. A **contraceptive** is the measure taken or device used to lessen the likelihood of conception and pregnancy.

- **Hormone replacement therapy (HRT)** is used to replace the estrogen and progesterone that are no longer produced during perimenopause and after menopause.

- A **Papanicolaou test** (pap-ah-**nick**-oh-**LAY**-ooh), also known as a **Pap smear,** is an exfoliative biopsy for the detection and diagnosis of conditions of the cervix and surrounding tissues (Figure 14.14). As used here, *exfoliative* (ecks-**FOH**-lee-**ay**-tiv) means that cells are scraped from the tissue and examined under a microscope.

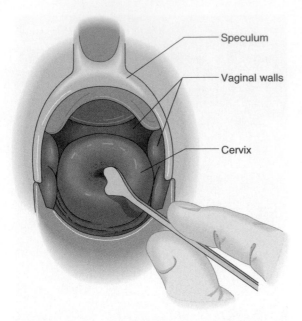

FIGURE 14.14 Performing a Pap smear. A speculum is used to spread the vaginal walls. A disposable Ayer blade, similar to a tongue depressor, is used to scrape away a few cells. These are fixed on a glass slide and sent to a laboratory for examination.

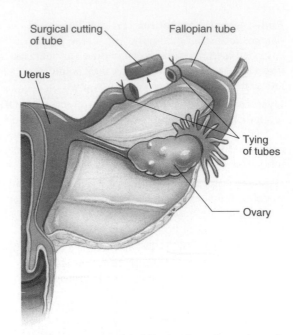

FIGURE 14.15 Tubal ligation is performed as a form of female sterilization.

THE OVARIES AND FALLOPIAN TUBES

- An **oophorectomy** (oh-ahf-oh-**RECK**-toh-mee), also known as **ovariectomy** (oh-vay-ree-**ECK**-toh-mee), is the surgical removal of an ovary (**oophor** means ovary and **-ectomy** means surgical removal).

- A **salpingectomy** (sal-pin-**JECK**-toh-mee) is the surgical removal of a fallopian tube (**salping** means tube and **-ectomy** means surgical removal).

- **Tubal ligation** is a surgical procedure performed for purpose of female sterilization. Each fallopian tube is ligated and a section is removed to prevent the ovum from reaching the uterus. *Ligate* means to bind or tie (Figure 14.15).

THE UTERUS, CERVIX, AND VAGINA

- A **cervicectomy** (ser-vih-**SECK**-toh-mee) is surgical removal of the cervix (**cervic** means cervix and **-ectomy** means surgical removal).

- A **colpopexy** (**KOL**-poh-**peck**-see) is the surgical fixation of the vagina to a surrounding structure (**colp/o** means vagina and **-pexy** means surgical fixation in place).

- **Conization** (kon-ih-**ZAY**-shun *or* koh-nih-**ZAY**-shun), also known as a **cone biopsy,** is the surgical removal of a cone-shaped section of tissue from the cervix. This may be performed as a diagnostic procedure or to remove an abnormal area.

- **Colporrhaphy** (kol-**POR**-ah-fee) means suturing the vagina (**colp/o** means vagina and **-rrhaphy** means to suture).

- **Dilation and curettage (D & C)** is the dilation of the cervix and curettage of the uterus. **Dilation** (dye-**LAY**-shun) is the expansion of an opening, and **curettage** (kyou-reh-**TAHZH**) is the removal of material from the surface. This may be removed by scraping with a **curette** or by the use of suction. This procedure may be performed as a diagnostic or treatment procedure (Figure 14.16).

- A **hysteropexy** (**HISS**-ter-oh-**peck**-see) is the surgical fixation of a misplaced or abnormally movable uterus (**hyster/o** means uterus and **-pexy** means surgical fixation).

- **Vaginoplasty** (vah-**JIGH**-noh-**plas**-tee) is the surgical repair of the vagina (**vagin/o** means vagina and **-plasty** means surgical repair).

Hysterectomies

- A **hysterectomy** (hiss-teh-**RECK**-toh-mee) is the surgical removal of the uterus and may or may not include the cervix (**hyster** means uterus and **-ectomy** means surgical removal) (Figure 14.17).

- A **vaginal hysterectomy (VH)** is performed through the vagina (Figure 14.17A).

- A **total abdominal hysterectomy** is performed through an incision in the abdomen. Because this procedure includes the removal of the uterus, cervix, fallopian tubes, and ovaries, its full name is a **total hysterectomy, plus bilateral salpingo-oophorectomy.**

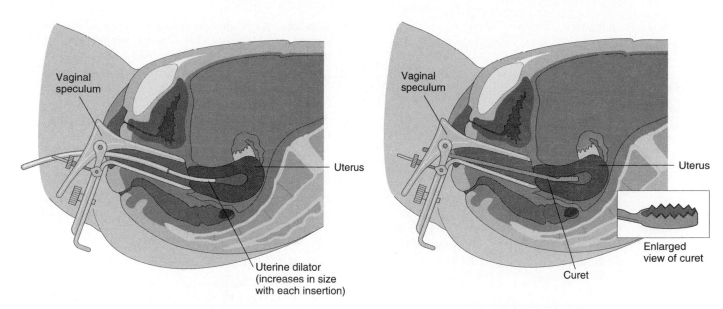

FIGURE 14.16 Dilation and curettage. (A) Dilation is the expansion of the cervical opening. (B) Curettage is the removal of material from the surface of the uterus.

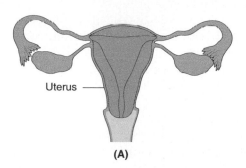

(A)

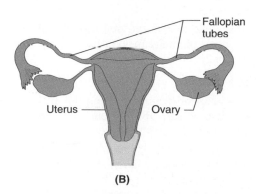

(B)

FIGURE 14.17 Types of hysterectomy. (A) In a vaginal hysterectomy, only the uterus and cervix are removed. (B) In a total hysterectomy (hysterosalpingo-oophorectomy), the cervix, uterus, tubes, and ovaries are removed.

- A **bilateral salpingo-oophorectomy** (sal-**ping**-goh oh-**ahf**-oh-**RECK**-toh-mee) **(SO)** is the surgical removal of both fallopian tubes and both ovaries (**salping/o** means tube, **oophor** means ovary, and **-ectomy** means surgical removal).

- A **bilateral hysterosalpingo-oophorectomy** (**hiss**-ter-oh-sal-**ping**-goh oh-**ahf**-oh-**RECK**-toh-

mee) is the surgical removal of the uterus and cervix, plus both fallopian tubes and both ovaries (**hyster/o** means uterus, **salping/o** means tube, **oophor** means ovary and **-ectomy** means surgical removal) (Figure 14.17B).

- A **radical hysterectomy** includes the surgical removal of the uterus, tubes, ovaries, adjacent lymph nodes, and part of the vagina. This surgery is performed as part of the treatment of cancer in any of these organs.

THE BREASTS

- **Mastectomy** as treatment of breast cancer is discussed in Chapter 6.

- **Mammoplasty** (**MAM**-oh-**plas**-tee), also spelled **mammaplasty,** is the surgical repair or restructuring of the breast (**mamm/o** means breast and **-plasty** means surgical repair).

- **Breast augmentation** is mammoplasty to increase breast size.

- **Mastopexy** (**MAS**-toh-**peck**-see) is surgery to affix sagging breasts in a more elevated position (**mast/o** means breast and **-pexy** means surgical fixation).

ASSISTED REPRODUCTION

Infertility is the inability of a couple to achieve pregnancy after one year of regular, unprotected intercourse or the inability of a woman to carry a pregnancy to a live birth.

- An infertile couple may seek the help of an **infertility specialist,** also known as a **fertility specialist,** who diagnoses and treats problems associated with conception and maintaining pregnancy.

Table 14.2 summarizes the abbreviations and terms commonly associated with assisted reproduction.

Table 14.2

ABBREVIATIONS AND TERMS RELATED TO ASSISTED FERTILIZATION	
AMA	**Advanced maternal age** decreases the possibility of pregnancy. This term is applied to women in their late thirties to middle forties.
ART	**Assisted reproductive technology** is the term used to describe techniques used to aid an infertile couple in achieving a viable pregnancy.
GIFT	**Gamete intrafallopian transfer** is a procedure in which ovum and sperm are mixed outside of the body then transferred by laparoscopic surgery into the fallopian tube, where hopefully fertilization will occur.
ICSI	**Intracytoplasmic sperm injection,** which is pronounced *icksy,* is a procedure outside of the body in which one sperm is placed into one egg, thereby fertilizing it. This procedure is used in the case of severe male factor infertility.
IVF	**In vitro fertilization** is a procedure in which mature ova are removed from the mother and fertilized outside of the body. The resulting embryos are transferred into the uterus with the hope that they will implant and continue to develop as in a normal pregnancy.
ZIFT	**Zygote intrafallopian transfer** is a laparoscopic procedure in which a zygote is placed in the fallopian tube, allowing it to travel down the tube to the uterus, where it implants.

PREGNANCY AND CHILDBIRTH

OVULATION

Ovulation (**ov**-you-**LAY**-shun) is the release of a mature egg from the follicle on the surface of the ovary.

- After the ovum is released, it is caught up by the fimbriae of the fallopian tube. There, wavelike peristaltic actions move the ovum down the fallopian tube toward the uterus.

- It usually takes an ovum about five days to pass through the fallopian tube. If sperm are present, fertilization occurs within the fallopian tube.

- After the ovum has been released, the ruptured follicle enlarges, takes on a yellow fatty substance, and becomes the corpus luteum.

- The **corpus luteum** (**KOR**-pus **LOO**-tee-um) secretes the hormone progesterone during the second half of the menstrual cycle. This maintains the growth of the uterine lining in preparation for the fertilized egg.

- If the ovum is not fertilized, the corpus luteum dies and the endometrium sloughs off as the menstrual flow.

FERTILIZATION

- During **coitus** (**KOH**-ih-tus), also known as **copulation** (kop-you-**LAY**-shun) or **sexual intercourse,** the male **ejaculates** approximately 100 million sperm cells into the female's vagina. The sperm travel upward through the vagina, into the uterus, and on into the fallopian tube.

- When a sperm penetrates the descending ovum, **fertilization,** also known as **conception,** occurs and a new life begins.

- After fertilization occurs in the fallopian tube, the fertilized egg, which is now called a **zygote** (**ZYE**-goht), travels to the uterus.

- **Implantation** is the embedding of the zygote into the endothelial lining of the uterus.

- From implantation through the eighth week of pregnancy, the developing child is known as an **embryo** (**EM**-bree-oh).

- A **fetus** (**FEE**-tus) is the developing child from the ninth week of pregnancy to the time of birth (see Figure 14.20).

Multiple Births

- If more than one egg is passing down the fallopian tube when sperm are present, the fertilization of more than one egg is possible.

- **Fraternal twins** result from the fertilization of separate ova by separate sperm cells. These develop into two separate embryos.

- **Identical twins** are formed from the fertilization of a single egg cell by a single sperm. As the fertilized egg cell divides, it separates into two parts, and each part forms a separate embryo.

THE CHORION AND PLACENTA

- The **chorion** (**KOR**-ee-on) is the outer membrane that encloses the fetus. It contributes to the formation of the placenta (Figure 14.18).

- The **placenta** (plah-**SEN**-tah) is a temporary organ that forms within the uterus to allow the exchange of

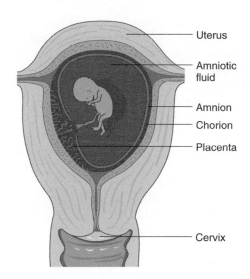

FIGURE 14.18 Structures related to the developing fetus.

nutrients, oxygen, and waste products between the mother and fetus without allowing maternal blood and fetal blood to mix. The placenta also produces hormones necessary to maintain the pregnancy (Figure 14.19).

● At delivery, the placenta is expelled as the **after-birth.**

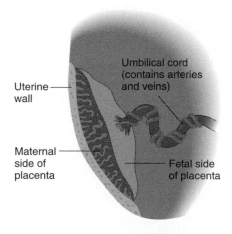

FIGURE 14.19 The placenta allows the exchange of nutrients and waste materials between mother and fetus without intermingling blood.

THE AMNION

The **amnion** (**AM**-nee-on), also known as the **amniotic sac,** is the innermost of the membranes that surround the embryo in the uterus and form the **amniotic cavity** (am-nee-OT-ick).

● **Amnionic fluid** (am-nee-ON-ick), also known as **amniotic fluid,** is the liquid in which the fetus floats and is protected (see Figure 14.18).

The Umbilical Cord

The **umbilical cord** (um-**BILL**-ih-kal) is the structure that connects the fetus to the placenta.

● After birth, the **navel,** also known as the **belly button,** is formed where the umbilical cord was attached to the fetus.

GESTATION

Gestation (jes-**TAY**-shun), which lasts approximately 280 days, is the period of development of the child in the mother's uterus.

● The term **pregnancy,** which is often used interchangeably with gestation, means the condition of having a developing child in the uterus.

● Pregnancy is described in terms of the number of weeks of gestation (40 total), or it may be divided into three **trimesters** of three months each (Figure 14.20).

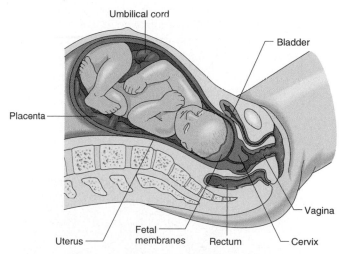

FIGURE 14.20 The fetus in normal position at term.

● The **due date,** or **estimated date of confinement (EDC),** is calculated from the first day of the **last menstrual period (LMP).**

● **Quickening** is the first movement of the fetus felt in the uterus. This usually occurs during the sixteenth to twentieth week of pregnancy.

● The fetus is **viable** when it is capable of living outside the mother. Viability depends on the developmental age, birth weight, and developmental stage of the lungs of the fetus.

THE MOTHER

● A **nulligravida** (null-ih-**GRAV**-ih-dah) is a woman who has never been pregnant (**nulli-** means none and **-gravida** means pregnant).

● A **nullipara** (nuh-**LIP**-ah-rah) is a woman who has never borne a viable child (**nulli-** means none and **-para** means to bring forth).

- A **primigravida** (**prye**-mih-**GRAV**-ih-dah) is a woman during her first pregnancy (**primi-** means first and **-gravida** means pregnant).

- A **primipara** (prye-**MIP**-ah-rah) is a woman who has borne one child (**primi-** means first and **-para** means to bring forth).

- **Multiparous** (mul-**TIP**-ah-rus) means a woman who has given birth two or more times (**multi-** means many and **-parous** means having borne one or more children).

CHILDBIRTH

Parturition (**par**-tyou-**RISH**-un), also known as **labor** and **childbirth,** is the act of giving birth to an offspring. The term **antepartum** means before the onset of labor with reference to the mother.

- **Labor and delivery (L & D)** occur in three stages (Figure 14.21).

- The first stage begins with contractions of the uterus and gradual **dilatation** (enlargement) of the cervix. During this stage, **effacement** (eh-**FAYSS**-ment) is the thinning and shortening of the cervix.

- The second stage is the delivery of the infant. The **amniotic sac,** also known as the **bag of waters,** ruptures. Then the uterine contractions become stronger and more frequent until the child is expelled.

- **Presentation** is the term used to describe the portion of the fetus that can be touched by the examining finger during labor.

- Normally, the head presents first, and the stage at which the head can be seen at the vaginal orifice is called **crowning.**

- The third stage is the expulsion of the placenta as the **afterbirth.** The term **delivery** means the expulsion of the infant and afterbirth.

POSTPARTUM

The term **postpartum** (pohst-**PAR**-tum) means after childbirth.

The Mother

- For the mother, **puerperium** (**pyou**-er-**PEE**-ree-um) is the period of three to six weeks after childbirth until the uterus returns to its normal size.

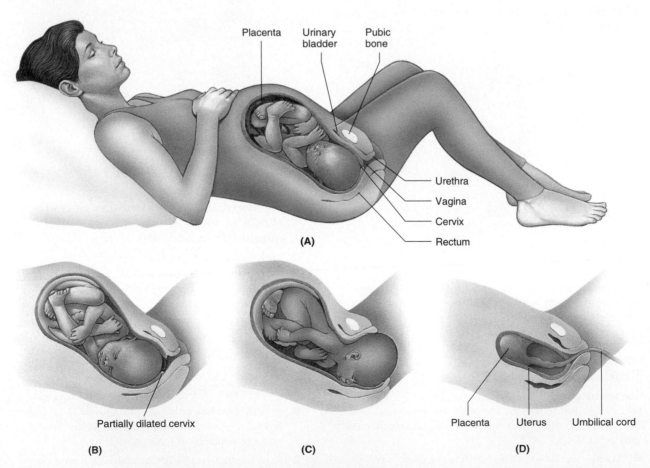

FIGURE 14.21 The stages of labor. (A) Position of the fetus before labor. (B) First stage of labor, cervical dilation. (C) Second stage of labor, fetal delivery. (D) Third stage of labor, delivery of the placenta.

- **Colostrum** (kuh-**LOS**-trum) is the fluid secreted by the breasts during the first days postpartum. This fluid is rich in antibodies and confers passive immunity to the newborn.
- **Lactation** (lack-**TAY**-shun) is the process of forming and secreting milk from the breasts as nourishment for the infant.
- **Lochia** (**LOH**-kee-ah) is the vaginal discharge during the first week or two after childbirth. It consists of blood, tissue, and mucus.
- **Uterine involution** is the return of the uterus to its normal size and former condition.

The Baby

- The newborn infant is known as a **neonate** (**NEE**-oh-nayt) during the first four weeks after birth.
- **Meconium** (meh-**KOH**-nee-um) is a greenish material that collects in the intestine of a fetus and forms the first stools of a newborn.

PATHOLOGY OF PREGNANCY AND CHILDBIRTH

Pregnancy

- An **abortion** (ah-**BOR**-shun) **(AB)** is the interruption or termination of pregnancy before the fetus is viable. A **spontaneous abortion (SAB),** also known as a **miscarriage,** occurs without outside action. An **induced abortion,** also known as a **therapeutic abortion (TAB),** is deliberately caused by human action for medical purposes.
- An **ectopic pregnancy** (eck-**TOP**-ick), also known as an **extrauterine pregnancy,** is a pregnancy in which the fertilized egg is implanted and begins to develop outside of the uterus. *Ectopic* means out of place.
- A **tubal pregnancy** is an ectopic pregnancy in which the embryo is implanted within the fallopian tube rather than the uterus.
- **Preeclampsia** (pree-ee-**KLAMP**-see-ah), also known as **toxemia of pregnancy,** is a complication of pregnancy characterized by hypertension (high blood pressure), edema (swelling), and proteinuria. *Proteinuria* (**proh**-tee-in-**YOU**-ree-ah) is an abnormally high level of protein in the urine.
- **Eclampsia** (eh-**KLAMP**-see-ah), a more serious form of preeclampsia, is characterized by convulsions and sometimes coma.

The Rh Factor

- When the mother's blood is **Rh-negative (Rh-)** and the father's is **Rh-positive (Rh+),** the baby may inherit the Rh+ factor from the father. (The Rh factor is discussed further in Chapter 5.)
- During labor or a miscarriage, some of the baby's blood may enter the mother's circulation. Entry of the baby's Rh+ blood sensitizes the mother to the Rh+ factor and causes her body to develop Rh+ antibod-

ies. These antibodies can cause a problem during her *next* pregnancy.
- Blood tests of the parents can identify this potential problem, and, if it exists, the mother is vaccinated with Rh immune globulin to prevent the development of these antibodies (Figure 14.22).

Childbirth

- **Abruptio placentae** (ab-**RUP**-shee-oh plah-**SEN**-tee) is an abnormal condition in which the placenta separates from the uterine wall prematurely before the birth of the fetus.
- **Breech presentation** is when the buttocks or feet of the fetus are presented first.
- **Placenta previa** (plah-**SEN**-tah **PREE**-vee-ah) is the abnormal implantation of the placenta in the lower portion of the uterus. Symptoms include painless sudden-onset bleeding during the third trimester. Treatment ranges from bed rest to immediate delivery by cesarean section.
- A **premature infant,** also known as a **preemie,** is any neonate born before the thiry-seventh week of gestation.
- **Stillbirth** is the birth of a fetus that died before or during delivery.

DIAGNOSTIC PROCEDURES RELATED TO PREGNANCY

- **Amniocentesis** (**am**-nee-oh-sen-**TEE**-sis) is a surgical procedure in which a needle is passed through the abdominal and uterine walls to obtain a specimen of amniotic fluid (**amnio** means amnion and fetal membrane, and **-centesis** means a surgical puncture to remove fluid). This specimen, which is obtained after the sixteenth week of pregnancy, is used to evaluate fetal health and to diagnose certain congenital disorders (Figure 14.23).
- **Chorionic villus sampling (CVS)** is the retrieval of chorionic cells from the placenta between the eighth to tenth weeks of pregnancy. These cells are evaluated to test for genetic abnormalities in the developing child.
- An **electronic fetal monitor** is a device that allows observation of the fetal heart rate and the maternal uterine contractions during labor.
- **Fetal ultrasound** is a noninvasive procedure used to evaluate fetal development. (Diagnostic ultrasound is discussed further in Chapter 15).
- **Pelvimetry** (pel-**VIM**-eh-tree) is the measurement of the dimensions of the pelvis to determine its capacity to allow passage of the fetus through the birth canal.
- A **pregnancy test** is performed on either a blood or urine specimen to determine human chorionic gonadotropin (HCG) levels. An unusually high level usually indicates pregnancy.

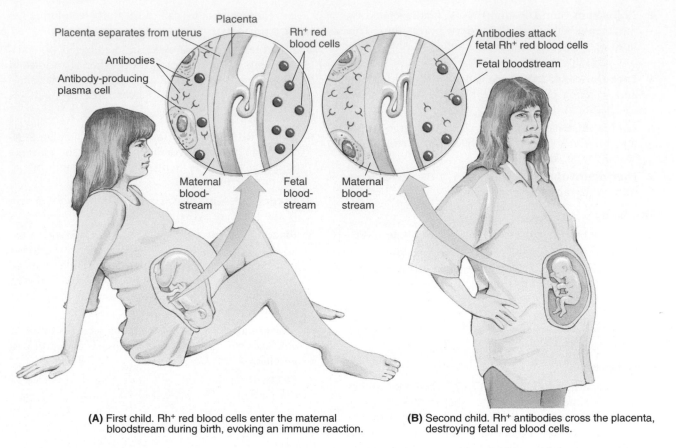

(A) First child. Rh⁺ red blood cells enter the maternal bloodstream during birth, evoking an immune reaction.

(B) Second child. Rh⁺ antibodies cross the placenta, destroying fetal red blood cells.

FIGURE 14.22 Rh incompatibility can cause problems for the fetus during a second pregnancy.

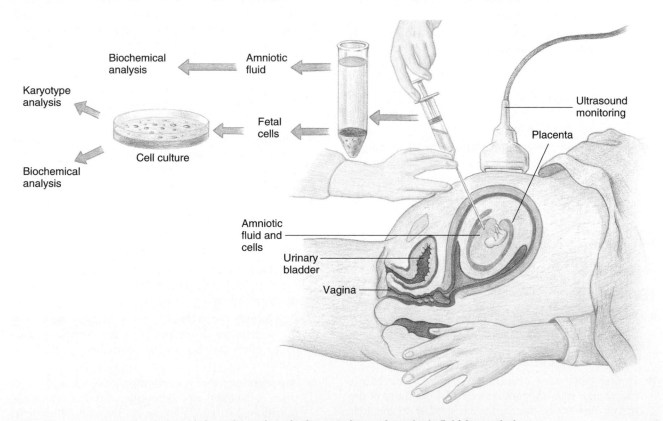

FIGURE 14.23 Amniocentesis is performed to obtain a specimen of amnionic fluid for analysis.

TREATMENT PROCEDURES RELATED TO PREGNANCY AND CHILDBIRTH

- An **Apgar score** is an evaluation of a newborn infant's physical status by assigning numerical values (0 to 2) to each of five criteria: (1) heart rate, (2) respiratory effort, (3) muscle tone, (4) response stimulation, and (5) skin color. The newborn is evaluated at one and five minutes after birth, and a total score of 8 to 10 indicates the best possible condition.

- A **cesarean delivery,** also known as a **cesarean section** (seh-**ZEHR**-ee-un **SECK**-shun) or **C-section,** is the delivery of the child through an incision in the maternal abdominal and uterine walls.

- The vaginal delivery of a subsequent child after a cesarean birth is referred to as a **VBAC** (vaginal birth after cesarean).

- An **episiotomy** (eh-**piz**-ee-**OT**-oh-mee) is a surgical incision of the perineum and vagina to facilitate delivery and prevent laceration of the tissues (**episi** means vulva and **-otomy** means a surgical incision). A *laceration* is a jagged tear of the tissue.

- An **episiorrhaphy** (eh-**piz**-ee-**OR**-ah-fee) is a sutured repair of an episiotomy (**episi/o** means vulva and **-rrhaphy** means to suture).

Career Opportunities

In addition to the medical specialties already discussed, some of the health occupations involving the treatment of the reproductive systems include

- **Midwife:** assists in labor and delivery. A certified nurse midwife (CNM) is an RN with specialized training in obstetrics and gynecology who provides primary care in normal pregnancies and deliveries.

- **Doula:** provides emotional, physical, and informational support to the mother before and during labor and delivery

- **Sonographer** or **ultrasound technologist:** conducts ultrasound tests to show the development and condition of the fetus

- **Registered nurse mother/baby unit (RN-MBU):** an RN who specializes in maternity and newborn care

- **Childbirth educator:** teaches expectant parents about prenatal care, childbirth, and infant care

- **Mammographer:** a radiographer who specializes in performing mammograms

- **Genetics counselor:** works with members of a healthcare team to provide information and support to families regarding the risks of birth defects or genetic disorders

Health Occupation Profile: CERTIFIED NURSE MIDWIFE

Maureen Darcey is a certified nurse midwife. "I started out as a nurse in orthopedics at a small hospital. When I became the night supervisor, I was often needed in labor and delivery. Doctors sometimes couldn't get to the hospital in time, so I would help women in labor and even catch their babies. I loved supporting these women through their labor and being present with them at such a defining moment in their lives. I decided to enroll in the SUNY Downstate Medical Center midwifery program and became a certified nurse midwife.

"Midwives believe that women deserve to have both a choice and a voice in their health care. Midwives are able to function independently and to offer complete well-woman health care throughout a woman's life—from a young girl's first menses through and beyond menopause. The primary focus is on obstetrical care: prenatal, labor and delivery, and postpartum. Midwives approach birth as a natural process and invite a woman to trust her own body. Midwives do not independently handle high-risk birth situations requiring medical intervention, but for a birth without complications, we help create a homelike environment where birth is honored as a special family event."

STUDY BREAK

The period of *gestation* for the development of a human fetus in the uterus is usually around nine months (253–300 days). The fact that women are limited to about one pregnancy a year is an important factor in determining human population growth.

Imagine how many people there might be on the planet if the human gestation period were that of a

- Wolf (60–63 days)
- Rabbit (30–35 days)
- Mouse (19–30 days)

Another factor limiting human population is the relatively low number of children born to most mothers. Our population would truly explode if every mother matched the record set by Mrs. Feodor Vassilyev of Russia in the eighteenth century: 69 children, including 16 pairs of twins, 7 sets of triplets and 4 sets of quadruplets!

Review Time

Write the answers to the following questions on a separate piece of paper or in your notebook. In addition, be prepared to take part in the classroom discussion.

1. **Written assignment:** Describe why **sexually transmitted diseases** are sometimes referred to as **venereal diseases.**

   Discussion assignment: What are the most common STDs?

2. **Written assignment:** Using terms a physician would understand, describe the **male** and **female sterilization procedures.**

   Discussion assignment: How would you explain each of these procedures to a patient?

3. **Written assignment:** Describe the phase of the menstrual cycle during which the female is most likely to **become pregnant.**

   Discussion assignment: How would you explain this concept to a couple who want this information to help with birth control planning?

4. **Written assignment:** Using terms a patient would understand, describe the difference between **preeclampsia** and **eclampsia.**

   Discussion assignment: Why is prenatal care so important in detecting and controlling these conditions?

5. **Written assignment:** Report on your research about the person for whom **Apgar scores** were named. Include in your report his or her full name and dates.

   Discussion assignment: How are these scores used to evaluate the physical status of a newborn?

Optional Internet Activity

*The goal of this activity is to help you learn more about medical terminology while improving your Internet skills. Select **one** of these two options and follow the instructions.*

1. **Internet Search:** Search for information about **PMS.** Write a brief (one- or two-paragraph) report on something new you learned here and include the address of the web site where you found this information.

2. **Web Site:** To learn more about **sexually transmitted diseases,** go to this web address: **http://www.4woman.gov/.** Search on Frequently Asked Questions and find Sexually Transmitted Diseases. Write a brief (one- or two-paragraph) report on something new you learned here.

The Human Touch: Critical Thinking Exercise

The following story and questions are designed to stimulate critical thinking through class discussion or as a brief essay response. There are no right or wrong answers to these questions.

"But Sam, you promised!" Jamie Chu began.

"Please don't get so upset," her husband interrupted. "I know I agreed to a vasectomy, but Grandmother may have a point. I do not have a son. Our family name has to be considered. I just feel that we should think about this."

"But Sam, we already discussed it. You're scheduled for the procedure." It seemed to Jamie that they had already spent plenty of time considering the number of children they wanted and talking about various contraceptive methods. Jamie had problems taking the pill, and Sam didn't like using a condom. A tubal ligation could have been the answer, but Jamie had a fear of not waking up from the anesthesia. Besides, she had been the one to go through two pregnancies and childbirths. Sam had reluctantly agreed that it was his turn to take responsibility for family planning.

Their two daughters, two-year-old Nanyn and her big sister Nadya, made the perfect size family, Jamie thought. She had grown up in a large family. A lot of her childhood was spent taking care of her brothers and sisters, and she rarely had her mother's undivided attention. She didn't want that for her children.

Sam's story was different. Before his parents immigrated to America they had had four daughters. His father was so proud when he was born, a son to carry on the family tradition.

It had taken quite a long time to convince Sam that a family of only daughters could be considered complete. And now Grandmother was questioning that decision.

Suggested Discussion Topics

1. Which partner is responsible for birth control and why?
2. If a couple cannot agree about family size or birth control methods, what should they do?
3. Compare large families to small families. Discuss the good and bad points of each.
4. Discuss how cultural differences and religious beliefs influence choices like family size and birth control.
5. Why do some cultures value male children over female children?

Student Workbook and Student Activity CD-ROM

1. Go to your **Student Workbook** and complete the Learning Exercises for this chapter.
2. Go to the **Student Activity CD-ROM** and have fun with the exercises and games for this chapter.

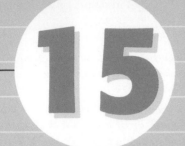
Diagnostic Procedures and Pharmacology

● **Overview of Diagnostic Procedures and Pharmacology**

Basic diagnostic procedures	Vital signs
	Auscultation
	Palpation and percussion
	Basic examination instruments
	Basic examination positions
Laboratory tests	Blood tests
	Urinalysis
Endoscopy	Visual examination
	Endoscopic surgery
Imaging techniques	Radiography (x-ray)
	Computed tomography (CT)
	Magnetic resonance imaging (MRI)
	Fluoroscopy
	Diagnostic ultrasound
Nuclear medicine	Nuclear medicine
Radiographic projections and positioning	Projections
	Positioning
	Basic radiographic projections
Pharmacology	Terms related to pharmacology
	Routes of administration

Vocabulary Related to Diagnostic Procedures and Pharmacology

Terms marked with the ❖ symbol are pronounced on the Student Activity CD-ROM that accompanies this text.

KEY WORD PARTS

☐ albumin/o
☐ calc/i
☐ cin/e
☐ fluor/o
☐ glycos/o
☐ -graph
☐ -graphy
☐ hemat/o
☐ -ous
☐ per-
☐ phleb/o
☐ radi/o
☐ -scope
☐ -scopy
☐ -uria

KEY MEDICAL TERMS

☐ abdominocentesis
  (ab-**dom**-ih-noh-sen-**TEE**-sis) ❖
☐ addiction
☐ adverse drug reaction
☐ agglutination (ah-**gloo**-tih-**NAY**-shun) ❖
☐ albuminuria (**al**-byou-mih-**NEW**-ree-ah) ❖
☐ assay (**ASS**-ay) ❖
☐ assessment
☐ auscultation (**aws**-kul-**TAY**-shun) ❖
☐ bacteriuria (back-**tee**-ree-**YOU**-ree-ah) ❖
☐ blood urea nitrogen (you-**REE**-ah)
☐ bruit (**BREW** ee or **BROOT**) ❖
☐ calciuria (**kal**-sih-**YOU**-ree-ah) ❖
☐ cardiocentesis (**kar**-dee-oh-sen-**TEE**-sis) ❖
☐ centesis (sen-**TEE**-sis) ❖
☐ cineradiography (sin-eh-**ray**-dee-**OG**-rah-fee) ❖
☐ compliance
☐ computed tomography (toh-**MOG**-rah-fee) ❖
☐ contraindication
☐ creatinuria (kree-**at**-ih-**NEW**-ree-ah) ❖
☐ decubitus (dee-**KYOU**-bih-tus) ❖
☐ endoscopy (en-**DOS**-koh-pee) ❖
☐ extraoral radiography
☐ fluoroscopy (**floo**-or-**OS**-koh-pee) ❖
☐ glycosuria (**glye**-koh-**SOO**-ree-ah) ❖
☐ hematocrit (hee-**MAT**-oh-krit) ❖
☐ hematuria (**hee**-mah-**TOO**-ree-ah or
  hem-ah-**TOO**-ree-ah) ❖
☐ hypodermic (**high**-poh-**DER**-mick) ❖
☐ idiosyncratic (**id**-ee-oh-sin-**KRAT**-ick) ❖
☐ immunofluorescence
  (im-you-noh-**floo**-oh-**RES**-ens) ❖

☐ intradermal injection
☐ intramuscular injection
☐ intraoral radiography
☐ intravenous injection
☐ ketonuria (**kee**-toh-**NEW**-ree-ah) ❖
☐ lithotomy (lih-**THOT**-oh-mee)
☐ lymphangiography (lim-**fan**-jee-**OG**-rah-fee) ❖
☐ magnetic resonance imaging ❖
☐ ophthalmoscope (ahf-**THAL**-moh-skope) ❖
☐ otoscope (**OH**-toh-skope) ❖
☐ palliative (**PAL**-ee-**ay**-tiv or **PAL**-ee-ah-tiv) ❖
☐ palpation (pal-**PAY**-shun) ❖
☐ parenteral (pah-**REN**-ter-al) ❖
☐ percussion (per-**KUSH**-un) ❖
☐ percutaneous (**per**-kyou-**TAY**-nee-us) ❖
☐ perfusion (per-**FYOU**-zuhn)
☐ pericardiocentesis
  (**pehr**-ih-**kar**-dee-oh-sen-**TEE**-sis) ❖
☐ phlebotomist (fleh-**BOT**-oh-mist) ❖
☐ phlebotomy (fleh-**BOT**-oh-mee) ❖
☐ placebo (plah-**SEE**-boh) ❖
☐ positron emission tomography ❖
☐ potentiation (poh-**ten**-shee-**AY**-shun) ❖
☐ proteinuria (**proh**-tee-in-**YOU**-ree-ah) ❖
☐ prothrombin (proh-**THROM**-bin) ❖
☐ pyuria (pye-**YOU**-ree-ah) ❖
☐ radioimmunoassay
  (**ray**-dee-oh-**im**-you-noh-**ASS**-ay) ❖
☐ radiologist (**ray**-dee-**OL**-oh-jist) ❖
☐ radiolucent (**ray**-dee-oh-**LOO**-sent) ❖
☐ radionuclide imaging
  (**ray**-dee-oh-**NEW**-klyd) ❖
☐ radiopaque (**ray**-dee-oh-**PAYK**) ❖
☐ radiopharmaceuticals
☐ rale (**RAHL**) ❖
☐ recumbent (ree-**KUM**-bent) ❖
☐ regimen (**REJ**-ih-men) ❖
☐ rhonchus (**RONG**-kus) ❖
☐ single photon emission computed
  tomography ❖
☐ speculum (**SPECK**-you-lum) ❖
☐ sphygmomanometer
  (**sfig**-moh-mah-**NOM**-eh-ter) ❖
☐ stethoscope (**STETH**-oh-skope) ❖
☐ stridor (**STRYE**-dor) ❖
☐ subcutaneous injection
☐ supine (**SUE**-pine) ❖
☐ thoracentesis (**thoh**-rah-sen-**TEE**-sis) ❖
☐ ultrasonography (**ul**-trah-son-**OG**-rah-fee) ❖
☐ urinalysis (**you**-rih-**NAL**-ih-sis) ❖
☐ venipuncture (**VEN**-ih-**punk**-tyour) ❖

Objectives

Upon completion of this chapter, you should be able to:

1. Describe the four vital signs recorded for most patients.

2. Recognize, define, spell, and pronounce the terms associated with basic examination procedures.

3. Identify and describe the basic examination positions.

4. Recognize, define, spell, and pronounce terms associated with frequently performed blood and urinalysis laboratory tests.

5. Recognize, define, spell, and pronounce terms associated with radiography and other imaging techniques.

6. Differentiate between projection and position and describe basic radiographic projections.

7. Recognize, define, spell, and pronounce the pharmacology terms introduced in this chapter.

BASIC EXAMINATION PROCEDURES

Basic examination procedures are performed during the assessment of the patient's condition. As used in medicine, **assessment** means the evaluation or appraisal of a condition. This information is used in reaching a diagnosis and in formulating a patient care plan.

VITAL SIGNS

Four vital signs are recorded for most patients. These are temperature, pulse, respiration, and blood pressure.

- **Temperature (T).** An average normal temperature is 98.6°F (Fahrenheit) or 37.0°C (Celsius) (Figure 15.1).

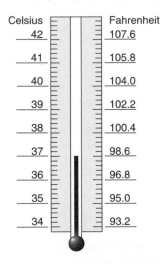

Celsius	Fahrenheit
42	107.6
41	105.8
40	104.0
39	102.2
38	100.4
37	98.6
36	96.8
35	95.0
34	93.2

FIGURE 15.1 The average normal temperature is 98.6°F (Fahrenheit) or 37.0°C (Celsius).

- **Pulse (P).** The pulse rate is the number of times the heart beats each minute. The pulse may be measured at different points on the body (Figure 15.2). A normal adult pulse ranges from 50 to 80 beats per minute (bpm).

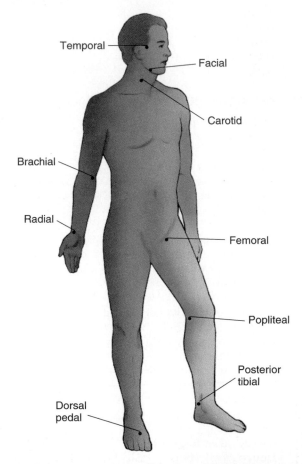

FIGURE 15.2 Major sites where arterial pulses may be detected.

- **Respiration rate (RR).** The rate is recorded as the number of respirations each minute. (A single respiration is one inhalation and one exhalation.) The average respiratory rate for an adult ranges from 12 to 20 breaths per minute.

- **Blood pressure (BP).** A **sphygmomanometer** (sfig-moh-mah-**NOM**-eh-ter) is an instrument used to mea-

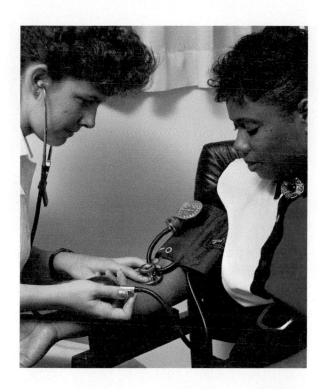

FIGURE 15.3 A sphygmomanometer and stethoscope are being used to measure blood pressure.

sure blood pressure. A **stethoscope** (**STETH**-oh-skope) is used to listen to sounds within the body and during the measurement of blood pressure (Figure 15.3). Blood pressure is discussed in Chapter 5.

AUSCULTATION SOUNDS

Auscultation (**aws**-kul-**TAY**-shun) is listening through a stethoscope for sounds within the body to determine the condition of the lungs, pleura, heart, and abdomen (Figure 15.4). Table 15.1 contains tips for remembering some of the auscultation sounds.

Table 15.1

AN AID TO REMEMBERING AUSCULTATION SOUNDS

To remember the meaning of these terms, say each out loud so it resembles the sound heard from the body.

- A **bruit** sounds "murmury."
- A **rale** sounds "rattley."
- **Rhonchus** sounds musical.
- **Stridor** sounds harsh.

- A **bruit** (**BREW**-ee *or* **BROOT**) is an abnormal sound or murmur heard in auscultation.
- A **rale** (**RAIL**) is an abnormal rattle or crackle-like respiratory sound heard during inspiration (breathing in).
- **Rhonchus** (**RONG**-kus), also known as **wheezing,** is an added sound with a musical pitch occurring during inspiration or expiration that results from a partially obstructed airway caused by inflammation, spasm of smooth muscles, or the presence of mucus in the airways (plural, **rhonchi**).
- **Stridor** (**STRYE**-dor) is an abnormal, high-pitched, harsh or crowing sound heard during inspiration that results from a partial blockage of the pharynx, larynx, and trachea.

PALPATION AND PERCUSSION

- **Palpation** (pal-**PAY**-shun) is an examination technique in which the examiner's hands are used to feel the texture, size, consistency, and location of certain body parts (Figure 15.5).

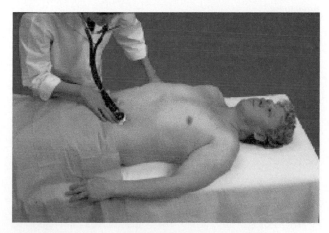

FIGURE 15.4 Auscultation is listening through a stethoscope to sounds within the body.

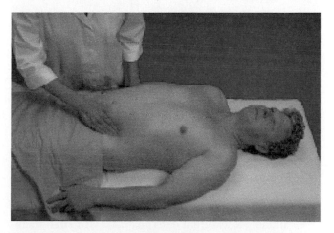

FIGURE 15.5 Palpation is the use of the fingertips to detect tenderness and to determine structure size.

- **Percussion** (per-**KUSH**-un) is a diagnostic procedure to determine the density of a body area by the sound produced by tapping the surface with the finger or instrument (Figure 15.6).

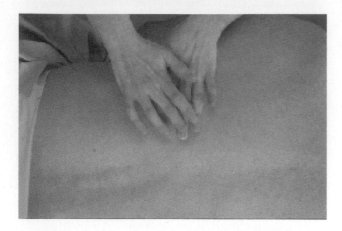

FIGURE 15.6 Percussion is the use of the fingers in a tapping motion to evaluate air content in the lungs and over the abdomen to detect air in the loops of intestine.

ADDITIONAL EXAMINATION PROCEDURES

- An **ophthalmoscope** (ahf-**THAL**-moh-skope) is used to examine the interior of the eye (**ophthalm/o** means eye and **-scope** means instrument for visual examination). See Figure 15.7.

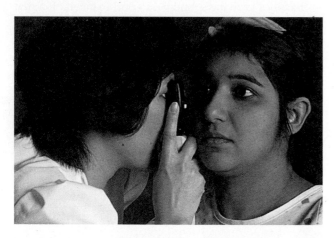

FIGURE 15.7 An ophthalmoscope is used to examine the interior of the eye.

- The abbreviation **PERRLA** means "pupils are equal, round, responsive to light and accommodation." This is a diagnostic observation, and any abnormality might indicate a head injury or damage to the brain.
- An **otoscope** (**OH**-toh-skope) is used to visually examine the external ear canal and tympanic membrane (**ot/o** means ear and **-scope** means instrument for visual examination). See Figure 15.8.

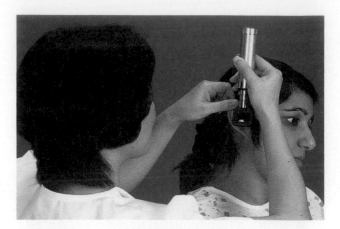

FIGURE 15.8 An otoscope is used to examine the ear canal and tympanic membrane.

- A **speculum** (**SPECK**-you-lum) is used to enlarge the opening of any canal or cavity to facilitate inspection of its interior (Figure 15.9).

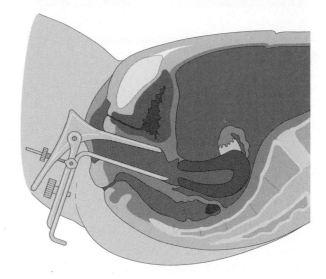

FIGURE 15.9 A speculum in place for inspection of the vagina.

BASIC EXAMINATION POSITIONS

RECUMBENT POSITION

The term **recumbent** (ree-**KUM**-bent) may be used to describe any position in which the patient is lying down either on the back, front, or side.

- The term **decubitus** (dee-**KYOU**-bih-tus) also means the act of lying down or the position assumed in lying down.
- In radiography, the term **decubitus** is used to describe the position of the patient when lying in a recumbent position. However, *decubitus* is most

commonly used to describe a decubitus ulcer, which is also known as a bedsore (see Chapter 12).

PRONE POSITION

In a **prone position,** the recumbent patient is lying on the belly *face down.* The arms may be placed under the head for comfort (Figure 15.10). This position is used for the examination and treatment of the back and buttocks.

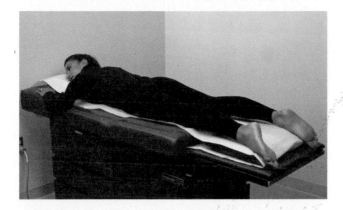

FIGURE 15.10 The prone position.

SUPINE POSITION

In the **supine position** (SUE-pine), also known as the **horizontal recumbent position,** the patient is lying on the back with the *face up* (Figure 15.11). This position is used for examination and treatment of the anterior surface of the body and for x-rays.

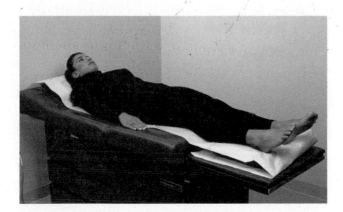

FIGURE 15.11 The horizontal recumbent (supine) position.

DORSAL RECUMBENT POSITION

In the **dorsal recumbent position,** the patient is supine (lying on the back) with the knees bent (Figure 15.12). This position is used for the examination and treatment of the abdominal area and for vaginal or rectal examinations.

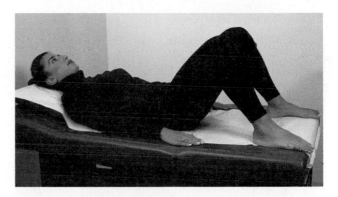

FIGURE 15.12 The dorsal recumbent position.

SIMS' POSITION

In the **Sims' position,** the patient is lying on the left side with the right knee and thigh drawn up with the left arm placed along the back (Figure 15.13). This position is used in the examination and treatment of the rectal area.

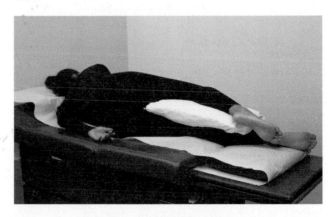

FIGURE 15.13 The Sims' position.

KNEE-CHEST POSITION

In the **knee-chest position,** the patient is lying face down with the hips flexed (bent) so the knees and chest rest on the table (Figure 15.14). This position is used for rectal examinations.

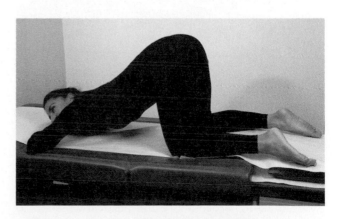

FIGURE 15.14 The knee-chest position.

LITHOTOMY POSITION

In the **lithotomy position** (lih-**THOT**-oh-mee) the patient is supine with the feet and legs raised and supported in stirrups (Figure 15.15). This position is used for vaginal and rectal examinations.

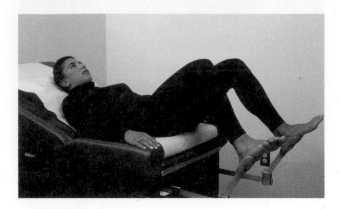

FIGURE 15.15 The lithotomy position.

● *Lithotomy* also means a surgical incision for the removal of a stone, usually from the urinary bladder. This is discussed in Chapter 9.

TRENDELENBURG POSITION

In the **Trendelenburg position,** the patient is lying on the back with the pelvis higher than the head; the knees are slightly bent; and the legs are hanging off the end of the table (Figure 15.16). This position is used for pelvic surgery and for some radiographic examinations.

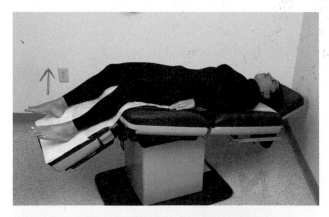

FIGURE 15.16 The Trendelenburg position.

The **modified Trendelenburg position**, which is not shown here, is used in the treatment of shock. The patient is positioned lying flat on the back with the legs elevated 12–16 inches above the head in an effort to improve the blood flow to the brain.

LABORATORY TESTS

● When used in regard to laboratory tests, the term **profile** means tests that are frequently performed as a group on automated multichannel laboratory testing equipment.

● When a laboratory test is ordered **stat** the results are needed immediately, and the tests should have top priority in the laboratory. (*Stat* comes from the Latin word meaning immediately.)

BLOOD TESTS

Obtaining Specimens

● **Phlebotomy** (fleh-**BOT**-oh-mee) is the puncture of a vein for the purpose of drawing blood (**phleb** means vein and **-otomy** means a surgical incision). This is also known as **venipuncture** (**VEN**-ih-**punk**-tyour).

● A **phlebotomist** (fleh-**BOT**-oh-mist) is an individual trained and skilled in phlebotomy.

● A **capillary puncture** is the technique used when only a small amount of blood is needed as a specimen for a blood test. Named for where it is performed, it may be a fingerstick, heelstick, or earlobe stick.

Complete Blood Cell Counts

A **complete blood cell count (CBC)** is a series of tests performed as a group to evaluate several blood conditions.

● **Erythrocyte sedimentation rate** (eh-**RITH**-roh-site) **(ESR),** also known as **sed rate,** is a test based on the rate at which the red blood cells separate from the plasma and settle to the bottom of the container. An elevated count indicates the presence of inflammation in the body.

● A **hematocrit test** (hee-**MAT**-oh-krit) **(Hct or HCT)** measures the percentage by volume of packed red blood cells in a whole blood sample (**hemat/o** means blood and **-crit** means to separate). This test is used to diagnose abnormal states of **hydration** (fluid level in the body), **polycythemia** (excess red blood cells), and **anemia** (deficient red blood cells).

● A **platelet count (PLC)** measures the number of platelets in a specified amount of blood. This test is used to assess the effects of chemotherapy and radiation therapy and to aid in the diagnosis of **thrombocytopenia** (an abnormal decrease in the number of platelets).

● A **red blood cell (RBC) count** is a determination of the number of erythrocytes in the blood. A depressed count may indicate anemia or a hemorrhage lasting more than 24 hours.

● A **total hemoglobin (Hb) test** measures the amount of hemoglobin found in whole blood (**hem/o** means blood and **-globin** means protein). Test results measure the severity of anemia or polycythemia and monitor the response to therapy.

- A **white blood cell (WBC) count** is a determination of the number of leukocytes in the blood. An elevated count may be an indication of infection or inflammation.

- A **white blood cell differential** determines what percentage of the total WBC count is composed of each of the five types of leukocyte. This test provides information about the patient's immune system, detects certain types of leukemia, and determines the severity of infection.

Additional Blood Tests

- **Agglutination testing** (ah-**gloo**-tih-**NAY**-shun) includes a variety of tests that involve the clumping together of cells or particles when mixed with incompatible serum. These tests are performed to determine the patient's blood type and to check compatibility of donor and recipient blood before a transfusion.

- **Blood urea nitrogen** (you-**REE**-ah) **(BUN)** is the amount of urea present in the blood. *Urea* is the major end product of protein metabolism found in urine and blood, and this test is a rough indicator of kidney function.

- **Lipid tests,** also known as a **lipid panel,** measure the amounts of total cholesterol, high-density lipoprotein (HDL), low-density lipoprotein (LDL), and triglycerides in a blood sample.

- **Prothrombin time** (proh-**THROM**-bin), also known as **pro time,** is a test used to diagnose conditions associated with abnormal bleeding and to monitor anticoagulant therapy.

- **Serum enzyme tests** are used to measure the blood enzymes. These tests are useful as evidence of a myocardial infarction.

- The **serum bilirubin test** measures how well red blood cells are being broken down. Elevated levels of bilirubin, which cause jaundice, may indicate liver problems or gallstones.

- A **thyroid-stimulating hormone assay** measures circulating blood levels of thyroid-stimulating hormone (TSH) that may indicate abnormal thyroid activity.

URINALYSIS

Urinalysis (**you**-rih-**NAL**-ih-sis) is the examination of the physical and chemical properties of urine to determine the presence of abnormal elements. Routine urinalysis is performed to screen for urinary and systemic disorders.

- For routine analysis, a **dipstick** is used (Figure 15.17). Chemicals impregnated on this plastic strip react with substances in the urine and change color when abnormalities are present.

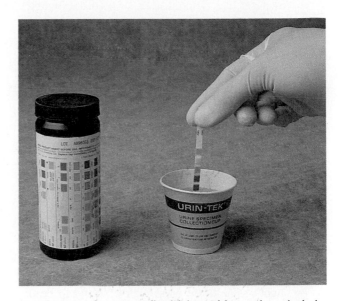

FIGURE 15.17 A dipstick is used for routine urinalysis.

- More detailed testing requires **microscopic examination** of the specimen. For example, casts are identified through microscopic examination. **Casts** are fibrous or protein materials, such as pus and fats, that are thrown off into the urine in kidney disease.

- The average normal **pH** range of urine is from 4.5 to 8.0. A pH value *below* 7 indicates acid urine and is an indication of acidosis. A pH value *above* 7 indicates alkaline urine and may indicate conditions including a urinary tract infection. (The abbreviation **pH** describes the degree of acidity or alkalinity of a substance. A pH of 7 is neutral—that is, neither acid nor alkaline. Maximum acidity is 0 pH, and maximum alkalinity is pH 14.)

- The **specific gravity** reflects the amount of wastes, minerals, and solids in the urine. Low specific gravity (dilute urine) is characteristic of diabetes insipidus. High specific gravity (concentrated urine) occurs in conditions such as dehydration, liver failure, and shock.

Conditions Identified through Urinalysis

- **Acetone** (**ASS**-eh-tohn), which has a sweet fruity odor, is found in small quantities in normal urine and in larger amount in diabetic urine.

- **Albuminuria** (al-byou-mih-**NEW**-ree-ah) is the presence of the serum protein albumin in the urine and is a sign of impaired kidney function (**albumin** means albumin or protein and **-uria** means urine).

- **Bacteriuria** (back-**tee**-ree-**YOU**-ree-ah) is the presence of bacteria in the urine (**bacteri** means bacteria and **-uria** means urine).

- **Calciuria** (**kal**-sih-**YOU**-ree-ah) is the presence of calcium in the urine (**calci** means calcium and **-uria** means urine). Abnormally high levels may be diagnostic for hyperparathyroidism. Lower than normal levels may indicate osteomalacia.

- **Creatinuria** (kree-at-ih-**NEW**-ree-ah) is an increased concentration of creatine in the urine (**creatin** means creatinine and **-uria** means urine). **Creatinine,** a waste product of muscle metabolism, is normally removed by the kidneys. Its presence in urine is an indication of increased muscle breakdown or a disruption of kidney function.

- **Glycosuria** (glye-koh-**SOO**-ree-ah) is the presence of glucose in the urine and is most commonly caused by diabetes (**glycos** means glucose and **-uria** means urine).

- **Hematuria** (**hee**-mah-**TOO**-ree-ah *or* **hem**-ah-**TOO**-ree-ah) is the presence of blood in the urine (**hemat** means blood and **-uria** means urine). This condition may be caused by kidney stones, infection, damage to the kidney, or bladder cancer.

- In **gross hematuria** the urine may look pink, brown, or bright red, and the presence of blood can be detected without magnification. In **microscopic hematuria** the urine is clear, but blood cells can be seen under a microscope.

- **Ketonuria** (kee-toh-**NEW**-ree-ah) is the presence of ketones in the urine (**keton** means ketones and **-uria** means urine). **Ketones** are formed when the body breaks down fat. Their presence in urine may indicate starvation or uncontrolled diabetes.

- **Proteinuria** (**proh**-tee-in-**YOU**-ree-ah) is an excess of serum protein in the urine and is usually a sign of kidney disease (**protein** means protein and **-uria** means urine).

- **Pyuria** (pye-**YOU**-ree-ah) is the presence of pus in the urine (**py** means pus and **-uria** means urine).

- **Urine culture and sensitivity** is an additional laboratory test to identify the cause of a urinary tract infection and to determine which antibiotic would be the most effective treatment.

ENDOSCOPY

Endoscopy (en-**DOS**-koh-pee) is the visual examination of the interior of a body cavity (**endo-** means within and **-scopy** means visual examination). The fiber optic instrument used in this examination is an **endoscope.**

ENDOSCOPIC SURGERY

The term *endoscopy* also describes surgical procedures requiring only very small incisions. Examples of these procedures include reconstructive knee surgery, laparoscopic cholecystectomy (gallbladder removal), bladder cancer treatment, hysterectomy, appendectomy, and lung biopsy.

The procedures and instruments are named for the body parts involved. For example, Figure 15.18 shows an **arthroscope** being used to perform knee surgery.

CENTESIS

Centesis (sen-**TEE**-sis) is a surgical puncture to remove fluid for diagnostic purposes or to remove excess fluid.

- **Abdominocentesis** (ab-**dom**-ih-noh-sen-**TEE**-sis) is the surgical puncture of the abdominal cavity (**abdomin/o** means abdomen, and **-centesis** means a surgical puncture to remove fluid).

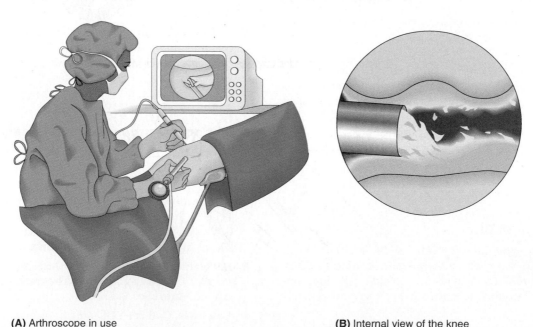

(A) Arthroscope in use

(B) Internal view of the knee during arthroscopy

FIGURE 15.18 Arthroscopic surgery. (A) The physician views progress on a monitor. (B) Internal view as diseased tissue is removed during surgery.

- **Amniocentesis** (**am**-nee-oh-sen-**TEE**-sis) is a diagnostic test to evaluate fetal health and is discussed in Chapter 14.

- **Cardiocentesis** (**kar**-dee-oh-sen-**TEE**-sis), also known as **cardiopuncture,** is the puncture of a chamber of the heart for diagnosis or therapy (**cardi/o** means heart and **-centesis** means a surgical puncture to remove fluid).

- **Pericardiocentesis** (**pehr**-ih-**kar**-dee-oh-sen-**TEE**-sis) is the drawing of fluid from the pericardial sac (**peri-** means surrounding, **cardi/o** means heart, and **-centesis** means a surgical puncture to remove fluid).

- **Thoracentesis** (**thoh**-rah-sen-**TEE**-sis) is the puncture of the chest wall to obtain fluid for diagnostic purposes, to drain pleural effusions, or to reexpand a collapsed lung.

IMAGING TECHNIQUES

Imaging techniques are used to visualize and examine internal body structures. The three most commonly used techniques are compared in Table 15.2 and Figure 15.19.

Two of these techniques involve the use of ionizing radiation, commonly known as **x-rays,** which is invisible, has no odor, and cannot be felt. This radiation is beneficial in producing images and in treating cancer; however, excessive exposure is dangerous and can cause death.

CONTRAST MEDIUM

A **radiographic contrast medium** is a substance used to make visible structures that are otherwise hard to see.

- A **radiopaque contrast medium** (ray-dee-oh-**PAYK**), such as barium sulfate, *does not* allow the x-rays to pass through and appears white or light gray on the resulting film.

- A **radiolucent contrast medium** (ray-dee-oh-**LOO**-sent), such as air or nitrogen gas, *does* allow the x-rays to pass through and appears black or dark gray on the resulting film.

Barium

Barium (Ba) is a radiopaque contrast medium used primarily to visualize the gastrointestinal (GI) system (Figure

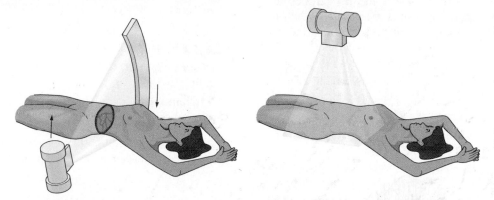

FIGURE 15.19 (Left) Computed tomography provides cross-sectional images. (Right) Conventional x-rays superimpose anatomy and can capture images in only one plane.

Table 15.2

IMAGING SYSTEMS COMPARED

Method	How It Works
Conventional radiography (x-ray)	Uses radiation (x-rays) passing through the patient to expose a film that shows the body in profile. Hard tissues are light; soft tissues appear as shades of gray; and air is black.
Computed tomography (CT)	Uses radiation (x-rays) with computer assistance to produce multiple cross-sectional views of the body. Hard tissues are light, and soft tissues appear as shades of gray.
Magnetic resonance imaging (MRI)	Uses a combination of radio waves and a strong magnetic field to produce images. Hard tissues are dark, and soft tissues appear as shades of gray.

15.20). It is administered orally as a barium swallow (upper GI study) or rectally as a barium enema (lower GI study). X-rays and fluoroscopy are used to trace the flow of the barium.

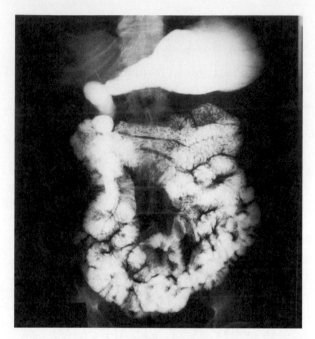

FIGURE 15.20 A radiograph after a barium swallow. The stomach and a portion of the small intestine are visible.

Intravenous Contrast Medium

An **intravenous contrast medium** is injected into the vein to make visible the flow of blood through blood vessels and organs (see Figure 5.17). These techniques are usually named for the vessels or organs involved.

- For example, **lymphangiography** (lim-**fan**-jee-**OG**-rah-fee) is the radiographic examination of the lymphatic vessels after the injection of a contrast medium (**lymphangi/o** means lymph vessel, and **-graphy** means process of recording).

RADIOLOGY

- A **radiologist** (**ray**-dee-**OL**-oh-jist) is a physician who specializes in diagnosing and treating diseases and disorders with x-rays and other forms of radiant energy (**radi** means radiation and **-ologist** means specialist).

- In conventional **radiology,** also known as **x-ray** or **radiography,** an image of hard-tissue internal structures is created by the exposure of sensitized film to x-radiation (**radi/o** means radiation and **-graphy** means the process of recording). The resulting film is known as an **x-ray** or a **radiograph** (**radi/o** means radiation and **-graph** means the resulting record).

- Radiographs are made up of shades of gray. Radiopaque hard tissues, such as bone and tooth

enamel, *do not* permit x-rays to pass through, and they appear white or light gray on the radiograph.

- Radiolucent air and soft tissues *do* permit x-rays to pass through, and they appear as shades of gray to black on the radiograph (Figure 15.21).

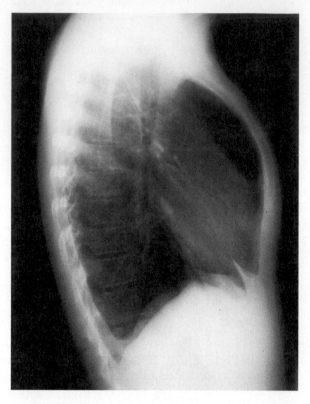

FIGURE 15.21 A posteroanterior chest x-ray. Bones of the spine are white, and the soft tissues are shades of gray.

RADIOGRAPHIC POSITIONING AND PROJECTIONS

POSITIONING

The term **positioning** describes the body placement and the part of the body closest to the film. For example, in a left lateral position, the left side of the body is placed nearest the film.

- The basic projections described in the next section may be used for most body parts (Figure 15.22). These projections may be exposed with the patient in a standing or recumbent position.

PROJECTIONS

The term **projection** describes the path that the x-ray beam follows through the body from entrance to exit.

- When the name of the projection combines two terms into a single word, the term listed first is the one that the x-ray penetrates first. For example, in a

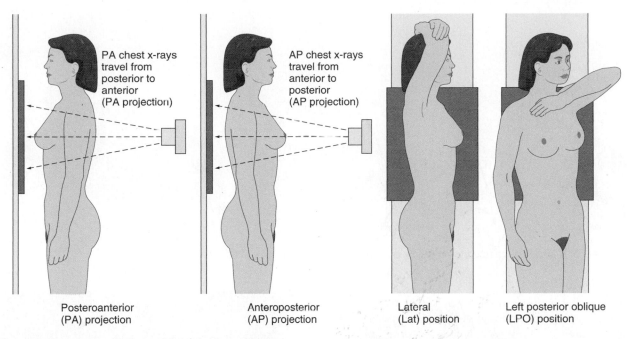

Posteroanterior
(PA) projection

Anteroposterior
(AP) projection

Lateral
(Lat) position

Left posterior oblique
(LPO) position

FIGURE 15.22 Radiographic projection positions.

posteroanterior projection, the x-rays travel through the body from the posterior (back) toward the anterior (front) to expose the film (see Figure 15.22).

Basic Radiographic Projections

● An **anteroposterior projection (AP)** has the patient positioned with the back parallel to the film. The x-ray beam travels from anterior (front) to posterior (back).

● A **posteroanterior projection (PA)** has the patient positioned facing the film and parallel to it. The x-ray beam travels through the body from posterior to anterior.

● A **lateral projection (Lat),** also known as a **side view,** has the patient positioned at right angles to the film. This view is named for the side of the body nearest the film.

● An **oblique projection (Obli)** has the patient positioned so the body is slanted sideways to the film. This is halfway between a parallel and a right angle position. This view is named for the side of the body nearest the film. *Oblique* means slanted sideways, and these projections are named for the portion of the body nearest the film.

DENTAL RADIOGRAPHY

Specialized techniques and equipment are used in obtaining dental radiographs.

Extraoral Radiography

Extraoral radiography, as used in dentistry, means that the film is placed outside of the mouth. Figure 15.23 is a **panoramic radiograph,** which is also known as a **Panorex.**

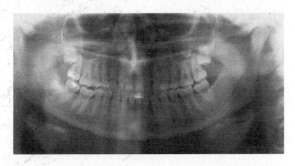

FIGURE 15.23 A Panorex radiograph shows all of the teeth and surrounding structures of the upper and lower dental arches on a single film.

Intraoral Radiography

Intraoral radiography, as used in dentistry, means that the film is placed within the mouth (Figure 15.24).

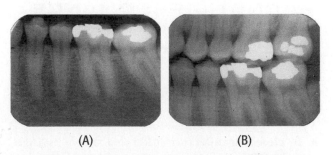

(A)　　　　　(B)

FIGURE 15.24 Intraoral dental radiographs. (A) A periapical film shows the entire length of a tooth and some of the tissues surrounding the root. (B) A bitewing film shows the crowns of the upper and lower teeth in one area of both jaws. The white areas on these teeth are amalgam (silver) fillings.

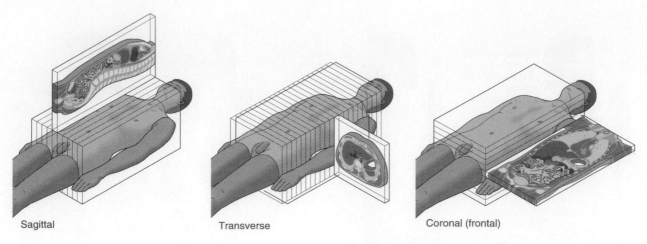

Sagittal   Transverse   Coronal (frontal)

FIGURE 15.25 Computed tomography provides cross-sectional views of different body planes.

- **Periapical radiographs,** which show the entire tooth and some surrounding tissue, are used to detect abnormalities, such as an abscess, at the tip of the root (**peri-** means surrounding, **apic** means apex, and **-al** means pertaining to).

- **Bitewing radiographs,** which show the crowns of teeth in both arches, are used primarily to detect decay (cavities) between the teeth.

COMPUTED TOMOGRAPHY

Computed tomography (toh-**MOG**-rah-fee), also known as **CT** or **computed axial tomography (CAT),** uses a thin, fan-shaped x-ray beam that rotates around the patient to produce multiple cross-sectional views of the body (Figure 15.25).

- Information gathered by radiation detectors is downloaded to a computer, analyzed, and converted into gray-scale images corresponding to anatomic slices of the body (Figure 15.26). These images are viewed on a monitor or printed as hard copy (films).

MAGNETIC RESONANCE IMAGING

Magnetic resonance imaging (MRI) uses a combination of radio waves and a strong magnetic field to create signals that are sent to a computer and converted into images of any plane through the body. In an MRI, hard tissues appear dark, and soft tissues are bright (Figure 15.27, see also Figure 10.14).

- In **closed architecture MRI,** also known as **high-field MRI,** patients may be uncomfortable because of the noise generated by the machine and the feeling of being closed in. In **open architecture MRI,** the design of the equipment is less confining and more comfortable for some patients.

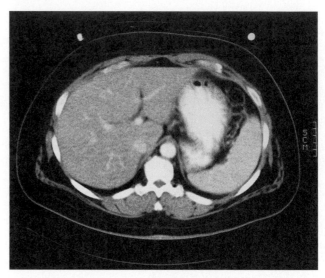

FIGURE 15.26 An abdominal CT scan in which the liver is predominant in the upper left and the stomach is visible in the upper right.

- **Magnetic resonance angiography (MRA),** also known as **MR angio,** shows veins and arteries without the injection of contrast material or dye.

- Because of the strong magnetic field, patients with pacemakers or other implanted electronic devices cannot be examined using these techniques.

FLUOROSCOPY

Fluoroscopy (floo-or-**OS**-koh-pee) is used to visualize body parts in motion by projecting x-ray images on a luminous fluorescent screen (**fluor/o** means glowing and **-scopy** means visual examination).

- **Cineradiography** (**sin**-eh-**ray**-dee-**OG**-rah-fee) is the recording of images as they appear in motion on a fluorescent screen (**cine** means relationship to movement, **radio** means radiation, and **-graphy** means process of recording).

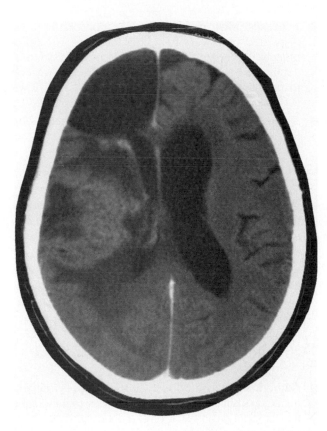

FIGURE 15.27 An MRI of the brain with a tumor visible in the upper left.

● Fluoroscopy may also be used in conjunction with conventional x-ray techniques to capture a record of parts of the examination.

DIAGNOSTIC ULTRASOUND

Diagnostic ultrasound, also known as **ultrasonography** (**ul**-trah-son-**OG**-rah-fee), is imaging of deep body structures by recording the echoes of pulses of sound waves above the range of human hearing. The resulting record is called a **sonogram** (**SOH**-noh-gram).

● Ultrasound is most effective for viewing solid organs of the abdomen and soft tissues where the signal is not stopped by intervening bone or air. Shown in Figure 15.28 is an echocardiogram, which is a specialized type of ultrasonography. In this image, which is enhanced with color Doppler, a large area of red shows an abnormal opening and blood flow between the aorta and the right atrium.

NUCLEAR MEDICINE

Nuclear medicine (NM), also known as **radionuclide imaging** (**ray**-dee-oh-**NEW**-klyd), is used for both diagnosis and treatment. Although other imaging techniques focus on the anatomic structures, NM looks at physiological processes to determine how well body organs or systems are functioning.

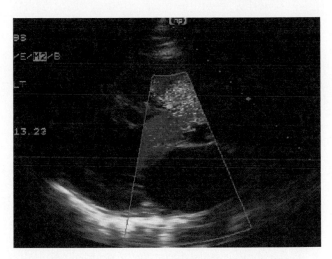

FIGURE 15.28 An echocardiogram enhanced with color Doppler.

● Nuclear medicine involves the use of **radiopharmaceuticals** that arc injected or inhaled into the body and taken up (absorbed) by a particular organ.

● Each radiopharmaceutical contains a **radionuclide tracer,** also known as a **radioactive tracer,** which is specific to the body system being examined.

● A **gamma-ray camera** attached to a computer is used to generate an image showing the pattern of absorption. It is the pattern of absorption that indicates pathology.

NUCLEAR SCANS

A **nuclear scan,** also known as a **scintigram** (**SIN**-tih-gram), uses nuclear medicine technology to gather information about the structure and function of organs or systems that cannot be seen on conventional x-rays.

Bone Scans

In a **bone scan** the radionuclide tracer is injected into the bloodstream, and then the patient waits while the material travels through the body tissues. Only pathology in the bones absorbs the radionuclide, and these are visible as dark areas on the scan (Figure 15.29).

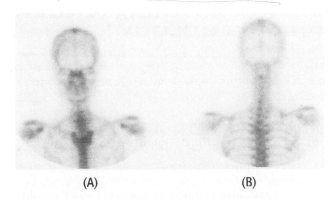

(A)   (B)

FIGURE 15.29 A bone scan of the head, shoulders, and upper spine. (A) Anterior view. (B) Posterior view.

Thyroid Scans

For a **thyroid scan,** a radiopharmaceutical containing radioactive iodine is administered. The rate of iodine uptake by the thyroid is an indicator of thyroid function.

SINGLE PHOTON EMISSION COMPUTED TOMOGRAPHY

Single photon emission computed tomography (SPECT) is a nuclear imaging technique in which pictures are taken by one to three gamma cameras after a radionuclide tracer has been injected into the blood.

- In SPECT, these **gamma cameras,** also known as **detectors,** rotate around the patient's body, collecting data and producing images on a variety of planes.

- This technique is used to study myocardial perfusion. **Perfusion** (per-**FYOU**-zuhn) is the flow of blood through the vessels of an organ (see Chapter 5).

POSITRON EMISSION TOMOGRAPHY

Positron emission tomography (PET) combines tomography with radionuclide tracers to produce enhanced images of selected body organs or areas. PET is used to determine cardiac or cerebral perfusion and for brain imaging to aid in the diagnosis of epilepsy, dementia, and recurrent brain tumors.

RADIOIMMUNOASSAY

Radioimmunoassay (**ray**-dee-oh-**im**-you-noh-**ASS**-ay), also known as **radioassay,** is a laboratory technique in which a radioactively labeled substance is mixed with a blood specimen.

- **Assay** (**ASS**-ay) means to determine the amount of a particular substance in a mixture. These techniques can be used to evaluate function of the pituitary and thyroid glands.

- **Immunofluorescence** (**im**-you-noh-**floo**-oh-**RES**-ens) is a method of tagging antibodies with a fluorescent dye to detect or localize antigen-antibody combinations.

PHARMACOLOGY

Pharmacology is the study of the nature, uses, and effects of drugs for medical purposes. A **pharmacist** is a specialist who is licensed in formulating and dispensing medications.

PRESCRIPTION AND OVER-THE-COUNTER DRUGS

- A **prescription (R$_x$)** is an order for medication, therapy, or a therapeutic device given (usually in writing) by an authorized person to a person properly authorized to dispense or perform the order.

- A **prescription drug** is a medication that may be dispensed only with a prescription from an appropriately licensed professional such as a physician or dentist. The abbreviations commonly used in relation to prescriptions and drug administration are shown in Table 15.3.

- An **over-the-counter drug (OTC)** is a medication that may be dispensed without a written prescription.

GENERIC AND BRAND NAME DRUGS

- A **generic drug** is usually named for its chemical structure and is not protected by a brand name or trademark. For example, *diazepam* is the generic name of a drug frequently used as a muscle relaxant.

- A **brand name** drug is sold under the name given the drug by the manufacturer. A brand name is always spelled with a capital letter. For example, *Valium* is the brand name for diazepam.

TERMINOLOGY RELATED TO PHARMACOLOGY

- **Addiction** is compulsive, uncontrollable dependence on a substance, habit, or practice to the degree that stopping causes severe emotional, mental, or physiologic reactions.

- An **adverse drug reaction (ADR),** also known as a **side effect** or an **adverse drug event (ADE),** is an undesirable drug response that accompanies the principal response for which the drug was taken.

- **Compliance** is the patient's consistency and accuracy in following the regimen prescribed by a physician or other healthcare professional. As used here, **regimen** (**REJ**-ih-men) means directions or rules.

- A **contraindication** is a factor in the patient's condition that makes the use of a drug dangerous or ill advised.

- A **drug interaction** occurs when the effect of one drug is modified (changed) when it is administered at the same time as another drug.

- An **idiosyncratic reaction** (**id**-ee-oh-sin-**KRAT**-ick) is an unexpected reaction to a drug.

- A **palliative** (**PAL**-ee-**ay**-tiv *or* **PAL**-ee-ah-tiv) is a substance that eases the pain or severity of a disease but does not cure it.

- A **placebo** (plah-**SEE**-boh) is a substance containing no active ingredients that is given for its suggestive effects. In research, a placebo identical in appearance with the material being tested is administered to distinguish between drug action and suggestive effect of the material under study.

- **Potentiation** (poh-**ten**-shee-**AY**-shun), also known as **synergism** (**SIN**-er-jizm), is a drug interaction that occurs when the effect of one drug is potentiated (increased) by another drug.

Table 15.3

FREQUENTLY USED DRUG ADMINISTRATION ABBREVIATIONS AND SYMBOLS

Abbreviation	Meaning
@	at
a.c.	before meals
ad lib	as desired
b.i.d.	twice a day
c̄	with
NPO	nothing by mouth
p.c.	after meals
p.r.n.	as needed
p.o.	by mouth
qd	every day
q.h	every hour
q.i.d.	four times a day
>	greater than
<	less than
t.i.d.	three times a day

ROUTES OF DRUG ADMINISTRATION

- **Inhalation administration** refers to vapor and gases taken in through the nose or mouth and absorbed into the bloodstream through the lungs. For example, the gases used for general anesthesia are administered by inhalation.

- **Oral administration** refers to drugs taken by mouth to be absorbed from the stomach or small intestine. These drugs may be in forms such as liquids, pills, or capsules. An **enteric coating** is applied to some tablets or capsules to prevent the release and absorption of their contents until they reach the small intestine.

- **Percutaneous treatment** (**per**-kyou-**TAY**-nee-us) means a procedure performed through the skin (**per-** means through, **cutane** means skin, and **-ous** means pertaining to). For example, a needle passed through the skin is used to aspirate fluid from a space below the skin.

- **Rectal administration** is the insertion of medication in the rectum by use of either suppositories or liquid solutions. A *suppository* is medication in a semisolid form that is introduced into the rectum. The suppository melts at body temperature, and the medication is absorbed through the surrounding tissues.

- With **sublingual administration,** the medication is placed under the tongue and allowed to dissolve slowly. Once dissolved, the medication is quickly absorbed through the sublingual tissue directly into the bloodstream.

- **Topical administration** refers to the drugs, such as lotions, ointments, and eyedrops, that are applied for local action.

- **Transdermal delivery** is a method of applying a drug to unbroken skin via a patch worn on the patient's skin. The drug is absorbed through the skin and into systemic circulation.

Parenteral Administration

- **Parenteral administration** (pah-**REN**-ter-al) is the administration of medication by injection through a **hypodermic syringe** (**high**-poh-**DER**-mick) (Figure 15.30).

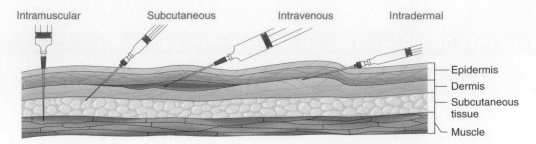

FIGURE 15.30 Types of injections.

- An **intramuscular injection (IM)** is made directly into muscle tissue.
- A **subcutaneous injection (SC)** is made into the fatty layer just below the skin.
- An **intravenous injection (IV)** is made directly into a vein.
- An **intradermal injection (ID)** is made into the middle layers of the skin.

Career Opportunities

In addition to the medical specialties already discussed, some of the health occupations involving diagnostic procedures and pharmacology include:

- **Medical laboratory technologist (MT)** or **clinical laboratory technologist:** works under the supervision of a pathologist to study tissues, fluids, and cells of the human body to help determine the presence and/or cause of disease. Specialties include

  clinical chemistry   microbiology

  blood bank technology   immunology
  and hematology

- **Medical laboratory technician (MLT):** works under the supervision of an MT or pathologist, performing many of the routine tests that do not require advanced knowledge

- **Histologic technician:** works under the supervision of an MT to cut and stain tissue specimens for microscopic examination

- **Medical laboratory assistant:** prepares specimens for testing and helps clean and maintain laboratory equipment

- **Pharmacy technician:** works under the supervision of a pharmacist to prepare medications for dispensing to patients, label medications, prepare IV solutions, maintain records, and order supplies

- **Radiologic technologist (RT)** or **X-ray technician:** works under the supervision of a radiologist to take x-rays for diagnostic purposes, administer radiation, and use nuclear medicine, ultrasound, and magnetic resonance for the diagnosis and treatment of disease

- **MRI technologist:** an RT who works with magnetic resonance imaging

- **Radiation therapy technologist:** prepares cancer patients for treatment and administers prescribed doses of ionizing radiation to specific body parts

- **Sonographer** or **ultrasound technologist:** conducts ultrasound tests. Specialties include

  abdominal   obstetrics and
  sonography   gynecology

  echocardiography   ophthalmology
  (heart)   (eyes)

  neurosonography   vascular sonography
  (brain)   (blood vessels)

STUDY BREAK

Everyone knows that one of the most important *vital signs* is body temperature. One of the most obvious indications of illness is an elevated body temperature, or fever, as the body attempts to kill certain viruses and bacteria that are sensitive to heat.

But is the body always the same temperature?

No. Not every person has 98.6°F as the normal temperature. And most individuals find that their temperature rises during the late afternoon and drops at night. When we go outside, our body temperature may lower when it is cold outside or raise if it is hot. The body will attempt to equalize this change in temperature through shivering, sweating, and other adjustments to the skin.

Women also have a slight change in body temperature throughout their menstrual cycle. That is why women who are trying to get pregnant will sometimes take a daily temperature reading upon awakening and will try to have intercourse when a dip in body temperature indicates that they may be about to ovulate.

Health Occupation Profile: MEDICAL TECHNOLOGIST

Laurie Howland has been a medical technologist, or clinical laboratory scientist, for 30 years. "A love of science and math first led me to the clinical laboratory field. I was fascinated by biology and chemistry labs, wanted an active job where I could do things with my hands, and did not want to be chained to a desk. I can report that my career definitely meets these objectives. I've been pleased with a healthcare profession that is 'behind the scenes,' yet still critical to the care of patients, and always on the leading edge of new treatments and advances in medicine."

"I've had the opportunity to work in the endocrinology, radioimmunoassay, and chemistry departments. I now focus my efforts on a computer system unique to hospital laboratories. This is a very good profession for full-time or flexible, part-time work. There are also opportunities to stretch beyond the hospital or clinic. I have colleagues who work in the pharmaceutical field and for laboratory instrumentation, computer, and agricultural businesses."

Review Time

Write the answers to the following questions on a separate piece of paper or in your notebook. In addition, be prepared to take part in the classroom discussion.

1. **Written assignment:** Describe the differences between **palpation** and **percussion.**

   Discussion assignment: How are these examination techniques used?

2. **Written assignment:** Using terms a physician would understand, identify three conditions a **hematocrit** (Hct) test would be used to diagnose.

   Discussion assignment: How would you explain to a patient the need for this test?

3. **Written assignment:** Describe the difference between **gross hematuria** and **microscopic hematuria.**

   Discussion assignment: What conditions might cause blood to be present in the urine?

4. **Written assignment:** Describe the differences between **computed tomography** and **magnetic resonance imaging.**

   Discussion assignment: Why are some patients uncomfortable about undergoing a closed architecture MRI?

5. Dr. Vaughn instructs you to position the patient for a vaginal examination.

   Written assignment: Name the examination position you would use and describe how the patient would be placed.

   Discussion assignment: What steps should be taken to maintain patient modesty in each of the commonly used examination positions?

Optional Internet Activity

*The goal of this activity is to help you learn more about medical terminology while improving your Internet skills. Select **one** of these two options and follow the instructions.*

1. **Internet Search:** Search for information about a bone scan. Write a brief (one- or two-paragraph) report on something new you learned here and include the address of the web site where you found this information.

2. **Web Site:** To learn more about **radiology,** go to this web address: **http://www.rad.uab.edu/.** Search under Teaching File and explore the films of greatest interest to you. Write a brief (one- or two-paragraph) report on something new you learned here.

The Human Touch: Critical Thinking Exercise

The following story and questions are designed to stimulate critical thinking through class discussion or as a brief essay response. There are no right or wrong answers to these questions.

Seth and Hiroshi grew up at the beach, surfing and playing the party scene. After high school, Hiroshi studied law enforcement and joined the police department. Seth bummed around the world chasing waves for a few more years before going to computer school and getting a job at Sebring Software.

One night while they were watching the game at the Tradewinds Sports Bar, Seth said to his old friend, "You'll never guess what Sebring's security is doing now." Seth's employer was always worried that an employee would steal programming ideas and market them to the competition.

"Don't tell me," Hiroshi smirked. "A guard makes surprise raids on your home computer to see if you've downloaded any Sebring secrets."

"Not that," Seth spoke seriously, "but just as bad. They're going to do random drug testing. Whether a person does a little weed at night to relax is nobody else's business!"

"Our department does drug testing all the time," Hiroshi pointed out.

"Yeah, but you carry guns. I wouldn't want to be pulled over by some drugged-out cop waving a weapon. Someone could get hurt!"

Hiroshi thought a moment and finished his drink. "Seth, you design programs that operate traffic lights. What would happen if you messed up?"

Suggested Discussion Topics

1. Drug testing by urine sample is a common practice at many places of employment. Discuss how you would feel if it were required of you.

2. Some drugs can be detected in urine 72 hours after they have been taken. Should an employer be able to reprimand employees for something they did on their own time? Why?

3. What types of jobs do you think should have mandatory drug testing? Why?

4. If someone were taking recreational drugs and wanted to hide that fact, is there any way he or she could avoid testing positive?

5. Do you think mandatory drug testing makes the workplace or job safer? If so, why?

Student Workbook and Student Activity CD-ROM

1. Go to your **Student Workbook** and complete the Learning Exercises for this chapter.

2. Go to the **Student Activity CD-ROM** and have fun with the exercises and games for this chapter.

Appendix A
Prefixes, Word Roots (Combining Forms), and Suffixes

	Pertaining to			Abnormal Conditions
-ac	pertaining to		-ago	abnormal condition, disease
-al	pertaining to		-esis	abnormal condition, disease
-ar	pertaining to		-ia	abnormal condition, disease
-ary	pertaining to		-iasis	abnormal condition, disease
-eal	pertaining to		-ion	condition
-ical	pertaining to		-ism	condition, state of
-ial	pertaining to		-osis	abnormal condition, disease
-ic	pertaining to			

				Noun Endings
-ine	pertaining to		-a	noun ending
-ior	pertaining to		-e	noun ending
-ory	pertaining to		-um	singular noun ending
-ous	pertaining to		-us	singular noun ending
-tic	pertaining to		-y	noun ending

A

a-	no, not without, away from, negative
-a	noun ending
ab-	away from, negative absent
abdomin/o	abdomen
-able	capable of, able to
abort/o	premature expulsion of a nonviable fetus
abrad/o, abras/o	rub or scrape off
abrupt/o	broken away from
abs-	away from
abscess/o	going away, collection of pus
absorpt/o	suck up, suck in
-ac	pertaining to
acanth/o	spiny, thorny
acetabul/o	acetabulum (hip socket)
-acious	characterized by
acne/o	point or peak
acous/o, acoust/o	hearing, sound
acquir/o	get, obtain
acr/o	extremities (hands and feet), top, extreme point

acromi/o	acromion, point of shoulder blade
actin/o	light
acu/o	sharp, severe, sudden
acuit/o, acut/o	sharp, sharpness
acust/o, -acusia, -acusis	hearing, sense of hearing
ad-	toward, to, in direction of
aden/o	gland
adenoid/o	adenoids
adhes/o	stick to, cling to
adip/o	fat
adnex/o	bound to
adren/o, adrenal/o	adrenal glands
aer/o	air, gas
aesthet/o	sensation, sense of perception
af-	toward, to
affect/o	exert influence on
agglutin/o	clumping, stick together
aggress/o	attack, step forward
-ago	abnormal condition, disease
agor/a	marketplace
-agra	excessive pain, seizure, attack of severe pain
-aise	comfort, ease
-al	pertaining to
alb/i, alb/o, albin/o	white
albumin/o	albumin, protein
alg/e, algi/o, alg/o, algesi/o	relationship to pain
-algesia, -algesic	painful, pain sense
-algia	pain, painful condition
align/o	bring into line or correct position
aliment/o	to nourish
all/o, all-	other, different from normal, reversal
alopec/o	baldness, mangy
alveol/o	alveolus, air sac, small sac
ambi-	both sides, around or about, double
ambly/o	dull, dim
ambul/o, ambulat/o	walk
ametr/o	out of proportion
-amine	nitrogen compound
amni/o	amnion, fetal membrane
amph-	around, on both sides, doubly
amput/o, amputat/o	cut away, cut off a part of the body
amyl/o	starch
an-	no, not, without
an-, ana-	up, apart, backward, excessive
an/o	anus, ring
-an	characteristic of, pertaining to
-ancy	state of
andr/o	relationship to the male
aneurysm/o	aneurysm
angi/o	blood or lymph vessels
angin/o	angina, choking, strangling
anis/o	unequal
ankyl/o	crooked, bent, stiff
anomal/o	irregularity
ante-	before, in front of
anter/o	before, front
anthrac/o	coal, coal dust
anti-	against
anxi/o, anxiet/o	uneasy, anxious
aort/o	aorta
ap-	toward, to
-apheresis	removal
aphth/o	ulcer
apic/o	apex
aplast/o	defective development, lack of development
ap-, apo-	separation, away from, opposed, detached
aponeur/o	aponeurosis (type of tendon)
apoplect/o	a stroke
append/o, appendic/	appendix
aqu/i, aqu/o, aque/o	water
-ar	pertaining to
arachn/o	spider web, spider
arc/o	bow, arc or arch
-arche	beginning
areat/o	occurring in patches or circumscribed areas
areol/o	little open space
-aria	connected with
arrect/o	upright, lifted up, raised
arter/o, arteri/o	artery
arthr/o	joint
articul/o	joint
-ary	pertaining to

as-	toward, to
-ase	enzyme
aspir/o, aspirat/o	to breathe in
asthen-, -asthenia	weakness, lack of strength
asthmat/o	gasping, choking
astr/o	star, star-shaped
at-	toward, to
atel/o	incomplete, imperfect
ather/o	plaque, fatty substance
athet/o	uncontrolled
atop/o	strange, out of place
atres/i	without an opening
atri/o	atrium
attenuat/o	diluted, weakened
aud-, audi/o, audit/o	ear, hearing, the sense of hearing
aur/i, aur/o	ear, hearing
auscult/o	listen
aut/o	self
-ax	noun ending
ax/o	axis, main stem
axill/o	armpit
azot/o	urea, nitrogen

B

bacill/o	rod-shaped bacterium (plural, *bacteria*)
bacteri/o	bacteria (singular, *bacterium*)
balan/o	glans penis
bar/o	pressure, weight
bartholin/o	Bartholin's gland
bas/o	base, opposite of acid
bi-, bis-	twice, double, two
bio-	life
bifid/o	split, divided into two parts
bifurcat/o	divide or fork into two branches
bil/i	bile, gall
bilirubin/o	bilirubin
bin-	two by two
-blast	embryonic, immature, formative element
blephar/o	eyelid
borborygm/o	rumbling sound
brachi/o	arm
brachy-	short
brady-	slow
brev/i, brev/o	short

bronch/i, bronchi/o, bronch/o	bronchial tube, bronchus
bronchiol/o	bronchiole, bronchiolus
brux/o	grind
bucc/o	cheek
burs/o	bursa, sac of fluid near joint
byssin/o	cotton dust

C

cadaver/o	dead body, corpse
calc/i	calcium, lime, the heel
calci-, calc/o	calcium
calcane/o	calcaneus, heel bone
calcul/o	stone, little stone
cali/o, calic/o	cup, calyx
call/i, callos/o	hard, hardened and thickened
calor/i	heat
canalicul/o	little canal or duct
canth/o	corner of the eye
capill/o	hair
capit/o	head
capn/o	carbon dioxide, sooty or smoky appearance
capsul/o	little box
carb/o	carbon
carbuncl/o	carbuncle
carcin/o	cancerous
cardi/o, card/o	heart
cari/o	rottenness, decay
carot/o	stupor, sleep
carp/o	wrist bones
cartilag/o	cartilage, gristle
caruncul/o	bit of flesh
cat-, cata-, cath-	down, lower, under, downward
catabol/o	a breaking down
cathart/o	cleansing, purging
cathet/o	insert, send down
caud/o	lower part of body, tail
caus/o, caust/o	burning, burn
cauter/o, caut/o	heat, burn
cav/i, cav/o	hollow, cave
cavern/o	containing hollow spaces
cec/o	cecum
-cele	hernia, tumor, swelling
celi/o, cel/o	abdomen, belly
cement/o	cementum, a rough stone
cent-	hundred

-centesis	surgical puncture to remove fluid
cephal/o, -ceps	head
cera-	wax
cerebell/o	cerebellum
cerebr/o	cerebrum, brain
cerumin/o	cerumen, earwax
cervic/o	neck, cervix (neck of uterus)
cheil/o	lip
cheir/o	hand
chem/i, chem/o, chemic/o	drug, chemical
chir/o	hand
chlor/o	green
chlorhydr/o	hydrochloric acid
chol/e	bile, gall
cholangi/o	bile duct
cholecyst/o	gallbladder
choledoch/o	common bile duct
cholesterol/o	cholesterol
chondr/o	cartilage
chord/o	spinal cord, cord
chore/o	dance
chori/o, chorion/o	chorion, membrane
choroid/o	choroid layer of eye
chrom/o, chromat/o	color
chron/o	time
chym/o	to pour, juice
cib/o	meal
cicatric/o	scar
-cidal	pertaining to killing
-cide	causing death
cili/o	eyelashes, microscopic hair-like projections
cine-	relationship to movement
circ/i	ring or circle
circulat/o	circulate, go around in a circle
circum-	around, about
circumcis/o	cutting around
circumscrib/o	confined, limited in space
cirrh/o	orange-yellow, tawny
cis/o	cut
clasis, -clast	break down
claudicat/o	limping
claustr/o	barrier
clav/i	key
clavicul/o, cleid/o	clavicle, collar bone
climacter/o	crisis, rung of a ladder
clitor/o	clitoris
-clonus	violent action
clus/o	shut or close
-clysis	irrigation, washing
co-	together, with
coagul/o, coagulat/o	clotting, coagulation
coarct/o, coarctat/o	press together, narrow
cocc/i, cocc/o, -coccus	spherical bacteria
coccyg/o	coccyx, tailbone
cochle/o	spiral, snail, snail shell
coher/o, cohes/o	cling, stick together
coit/o	a coming together
col/o	colon, large intestine
coll/a	glue
colon/o	colon, large intestine
colp/o	vagina
column/o	pillar
com-	together, with
comat/o	deep sleep
comminut/o	break into pieces
communic/o	share, to make common
compatibil/o	sympathize with
con-	together, with
concav/o	hollow
concentr/o	condense, intensify, remove excess water
concept/o	become pregnant
conch/o	shell
concuss/o	shaken together, violently agitated
condyl/o	knuckle, knob
confus/o	confusion, disorder
coni/o	dust
conjunctiv/o	onjunctiva, joined together, connected
consci/o	aware, awareness
consolid/o	become firm or solid
constipat/o	pressed together, crowded together
constrict/o	draw tightly together
-constriction	narrowing
contact/o	touched, infected
contagi/o	infection, unclean, touching of something
contaminat/o	render unclean by contact, pollute

contine/o, continent/o	keep in, contain, hold back, restrain
contra-	against, counter, opposite
contracept/o	prevention of conception
contus/o	bruise
convalesc/o	recover, become strong
convex/o	arched, vaulted
convolut/o	coiled, twisted
convuls/o	pull together
copi/o	plentiful
copulat/o	joining together, linking
cor/o	pupil
cord/o	cord, spinal cord
cordi/o	heart
core/o, cor/o	pupil
cori/o	skin, leather
corne/o	cornea
coron/o	coronary, crown
corp/u, corpor/o	body
corpuscul/o	little body
cort-	covering
cortic/o	cortex, outer region
cost/o	rib
cox/o	hip, hip joint
crani/o	skull
-crasia	a mixture or blending
creatin/o	creatine
crepit/o, crepitat/o	crackling, rattling
crin/o, -crine	secrete
cris/o, critic/o	turning point
-crit	to separate
cry/o	cold
crypt/o	hidden
cubit/o	elbow
cuboid/o	cubelike
culd/o	cul-de-sac, blind pouch
cult/o	cultivate
-cusis	hearing
cusp/i	point, pointed flap
cutane/o	skin
cyan/o	blue
cycl/o	ciliary body of eye, cycle
-cyesis	pregnancy
cyst-, -cyst	bladder, bag
cyst/o	urinary bladder, cyst, sac of fluid
cyt/o, -cyte	cell
-cytic	pertaining to a cell
-cytosis	condition of cells

D

dacry/o	tear, lacrimal duct (tear duct)
dacryocyst/o	lacrimal sac (tear sac)
dactyl/o	fingers, toes
de-	down, lack of, from, not, removal
debrid/e	open a wound
deca-, deci-	ten, tenth
decidu/o	shedding, falling off
decubit/o	lying down
defec/o, defecat/o	free from waste, clear
defer/o	carrying down or out
degenerat/o	gradual impairment, breakdown, diminished function
deglutit/o	swallow
dehisc/o	burst open, split
deliri/o	wandering in the mind
delt/o	Greek letter delta, triangular shape
delus/o	delude, mock, cheat
dem/o	people, population
-dema	swelling (fluid)
demi-	half
dendr/o	branching, resembling a tree
dent/i, dent/o	tooth, teeth
depilat/o	hair removal
depress/o	press down lower, pressed or sunk down
derma-, dermat/o, derm/o	skin
desic/o	drying
-desis	surgical fixation of bone or joint, to bind, tie together
deteriorat/o	worsening or gradual impairment
dextr/o	right side
di-	twice, twofold, double
dia-	through, between, apart, complete
diaphor/o	sweat
diaphragmat/o	diaphragm, wall across
diastol/o	standing apart, expansion
didym/o	testes, twins, double
diffus/o	pour out, spread apart
digest/o	divide, distribute
digit/o	finger or toe
dilat/o, dilatat/o	spread out, expand
-dilation	widening, stretching, expanding
dilut/o	dissolve, separate

diphther/o	membrane
dipl/o	double
dips/o, -dipsia	thirst
dis-	negative, apart, absence of
dislocat/o	displacement
dissect/o	cutting apart
disseminat/o	widely scattered
dist/o	far
distend/o, distent/o	stretch apart, expand
diur/o, diuret/o	tending to increase urine output
divert/i	turning aside
domin/o	controlling, ruling
don/o	give
dors/i, dors/o	back of body
-dote	what is given
-drome	to run, running
-duct	opening
duct/o	to lead, carry
duoden/i, duoden/o	duodenum
dural	pertaining to dura mater
-dynia	pain
dys-	bad, difficult, painful

E

e-	out of, from
-e	noun ending
-eal	pertaining to
ec-	out, outside
ecchym/o	pouring out of juice
ech/o	sound
eclamps/o, eclampt/o	flashing or shining forth
ectasia, -ectasis	stretching, dilation, enlargement
ecto-	out, outside
-ectomy	surgical removal, cutting out, excision
-ectopy	displacement
eczemat/o	eruption
-edema	swelling
edem-, edemat/o	swelling, fluid, tumor
edentul/o	without teeth
ef-	out
effect/o	bring about a response, activate
effus/o	pouring out
ejaculat/o	throw or hurl out

electr/o	electricity, electric
eliminat/o	expel from the body
em-	in
emaciat/o	wasted by disease
embol/o	something inserted or thrown in
embry/o	fertilized ovum, embryo
-emesis	vomiting
emet/o	vomit
-emia	blood, blood condition
emmetr/o	in proper measure
emolli/o	make soft, soften
en-	in, within, into
encephal/o	brain
end-, endo-	in, within, inside
endocrin/o	secrete within
enem/o	end in, inject
enter/o	small intestine
ento-	within
enzym/o	leaven
eosin/o	red, rosy
epi-	above, upon, on
epidemi/o	among the people, an epidemic
epididym/o	epididymis
epiglott/o	epiglottis
episi/o	vulva
epithel/i, epitheli/o	epithelium
equin/o	pertaining to a horse
-er	one who
erect/o	upright
erg/o, -ergy	work
erot/o	sexual love
eruct/o, eructat/o	belch forth
erupt/o	break out, burst forth
erythem/o, erythemat/o	flushed, redness
erythr/o	red
es-	out of, outside, away from
-esis	abnormal condition, disease
eso-	inward
esophag/o	esophagus
-esthesia, esthesi/o	sensation, feeling
esthet/o	feeling, nervous sensation, sense of perception
estr/o	female
ethm/o	sieve
eti/o	cause
eu-	good, normal, well, easy

-eurysm	widening
evacu/o, evacuat/o	empty out
ex-	out of, outside, away from
exacerbat/o	aggravate, irritate
exanthemat/o	rash
excis/o	cutting out
excori/o, excoriat/o	abrade or scratch
excret/o	separate, discharge
excruciat/o	intense pain, agony
exhal/o, exhalat/o	breathe out
exo-	out of, outside, away from
exocrin/o	secrete out of
expector/o	cough up
expir/o, expirat/o	breathe out
exstroph/o	turned or twisted out
extern/o	outside, outer
extra-	on the outside, beyond, outside
extrem/o, extremit/o	extremity, outermost
extrins/o	from the outside, contained outside
exud/o, exudat/o	to sweat out

F

faci/o	face, form
-facient	making, producing
fasci/o	fascia, fibrous band
fascicul/o	little bundle
fatal/o	pertaining to fate, death
fauc/i	narrow pass, throat
febr/i	fever
fec/i, fec/o	dregs, sediment, waste
femor/o	femur, thigh bone
fenestr/o	window
fer/o	bear, carry
-ferent	carrying
-ferous	bearing, carrying, producing
fertil/o	fertile, fruitful, productive
fet/i, fet/o	fetus, unborn child
fibr/o	fiber
fibrill/o	muscular twitching
fibrin/o	fibrin, fibers, threads of a clot
fibros/o	fibrous connective tissue
fibul/o	fibula
-fic, fic/o	making, producing, forming
-fication	process of making
-fida	split

filtr/o, filtrat/o	filter, to strain through
fimbri/o	fringe
fiss/o, fissur/o	crack, split, cleft
fistul/o	tube or pipe
flamme/o	flame colored
flat/o	flatus, breaking wind, rectal gas
flex/o	bend
flu/o	flow
fluor/o	luminous, glowing
foc/o	focus, point
foll/i	bag, sac
follicul/o	follicle, small sac
foramin/o	opening, foramen
fore-	before, in front of
-form, form/o	resembling, in the shape of
fornic/o	arch, vault, brothel
foss/o	ditch, shallow depression
fove/o	pit
fract/o	break, broken
fren/o	device that limits movement
frigid/o	cold
front/o	forehead, brow
-fuge	to drive away
funct/o, function/o	perform, function
fund/o	bottom, base, ground
fung/i	fungus
furc/o	forking, branching
furuncul/o	furunculus, a boil, an infection
-fusion	pour

G

galact/o	milk
gamet/o	wife or husband, egg or sperm
gangli/o, ganglion/o	ganglion
gangren/o	eating sore, gangrene
gastr/o	stomach, belly
gastrocnemi/o	gastrocnemius, calf muscle
gemin/o	twin, double
gen-, gen/o, -gen	producing, forming
-gene	production, origin, formation
-genic, -genesis	creation, reproduction
genit/o	produced by, birth, reproductive organs
-genous	producing

ger/i	old age
germin/o	bud, sprout, germ
geront/o	old age
gest/o, gestat/o	bear, carry young or off-spring
gigant/o	giant, very large
gingiv/o	gingival tissue, gums
glauc/o	gray
glen/o	socket or pit
gli/o	neurologic tissue, supportive tissue of nervous system
globin/o, -globulin	protein
globul/o	little ball
glomerul/o	glomerulus
gloss/o	tongue
glott/i, glott/o	back of the tongue
gluc/o	glucose, sugar
glute/o	buttocks
glyc/o, glycos/o	glucose, sugar
glycer/o	sweet
glycogen/o	glycogen, animal starch
gnath/o	jaw
-gnosia	knowledge, to know
-gog, -gogue	make flow
goitr/o	goiter, enlargement of the thyroid gland
gon/e, gon/o	seed
gonad/o	gonad, sex glands
goni/o	angle
gracil/o	slender
grad/i	move, go, step, walk
-grade	go
-gram	resulting record
granul/o	granule(s)
-graph	resulting record
-graphy	process of recording
gravid/o	pregnancy
-gravida	pregnant
gynec/o	woman, female
gyr/o	turning, folding

H

hal/o, halit/o	breath
halluc/o	great or large toe
hallucin/o	hallucination, to wander in the mind
hem/e	deep red iron-containing pigment
hem/o, hemat/o	blood, relating to the blood

hemangi/o	blood vessel
hemi-	half
hemoglobin/o	hemoglobin
hepat/o	liver
hered/o, heredit/o	inherited, inheritance
herni/o	hernia
herpet/o	creeping
heter/o	other, different
-hexia	habit
hiat/o	opening
hidr/o	sweat
hil/o	hilum, notch or opening from a body part
hirsut/o	hairy, rough
hist/o, histi/o	tissue
holo-	all
hom/o	same, like, alike
home/o	sameness, unchanging, constant
hormon/o	hormone
humer/o	humerus (upper arm bone)
hydr/o, hydra-	relating to water
hygien/o	healthful
hymen/o	hymen, a membrane
hyper-	excessive, increased
hyph-	under
hypn/o	sleep
hypo-	deficient, decreased
hyster/o	uterus

I

-ia	abnormal condition, disease, plural of -ium
-ial	pertaining to
-ian	specialist
-iasis	abnormal condition, disease
iatr/o	physician, treatment
-iatrics	field of medicine, healing
-iatrist	specialist
-iatry	field of medicine
-ible	capable of, able to
-ic	pertaining to
ichthy/o	dry, scaly
-ician	specialist
icter/o	jaundice
idi/o	peculiar to the individual or organ, one, distinct
-iferous	bearing, carrying, producing
-ific	making, producing

-iform	shaped or formed like, resembling
-igo	attack, diseased condition
-ile	capable of
ile/o	ileum, small intestine
ili/o	ilium, hip bone
illusi/o	deception
im-	not
immun/o	immune, protection, safe
impact/o	pushed against, wedged against, packed
impress/o	pressing into
impuls/o	pressure or pushing force, drive, urging on
in-	in, into, not, without
-ine	pertaining to
incis/o	cutting into
incubat/o	incubation, hatching
indurat/o	hardened
infarct/o	filled in, stuffed
infect/o	infected, tainted
infer/o	below, beneath
infest/o	attack, assail, molest
inflammat/o	flame within, set on fire
infra-	below, beneath, inferior to
infundibul/o	funnel
ingest/o	carry or pour in
inguin/o	groin
inhal/o, inhalat/o	breathe in
inject/o	to force or throw in
innominat/o	unnamed, nameless
inocul/o	implant, introduce
insipid/o	tasteless
inspir/o, inspirat/o	breathe in
insul/o	island
insulin/o	insulin
intact/o	untouched, whole
inter-	between, among
intermitt/o	not continuous
intern/o	within, inner
interstiti/o	the space between things
intestin/o	intestine
intim/o	innermost
intoxic/o	put poison in
intra-	within, inside
intrins/o	contained within
intro-	within, into, inside
introit/o	entrance or passage
intussuscept/o	take up or receive within
involut/o	rolled up, curled inward
iod/o	iodine
-ion	action, process, state or condition
ion/o	ion, to wander
-ior	pertaining to
ipsi-	same
ir-	in
ir/i, ir/o, irid/o, irit/o	iris, colored part of eye
is/o	same, equal
isch/o	to hold back
ischi/o	ischium
-is	noun ending
-ism	condition, state of
iso-	equal
-ist	a person who practices, specialist
-itis	inflammation
-ium	structure, tissue
-ize	to make, to treat

J

jejun/o	jejunum
jugul/o	throat
juxta-	beside, near, nearby

K

kal/i	potassium
kary/o	nucleus, nut
kata-, kath-	down
kel/o	growth, tumor
kera-	horn, hardness
kerat/o	horny, hard, cornea
ket/o, keton/o	ketones, acetones
kines/o, kinesi/o, -kinesia	movement
-kinesis	motion
klept/o	to steal
koil/o	hollow or concave
kraur/o	dry
kyph/o	bent, hump

L

labi/o	lip
labyrinth/o	maze, labyrinth, the inner ear
lacer/o, lacerat/o	torn, mangled
lacrim/o	tear, tear duct, lacrimal duct

lact/i, **lact/o**	milk
lactat/o	secrete milk
lamin/o	lamina
lapar/o	abdomen, abdominal wall
laps/o	slip, fall, slide
-lapse	to slide, fall, sag
laryng/o	larynx, throat
lat/i, **lat/o**	broad
later/o	side
lav/o, **lavat/o**	wash, bathe
lax/o, **laxat/o**	loosen, relax
leiomy/o	smooth (visceral) muscle
lemm/o	husk, peel, bark
-lemma	sheath, covering
lent/i	the lens of the eye
lenticul/o	shaped like a lens, pertaining to a lens
-lepsy	seizure
lept/o	thin, slender
-leptic	to seize, take hold of
lepto-	small, soft
letharg/o	drowsiness, oblivion
leuk/o	white
lev/o, **levat/o**	raise, lift up
lex/o, **-lexia**	word, phrase
libid/o, **libidin/o**	sexual drive, desire, passion
ligament/o	ligament
ligat/o	binding or tying off
lingu/o	tongue
lipid/o, **lip/o**	fat, lipid
-listhesis	slipping
lith/o, **-lith**	stone, calculus
lithiasis	presence of stones
lob/i, **lob/o**	lobe, well-defined part of an organ
loc/o	place
loch/i	childbirth, confinement
-logy	study of
longev/o	long-lived, long life
lord/o	curve, swayback bent
lumb/o	lower back, loin
lumin/o	light
lun/o, **lunat/o**	moon
lunul/o	crescent
lup/i, **lup/o**	wolf
lute/o	yellow
lux/o	to slide
lymph/o	lymph, lymphatic tissue
lymphaden/o	lymph gland
lymphangi/o	lymph vessel
-lysis	breakdown, separation, setting free, destruction, loosening
-lyst	agent that causes lysis or loosening
-lytic	to reduce, destroy

M

macro-	large, abnormal size or length, long
macul/o	spot
magn/o	great, large
major/o	larger
mal-	bad, poor, evil
-malacia	abnormal softening
malign/o	bad, evil
malle/o	malleus, hammer
malleol/o	malleolus, little hammer
mamm/o	breast
man/i	madness, rage
man/i, **man/o**	hand
mandibul/o	mandible, lower jaw
-mania	obsessive preoccupation
manipul/o	use of hands
manubri/o	handle
masset/o	chew
mast/o	breast
mastic/o, **masticat/o**	chew
mastoid/o	mastoid process
matern/o	maternal, of a mother
matur/o	ripe
maxill/o	maxilla (upper jaw)
maxim/o	largest, greatest
meat/o	opening or passageway
medi/o	middle
mediastin/o	mediastinum, middle
medic/o	medicine, physician, healing
medicat/o	medication, healing
medull/o	medulla (inner section), middle, soft, marrow
mega-	large, great
-megaly	enlargement
mei/o	less, meiosis
melan/o	black, dark
mellit/o	honey, honeyed
membran/o	membrane, thin skin
men/o	menstruation, menses

mening/o, meningi/o	membranes, meninges
menisc/o	meniscus, crescent
mens/o	menstruate, menstruation, menses
menstru/o, menstruat/o	occurring monthly
ment/o	mind, chin
mes-, meso-	middle
mesenter/o	mesentery
mesi/o	middle, median plane
meta-	change, beyond, subsequent to, behind, after or next
metabol/o	change
metacarp/o	metacarpals, bones of the hand
metatars/o	bones of the foot between the tarsus and toes
-meter	measure, instrument used to measure
metr/i, metr/o, metri/o	uterus
-metrist	one who measures
-metry	to measure
mio-	smaller, less
micr/o, micro-	small
mictur/o, micturit/o	urinate
mid-	middle
midsagitt/o	from front to back, at the middle
milli-	one-thousandth
-mimetic	mimic, copy
mineral/o	mineral
minim/o	smallest, least
minor/o	smaller
-mission	to send
mit/o	a thread
mitr/o	a miter having two points on top
mobil/o	capable of moving
mono-	one, single
monil/i	string of beads, genus of parasitic mold or fungus
morbid/o	disease, sickness
moribund/o	dying
morph/o	shape, form
mort/i, mort/o, mort/u	death, dead
mortal/i	pertaining to death, subject to death

mot/o, motil/o	motion, movement
mu/o	close, shut
muc/o, mucos/o	mucus
multi-	many, much
muscul/o	muscle
mut/a	genetic change
mut/o	unable to speak, inarticulate
mutagen/o	causing genetic change
my/o	muscle
myc/e, myc/o	fungus
mydri/o	wide
mydrias/i	dilation of the pupil
myel/o	spinal cord, bone marrow
myocardi/o	myocardium, heart muscle
myom/o	muscle tumor
myos/o	muscle
myring/o	tympanic membrane, eardrum
myx/o, myxa-	mucus

N

nar/i	nostril
narc/o	numbness, stupor
nas/i, nas/o	nose
nat/i	birth
natr/o	sodium
nause/o	nausea, seasickness
neo-	new, strange
necr/o	death
-necrosis	tissue death
nect/o	bind, tie, connect
nephr/o	kidney
nerv/o, neur/i, neur/o	nerve, nerve tissue
neutr/o	neither, neutral
nev/o	birthmark, mole
nid/o	next
niter-, nitro-	nitrogen
noct/i	night
nod/o	knot, swelling
nodul/o	little knot
nom/o	law, control
non-	no
nor-	chemical compound
norm/o	normal or usual
nuch/o	the nape
nucle/o	nucleus
nucleol/o	little nucleus, nucleolus

nulli-	none
numer/o	number, count
nunci/o	messenger
nutri/o, nutrit/o	nourishment, food, nourish, feed
nyct/o, nyctal/o	night

O

ob-	against
obes/o	obese, extremely fat
obliqu/o	slanted, sideways
oblongat/o	oblong, elongated
obstetr/i, obstetr/o	midwife, one who stands to receive
occipit/o	back of the skull, occiput
occlud/o, occlus/o	shut, close up
occult/o	hidden, concealed
ocul/o	eye
odont/o	tooth
-oid	like, resembling
-ole	little, small
olecran/o	elbow, olecranon
olfact/o	smell, sense of smell
olig/o	scanty, few
-ologist	specialist
-ology	the science or study of
-oma	tumor, neoplasm
om/o	shoulder
oment/o	omentum, fat
omphal/o	umbilical cord, the navel
onc/o	tumor
-one	hormone
onych/o	fingernail or toenail
o/o, oo/o	egg
oophor/o	ovary
-opaque	obscure
opac/o, opacit/o	shaded, dark, impenetrable to light
oper/o, operat/o	perform, operate, work
opercul/o	cover or lid
ophthalm/o	eye, vision
-opia	vision condition
opisth/o	backward
-opsia, -opsis, -opsy	vision, view of
opt/i, opt/o, optic/o	eye, vision
or/o	mouth, oral cavity
orbit/o	orbit, bony cavity or socket

orch/o, orchid/o, orchi/o	testicles, testis, testes
-orexia	appetite
organ/o	organ
orgasm/o	swell, be excited
orth/o	straight, normal, correct
-ory	pertaining to
os-	mouth, bone
-ose	full of, pertaining to, sugar
-osis	abnormal condition, disease
osm/o	pushing, thrusting
-osmia	smell, odor
oss/e, oss/i, oste/o, ost/o	bone
ossicul/o	ossicle (small bone)
-ostomy	surgically creating an opening
-ostosis	condition of bone
ot/o	ear, hearing
-otia	ear condition
-otomy	cutting, surgical incision
ov/i, ov/o	egg, ovum
ovari/o	ovary
ovul/o	egg
-oxia	oxygen condition
ox/i, ox/o, ox/y	oxygen
oxid/o	containing oxygen
oxy-	swift, sharp, acid,
oxysm/o	sudden

P

pachy-	heavy, thick
palat/o	palate, roof of mouth
pall/o, pallid/o	pale, lacking or drained of color
palliat/o	cloaked, hidden
palm/o	palm of the hand
palpat/o	touch, feel, stroke
palpebr/o	eyelid
palpit/o	throbbing, quivering
pan-	all, entire, every
pancreat/o	pancreas
papill/i, papill/o	nipple-like
papul/o	pimple
par-, para-	beside, near, beyond, abnormal, apart from opposite, along side of
par/o	to bear, bring forth, labor
-para	to give birth

paralys/o, paralyt/o	disable
parasit/o	parasite
parathyroid/o	parathyroid glands
pares/i	to disable
-paresi	partial or incomplete paralysis
paret/o	to disable
-pareunia	sexual intercourse
pariet/o	wall
parotid/o	parotid gland
-parous	having borne one or more children
paroxysm/o	sudden attack
-partum, parturit/o	childbirth, labor
patell/a, patell/o	patella, kneecap
path/o, -pathy	disease, suffering, feeling, emotion
paus/o	cessation, stopping
-pause	stopping
pector/o	chest
ped/o	child, foot
pedi/a	child
pedicul/o	louse (singular), lice (plural)
pelv/i, pelv/o	pelvic bone, pelvic cavity, hip
pen/i	penis
pendo	to hang
-penia	deficiency, lack, too few
peps/i, -pepsia, pept/o	digest, digestion
per-	excessive, through
percept/o	become aware, perceive
percuss/o	strike, tap, beat
peri-	surrounding, around
perine/o	perineum
peristals/o, peristalt/o	constrict around
peritone/o	peritoneum
perme/o	to pass or go through
pernici/o	destructive, harmful
perone/o	fibula
perspir/o	perspiration
pertuss/i	intensive cough
petechi/o	skin spot
-pexy	surgical fixation
phac/o	lens of eye
phag/o	eat, swallow
-phage	a cell that destroys, eat, swallow

-phagia	eating, swallowing
phak/o	lens of eye
phalang/o	phalanges, finger and toe
phall/o	penis
pharmac/o, pharmaceut/o	drug
pharyng/o	throat, pharynx
phas/o	speech
-phasia	speak or speech
phe/o	dusky
pher/o	to bear or carry
-pheresis	removal
phil/o, -phila, -philia	attraction to, like, love
phleb/o	vein
phlegm/o	thick mucus
phob/o, -phobia	abnormal fear
phon/o, -phonia	sound, voice
phor/o	carry, bear, movement
-phoresis	carrying, transmission
-phoria	to bear, carry, feeling, mental state
phot/o	light
phren/o	diaphragm, mind
-phthisis	wasting away
-phylactic	protective, preventive
-phylaxis	protection
physi/o, physic/o	nature
-physis	to grow
phyt/o, -phyte	plant
pigment/o	pigment, color
pil/i, pil/o	hair
pineal/o	pineal gland
pinn/i	external ear, auricle
pituit/o, pituitar/o	pituitary gland
plac/o	flat plate or patch
placent/o	placenta, round flat cake
plak/o, -plakia	plaque, plate, thin flat layer or scale
plan/o	flat
plant/i, plant/o	sole of foot
plas/i, plas/o	development, growth, formation
plas/o, -plasia	development, formation, growth
-plasm	formative material of cells
plasm/o	something molded or formed
plast/o	growth, development, mold
-plastic	pertaining to formation

-plasty	surgical repair
ple/o	more, many
-plegia	paralysis, stroke
-plegic	one affected with paralysis
pleur/o	pleura, side of the body
plex/o	plexus, network
plic/o	fold or ridge
-pnea	breathing
-pneic	pertaining to breathing
pne/o-	breath, breathing
pneum/o, pneumon/o	lung, air
pod/o	foot
-poiesis	formation, to make
poikil/o	varied, irregular
pol/o	extreme
poli/o	gray matter of brain and spinal cord
pollic/o	thumb
poly-	many
polyp/o	polyp, small growth
pont/o	pons (a part of the brain), bridge
poplit/o	back of the knee
por/o	pore, small opening
-porosis	lessening in density, porous condition
port/i	gate, door
post-	after, behind
poster/o	behind, toward the back
potent/o	powerful
pract/i, practic/o	practice, pursue an occupation
prandi/o, -prandial	meal
-praxia	action, condition concerning the performance of movements
-praxis	act, activity, practice use
pre-	before, in front of
precoc/i	early, premature
pregn/o	pregnant, full of
prematur/o	too early, untimely
preputi/o	foreskin, prepuce
presby/o	old age
press/o	press, draw
priap/o	penis
primi-	first
pro-	before, in behalf of
process/o	going forth
procident/o	fall down or forward

procreat/o	reproduce
proct/o	anus and rectum
prodrom/o	running ahead, precursor
product/o	lead forward, yield, produce
prolaps/o	fall downward, slide forward
prolifer/o	reproduce, bear offspring
pron/o, pronat/o	bent forward
pros-	before
prostat/o	prostate gland
prosth/o, prosthet/o	addition, appendage
prot/o, prote/o	first
protein/o	protein
proxim/o	near
prurit/o	itching
pseud/o	false
psor/i, psor/o	itch, itching
psych/o	mind
ptomat/o	a fall
-ptosis	droop, sag, prolapse, fall
-ptyal/o	saliva
-ptysis	spitting
pub/o	pubis, part of hip bone
pubert/o	ripe age, adult
pudend/o	pudendum
puerper/i	childbearing, labor
pulm/o, pulmon/o	lung
pulpos/o	fleshy, pulpy
puls/o	beat, beating, striking
punct/o	sting, prick, puncture
pupill/o	pupil
pur/o	pus
purpur/o	purple
purul/o	pus-filled
pustul/o	infected pimple
py/o	pus
pyel/o	renal pelvis, bowl of kidney
pylor/o	pylorus, pyloric sphincter
pyr/o, pyret/o	fever, fire
pyramid/o	pyramid-shaped

Q

quadr/i, quadr/o	four

R

rabi/o	madness, rage
rachi/o	spinal column, vertebrae

radi/o	radiation, x-rays, radius (lateral lower arm bone)
radiat/o	giving off rays or radiant energy
radicul/o	nerve root
raph/o	seam, suture
re-	back, again
recept/o	receive, receiver
recipi/o	receive, take to oneself
rect/o	rectum, straight
recticul/o	network
recuperat/o	recover, regain health
reduct/o	bring back together
refract/o	bend back, turn aside
regurgit/o	flood or gush back
remiss/o	give up, let go, relax
ren/o	kidney
restor/o	rebuild, put back, restore
resuscit/o	revive
retent/o	hold back
reticul/o	network
retin/o	retina, net
retro-	behind, backward, back of
retract/o	draw back or in
rhabdomy/o	striated muscle
rheum/o, rheumat/o	watery flow, subject to flow
rhin/o	nose
rhiz/o	root
rhonc/o	snore, snoring
rhythm/o	rhythm
rhythm/o	rhythm
rhytid/o	wrinkle
rigid/o	stiff
ris/o	laugh
roentgen/o	x-ray
rotat/o	rotate, revolve
-rrhage, -rrhagia	bleeding, abnormal excessive fluid discharge
-rrhaphy	to suture
-rrhea	abnormal flow, discharge
-rrhexis	rupture
rube-	red
rug/o	wrinkle, fold

S

sacc/i, sacc/o	sac
sacchar/o	sugar
sacr/o	sacrum

saliv/o	saliva
salping/o	uterine (fallopian) tube, auditory (eustachian) tube
-salpinx	uterine (fallopian) tube
san/o	sound, healthy, sane
sangu/i, sanguin/o	blood
sanit/o	soundness, health
saphen/o	clear, apparent, manifest
sapr/o	decaying, rotten
sarc/o	flesh, connective tissue
scalp/o	carve, scrape
scapul/o	scapula, shoulder blade
schiz/o	division, split
scintill/o	spark
scirrh/o	hard
scler/o	sclera, white of eye, hard
-sclerosis	abnormal hardening
scoli/o	curved, bent
-scope	instrument for visual examination
-scopic	pertaining to visual examination
-scopy	visual examination
scot/o	darkness
scrib/o, script/o	write
scrot/o	bag or pouch
seb/o	sebum
secret/o	produce, separate out
sect/o, secti/o	cut, cutting
segment/o	pieces
sell/o	saddle
semi-	half
semin/i	semen, seed, sperm
sen/i	old
senesc/o	grow old
senil/o	old age
sens/i	feeling, sensation
sensitiv/o	sensitive to, affected by
seps/o	infection
sept/o	infection, partition
ser/o	serum
seros/o	serous
sial/o	saliva
sialaden/o	salivary gland
sider/o	iron
sigm/o	Greek letter sigma
sigmoid/o	sigmoid colon
silic/o	glass
sin/o, sin/u	hollow, sinus

sinistr/o	left, left side
sinus/o	sinus
-sis	abnormal condition, disease
sit/u	place
skelet/o	skeleton
soci/o	companion, fellow being
-sol	solution
solut/o, solv/o	loosened, dissolved
soma-, somat/o	body
somn/i, somn/o	sleep
son/o	sound
sopor/o	sleep
spad/o	draw off, draw
-spasm, spasmod/o	sudden involuntary contraction, tightening or cramping
spec/i	look at, a kind or sort
specul/o	mirror
sperm/o, spermat/	sperm, spermatozoa, seed
sphen/o	sphenoid bone, wedge
spher/o	round, sphere, ball
sphincter/o	tight band
sphygm/o	pulse
spin/o	spine, backbone
spir/o	to breathe
spirill/o	little coil
spirochet/o	coiled microorganism
splen/o	spleen
spondyl/o	vertebrae, vertebral column, backbone
spontane/o	unexplained, of one's own accord
spor/o	seed, spore
sput/o	sputum, spit
squam/o	scale
-stalsis	contraction, constriction
staped/o, stapedi/o	stapes (middle ear bone)
staphyl/o	clusters, bunch of grapes
-stasis, -static	control, maintenance of a constant level
steat/o	fat, lipid, sebum
sten/o	narrowing, contracted
-stenosis	abnormal narrowing
ster/o	solid structure
stere/o	solid, three-dimensional
steril/i	sterile
stern/o	sternum, the breastbone
stert/o	snore, snoring
steth/o	chest
-sthenia	strength
stigmat/o	point, spot
stimul/o	goad, prick, incite
stol/o	send or place
stomat/o	mouth
-stomosis, -stomy	furnish with a mouth or outlet, new opening
strab/i	squint, squint-eyed
strat/i	layer
strept/o	twisted chain
striat/o	stripe, furrow, groove
stric-	narrowing
strict/o	draw tightly together, bind or tie
strid/o	harsh sound
stup/e	benumbed, stunned
styl/o	pen, pointed instrument
sub-	under, less, below
subluxat/o	partial dislocation
sucr/o	sugar
sudor/i	sweat
suffoc/o, suffocat/o	choke, strangle
sulc/o	furrow, groove
super-, super/o	above, excessive, higher than
superflu/o	overflowing, excessive
supin/o	lying on the back
supinat/o	bend backward, place on the back
suppress/o	press down
suppur/o, x rheumat/o	to form pus
supra-	above, upper, excessive
supraren/o	above or on the kidney, suprarenal gland
sutur/o	stitch, seam
sym-	with, together, joined together
symptomat/o	falling together, symptom
syn-	together, with, union, association
synaps/o, synapt/o	point of contact
syncop/o	to cut short, cut off
-syndesis	surgical fixation of vertebrae
syndesm/o	ligament
syndrom/o	running together
synovi/o, synov/o	synovial membrane, synovial fluid
syphil/i, syphil/o	syphilis

syring/o	tube	tinnit/o	ringing, buzzing, tinkling
system/o, systemat/o	body system	-tion	process, state or quality of
systol/o	contraction	toc/o, -tocia, -tocin	labor, birth
		tom/o	cut, section, slice
		-tome	instrument to cut
T		-tomy	process of cutting
-thorax	chest, pleural cavity	ton/o	tension, tone, stretching
tachy-	fast, rapid	tone/o	to stretch
tact/i	touch	tonsill/o	tonsil, throat
talip/o	foot and ankle deformity	top/o	place, position, location
tars/o	tarsus (ankle bone), instep, edge of the eyelid	tors/o	twist, rotate
		tort/i	twisted
tax/o	coordination, order	tox/o, toxic/o	poison, poisonous
techn/o, techni/o	skill	trabecul/o	little beam marked with cross bars or beams
tectori/o	covering, rooflike		
tele/o	distant, far	trache/i, trache/o	trachea, windpipe
tempor/o	temporal bone, temple	trachel-	neck
ten/o, tend/o	tendon, stretch out, extend, strain	tract/o	draw, pull, path, bundle of nerve fibers
tenac/i	holding fast, sticky	tranquil/o	quiet, calm, tranquil
tendin/o	tendon	trans-	across, through
tens/o	stretch out, extend, strain	transfus/o	pour across, transfer
terat/o	malformed fetus	transit/o	changing
termin/o	end, limit	transvers/o	across, crosswise
test/i, test/o, testicul/o	testis, testicle	traumat/o	injury
		trem/o	shaking, trembling
tetan/o	rigid, tense	tremul/o	fine tremor or shaking
tetra-	four	treponem/o	coiled, turning microbe
thalam/o	thalamus, inner room	-tresia	opening
thalass/o	sea	tri-	three
thanas/o, thanat/o	death	trich/o	hair
the/o	put, place	trigon/o	trigone
thec/o	sheath	-tripsy	to crush
thel/o	nipple	-trite	instrument for crushing
therap/o, therapeut/o	treatment	trochle/o	pulley
		trop/o, -tropia	turn, change
therm/o	heat	troph/o, -trophy	development, nourishment
thio-	sulfur	-tropic	turning
thora/o, thorac/o	chest	-tropin	stimulate, act on
thromb/o	clot	tub/i, tub/o	tube, pipe
thym/o	thymus gland, soul	tubercul/o	little knot, swelling
-thymia	mind	tunic/o	covering, cloak, sheath
-thymic	pertaining to the mind	turbinat/o	coiled, spiral shaped
thyr/o, thyroid/o	thyroid gland	tuss/i	cough
tibi/o	tibia (shin bone)	tympan/o	tympanic membrane, eardrum
-tic	pertaining to		
tine/o	gnawing worm, ringworm	-type	classification, picture

U

-ula	small, little
-ule	small one
ulcer/o	sore, ulcer
uln/o	ulna (medial lower arm bone)
ultra-	beyond, excess
-um	singular noun ending
umbilic/o	navel
un-	not
ungu/o	nail
uni-	one
ur/o	urine, urinary tract
-uresis	urination
ureter/o	ureter
urethr/o	urethra
urg/o	press, push
-uria	urination, urine
urin/o	urine or urinary organs
urtic/o	nettle, rash, hives
-us	thing, singular noun ending
uter/i, uter/o	uterus
uve/o	iris, choroid, ciliary body, uveal tract
uvul/o	uvula, little grape

V

vaccin/i, vaccin/o	vaccine
vacu/o	empty
vag/o	vagus nerve, wandering
vagin/o	vagina
valg/o	bent or twisted outward
valv/o, valvul/o	valve
var/o	bent or twisted inward
varic/o	varicose veins, swollen or dilated vein
vas/o	vas deferens, vessel
vascul/o	blood vessel, little vessel
vast/o	vast, great, extensive
vect/o	carry, convey
ven/o	vein
vener/o	sexual intercourse
venter-	abdomen
ventilat/o	expose to air, fan
ventr/o	in front, belly side of body

ventricul/o	ventricle of brain or heart, small chamber
venul/o	venule, small vein
verg/o	twist, incline
verm/i	worm
verruc/o	wart
-verse, -version	to turn
vers/o, vert/o	turn
vertebr/o	vertebra, backbone
vertig/o, vertigin/o	whirling round
vesic/o	urinary bladder
vesicul/o	seminal vesicle, blister, little bladder
vestibul/o	entrance, vestibule
vi/o	force
vill/i	shaggy hair, tuft of hair
vir/o	poison, virus
viril/o	masculine, manly
vis/o	seeing, sight
visc/o	sticky
viscer/o	viscera, internal organ
viscos/o	sticky
vit/a, vit/o	life
viti/o	blemish, defect
vitre/o	glassy, made of glass
voc/i	voice
vol/o	palm or sole
volv/o	roll, turn
vulgar/i	common
vulv/o	vulva, covering

X

xanth/o	yellow
xen/o	strange, foreign
xer/o	dry
xiph/i, xiph/o	sword

Y

-y	noun ending

Z

zo/o	animal life
zygomat/o	cheek bone, yoke
zygot/o	joined together

Appendix B
Abbreviations and Meanings

A

A2 or A$_2$	aortic valve closure
A	accommodation; age; anterior
AAA	abdominal aortic aneurysm
AAL	anterior axillary line
AAV	adeno-associated virus
Ab	antibody
AB, ab	abortion
abd	abdomen
AB, Abnl	abnormal
A/B	acid-base ratio
ABC	aspiration; biopsy; cytology
ABE	acute bacterial endocarditis
ABG	arterial blood gases
ABP	arterial blood pressure
ABR	auditory brainstem response
AC	acromioclavicular; air conduction
ac	acute
AC, ac	before meals
Acc	accommodation
ACD	acid-citrate-dextrose; anterior chest diameter
ACG	angiocardiography; apex cardiogram
ACH	adrenocortical hormone
ACL	anterior cruciate ligament
ACLS	advanced cardiac life support
ACP	acid phosphatase
ACTH	adrenocorticotropic hormone
ACVD	acute cardiovascular disease
AD	abdominal diaphragmatic breathing; adenovirus; Alzheimer's disease; right ear
ADD	attention deficit disorder
ADE	adverse drug event
ADH	antidiuretic hormone
ADHD	attention deficit hyperactivity disorder
ADL	activities of daily living
ad lib	as desired
adm	admission
ADS	antibody deficiency syndrome
ADR	adverse drug reaction
ADT	admission; discharge; transfer

AE	above elbow
AED	automated external defibrillation
AF	acid-fast; atrial fibrillation
AFB	acid-fast bacilli
A fib	atrial fibrillation
AFP	alpha-fetoprotein
Ag	antigen
AG, A/G	albumin/globulin ratio
AH	abdominal hysterectomy
AHD	arteriosclerotic heart disease; autoimmune hemolytic disease
AHF	antihemophilic factor VIII
AHG	antihemophilic globulin factor VIII
AI	aortic insufficiency; atherogenic index
AID	acute infectious disease; artificial insemination donor
AIDS	acquired immune deficiency syndrome
AIH	artificial insemination homologous
AIHA	autoimmune hemolytic anemia
aj	ankle jerk
AK	above knee
AKA	above-knee amputation; also known as
alb	albumin
ALG	antilymphocytic globulin
alk	alkaline
alk phos	alkaline phosphatase
ALL	acute lymphoblastic leukemia; acute lymphocytic leukemia
ALND	axillary lymph node dissection
ALP	alkaline phosphatase
ALS	aldolase; amyotrophic lateral sclerosis; antilymphocytic serum
ALT	alanine transaminase (liver and heart enzyme)
alt dieb	alternate days; every other day
alt hor	alternate hours
alt noct	alternate nights
AMA	advanced maternal age; against medical advice; American Medical Association
amb	ambulate; ambulatory
AMD	age-related macular degeneration

AMI	acute myocardial infarction
AML	acute myeloblastic leukemia; acute myelocytic leukemia
amp	ampule
AMS	amylase
amt	amount
AN	anesthesiology
ANA	antinuclear antibodies
ANF	antinuclear factor
ANLL	acute nonlymphocytic leukemia
ANS	autonomic nervous system
ant	anterior
AOD	adult-onset diabetes; arterial occlusive disease
AOM	acute otitis media
A & P	anterior and posterior; auscultation and percussion
AP	angina pectoris; anteroposterior; anterior-posterior
APLD	aspiration percutaneous lumbar diskectomy
aq	aqueous; water
ARD	acute respiratory disease
ARDS	adult respiratory distress syndrome
ARF	acute renal failure; acute respiratory failure
ARM	artificial rupture of membranes
ART	assisted reproductive technology
AS	ankylosing spondylitis; aortic stenosis; left ear
ASA	aspirin
ASAP	as soon as possible
ASCVD	arteriosclerotic cardiovascular disease
ASD	atrial septal defect
ASH	asymmetrical septal hypertrophy
ASHD	arteriosclerotic heart disease
ASIS	anterior superior iliac spine
ASO	arteriosclerosis obliterans
ASS	anterior superior spine
AST	aspartate aminotransferase
as tol	as tolerated
ATP	adenosine triphosphate
Au	gold
AU	aures unitas; both ears
AUL	acute undifferentiated leukemia
ausc	auscultation
A-V	aortic valve; artificial ventilation; atrioventricular; arteriovenous
AVM	arteriovenous malfunction
AVN	atrioventricular node
AVR	aortic valve replacement
Ax	axillary
AZT	Aschheim-Zondek test

B

B/A	backache
BA	bronchial asthma
Ba	barium
BAC	blood alcohol concentration
BaE	barium enema
BAO	basal acid output
bas	basophils
BBB	blood-brain barrier; bundle branch block
BBT	basal body temperature
BC	bone conduction
BCC	basal cell carcinoma
BE	barium enema; below elbow
BEAM	brain electrical activity map
BED	binge eating disorder
BFP	biologic false positive
BID, bid, b.i.d.	bis in die; twice a day
bil	bilateral
BIN, bin	twice a night
BK	below knee
BKA	below-knee amputation
Bld	blood
BJ	Bence Jones
BM	bone marrow; bowel movement
BMD	Becker's muscular dystrophy; bone mineral density
BMI	body mass index
BMR	basal metabolic rate
BMT	barium meal test; bone marrow transplant
BNO	bladder neck obstruction
BNR	bladder neck resection
BOM	bilateral otitis media
B/P, BP	blood pressure
BP&P	blood pressure and pulse
BPH	benign prostatic hyperplasia; benign prostatic hypertrophy
BPM, bpm	beats per minute; breaths per minute
BPPV	benign paroxysmal positional vertigo

BR	bed rest
BRBPR	bright red blood per rectum
Bronch	bronchoscopy
BRP	bathroom privileges
BS	blood sugar; bowel sounds; breath sounds
BSE	breast self-examination
BSO	bilateral salpingo-oophorectomy
BT	bleeding time
BUN	blood urea nitrogen
BV	bacterial vaginosis; blood volume
Bx, bx	biopsy

C

C1–C7	cervical vertebrae
C	centigrade; Celsius
c	centimeter
c̄	with
c̲	without
Ca	calcium
CA, Ca	cancer; cardiac arrest; carcinoma; chronological age
CAB	coronary artery bypass
CABG	coronary artery bypass grafting
CAD	computer-assisted diagnosis; coronary artery disease
cal	calorie
cap, caps	capsule
CAPD	continuous ambulatory peritoneal dialysis
CAT	computerized axial tomography
cath	catheter; catheterize
CAVH	continuous arteriovenous hemofiltration
CBC, cbc	complete blood count
CBF	capillary blood flow; coronary blood flow
CBI	continuous bladder irrigation
CBR	complete bedrest
CBS	chronic brain syndrome
CC	chief complaint; colony count; cardiac cycle; cardiac catherization; creatinine clearance
cc	cubic centimeter (1/1000 liter)
CCA	circumflex coronary artery
CCCR	closed chest cardiopulmonary resuscitation
CCPD	continuous cycle peritoneal dialysis

CCr	creatinine clearance
CCT	cranial computed tomography
CCU	coronary care unit
CDC	calculated date (day) of confinement; Centers for Disease Control and Prevention
CDE	common duct exploration
CDH	congenital dislocation of the hip
CDT	cumulative trauma disorders
CEA	carcinoembryonic antigen
CF	complete fixation; counting fingers; cystic fibrosis
CFS	chronic fatigue syndrome
C gl	with correction; with glasses
CGL	chronic granulomatous leukemia
Ch	cholesterol
CHB	complete heart block
CHD	congenital heart defects; coronary heart disease
CHF	congestive heart failure
CHO	carbohydrate
chol	cholesterol
chr	chronic
CI	coronary insufficiency
cib	food
CID	cytomegalic inclusion disease
CIE	counter immunoelectrophoresis
CIN	cervical intraepithelial neoplasia
circ	circumcision
CIS	carcinoma in situ
CIT	conventional insulin treatment
CK	creatine kinase
ck	check
Cl, cl	clinic; chloride
CL	cholelithiasis; chronic leukemia; cirrhosis of the liver; cleft lip; corpus luteum
CLD	chronic liver disease
CLL	chronic lymphocytic leukemia
cl liq	clear liquid
cm	centimeter (1/100 meter)
cm³	cubic centimeter
CME	cystoid macular edema
CMG	cystometrogram
CML	chronic myelocytic leukemia
CMM	cutaneous malignant melanoma
CMV	controlled mechanical ventilation; cystometrogram; cytomegalovirus

CNS	central nervous system; cutaneous nerve stimulation
c/o, C/O	complains of
Co	cobalt
CO	carbon monoxide; coronary occlusion; coronary output
CO_2	carbon dioxide
COD	cause of death
COH	carbohydrate
COLD	chronic obstructive lung disease
comp	compound
cond	condition
contra	against
COPD	chronic obstructive pulmonary disease
CP	cardiopulmonary; cerebral palsy
CPA	carotid phonoangiograph
CPAP	continuous positive airway pressure
CPC	clinicopathologic conference
CPD	cephalopelvic disproportion
CPE	cytopathic effect
CPK	creatine phosphokinase
CPN	chronic pyelonephritis
CPPB	continuous positive-pressure breathing
CPR	cardiopulmonary resuscitation
CPS	cycles per second
CRD	chronic respiratory disease
CRF	chronic renal failure
creat	creatinine
CR	conditioned reflex; complete response
CRF	chronic renal failure
CS	central supply; cesarean section; complete stroke; conditioned stimulus; Cushing's syndrome
C & S	culture and sensitivity
CSAP	cryosurgical ablation of the prostate
CSF	cerebrospinal fluid
CSR	central supply room; Cheyne-Stokes respiration
CT	computed tomography
CTCL	cutaneous T-cell lymphoma
CTS	carpal tunnel syndrome
CTT	computed transaxial tomography
CTZ	chemoreceptor trigger zone
cu	cubic
CUC	chronic ulcerative colitis
CUG	cystourethrogram
CV	cardiovascular
CVA	cardiovascular accident; cerebrovascular accident; costovertebral angle
CVD	cardiovascular disease
CVL	central venous line
CVP	central venous pressure; Cytoxan, vincristine, prednisone
CVS	chorionic villus sampling
CWP	childbirth without pain; coal workers' pneumoconiosis
Cx	cervix
CX, CXR	chest x-ray film
cysto	cystoscopic examination; cystoscopy

D

D	diopter (lens strength)
d	day
DAT	diet as tolerated
db	decibel
D & C	dilation and curettage
D/C, DC	discontinue
DCC	direct-current cardioversion
DCIS	ductal carcinoma in situ
DCR	direct cortical response
Ddx	differential diagnosis
D & E	dilation and evacuation
del	delivery
DES	diethylstilbestrol
DGE	delayed gastric emptying
DEXA	dual energy x-ray absorptiometry
DHEA	dehydroepiandrosterone
DHFS	dengue hemorrhagic fever shock syndrome
DI	diabetes insipidus
diag	diagnosis
DIC	diffuse intravascular coagulation
diff	differential
DIP	distal interphalangeal
disch	discharge
DJD	degenerative joint disease
DKA	diabetic ketoacidosis
DL	danger list
DLE	discoid lupus erythematosus
DM	dermatomyositis; diabetes mellitus; diastolic murmur
DMD	Duchenne's muscular dystrophy

DNA	deoxyribonucleic acid
DNR	do not resuscitate
DNS	deviated nasal septum
DOA	dead on arrival
DOB	date of birth
DOC	date of conception
DOE	dyspnea on exertion
DOMS	delayed-onset muscle soreness
DOT	directly observed therapy
DQ	developmental quotient
DPT	diphtheria-pertussis-tetanus
dr	dram; dressing
DR	diabetic retinopathy; digital radiography; doctor
DRE	digital rectal exam
DRG	diagnosis-related group
D/S	dextrose in saline
DSA	digital subtraction angiography
DSD	dry sterile dressing
dsg	dressing
DT	diphtheria and tetanus toxoids
DTP	diphtheria, tetanus toxoids, and pertussis vaccine
DTs	delirium tremens
DTR	deep tendon reflex
DUB	dysfunctional uterine bleeding
DVA	distance visual acuity
DVI	digital vascular imaging
DW	distilled water
D/W	dextrose in water
Dx	diagnosis

E

E	enema
EBL	estimated blood loss
EBP	epidural blood patch
EBV	Epstein-Barr virus
ECC	endocervical curettage; extracorporeal circulation
ECCE	extracapsular lens extraction
ECG	electrocardiogram; electrocardiography
ECHO	echocardiogram; echocardiography
ECOM	extracorporeal membrane oxygenator
ECT	electroconvulsive therapy
ED	effective dose
EDC	estimated date (day) of confinement

EDD	end-diastolic dimension
EDG	electrodynogram
EDV	end-diastolic volume
EEG	electroencephalogram; electroencephalography
EENT	eye, ear, nose, and throat
EFM	electronic fetal monitor
EIA	enzyme immunoassay
EIB	exercise-induced bronchospasm
Ej	elbow jerk
EKG	electrocardiogram; electrocardiography
ELISA	enzyme-linked immunoassay; enzyme-linked immunosorbent assay
elix	elixir
EM	electron microscope; emmetropia
EMG	electromyogram; electromyography
EMR	educable mentally retarded; electronic medical record; eye movement record
EMS	early morning specimen; electromagnetic spectrum
ENG	electronystagmography
ENT	ear, nose, and throat
EOG	electro-oculogram
EOM	extraocular muscles; extraocular movement
Eos, eosins	eosinophils
EP	ectopic pregnancy; evoked potential
EPF	early pregnancy factor; exophthalmos-producing factor
EPO	erythropoietin
EPR	electron paramagnetic resonance; emergency physical restraint
EPS	extrapyramidal symptoms; exophthalmos-producing substance
ER	emergency room; epigastric region
ERCP	endoscopic retrograde cholangiopancreatography
ERG	electroretinogram
ERPF	effective renal plasma flow
ERT	estrogen replacement therapy; external radiation therapy
ERV	expiratory reserve volume
ESD	end-systolic dimension
ESPF	end-stage pulmonary fibrosis
ESR	erythrocyte sedimentation rate
ESRD	end-stage renal disease

ESWL	extracorporeal shock-wave lithotripsy		**FS**	frozen section
EST	electric shock therapy		**FSH**	follicle-stimulating hormone
ESV	end-systolic volume		**FSP**	fibrin-fibrinogen split products
ET	embryo transfer; enterically transmitted; esotropia		**FSS**	functional endoscopic sinus surgery
et	and		**FT**	family therapy
ETF	eustachian tube function		**FTA**	fluorescent treponemal antibody
etiol	etiology		**FTI**	free thyroxine index
ETT	endotracheal tube; exercise tolerance test		**FTND**	full-term normal delivery
EU	Ehrlich units; emergency unit; etiology unknown		**FTT**	failure to thrive
			FU, F/U	follow-up; follow up
EWB	estrogen withdrawal bleeding		**FUO**	fever of unknown origin
ex	excision; exercise		**FX, Fx**	fracture
exam	examination			
exp	expiration		**G**	
ext	extraction; external		**g**	gram
			g1	gravida (pregnancy)
F			**ga**	gallium
F	Fahrenheit		**GA**	gastric analysis; general anesthesia
FA	fluorescent antibody		**GB**	gallbladder
FAS	fetal alcohol syndrome		**GBM**	glomerular basement membrane
FB	foreign body		**GBS**	gallbladder series; Guillain-Barré syndrome
FBS	fasting blood sugar		**G-Cs**	glucocorticoids
FCD	fibrocystic disease		**GC**	gonorrhea
FDP	fibrin-fibrinogen degradation products		**G&D**	growth and development
Fe	iron		**GDM**	gestational diabetes mellitus
FECG	fetal electrocardiogram		**GER**	gastroesophageal reflux
FEF	forced expiratory flow		**GERD**	gastroesophageal reflux disease
FEV	forced expiratory volume		**GFR**	glomerular filtration rate
FFA	free fatty acids		**GG**	gamma globulin
FH	family history		**GGT**	gamma-glutamyl transferase
FHR	fetal heart rate		**GH**	growth hormone
FHS	fetal heart sounds		**GHb**	glycohemoglobin
FHT	fetal heart tones		**GIFT**	gamete intrafallopian transfer
FIA	fluorescent immunoassay; fluoroimmunoassay		**GIT**	gastrointestinal tract
			GLTT	glucose tolerance test
FME	full mouth extractions		**gm**	gram
fMRI	functional magnetic resonance imaging		**GMP**	guanosine monophosphate
			GOT	glutamic oxaloacetic transaminase
FMS	fibromyalgia syndrome		**GP**	general practice
FOBT	fecal occult blood test		**gr**	grain
FPG	fasting plasma glucose		**grav I**	pregnancy one; primigravida
FR	fibrin-fibrinogen related		**GS**	general surgery
fr	French (catheter size)		**GSW**	gunshot wound
FRC	functional residual capacity		**GT**	glucose tolerance
FROM	full range of motion		**GTP**	guanosine triphosphate
			GTT	glucose tolerance test

gtt	drops
GU	genitourinary
GVHD	graft-versus host disease
GxT	graded exercise test
GYN, Gyn	gynecology

H

h	hour
H	hydrogen; hypodermic
H & H	hemoglobin and hematocrit
HAA	hepatitis associated antigen; hepatitis Australia antigen
HAI	hemagglutination-inhibition immunoassay
HASHD	hypertensive arteriosclerotic heart disease
HAV	hepatitis A virus
HB	heart block; hemoglobin
HBE	His bundle electrocardiogram
HbF	fetal hemoglobin
HBP	high blood pressure
HbS	sickle cell hemoglobin
HBV	hepatitis B virus
HC	Huntington's cholera
HCD	heavy-chain disease
HCFA	Health Care Financing Administration
HCG	human chorionic gonadotropin
HCl	hydrochloric acid
HCL	hairy cell leukemia
HCPCS	Health Care Financing Administration Common Procedure Coding System
HCT, hct	hematocrit
HCV	hepatitis C virus
HCVD	hypertensive cardiovascular disease
HD	hearing distance; heart disease; hemodialysis; hip disarticulation; Hodgkin's disease; Huntington's disease
HDL	high-density lipoprotein
He	helium
H & E	hematoxylin and eosin stain
HDN	hemolytic disease of the newborn
HDS	herniated disk syndrome
HE	hereditary elliptocytosis
HEENT	head, eyes, ears, nose, throat
HF	heart failure
Hg	mercury

Hgb	hemoglobin
HGE	human granulocytic Ehrlichiosis
HI	hemagglutination-inhibition
HIE	hypoxic ischemic encephalopathy
HIV	human immunodeficiency virus
H & L	heart and lungs
HL	Hodgkin's lymphoma
HLA	human leukocyte antigen
HLR	heart-lung resuscitation
HM	hand motion
HMD	hyaline membrane disease
HMO	health maintenance organization
HNP	herniated nucleus pulposus
HO	hyperbaric oxygen
HOB	head of bed
H & P	history and physical
HP	hemipelvectomy; hyperparathyroidism
HPF	high-power field
HPL	human placental lactogen
HPN	hypertension
HPO	hypothalamic-pituitary-ovarian
HPS	hantavirus pulmonary syndrome
HPV	human papilloma virus
HR	heart rate
hr	hour
HRT	hormone replacement therapy
hs, h.s.	at bedtime; hour of sleep
HS	hereditary spherocytosis; herpes simplex
HSG	hysterosalpingogram
HSV	herpes simplex virus
ht	height; hematocrit
HT	hormone therapy
HTO	high tibial osteotomy
HV	hospital visit
HVD	hypertensive vascular disease
Hx	history
hypo	hypodermic
HZ	herpes zoster

I

I	intensity of magnetism; iodine
IABP	intra-aortic balloon pump
IACP	intra-aortic counterpulsation
IADH	inappropriate antidiuretic hormone
IASD	interatrial septal defect
IBC	iron-binding capacity

IBD	inflammatory bowel disease
IBS	irritable bowel syndrome
IC	inspiratory capacity
ICCE	intracapsular lens extraction
ICCU	intensive coronary care unit
ICD	implantable cardioverter defibrillator
ICF	intracellular fluid
ICP	intracranial pressure
ICS	intercostal space
ICSI	intracytoplasmic sperm injection
ICT	indirect Coombs' test; insulin coma therapy
ict ind	icterus index
ICU	intensive care unit
I & D	incision and drainage
ID	infectious disease; intradermal
IDC	infiltrating ductal carcinoma; invasive ductal carcinoma
IDD	insulin-dependent diabetes
IDDM	insulin-dependent diabetes mellitus
IDK	internal derangement of the knee
IDS	immunity deficiency state
I/E	inspiratory-expiratory ratio
IEMG	integrated electromyogram
IFG	impaired fasting glucose
Ig	immunoglobulin
IgA	immunoglobulin A
IgD	immunoglobulin D
IgE	immunoglobulin E
IgG	immunoglobulin G
IgM	immunoglobulin M
IGT	impaired glucose tolerance
IH	infectious hepatitis
IHD	ischemic heart disease
IHSS	idiopathic hypertrophic subaortic stenosis
IL	interleukin
ILC	infiltrating lobar carcinoma; invasive lobular carcinoma
IM	infectious mononucleosis; intramuscular
IMAG	internal mammary artery graft
IMF	idiopathic myelofibrosis
IMV	intermittent mandatory ventilation
IN	insulin
inf	inferior; infusion
I & O	intake and output

IO	intraocular
IOD	iron-overload disease (hemochromatosis)
IOL	intraocular lens
IOP	intraocular pressure
IPF	idiopathic pulmonary fibrosis
IPG	impedance plethysmography
IPPB	intermittent positive-pressure breathing
IQ	intelligence quotient
irrig	irrigation
IS	intercostal space
ISG	immune serum globulin
isol	isolation
ITP	idiopathic thrombocytopenic purpura
IU	international unit
IUD	intrauterine device
IUP	intrauterine pressure
IV	intravenous; intravenously
IVC	inferior vena cava
IVCP	inferior vena cava pressure
IVD	intervertebral disk
IVDA	intravenous drug abuse
IVF	in vitro fertilization
IVFA	intravenous fluorescein angiography
IVP	intravenous pyelogram
IVSD	interventricular septal defect
IVU	intravenous urogram

J

jct	junctions
JOD	juvenile-onset diabetes
JRA	juvenile rheumatoid arthritis
Jt	joint
JVP	jugular venous pressure; jugular venous pulse

K

K	potassium
KB	ketone bodies
KCF	key clinical findings
KCl	potassium chloride
KD	knee disarticulation
KE	kinetic energy
kg	kilogram
kj	knee jerk

KO	keep open
KOH	potassium hydrochloride
KS	Kaposi's sarcoma
KUB	kidney, ureter, bladder
KVO	keep vein open

L

l	liter
L1–L5	lumbar vertebrae
L & A	light and accommodation
LA	left atrium
lab	laboratory
lac	laceration
LAD	left anterior descending
LAP	leucine aminopeptidase
lap	laparotomy
laser	light amplification by stimulated emission of radiation
LASIK	laser in situ keratomileusis
lat	lateral
LAVH	laparoscopically assisted vaginal hysterectomy
lb	pound
LB	large bowel; low back
LBBB	left bundle branch block
LBW	low birth weight
LBBX	left breast biopsy and examination
LBP	low back pain
LCIS	lobular carcinoma in situ
L & D	labor and delivery
LD	lactic dehydrogenase
LDD	light-dark discrimination
LDH	lactic dehydrogenase
LDL	low-density lipoprotein
LE	left eye; life expectancy; lower extremity; lupus erythematosus
LES	lower esophageal sphincter
lg	large
LH	luteinizing hormone
LHBD	left heart bypass device
LHF	left-sided heart failure
LHR	leukocyte histamine release test
lig	ligament
liq	liquid
LLE	lower left extremity
LLL	left lower lobe
LLSB	left lower sternal border
LLQ	left lower quadrant

L/min	liters per minute
LMP	last menstrual period
LNMP	last normal menstrual period
LOC	level of consciousness; loss of consciousness
LOM	limitation of motion; loss of motion
LOS	length of stay
LP	light perception; lumbar puncture; lumboperitoneal
LPF	low-power field
LPS	lipase
LR	light reaction
LRDKT	living related donor kidney transplant
LSB	left sternal border
LSD	lysergic acid diethylamide
lt	left
LTB	laryngotracheobronchitis
LTC	long-term care
LTH	luteotropic hormone
LUE	left upper extremity
LUL	left upper lobe
LUQ	left upper quadrant
LV	left ventricle
LVH	left ventricle hypertrophy
lymphs	lymphocytes

M

M	meter; murmur
Mabs	monoclonal antibodies
MAO	maximal acid output; monoamine oxidase
MAR	multiple antibiotic resistant
MBC	maximal breathing capacity
MBD	minimal brain damage
mc	millicurie
mcg	microgram
MCH	mean corpuscular hemoglobin
MCHC	mean corpuscular hemoglobin concentration
MCT	mean circulation time
MCV	mean corpuscular volume
MD	macular degeneration; medical doctor; muscular dystrophy
MDS	myelodysplastic syndrome
MDR-TB	multidrug-resistant tuberculosis
ME	middle ear

MED	minimal effective dose; minimal erythema dose
mEq	milliequivalent
M & F	mother and father
MFT	muscle function test
mg	milligram
MG	myasthenia gravis
mgm	milligram
MH	malignant hyperpyrexia; malignant hyperthermia; marital history
MHA	microhemagglutination
MHC	major histocompatibility complex
MI	mitral insufficiency; myocardial infarction
MICU	medical intensive care unit; mobile intensive care unit
MID	multi-infarct dementia
MIDCAB	minimally invasive direct coronary artery bypass
MIP	maximal inspiratory pressure
ml, mL	milliliter
MLD	median lethal dose
mm	millimeter
mm Hg	millimeters of mercury
MM	multiple myeloma; malignant melanoma
MND	motor neuron disease
MNT	medical nutrition therapy
MODY	maturity-onset diabetes of the young
MOM	milk of magnesia
mono	monocytes
MP	metacarpal-phalangeal
MPD	myofascial pain dysfunction
MPJ	metacarpophalangeal joint
MR	mental retardation; metabolic rate; mitral regurgitation
MRD	medical record department
MRI	magnetic resonance imaging
MS	mitral stenosis; multiple sclerosis; musculoskeletal
MSH	melanocyte-simulating hormone
MSL	midsternal line
MT	medical technician; medical technologist
MTD	right eardrum
MTS	left eardrum
MTX	methotrexate
MV	mitral valve
MVP	mitral valve prolapse

MVPS	Medicare volume performance standard
MY	myopia
myel	myelogram
myop	myopia

N

N & T	nose and throat
N/C	no complaints
NA	not applicable; numerical aperture
Na	sodium
NaCl	sodium chloride
NAD	no acute disease; no apparent distress
NB	newborn
NBT	nitroblue tetrazolium
NCV	nerve conduction velocity
NED	no evidence of disease
NEG, neg	negative
neuro	neurology
NF	National Formulary; neurofibromatosis
N/G	nasogastric (tube)
ng	*Neisseria gonorrhoeae*
NGU	nongonococcal urethritis
NHL	non-Hodgkin's lymphoma
NICU	neurologic intensive care unit
NIDDM	non-insulin-dependent diabetes mellitus
NK	natural killer (cell)
NKA	no known allergies
NLP	neurolinguistic programming
NM	neuromuscular; nuclear medicine
N & M	nerves and muscles; night and morning
NMR	nuclear magnetic resonance
No	number
noc, noct	night
NOFTT	nonorganic failure to thrive
NPC	no point of convergence
NPH	neutral protamine Hagedorn
NPN	nonprotein nitrogen
NPO	nothing by mouth
NR	no response
NREM	no rapid eye movements
N/S	normal saline
NS	nephrotic syndrome; normal saline; not stated; not sufficient

NSAID	nonsteroidal anti-inflammatory drug
NSR	normal sinus rhythm
NSU	nonspecific urethritis
Nt	neutralization
NTD	neural tube defect
NTG	nitroglycerin
N & V	nausea and vomiting
NVA	near visual acuity
NVD	nausea, vomiting, and diarrhea; neck vein distention
NVS	neural vital signs
NYD	not yet diagnosed

O

OA	osteoarthritis
OB	obstetrics
OB-GYN	obstetrics and gynecology
obl	oblique
OBS	organic brain syndrome
Obs	obstetrics
OC	office call; oral contraceptive
OCC	occasional
OCD	obsessive compulsive disorder; oral cholecystogram
OCT	oral contraceptive therapy
OD	overdose; right eye (oculus dexter)
od	once a day
OGN	obstetric-gynecologic-neonatal
OGTT	oral glucose tolerance test
oint	ointment
OJD	osteoarthritic joint disease
OM	otitis media
OME	otitis media with effusion
OMR	optic mark recognition
OOB	out of bed
O & P	ova and parasites
OP	outpatient
OPD	outpatient department
OPG	oculoplethysmography
Ophth	ophthalmic
OPA	oropharyngeal airway
OPT	outpatient
OPV	oral poliovirus vaccine
OR	operating room
ORIF	open reduction internal fixation
ORT	oral rehydration therapy
Orth	orthopedics

OS	left eye (oculus sinister)
os	mouth
OSA	obstructive sleep apnea
OT	occupational therapy; old tuberculin
OTC	over-the-counter
Oto	otology
OU	each eye (oculus unitas)
oz	ounce
OXT	oxytocin

P

P, p	after; phosphorus; pulse
P & A	percussion and auscultation
PA	pernicious anemia; physician's assistant; posteroanterior; posterior-anterior; pulmonary artery
PABA	para-aminobenzoic acid
PAC	premature atrial contraction
PACAB	port-access coronary artery bypass
PADP	pulmonary artery diastolic pressure
PAMP	pulmonary arterial mean pressure
Pap	Papanicolaou smear
PAR	perennial allergic rhinitis; postanesthetic recovery
PARA (P_1)	full-term infants delivered
paren	parenterally
PASP	pulmonary artery systolic pressure
PAT	paroxysmal atrial tachycardia
Path	pathology
PBC	primary biliary cirrhosis
PBI	protein-bound iodine
PBP	progressive bulbar palsy
PBT4	protein-bound thyroxine
pc	after meals
PCO, PCOS	polycystic ovary syndrome
PCT	plasmacrit time
PCP	*Pneumocystis carinii* pneumonia
PCU	progressive care unit
PCV	packed cell volume
PD	interpupillary distance; Parkinson's disease; peritoneal dialysis
PDA	patent ductus arteriosus
PDD	pervasive developmental disorder
PDL	periodontal ligament
PE	physical examination
PEA	pulseless electrical activity
Pcds	pediatrics

PEEP	positive end-expiratory pressure	**PMS**	premenstrual syndrome
PEF	peak expiratory flow rate	**PMT**	premenstrual tension
PEG	pneumoencephalogram; pneumoencephalography	**PMVS**	prolapsed mitral valve syndrome
PEL	permissible exposure limit	**PND**	paroxysmal nocturnal dyspnea; postnasal drip
per	by; through	**PNH**	paroxysmal nocturnal hemoglobinuria
PERLA	pupils equally reactive (responsive) to light and accommodation	**PNS**	parasympathetic nervous system; peripheral nervous system
PERRLA	pupils equal, round, react (respond) to light and accommodation	**PO, p.o.**	by mouth; orally; phone order; postoperative
PET	positron emission tomography; preeclamptic toxemia	**POC**	products of conception
		polys	polymorphonuclear leukocytes
PFT	pulmonary function test	**POMR**	problem-oriented medical record
PG	pregnant; prostaglandin	**pos**	positive
PG, 2-h	post-load glucose (number indicates elapsed time)	**POS**	polycystic ovary syndrome
		post-op	postoperatively
PGH	pituitary growth hormone	**PP**	postpartum; postprandial (after meals); pulse pressure
PGL	persistent generalized lymphadenopathy	**PPA pos**	phenylpyruvic acid positive
pH	acidity; hydrogen ion concentration	**PPBS**	postprandial blood sugar
PH	past history; personal history; public health	**PPD**	purified protein derivative
		PPLO	pleuropneumonia-like organisms
PHN	postherpetic neuralgia	**PPS**	postperfusion syndrome; postpolio syndrome; progressive systemic sclerosis
PI	present illness		
PICU	pulmonary intensive care unit		
PID	pelvic inflammatory disease	**PPV**	positive-pressure ventilation
PIF	peak inspiratory flow	**PR**	peripheral resistance; pulse rate
PIP	proximal interphalangeal	**Pr**	presbyopia; prism
PK	pyruvate kinase; pyruvate kinase deficiency	**pr**	by rectum
		PRA	plasma renin activity
PKR	partial knee replacement	**PRBC**	packed red blood cells
PKU	phenylketonuria	**PRC**	packed red cells
PL	light perception	**PRE**	progressive restrictive exercise
PLC	platelet count	**preg**	pregnant
PLMS	periodic limb movements in sleep	**PRK**	photoreactive keratectomy
PLS	primary lateral sclerosis	**preop**	preoperative
PLTS	platelets	**prep**	prepare
PM	evening or afternoon; physical medicine; polymyositis; postmortem	**prn**	as needed
		proct	proctology
		prog	prognosis
PMA	progressive muscular atrophy	**PROM**	passive range of motion; premature rupture of membranes
PMH	past medical history		
PMI	point of maximal impulse	**pro time**	prothrombin time
PMN	polymorphonuclear neutrophils	**PRRE**	pupils round, regular, and equal
PMP	past menstrual period; previous menstrual period	**PSA**	prostate-specific antigen
		PSP	phenolsulfonphthalein
PMR	physical medicine and rehabilitation; polymyalgia rheumatica	**PSS**	progressive systemic sclerosis; physiologic saline solution

psych	psychiatry
PT	paroxysmal tachycardia; physical therapy; prothrombin time
pt	patient; pint
PTA	percutaneous transluminal angioplasty; plasma thromboplastin antecedent, factor XI
PPT	partial prothrombin time
PTB	patellar tendon bearing
PTC	percutaneous transhepatic cholangiography; plasma thromboplastic component, factor XI
PTCA	percutaneous transluminal coronary angioplasty
PTD	permanent and total disability
PTE	parathyroid extract
PTH	parathyroid hormone; parathormone
PTSD	posttraumatic stress disorder
PTT	partial thromboplastin time; prothrombin time
PU	peptic ulcer; pregnancy urine; prostatic urethra
PUD	peptic ulcer disease; pulmonary disease
pul	pulmonary
PV	peripheral vascular; plasma volume; polycythemia vera
P & V	pyloroplasty and vagotomy
PVC	premature ventricular contraction
PVD	peripheral vascular disease
PVE	prosthetic valve endocarditis
PVOD	peripheral vascular occlusive disease
PVS	persistent vegetative state
PVT	paroxysmal ventricular tachycardia
pvt	private
PWB	partial weight-bearing
PWP	pulmonary wedge pressure
Px	prognosis

Q

q	every
qd, q.d.	every day
qh, q.h	every hour
q 2 h	every 2 hours
QID, qid, q.i.d.	four times a day
qm	every morning
qn	every night

qns	quantity not sufficient
qod	every other day
qoh	every other hour
QOL	quality of life
qs	quantity sufficient
qt	quart; quiet
q.q.	each
quad	quadrant

R

R	rectal; respiration; right
RA	refractory anemia; rheumatoid arthritis; right arm; right atrium
Ra	radium
rad	radiation absorbed dose
RAF	rheumatoid arthritis factor
RAI	radioactive iodine
RAIU	radioactive iodine uptake determination
RAS	reticular activating system
RAST	radioallergosorbent
RAT	radiation therapy
RBBB	right bundle branch block
RBC	red blood cell; red blood count
RBCV	red blood cell volume
RBE	relative biologic effects
RCA	right coronary artery
RD	respiratory distress; retinal detachment
RDA	recommended daily allowance
RDS	respiratory distress syndrome
reg	regular
rehab	rehabilitation
RE	right eye
rem	roentgen-equivalent-man
REM	rapid eye movement
RER	renal excretion rate
RES	reticuloendothelial system
RBRVS	resource-based relative value scale
resp	respirations
RF	renal failure; rheumatoid factor; rheumatic fever
RFS	renal function study
RH	right hand
Rh neg	Rhesus factor negative
Rh pos	Rhesus factor positive
RHD	rheumatic heart disease
RIA	radioimmunoassay

RICE	rest, ice, compression, elevate	**RUE**	right upper extremity
RIF	right iliac fossa	**RUL**	right upper lobe
RIST	radioimmunosorbent	**RUQ**	right upper quadrant
RK	radial keratotomy	**RV**	residual volume; right ventricle
RL	right leg	**RVG**	radionuclide ventriculogram
RLC	residual lung capacity	**RVH**	right ventricular hypertrophy
RLD	related living donor	**RVS**	relative value schedule
RLE	right lower extremity	**RW**	ragweed
RLL	right lower lobe	**Rx**	prescription; take; therapy; treatment
RLQ	right lower quadrant		
RLS	restless legs syndrome		
RM	respiratory movement	**S**	
RML	right mediolateral	**s**	without
RMSF	Rocky Mountain spotted fever	**S-A**	sinoatrial node
RNA	ribonucleic acid	**S & A**	sugar and acetone
RND	radical neck dissection	**SA**	salicylic acid; sinoatrial; sperm analysis; surgeon's assistant
R/O	rule out		
ROA	right occipitis anterior	**SAAT**	serum aspartate aminotransferase
ROM	range of motion; rupture of membranes	**SAB**	spontaneous abortion
		SACH	solid ankle cushion heel
ROP	right occipitis posterior	**SACP**	serum acid phosphatase
ROPS	roll over protection structures	**SAFP**	serum alpha-fetoprotein
ROS	review of systems	**SALD**	serum aldolase
ROT	right occipitis transverse	**SAL**	sensorineural activity level; sterility assurance level; suction-assisted lipectomy
RP	relapsing polychondritis; retrograde pyelogram		
RPCF	Reiter protein complement fixation	**SALP**	salpingectomy; salpingography; serum alkaline phosphatase
RPF	renal plasma flow	**Salpx**	salpingectomy
RPG	retrograde pyelogram	**SAM**	self-administered medication program
rpm	revolutions per minute		
RPO	right posterior oblique	**SAS**	short arm splint; sleep apnea syndrome; social adjustment scale; subarachnoid space
RPR	rapid plasma reagin		
RQ	respiratory quotient		
R & R	rate and rhythm	**SB**	stillbirth
RR	recovery room; respiratory rate	**SBE**	subacute bacterial endocarditis
RSD	reflex sympathetic dystrophy	**SBO**	small bowel obstruction
RSHF	right-sided heart failure	**sc, SC**	subcutaneous
RSI	repetitive stress injuries	**SC**	spinal cord
RSR	regular sinus rhythm	**SCA**	sickle cell anemia
RSV	right subclavian vein	**SCC**	squamous cell carcinoma
rt	right; routine	**SCD**	sudden cardiac death
RT	radiation therapy; respiratory therapy	**SCI**	spinal cord injury
		schiz	schizophrenia
RTA	renal tubular acidosis	**SCID**	severe combined immune deficiency
rt lat	right lateral		
rtd	retarded	**SCPK**	serum creatine phosphokinase
RUL	right upper lobe	**SCT**	sickle cell trait
RU	roentgen unit; routine urinalysis	**SD**	septal defect; shoulder disarticulation; spontaneous delivery; sudden death

SDAT	senile dementia of Alzheimer's type
SDM	standard deviation of the mean
SDS	sudden death syndrome
sec	second
SED	sub-erythema dose
sed rate	sedimentation rate
seg	segmented neutrophils
SEM	scanning electron microscopy
semi	half
seq	sequela; sequestrum
SES	subcutaneous electric stimulation
sev	sever; severed
SF	scarlet fever; spinal fluid
SG	serum globulin; skin graft
SGA	small for gestational age
s gl	without correction; without glasses
SGGTP	serum gamma glutamyl transpeptidase
SGOT	serum glutamic oxaloacetic transaminase
SGPT	serum glutamic pyruvic transaminase
SH	serum hepatitis; sex hormone; social history
sh	shoulder
SI	saturation index
SICU	surgical intensive care unit
SIDS	sudden infant death syndrome
SIRS	systemic inflammatory response syndrome
SIS	saline infusion sonohysterography
SISI	short increment sensitivity index
SLAP	serum leucine aminopeptidase
SLE	St. Louis encephalitis; systemic lupus erythematosus
SLND	sentinel lymph node dissection
SLPS	serum lipase
SM	simple mastectomy
sm	small
SMA	sequential multiple analysis
SMAC	sequential multiple analysis computer
SMG	senile macular degeneration
SMR	submucous resection
SMRR	submucous resection and rhinoplasty
SNR	signal-to-noise ratio

SNS	sensory nervous system; sympathetic nervous system
SO	salpingo-oophorectomy
SOAP	symptoms, observations, assessments, plan; subjective, objective, assessment, plan
SOB	shortness of breath
SOM	serous otitis media
SONO	sonography
SOP	standard operating procedure
sos	if necessary
SPBI	serum protein-bound iodine
SPE	serum protein electrophoresis
spec	specimen
SPECT	single photon emission computed tomography
SPF	skin protective factor
sp gr	specific gravity
SPHI	serum phosphohexoisomerase
SPK	serum pyruvate kinase
SPP	suprapubic prostatectomy
SPR	scanned projection radiography
SQ	subcutaneous
SR	sedimentation rate; stimulus response; system review
Sr	strontium
SRS	smoker's respiratory syndrome
ss	half
SS	signs and symptoms; Sjögren's syndrome; soap solution
SSE	soap suds enema
SSU	sterile supply unit
ST	esotropia
staph	staphylococcus
stat	immediately
STD	sexually transmitted disease; skin test dose
STH	somatotropic hormone
STK	streptokinase
strep	streptococcus
STS	serologic test for syphilis
STSG	split thickness skin graft
subcu	subcutaneous
sub-Q	subcutaneous
SUI	stress urinary incontinence
supp	suppository
surg	surgical; surgery
SVC	superior vena cava

SVD	spontaneous vaginal delivery	**TKO**	to keep open
SVG	saphenous vein graft	**TKR**	total knee replacement
SVN	small volume nebulizer	**TLC**	tender loving care; total lung capacity
Sx	symptoms	**TLE**	temporal lobe epilepsy
Sz	seizure	**TM**	temporomandibular; tympanic membrane
T		**TMD**	temporomandibular disease; temporomandibular disorder
T	temperature	**TMJ**	temporomandibular joint
T1–T12	thoracic vertebrae	**TMs**	tympanic membranes
TA	therapeutic abortion	**Tn**	normal intraocular tension
T & A	tonsillectomy and adenoidectomy	**TND**	term normal delivery
tab	tablet	**TNF**	tumor necrosis factor
TAB	therapeutic abortion	**TNI**	total nodal irradiation
TACT	target air-enema computed tomography	**TNM**	tumor, nodes, metastases
TAF	tumor angiogenesis factor	**TO**	telephone order
TAH	total abdominal hysterectomy	**top**	topically
TAO	thromboangiitis obliterans	**TP**	testosterone propionate; total protein
TB	tuberculosis		
TBD	total body density	**TPA**	tissue plasminogen activator; *treponema pallidum* agglutination
TBF	total body fat		
TBG	thyroxine-binding globulin	**TPBF**	total pulmonary blood flow
TBI	thyroxine-binding index	**TPI**	*Treponema pallidum* immobilization
TBW	total body weight		
Tc	technetium	**TPN**	total parenteral nutrition
TCD	transcranial doppler	**TPR**	temperature, pulse, respiration
TCDB	turn, cough, deep breathe	**TPUR**	transperineal urethral resection
TCP	time care profile	**tr**	tincture
TD	total disability	**TR**	tuberculin residue
TDM	therapeutic drug monitoring	**trach**	tracheostomy
TDT	tone decay test	**TRBF**	total renal blood flow
TEE	transesophageal echocardiography	**TRH**	thyrotropin-releasing hormone
temp	temperature	**TS**	Tourette syndrome
TEN	toxic epidermal necrolysis	**TSD**	Tay-Sachs disease
TENS	transcutaneous electrical nerve stimulation	**TSE**	testicular self-examination
		TSH	thyroid-stimulating hormone
TES	treadmill exercise score	**TSP**	total serum protein
TF	tactile fremitus	**TSS**	toxic shock syndrome
TFS	thyroid function studies	**TST**	tuberculin skin test
TGA	transposition of great arteries	**TT**	thrombin time
THR	total hip replacement	**TTH**	thyrotropic hormone
TIA	transient ischemic attack	**TULIP**	transurethral ultrasound-guided laser-induced proctectomy
TIA-IR	transient ischemic attack incomplete recovery	**TUMT**	transurethral microwave therapy
TIBC	total iron-binding capacity	**TUR**	transurethral resection
TID, tid, t.i.d.	times interval difference; three times a day	**TURP**	transurethral resection of prostate; prostatectomy
tinct	tincture	**TV**	tidal volume; tricuspid valve

TVH	total vaginal hysterectomy
TW	tap water
TWE	tap water enema
Tx	traction; treatment

U

U	units
UA	urinalysis
UC	ulcerative colitis; urine culture; uterine contractions
UCD	usual childhood diseases
UCG	urinary chorionic gonadotropin; uterine chorionic gonadotropin
UCR	unconditioned reflex
UE	upper extremity
UFR	uroflowmeter; uroflowmetry
UG	upper gastrointestinal; urogenital
UGI	upper gastrointestinal
UK	unknown
UL	upper lobe
ULQ	upper left quadrant
umb	umbilicus
UN	urea nitrogen
ung	ointment
UOQ	upper outer quadrant
UP	uroporphyrin
UPP	urethral pressure profile
UR	upper respiratory
ur	urine
URD	upper respiratory disease
URI	upper respiratory infection
urol	urology
URQ	upper right quadrant
US	ultrasonic; ultrasonography
USP	United States Pharmacopeia
UTI	urinary tract infection
UV	ultraviolet
UVJ	ureterovesical junction

V

VA	vacuum aspiration; visual acuity
vag	vaginal
VB	viable birth
VBAC	vaginal birth after cesarean
VBP	ventricular premature beat
VC	acuity of color vision; vena cava; vital capacity

VCG	vectorcardiogram
VCUG	voiding cystourethrogram
VD	venereal disease
VDG	venereal disease, gonorrhea
VDH	valvular disease of heart
VDRL	Venereal Disease Research Laboratory
VDS	venereal disease, syphilis
VE	visual efficiency
VEP	visual evoked potential
VER	visual evoked response
VF	visual field; vocal fremitus
V fib	ventricular fibrillation
VG	ventricular gallop
VH	vaginal hysterectomy
VHD	valvular heart disease; ventricular heart disease
VI	volume index
vit cap	vital capacity
VLDL	very-low-density lipoprotein
VP	venipuncture; venous pressure
V & P	vagotomy and pyloroplasty
VPC	ventricular premature contraction
VPRC	volume of packed red cells
VS, vs	vital signs
VSD	ventricular septal defect
VTAs	vascular targeting agents
VZV	varicella-zoster virus (chickenpox)

W

W	water
WA	while awake
WB	weight-bearing; whole blood
WBC	white blood cell; white blood count
W/C, w/c	wheelchair
wd	wound
WD, w/d	well-developed
WDWN	well-developed, well-nourished
wf	white female
w/n	well nourished
WNL	within normal limits
w/o	without
WR, W.r.	Wassermann reaction
wt	weight
w/v	weight by volume

X

x	multiplied by; times
XDP	xeroderma pigmentosum
XM	cross-match
XR	x-ray
XT	exotropia
XU	excretory urogram

Y

y/o	year(s) old
YOB	year of birth
yr	year

Z

z	atomic number; no effect; zero

Appendix C
Glossary of Pathology and Procedures

A

abdominocentesis (ab-**dom**-ih-noh-sen-**TEE**-sis): Surgical puncture of the abdominal cavity to remove fluid for diagnostic purposes.

ablation (ab-**LAY**-shun): The removal or destruction of the function of a body part.

abortion (ah-**BOR**-shun): The interruption or termination of pregnancy before the fetus is viable.

abrasion (ah-**BRAY**-zhun): An injury in which superficial layers of skin are scraped or rubbed away; treatment involving scraping or rubbing away skin.

abruptio placentae (ab-**RUP**-shee-oh plah-**SEN**-tee): An abnormal condition in which the placenta separates from the uterine wall prematurely before the birth of the fetus.

abscess (**AB**-sess): A localized collection of purulent exudate (pus) within a circumscribed area.

accommodation (ah-**kom**-oh-**DAY**-shun): The process whereby the eyes make adjustments for seeing objects at various distances.

ACE inhibitors (angiotensin-converting enzyme inhibitors): Medications administered to treat hypertension and congestive heart failure.

acetone (**ASS**-eh-tohn): A substance with a sweet fruity odor that is found in small quantities in normal urine and in larger amounts in diabetic urine.

Achilles tendinitis (ten-dih-**NIGH**-tis): Inflammation of the Achilles tendon caused by excessive stress being placed on the tendon.

achlorhydria (**ah**-klor-**HIGH**-dree-ah): The absence of hydrochloric acid from gastric secretions.

acne vulgaris (**ACK**-nee vul-**GAY**-ris): A chronic inflammatory disease characterized by pustular eruptions of the skin in or near the sebaceous glands.

acquired immune deficiency syndrome: The advanced stage of HIV infection.

acromegaly (**ack**-roh-**MEG**-ah-lee): Enlargement of the extremities (hands and feet) caused by excessive secretion of the growth hormone *after* puberty.

acronym (**ACK**-roh-nim): A word formed from the initial letter or letters of the major parts of a compound term.

acrophobia (**ack**-roh-**FOH**-bee-ah): An excessive fear of being in high places.

actinic keratosis (ack-**TIN**-ick **kerr**-ah-**TOH**-sis): A precancerous skin lesion caused by excessive exposure to the sun.

acute nasopharyngitis (**nay**-zoh-**far**-in-**JIGH**-tis): Inflammation of the nose and throat; among the terms used to describe the common cold; also known as an upper respiratory infection.

acute respiratory distress syndrome: A type of lung failure resulting from many different disorders that cause pulmonary edema.

addiction: Compulsive, uncontrollable dependence on a substance, habit, or action to the degree that stopping causes severe emotional, mental, or physiologic reactions.

Addison's disease (**AD**-ih-sonz): A progressive disease in which the adrenal glands do not produce enough cortisol that if untreated can produce a life-threatening addisonian crisis.

adenectomy (**ad**-eh-**NECK**-toh-mee): Surgical removal of a gland.

adenitis (**ad**-eh-**NIGH**-tis): Inflammation of a gland.

adenocarcinoma (**ad**-eh-noh-**kar**-sih-**NOH**-mah): Any one of a large group of carcinomas derived from glandular tissue.

adenoidectomy (**ad**-eh-noid-**ECK**-toh-mee *or* **ad**-eh-noy-**DECK**-toh-mee): Surgical removal of the adenoids.

adenoma (**ad**-eh-**NOH**-mah): A benign tumor in which the cells form recognizable glandular structures.

adenoma, pituitary (**ad**-eh-**NOH**-mah): A benign tumor of the pituitary gland that causes excess hormone secretion. An ACTH-secreting tumor stimulates the excess production of cortisol that causes most cases of Cushing's syndrome.

adenoma, prolactin-producing: A benign tumor of the pituitary gland that causes it to produce too much prolactin; also known as a prolactinoma.

adenomalacia (**ad**-eh-noh-mah-**LAY**-shee-ah): Abnormal softening of a gland.

adenosclerosis (**ad**-eh-noh-skleh-**ROH**-sis): Abnormal hardening of a gland.

adenosis (**ad**-eh-**NOH**-sis): Any disease condition of a gland.

adhesion (ad-**HEE**-zhun): A band of fibrous tissue that holds structures together abnormally.

adrenalitis (ah-**dree**-nal-**EYE**-tis): Inflammation of the adrenal glands.

adrenitis (**ad**-reh-**NIGH**-tis): Inflammation of the adrenal glands.

adrenomegaly (ah-**dree**-noh-**MEG**-ah-lee): Enlargement of the adrenal glands.

adrenopathy (**ad**-ren-**OP**-ah-thee): Any disease of the adrenal glands.

aerophagia (**ay**-er-oh-**FAY**-jee-ah): The spasmodic swallowing of air followed by eructations.

agglutination testing (ah-**gloo**-tih-**NAY**-shun): Laboratory tests that involve the clumping together of cells or particles when mixed with incompatible serum. These tests are performed to determine the patient's blood type and to check compatibility of donor and recipient blood before a transfusion.

agoraphobia (**ag**-oh-rah-**FOH**-bee-ah): An overwhelming and irrational fear of leaving the familiar setting of home or venturing into the open.

albinism (**AL**-bih-niz-um): An inherited deficiency or absence of pigment in the skin, hair, and eyes due to an abnormality in production of melanin.

albuminuria (**al**-byou-mih-**NEW**-ree-ah): The presence of the serum protein albumin in the urine.

alcoholism (**AL**-koh-hol-izm): Chronic dependence on, or abuse of, alcohol with specific signs and symptoms of withdrawal.

aldosteronism (al-**DOSS**-teh-roh-**niz**-em *or* al-doh-**STER**-ohn-izm): An abnormality of electrolyte balance caused by excessive secretion of aldosterone.

allergen (**AL**-er-jen): An antigen capable of inducing an allergic response.

allergic rhinitis (rye-**NIGH**-tis): Commonly referred to as an **allergy,** is an allergic reaction to airborne allergens that causes an increased flow of mucus.

allergist (**AL**-er-jist): A specialist in diagnosing and treating conditions of allergic reactions and altered immunologic reactivity.

allergy: An overreaction by the body to a particular antigen; also known as hypersensitivity.

allogenic (**al**-oh-**JEN**-ick): Originating within another.

alopecia (**al**-oh-**PEE**-shee-ah): The partial or complete loss of hair; also known as baldness.

alopecia areata: A disease of unknown cause in which there are well-defined bald areas, usually on the scalp and face.

alopecia capitis totalis: A condition characterized by the loss of all the hair on the scalp.

alopecia universalis: The total loss of hair on all parts of the body.

Alzheimer's disease (**ALTZ**-high-merz): A group of disorders associated with degenerative changes in brain structure leading to characteristic symptoms including progressive memory loss, impaired cognition, and personality changes.

amblyopia (**am**-blee-**OH**-pee-ah): Dimness of vision or the partial loss of sight without detectable disease of the eye.

amebic dysentery (ah-**MEE**-bik **DIS**-en-ter-ee): An intestinal infection caused by *Entamoeba histolytica amoeba.*

amenorrhea (ah-**men**-oh-**REE**-ah *or* ay-**men**-oh-**REE**-ah): The absence of menstrual periods. This condition is normal only before puberty, during pregnancy, during breast-feeding, and after menopause.

ametropia (**am**-eh-**TROH**-pee-ah): An error of refraction in which only objects located a finite distance from the eye are focused on the retina.

amnesia (am-**NEE**-zee-ah): A disturbance in the memory marked by total or partial inability to recall past experiences.

amniocentesis (**am**-nee-oh-sen-**TEE**-sis): Surgical puncture to remove a specimen of amniotic fluid for diagnostic purposes

amobarbital (**am**-oh-**BAR**-bih-tal): A barbiturate used as a sedative and hypnotic.

amyotrophic lateral sclerosis (ah-**my**-oh-**TROH**-fick): A degenerative disease of the motor neurons in which patients become progressively weaker until they are completely paralyzed; also known as Lou Gehrig's disease.

analgesic (**an**-al-**JEE**-zick): A drug that relieves pain without affecting consciousness.

analgesic, narcotic: Medication, such as morphine and codeine, that is used to relieve severe pain but that may cause dependence or addiction.

analgesic, nonnarcotic: Medication, such as aspirin, that is used to relieve mild to moderate pain.

anaphylaxis (**an**-ah-fih-**LACK**-sis): A severe response to a foreign substance such as a drug, food, insect venom, or chemical.

anaplasia (**an**-ah-**PLAY**-zee-ah): Change in the structure of cells and in their orientation to each other.

anastomosis (ah-**nas**-toh-**MOH**-sis): A surgical connection between two hollow or tubular structures.

anemia (ah-**NEE**-mee-ah): A disorder characterized by lower than normal levels of red blood cells in the blood.

anemia, aplastic (ay-**PLAS**-tick ah-**NEE**-mee-ah): A marked absence of *all* formed blood elements.

anemia, Cooley's: A group of genetic disorders characterized by short-lived red blood cells lacking the normal ability to produce hemoglobin; also known as thalassemia.

anemia, hemolytic: A condition in which red blood cells are destroyed faster than the bone marrow can replace them.

anemia, megaloblastic (**MEG**-ah-loh-**blas**-tick ah-**NEE**-mee-ah): A form of anemia in which the bone marrow produces large abnormal red blood cells with a reduced capacity to carry oxygen.

anemia, pernicious: An autoimmune disorder resulting in the inability of the body to absorb vitamin B_{12} normally.

anemia, sickle cell: A genetic disorder that causes abnormal hemoglobin that results in the red blood cells' assuming an abnormal sickle shape.

anesthesia (**an**-es-**THEE**-zee-ah): The absence of normal sensation, especially sensitivity to pain.

anesthesia, epidural (**ep**-ih-**DOO**-ral): Regional anesthesia produced by injecting a local anesthetic into the epidural space of the lumbar or sacral region of the spine.

anesthesia, general: The total loss of body sensation and consciousness as induced by various anesthetic agents, given primarily by inhalation or intravenous injection.

anesthesia, local: The loss of sensation in a limited area produced by injecting an anesthetic solution near that area.

anesthesia, regional: The temporary interruption of nerve conduction produced by injecting an anesthetic solution near the nerves to be blocked.

anesthesia, spinal: Anesthesia produced by injecting an anesthetic into the subarachnoid space, which is located below the arachnoid membrane and above the pia mater that surrounds the spinal cord.

anesthesia, topical: An anesthetic that numbs only the tissue surface and is applied as a liquid, ointment, or spray.

anesthesiologist (**an**-es-**thee**-zee-**OL**-oh-jist): A physician who specializes in administering anesthetic agents before and during surgery.

anesthetic (**an**-es-**THET**-ick): The medication used to induce anesthesia. The anesthetic may be topical, local, regional, or general.

anesthetist (ah-**NES**-theh-tist): A specialist, other than a physician, trained in administering anesthesia.

aneurysm (**AN**-you-rizm): A localized weak spot or balloon-like enlargement of the wall of an artery.

aneurysmectomy (**an**-you-riz-**MECK**-toh-mee): Surgical removal of an aneurysm.

aneurysmorrhaphy (**an**-you-riz-**MOR**-ah-fee): To suture an aneurysm.

angiectomy (**an**-jee-**ECK**-toh-mee): Surgical removal of a blood vessel.

angiitis (**an**-je-**EYE**-tis): Inflammation of a blood or lymph vessel; also known as vasculitis.

angina pectoris (an-**JIGH**-nah *or* **AN**-jih-nuh **PECK**-toh-riss): Severe episodes of spasmodic choking or suffocating chest pain caused by an insufficient supply of oxygen to the heart muscle.

angiocardiography (**an**-jee-oh-**kar**-dee-**OG**-rah-fee): A radiographic study using x-rays and contrast medium to visualize the dimensions of the heart and large blood vessels.

angiogenesis (**an**-jee-oh-**JEN**-eh-sis): The ability of a tumor to support its growth by creating its own blood supply.

angiogram (**AN**-jee-oh-**gram**): The record produced by a radiographic study of blood vessels.

angiography (**an**-jee-**OG**-rah-fee): A radiographic study of blood vessels after the injection of a contrast medium.

angiomegaly (**an**-jee-oh-**MEG**-ah-lee): Abnormal enlargement of blood vessels.

angionecrosis (**an**-jee-oh-neh-**KROH**-sis): Death of the walls of blood vessels.

angiorrhaphy (**an**-jee-**OR**-ah-fee): A suture repair of any vessel, especially of a blood vessel.

angiosclerosis (**an**-jee-oh-skleh-**ROH**-sis): Abnormal hardening of the walls of blood vessels.

angiospasm (**AN**-jee-oh-**spazm**): Spasmodic contraction of the blood vessels.

angiostenosis (**an**-jee-oh-steh-**NOH**-sis): Abnormal narrowing of a blood vessel.

anhidrosis (**an**-high-**DROH**-sis): The condition of lacking or being without sweat.

anisocoria (**an**-ih-so-**KOH**-ree-ah): A condition in which the pupils are unequal in size.

ankylosing spondylitis (**ang**-kih-**LOH**-sing **spon**-dih-**LYE**-tis): Rheumatoid arthritis characterized by progressive stiffening of the spine caused by fusion of the vertebral bodies.

ankylosis (**ang**-kih-**LOH**-sis): Loss or absence of mobility in a joint due to disease, an injury, or a surgical procedure.

anomaly (ah-**NOM**-ah-lee): A deviation from what is regarded as normal.

anonychia (**an**-oh-**NICK**-ee-ah): Pertaining to the absence of fingernails or toenails.

anoplasty (**AY**-noh-**plas**-tee): Surgical repair of the anus.

anorchism (an-**OR**-kizm): The congenital absence of one or both testicles.

anorexia (**an**-oh-**RECK**-see-ah): The lack or loss of appetite for food.

anorexia nervosa: An eating disorder characterized by a refusal to maintain a minimally normal body weight and an intense fear of gaining weight.

anoscopy (ah-**NOS**-koh-pee): Visual examination of the anal canal and lower rectum using a short speculum called an anoscope.

anovulation (**an**-ov-you-**LAY**-shun): The failure to ovulate although menstruation may continue to occur.

anoxia (ah-**NOCK**-see-ah): The absence or almost complete absence of oxygen from inspired gases, arterial blood, or tissues.

anteflexion (**an**-tee-**FLECK**-shun): The normal position of the uterus.

anteversion (**an**-tee-**VER**-zhun): Abnormal tipping, tilting, or turning forward of the entire uterus, including the cervix.

anthracosis (**an**-thrah-**KOH**-sis): A form of pneumoconiosis caused by coal dust in the lungs; also known as black lung disease.

anti-angiogenesis: Treatment that cuts off the blood supply to a tumor.

antianxiety drugs: Medications administered to suppress anxiety and relax muscles; also known as tranquilizers.

antiarrhythmic (**an**-tih-ah-**RITH**-mick): Medication administered to control irregularities of the heartbeat.

antibiotic: A medication administered to combat bacterial infections.

anticoagulant (**an**-tih-koh-**AG**-you-lant): Medication administered to slow blood clotting and to prevent new clots from forming; also known as a thrombolytic.

anticonvulsant (**an**-tih-kon-**VUL**-sant): Medication administered to prevent seizures and convulsions.

antidepressant: Medication administered to prevent or relieve depression.

antiemetic (**an**-tih-ee-**MET**-ick): Medication administered to prevent or relieve nausea and vomiting.

antihypertensive (**an**-tih-**high**-per-**TEN**-siv): Medication administered to lower high blood pressure.

antineoplastic (**an**-tih-nee-oh-**PLAS**-tick): Medication that blocks the growth of neoplasms and is used to treat cancer.

antipsychotic (**an**-tih-sigh-**KOT**-ick): Medication administered to treat symptoms of severe psychiatric disorders.

antipyretic (**an**-tih-pye-**RET**-ick): Medication to reduce or relieve fever.

antisocial personality disorder: A pattern of disregard for, and violation of, the rights of others that brings the individual into continuous conflict with society.

antispasmodic: Medication that acts to control spasmodic activity of the smooth muscles such as those of the intestine.

antiviral (**an**-tih-**VYE**-ral); Medication used to treat viral infections or to provide temporary immunity.

anuresis (**an**-you-**REE**-sis): The complete suppression of urine formation by the kidneys; also known as anuria.

anuria (ah-**NEW**-ree-ah): See anuresis.

anxiety state: A feeling of apprehension, tension, or uneasiness that stems from the anticipation of danger, the source of which is largely unknown or unrecognized.

Apgar score: A system to evaluate a newborn infant's physical status.

aphakia (ah-**FAY**-kee-ah): The absence of the lens of an eye after cataract extraction.

aphasia (ah-**FAY**-zee-ah): A condition, often due to brain damage associated with a stroke, in which there is the loss of the ability to speak, write, or comprehend speech or the spoken word.

aphonia (ah-**FOH**-nee-ah): Loss of the ability to produce normal speech sounds.

aphthous ulcers (**AF**-thus): Recurrent blister-like sores that break and form lesions on the soft tissues lining the mouth; also known as canker sores.

aplasia (ah-**PLAY**-zee-ah): Lack of development of an organ or tissue.

apnea (**AP**-nee-ah *or* ap-**NEE**-ah): The absence of spontaneous respiration.

appendectomy (**ap**-en-**DECK**-toh-mee): The surgical removal of the appendix.

appendicitis (ah-**pen**-dih-**SIGH**-tis): Inflammation of the appendix.

arrhythmia, cardiac (ah-**RITH**-mee-ah): An irregularity or the loss of normal rhythm of the heartbeat; also known as dysrhythmia.

arteriectomy (**ar**-teh-ree-**ECK**-toh-mee): Surgical removal of part of an artery.

arteriogram (ar-**TEER**-ee-oh-gram): The record produced by arteriography.

arteriography (**ar**-tee-ree-**OG**-rah-fee): The process of recording a picture of an artery or arteries.

arteriomalacia (ar-**tee**-ree-oh-mah-**LAY**-shee-ah): Abnormal softening of the walls of an artery or arteries.

arterionecrosis (ar-**tee**-ree-oh-neh-**KROH**-sis): Tissue death of an artery or arteries.

arteriosclerosis (ar-**tee**-ree-oh-skleh-**ROH**-sis): Abnormal hardening of the walls of an artery or arteries.

arteriostenosis (ar-**tee**-ree-oh-steh-**NOH**-sis): Abnormal narrowing of an artery or arteries.

arteritis (**ar**-teh-**RYE**-tis): Inflammation of an artery or arteries.

arthralgia (ar-**THRAL**-jee-ah): Pain in a joint or joints.

arthrectomy (ar-**THRECK**-toh-mee): The surgical removal of a joint.

arthritis (ar-**THRIGH**-tis): Inflammation of one or more joints.

arthritis, gouty: Arthritis associated with the formation of uric acid crystals in the joint as the result of hyperuricemia. (Hyperuricemia means an abnormal level of uric acid in the blood.)

arthritis, juvenile rheumatoid: Arthritis that affects children with pain and swelling in the joints, skin rash, fever, slowed growth, and fatigue.

arthritis, rheumatoid: Autoimmune disorder in which the synovial membranes are inflamed and thicken.

arthrocentesis (**ar**-throh-sen-**TEE**-sis): Surgical puncture of the joint space to remove synovial fluid for analysis.

arthrodesis (**ar**-throh-**DEE**-sis): Surgical stiffening of a joint or joining of spinal vertebrae; also known as fusion or surgical ankylosis.

arthrolysis (ar-**THROL**-ih-sis): Surgical loosening of an ankylosed joint.

arthroplasty (**AR**-throh-**plas**-tee): Surgical repair of a joint; also surgical replacement of a joint.

arthrosclerosis (**ar**-throh-skleh-**ROH**-sis): Stiffness of the joints, especially in the elderly.

arthroscopy (ar-**THROS**-koh-pee): Visual examination and treatment of the internal structure of a joint using an arthroscope.

arthrotomy (ar-**THROT**-oh-mee): A surgical incision into a joint.

asbestosis (**ass**-beh-**STOH**-sis): A form of pneumoconiosis caused by asbestos particles found in the lungs of workers from the ship-building and construction trades.

asphyxia (ass-**FICK**-see-ah): Pathologic changes caused by a lack of oxygen in air that is inhaled.

asphyxiation (ass-**fick**-see-**AY**-shun): Any interruption of breathing that results in the loss of consciousness or death; also known as suffocation.

aspiration (ass-pih-**RAY**-shun): Inhaling or drawing a foreign substance into the upper respiratory tract; withdrawal by suction of fluids or gases from a body cavity.

assay (**ASS**-ay): To determine the amount of a particular substance in a mixture.

assessment: Evaluation or appraisal of a condition.

asthma (**AZ**-mah): A chronic allergic disorder characterized by episodes of severe breathing difficulty, coughing, and wheezing.

astigmatism (ah-**STIG**-mah-tizm): A condition in which the eye does not focus properly because of unequal curvatures of the cornea.

ataxia (ah-**TACK**-see-ah): Inability to coordinate the muscles in the execution of voluntary movement.

atelectasis (at-ee-**LEK**-tah-sis): A condition in which the lung fails to expand because air cannot pass beyond the bronchioles; also known as a collapsed lung.

atherectomy (ath-er-**ECK**-toh-mee): Surgical removal of plaque from the interior lining of an artery.

atheroma (ath-er-**OH**-mah): Fatty deposit within the wall of an artery.

atherosclerosis (ath-er-oh-skleh-**ROH**-sis): Hardening and narrowing of the arteries due to a buildup of cholesterol plaques.

atonic (ah-**TON**-ick): Lack of normal muscle tone.

atrophy (**AT**-roh-fee): Weakness and wasting away.

atropine (**AT**-roh-peen): Antispasmodic that may be administered preoperatively to relax smooth muscles.

attention deficit disorder: A condition in which a child has a short attention span and impulsiveness that are inappropriate for the child's developmental age.

attention deficit/hyperactivity disorder: A pattern of inattention and hyperactivity that are inappropriate for the child's developmental age.

audiologist (aw-dee-**OL**-oh-jist): A specialist in the measurement of hearing function and the rehabilitation of persons with hearing impairments.

audiometer (aw-dee-**OM**-eh-ter): An electronic device that produces acoustic stimuli of a known frequency and intensity.

auscultation (aws-kul-**TAY**-shun): Listening through a stethoscope for sounds within the body to determine the condition of the lungs, pleura, heart, and abdomen.

autism (**AW**-tizm): See autistic disorder.

autistic disorder (aw-**TISS**-tick): A disorder in which a young child cannot develop normal social relationships, behaves in compulsive and ritualistic ways, and frequently has poor communication skills; also known as an autism.

autoimmune disorder (aw-toh-ih-**MYOUN**): A disorder of the immune system in which the body attacks itself.

autologous (aw-**TOL**-uh-guss): Originating within an individual.

autopsy (**AW**-top-see): A postmortem (after death) examination.

azoospermia (ay-**zoh**-oh **SPER**-mee-ah): The absence of sperm in the semen.

B

bacilli (bah-**SILL**-eye): Rod-shaped spore-forming bacteria.

bacteria (back-**TEER**-ree-ah): A group of one-celled microscopic organisms, some of which cause disease in humans.

bactericide (back-**TEER**-ih-sighd): A substance that causes the death of bacteria.

bacteriostatic (bac-**tee**-ree-oh-**STAT**-ick): An agent that inhibits, slows, or retards the growth of bacteria.

bacteriuria (back-**tee**-ree-**YOU**-ree-ah): The presence of bacteria in the urine.

balanitis (**bal**-ah-**NIGH**-tis): Inflammation of the glans penis, usually associated with phimosis.

balloon angioplasty: A procedure in which a small balloon on the end of a catheter is used to open a partially blocked coronary artery; also known as percutaneous transluminal coronary angioplasty.

barbiturate (bar-**BIT**-you-rayt): A class of drugs whose major action is a calming or depressed effect on the central nervous system.

barium: A radiopaque contrast medium used primarily to visualize the digestive system.

Becker's muscular dystrophy (**BECK**-urz): A form of muscular dystrophy that is less severe than Duchenne's muscular distrophy and does not appear until early adolescence or adulthood.

Bell's palsy: Paralysis of the facial nerve (seventh cranial) that causes drooping only on the affected side of the face.

benign: Not recurring, nonmalignant, and with a favorable chance for recovery.

benign prostatic hypertrophy: An abnormal enlargement of the prostate gland.

beta-blockers: Medications administered to slow the heartbeat.

bilateral hysterosalpingo-oophorectomy (**hiss**-ter-oh-sal-**ping**-goh-oh-**ahf**-oh-**RECK**-toh-mee): Surgical removal of the uterus and cervix, plus both ovaries and both fallopian tubes.

bilateral salpingo-oophorectomy (sal-**ping**-goh-oh-**ahf**-oh-**RECK**-toh-mee): Surgical removal of both fallopian tubes and both ovaries.

binaural (bye-**NAW**-rul *or* bin-**AW**-rahl): Involving both ears.

biopsy (**BYE**-op-see): The removal of a small piece of living tissue for examination to confirm or establish a diagnosis.

biopsy, excisional: The removal of an entire tumor or lesion plus a margin of surrounding healthy tissue.

biopsy, incisional: The removal of a piece, but not all, of a tumor or lesion.

biopsy, needle: The use of a hollow needle to remove a core of tissue for examination.

bipolar disorder: A clinical course characterized by the occurrence of manic episodes alternating with depressive episodes; also known as a manic-depressive episode.

birthmark: See hemangioma and port-wine stain.

blastoma (blas-**TOH**-mah): A neoplasm composed of immature undifferentiated cells.

blepharedema (**blef**-ahr-eh-**DEE**-mah): Swelling of the eyelid.

blepharitis (**blef**-ah-**RYE**-tis): Inflammation of the eyelid.

blepharoplasty (**BLEF**-ah-roh-**plas**-tee): Surgical reduction of the upper and lower eyelids; also known as a lid lift.

blepharoptosis (**blef**-ah-roh-**TOH**-sis *or* **blef**-ah-rop-**TOH**-sis): Drooping of the upper eyelid.

blindness: The inability to see.

blood urea nitrogen (you-**REE**-ah): A laboratory test to determine the amount of urea present in the blood.

bone density testing: Radiographic tests to determine bone density.

bone marrow transplant: A treatment for cancers such as leukemia and lymphomas that affect bone marrow.

botulism (**BOT**-you-lizm): Food poisoning that is characterized by paralysis and is often fatal, caused by *Clostridium botulinum*.

brachytherapy (**brack**-ee-**THER**-ah-pee): Radioactive materials in contact with or implanted into the tissues to be treated.

bradycardia (**brad**-ee-**KAR**-dee-ah): An abnormally slow heartbeat.

bradykinesia (**brad**-ee-kih-**NEE**-zee-ah *or* **brad**-ee-kih-**NEE**-zhuh): Extreme slowness in movement.

bradypnea (**brad**-ihp-**NEE**-ah *or* **brad**-ee-**NEE**-ah): An abnormally slow rate of respiration, usually fewer than 10 breaths per minute.

brain tumor: An abnormal growth within the brain that may be either benign or malignant.

breast augmentation: Mammoplasty to increase breast size.

breast self-examination: An important self-care procedure for the early detection of breast cancer.

breech presentation: An abnormal birth position in which the buttocks or feet of the fetus are presented first.

bronchiectasis (**brong**-kee-**ECK**-tah-sis): Chronic dilation of bronchi or bronchioles resulting from an earlier lung infection that was not cured.

bronchitis (brong-**KYE**-tis): Inflammation of the bronchial walls.

bronchoconstrictor (**brong**-koh-kon-**STRICK**-tor): Medication that narrows the opening of the passages into the lungs.

bronchodilator (**brong**-koh-dye-**LAY**-tor): Medication that expands the opening of the passages into the lungs.

bronchoplasty (**BRONG**-koh-**plas**-tee): Surgical repair of a bronchial defect.

bronchoplegia (**brong**-koh-**PLEE**-jee-ah): Paralysis of the walls of the bronchi.

bronchopneumonia (**brong**-koh-new-**MOH**-nee-ah): A form of pneumonia that begins in the bronchioles.

bronchorrhagia (**brong**-koh-**RAY**-jee-ah): Bleeding from the bronchi.

bronchorrhea (**brong**-koh-**REE**-ah): An excessive discharge of mucus from the bronchi.

bronchoscopy (brong-**KOS**-koh-pee): Visual examination of the bronchi using a bronchoscope.

bruit (**BREW**-ee *or* **BROOT**): An abnormal sound or murmur heard in auscultation.

bruxism (**BRUCK**-sizm): Involuntary grinding or clenching of the teeth that usually occurs during sleep and is associated with tension or stress.

bulimia (byou-**LIM**-ee-ah *or* boo-**LEE**-mee-ah): An eating disorder characterized by episodes of binge eating followed by self-induced vomiting or misuse of laxatives; also known as bulimia nervosa.

bulla (**BULL**-ah): A blister that is *more than* 0.5 cm in diameter.

burn: An injury to body tissues caused by heat, flame, electricity, sun, chemicals, or radiation.

burn, first-degree: A burn that causes no blisters and only superficial damage to the epidermis; also known as a superficial burn.

burn, second-degree: A burn that causes blisters and superficial damage to the epidermis; also known as a partial-thickness burn.

burn, third-degree: A burn that damages the epidermis, dermis, and subcutaneous layers; also known as a full-thickness burn.

bursectomy (ber-**SECK**-toh-mee): Surgical removal of a bursa.

bursitis (ber-**SIGH**-tis): Inflammation of a bursa.

byssinosis (**biss**-ih-**NOH**-sis): A form of pneumoconiosis caused by cotton, flax, or hemp dust in the lungs; also known as brown lung disease.

C

calcium channel blockers: Medications administered to treat hypertension, angina, and arrhythmia.

calciuria (**kal**-sih-**YOU**-ree-ah): The presence of calcium in the urine.

callus (**KAL**-us): A thickening of part of the skin on the hands or feet caused by repeated rubbing; the bulging deposit that forms around the area of the break in a fractured bone.

capillary puncture: The technique used to draw a small amount of blood for testing; also known as a finger stick.

carbuncle (KAR-bung-kul): A cluster of furuncles that result in extensive sloughing of skin and scar formation.

carcinoma (kar-sih-**NOH**-mah): A malignant tumor that occurs in epithelial tissue.

carcinoma, basal cell: A malignant tumor of the basal cell layer of the epidermis.

carcinoma in situ: A malignant tumor in its original position that has not yet disturbed or invaded the surrounding tissues.

cardiac catheterization (KAR-dee-ack **kath**-eh-ter-eye-**ZAY**-shun): Placement of a catheter through a vein or artery and into the heart.

cardiocentesis (kar-dee-oh-sen-**TEE**-sis): A puncture of a chamber of the heart to remove fluid for diagnosis or therapy.

cardiologist (kar-dee-**OL**-oh-jist): A specialist in diagnosing and treating abnormalities, diseases, and disorders of the heart.

cardiomegaly (kar-dee-oh-**MEG**-ah-lee): Abnormal enlargement of the heart.

cardioplegia (kar-dee-oh-**PLEE**-jee-ah): Paralysis of the muscles of the heart.

cardiorrhaphy (kar-dee-**OR**-ah-fee): To suture the wall of the heart.

cardiorrhexis (kar-dee-oh-**RECK**-sis): Rupture of the heart.

cardiotomy (kar-dee-**OT**-oh-mee): A surgical incision into the heart.

cardioversion (kar-dee-oh-**VER**-zhun): The use of electrical shock to restore the heart's normal rhythm; also known as defibrillation.

carditis (kar-**DYE**-tis): Inflammation of the heart.

carpal tunnel syndrome (KAR-pul): Inflammation of the tendons passing through the carpal tunnel of the wrist.

castration (kas-**TRAY**-shun): Surgical removal or destruction of both testicles.

cataract (KAT-ah-rakt): Loss of transparency of the lens of the eye.

catatonic (kat-ah-**TON**-ick): Behavior marked by a lack of responsiveness, stupor, and a tendency to remain in a fixed posture.

catheterization (kath-eh-ter-eye-**ZAY**-shun): Insertion of a sterile catheter through the urethra and into the urinary bladder.

causalgia (kaw-**ZAL**-jee-ah): Intense burning pain after an injury to a sensory nerve.

cauterization (kaw-ter-eye-**ZAY**-zhun): The destruction of tissue by burning for therapeutic purposes.

cellulitis (sell-you-**LYE**-tis): A diffuse infection of connective tissue with severe inflammation within the layers of the skin.

centesis (sen-**TEE**-sis): A surgical puncture to remove fluid for diagnostic purposes or to remove excess fluid.

cephalalgia (sef-ah-**LAL**-jee-ah): Pain in the head; also known as a headache or cephalodynia.

cephalodynia: See cephalalgia.

cerebral palsy (SER-eh-bral or seh-**REE**-bral **PAWL**-zee): A condition caused by a brain injury that occurs during pregnancy, at birth, or soon after birth that is characterized by poor muscle control and other neurologic deficiencies.

cerebrovascular accident (ser-eh-broh-**VAS**-kyou-lar): Damage to the brain when the blood flow to the brain is disrupted because a blood vessel supplying it is blocked; also known as a stroke.

cervical radiculopathy (rah-**dick**-you-**LOP**-ah-thee): Nerve pain caused by pressure on the spinal nerve roots in the neck region.

cervicectomy (ser-vih-**SECK**-toh-mee): Surgical removal of the cervix.

cervicitis (ser-vih-**SIGH**-tis): Inflammation of the cervix.

cesarean section (seh-**ZEHR**-ee-un **SECK**-shun): The delivery of the child through an incision in the maternal abdominal and uterine wall; also known as a cesarean delivery or a C-section.

chalazion (kah-**LAY**-zee-on): A localized swelling of the eyelid resulting from obstruction of one of the oil-producing glands of the eyelid.

chemabrasion (keem-ah-**BRAY**-shun): The use of chemicals to remove the outer layers of skin to treat acne scaring, fine wrinkling, and general keratoses; also known as a chemical peel.

chemotherapy: The use of chemical agents and drugs to destroy malignant cells and tissues.

Cheyne-Stokes respiration (CHAYN-STOHKS): A pattern of alternating periods of hyperpnea (rapid breathing), hypopnea (slow breathing), and apnea (the absence of breathing).

chickenpox: An acute highly contagious viral disease caused by the herpes virus *Varicella zoster.*

chiropractor (KYE-roh-**prack**-tor): A specialist in manipulative treatment of disorders originating from misalignment of the spine.

chlamydia (klah-**MID**-ee-ah): A highly contagious sexually transmitted disease caused by the bacterium *Chlamydia trachomatis.*

chloasma (kloh-**AZ**-mah): A pigmentation disorder characterized by brownish spots on the face; also known as melasma or the mask of pregnancy.

cholecystalgia (koh-lee-sis-**TAL**-jee-ah): Pain in the gallbladder.

cholecystectomy (koh-lee-sis-**TECK**-toh-mee): Surgical removal of the gallbladder.

cholecystitis (koh-lee-sis-**TYE**-tis): Inflammation of the gallbladder.

choledocholithotomy (koh-**led**-oh-koh-lih-**THOT**-oh-mee): An incision in the common bile duct for the removal of gallstones.

cholelithiasis (**koh**-lee-lih-**THIGH**-ah-sis): The presence of gallstones in the gallbladder or bile ducts.

cholera (**KOL**-er-ah): An intestinal infection caused by the bacterium *Vibrio cholerae.*

cholesterol (koh-**LES**-ter-ol): Lipids that travel in the blood in packages called lipoproteins.

chondritis (kon-**DRY**-tis): Inflammation of cartilage.

chondroma (kon-**DROH**-mah): Benign tumor derived from cartilage cells.

chondromalacia (**kon**-droh-mah-**LAY**-shee-ah): Abnormal softening of the cartilage.

chondropathy (kon-**DROP**-ah-thee): A disease of the cartilage.

chondroplasty (**KON**-droh-**plas**-tee): Surgical repair of cartilage.

chorionic villus sampling: A diagnostic procedure using chorionic cells from the fetus to test for genetic abnormalities in the developing child.

chronic obstructive pulmonary disease: A general term used to describe a group of respiratory conditions characterized by chronic airflow limitations.

cicatrix (sick-**AY**-tricks): A "normal" scar resulting from the healing of a wound.

cineradiography (**sin**-eh-**ray**-dee-**OG**-rah-fee): The recording of images as they appear in motion on a fluorescent screen.

circumcision (**ser**-kum-**SIZH**-un): Surgical removal of the foreskin of the penis.

circumscribed (**SER**-kum-skrybed): Contained within a limited area.

cirrhosis (sih-**ROH**-sis): A progressive degenerative disease of the liver characterized by disturbance of structure and function of the liver.

claustrophobia (**klaws**-troh-**FOH**-bee-ah): An abnormal fear of being in narrow or enclosed spaces.

cleft lip: A congenital defect resulting in a deep fissure of the lip running upward to the nose; also known as a hare lip.

cleft palate: A congenital fissure of the palate that involves the upper lip, hard palate, and/or soft palate.

clubbing: Abnormal curving and shine on the nails that are often accompanied by enlargement of the fingertips. This condition can be hereditary or caused by changes associated with oxygen deficiencies related to coronary or pulmonary disease.

cognition (kog-**NISH**-un): The mental activities associated with thinking, learning, and memory.

colectomy (koh-**LECK**-toh-mee): Surgical removal of all or part of the colon.

colitis (koh-**LYE**-tis): Inflammation of the colon.

colonoscopy (**koh**-lun-**OSS**-koh-pee): Visual examination of the inner surface of the colon, from the rectum to the cecum.

colostomy (koh-**LAHS**-toh-mee): Surgical creation of an opening between the colon and the body surface.

colostrum (kuh-**LOS**-trum): The fluid secreted by the breasts during the first days postpartum.

colotomy (koh-**LOT**-oh-mee): A surgical incision into the colon.

colpitis (kol-**PYE**-tis): Inflammation of the lining of the vagina; also known as vaginitis.

colpopexy (**KOL**-poh-**peck**-see): Surgical fixation of the vagina to a surrounding structure.

colporrhaphy (kol-**POR**-ah-fee): Suturing of the vagina.

colporrhexis (**kol**-poh-**RECK**-sis): Laceration of the vagina.

colposcopy (kol-**POS**-koh-pee): The direct visual examination of the tissues of the cervix and vagina using a colposcope.

coma (**KOH**-mah): A profound state of unconsciousness marked by the absence of spontaneous eye movements, no response to painful stimuli, and no vocalization.

comatose (**KOH**-mah-tohs): The condition of being in a coma.

comedo (**KOM**-eh-doh): A lesion formed by the buildup of sebum and keratin in a hair follicle.

communicable (kuh-**MEW**-nih-kuh-bul): Any disease transmitted from one person to another by either direct or indirect contact.

complete blood cell count: A series of tests performed as a group to evaluate several blood conditions.

compliance: The patient's consistency and accuracy in following the regimen prescribed by a physician or other healthcare professional.

compulsions: Repetitive behaviors, the goal of which is to prevent or reduce anxiety or stress.

computed tomography (toh-**MOG**-rah-fee): An imaging technique that uses a thin, fan-shaped x-ray beam that rotates around the patient to produce multiple cross-sectional views of the body.

concussion (kon-**KUSH**-un): A violent shaking up or jarring of the brain

congenital disorder (kon-**JEN**-ih-tahl): An abnormal condition that exists at the time of birth and may be caused by a developmental disorder before birth, prenatal influences, premature birth, or injuries during birth.

congestive heart failure: A syndrome in which the heart is unable to pump enough blood to meet the body's needs for oxygen and nutrients.

conization (**kon**-ih-**ZAY**-shun *or* **koh**-nih-**ZAY**-shun): Surgical removal of a cone-shaped section of tissue from the cervix; also known as a cone biopsy.

conjunctivitis (kon-**junk**-tih-**VYE**-tis): Inflammation of the conjunctiva; also known as pinkeye.

conjunctivoplasty (**kon**-junk-**TYE**-voh-**plas**-tee): Surgical repair of the conjunctiva.

conscious: In a state of being awake, aware, and responding appropriately.

constipation: A decrease in frequency in the passage of stools, or difficulty in passing hard, dry stools.

contraceptive: A measure taken or device used to lessen the likelihood of conception and pregnancy.

contracture (kon-**TRACK**-chur): Abnormal shortening of muscle tissues, making the muscle resistant to stretching.

contraindication: A factor in the patient's condition that makes the use of a drug dangerous or ill advised.

contrast medium: A substance used in radiography to make visible structures that are otherwise hard to see.

contrast medium, radiolucent: A substance such as air that *does* allow x-rays to pass through and appears black or dark gray on the resulting film.

contrast medium, radiopaque: A substance that *does not* allow x-rays to pass through and appears white or light gray on the resulting film.

contusion (kon-**TOO**-zhun): An injury that does not break the skin and is characterized by swelling, discoloration, and pain.

contusion, cerebral: Bruising of brain tissue as a result of a head injury.

convergence (kon-**VER**-jens): The simultaneous inward movement of both eyes in an effort to maintain single binocular vision as an object comes nearer.

conversion disorder: A change in function, such as the paralysis of an arm, that suggests a physical disorder but has no physical cause.

convulsion: A sudden, violent, involuntary contraction of a group of muscles caused by a disturbance in brain function; also known as a seizure.

convulsion, clonic: A state marked by alternate contraction and relaxation of muscles resulting in jerking movements of the face, trunk, or extremities.

convulsion, tonic: A state of continuous muscular contraction that results in rigidity and violent spasms.

corneal abrasion: An injury, such as a scratch or irritation, to the outer layers of the cornea.

corneal transplant: The replacement of a scarred or diseased cornea with clear corneal tissue from a donor; also known as keratoplasty.

corneal ulcer: Pitting of the cornea caused by an infection or injury.

coronary artery bypass graft: A surgical procedure to replace a blocked coronary artery with a piece of vein from the leg; also known as bypass surgery.

coronary artery disease: Atherosclerosis of the coronary arteries that may cause angina pectoris, myocardial infarction, and sudden death.

coronary thrombosis (KOR-uh-**nerr**-ee throm-**BOH**-sis): Damage to the heart caused by a thrombus blocking a coronary artery.

corticosteroid (KOR-tih-koh-**STER**-oid): A hormone-like preparation used primarily as an anti-inflammatory and as an immunosuppressant.

cortisone (KOR-tih-sohn): The synthetic equivalent of corticosteroids produced by the body that is administered to suppress inflammation and as an immunosuppressant to prevent organ rejection by the body.

costectomy (kos-**TECK**-toh-mee): The surgical removal of a rib or ribs.

costotomy (kos-**TOT**-oh-mee): Surgical incision or division of a rib or ribs.

craniectomy (**kray**-nee-**EK**-toh-mee): Surgical removal of a portion of the skull.

craniocele (**KRAY**-nee-oh-**seel**): A congenital gap in the skull with herniation of brain substance; also known as an encephalocele.

craniomalacia (**kray**-nee-oh-mah-**LAY**-shee-ah): Abnormal softening of the skull.

cranioplasty (**KRAY**-nee-oh-**plas**-tee): Surgical repair of the skull.

craniotomy (**kray**-nee-**OT**-oh-mee): Surgical incision or opening into the skull that is performed to gain access to part of the brain; also known as a bone flap.

creatinuria (kree-**at**-ih-**NEW**-ree-ah): An increased concentration of creatine in the urine.

crepitation (**krep**-ih-**TAY**-shun): Crackling sensation that is felt and heard when the ends of a broken bone move together; also known as crepitus.

crepitus (**KREP**-ih-tus): See crepitation.

cretinism (**CREE**-tin-izm): A congenital lack of thyroid secretion.

Crohn's disease: A chronic autoimmune disorder involving any part of the gastrointestinal tract but most commonly resulting in scarring and thickening of the walls of the ileum, the colon, or both.

croup (**KROOP**): An acute respiratory syndrome in children and infants characterized by obstruction of the larynx, hoarseness, and a barking cough.

crust: A collection of dried serum and cellular debris on the skin.

cryosurgery: The elimination of abnormal tissue cells through the application of extreme cold.

cryptorchidism (krip-**TOR**-kih-dizm): A developmental defect in which one testis fails to descend into the scrotum; also known as an undescended testis.

curettage (**kyou**-reh-**TAHZH**): The removal of material from the surface by scraping or with the use of suction.

Cushing's syndrome (**KUSH**-ingz **SIN**-drohm): A condition caused by prolonged exposure to high levels of cortisol produced by the body or taken as medication.

cyanosis (**sigh**-ah-**NOH**-sis): Blue discoloration of the skin caused by a lack of adequate oxygen.

cyst: A closed sac or pouch containing fluid or semisolid material.

cystalgia (sis-**TAL**-jee-ah): Pain in the urinary bladder.

cystectomy (sis-**TECK**-toh-mee): Surgical removal of all or part of the urinary bladder.

cystic fibrosis (**SIS**-tick figh-**BROH**-sis): A genetic disorder in which the lungs are clogged with large quantities of abnormally thick mucus and the digestive system is

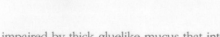

impaired by thick gluelike mucus that interferes with digestive juices.

cystitis (sis-**TYE**-tis): Inflammation of the bladder.

cystocele (**SIS**-toh-seel): A hernia of the bladder through the vaginal wall.

cystodynia (**sis**-toh-**DIN**-ee-ah): Pain in the urinary bladder.

cystography (sis-**TOG**-rah-fee): A radiographic examination of the bladder after instillation of a contrast medium via a urethral catheter.

cystolith (**SIS**-toh-lith): Presence of stones in the urinary bladder.

cystopexy (**sis**-toh-**peck**-see): Surgical fixation of the bladder to the abdominal wall.

cystoplasty (**SIS**-toh-**plas**-tee): Surgical repair of the bladder.

cystoptosis (**sis**-top-**TOH**-sis *or* **sis**-toh-**TOH**-sis): Prolapse of the bladder into the urethra.

cystorrhagia (**sis**-toh-**RAY**-jee-ah): Bleeding from the bladder.

cystorrhaphy (sis-**TOR**-ah-fee): To suture the bladder.

cystorrhexis (**sis**-toh-**RECK**-sis): Rupture of the bladder.

cystoscopy (sis-**TOS**-koh-pee): Visual examination of the urinary bladder using a cystoscope.

cystostomy (sis-**TOS**-toh-mee): Creation of an artificial opening between the urinary bladder and the exterior of the body.

cytomegalovirus (**sigh**-toh-**meg**-ah-loh-**VYE**-rus): An infection caused by a group of large herpes-type viruses with a wide variety of disease effects.

cytotoxic drug (**sigh**-toh-**TOK**-sick): Medication that kills or damages cells and is used as an immunosuppressant or an antineoplastic.

D

dacryocystitis (**dack**-ree-oh-sis-**TYE**-tis): An inflammation of the lacrimal sac that is associated with faulty tear drainage.

deafness: The complete or partial loss of the ability to hear.

debridement (day-breed-**MON**): The removal of dirt, foreign objects, damaged tissue, and cellular debris from a wound to prevent infection and to promote healing.

decubitus (dee-**KYOU**-bih-tus): The act of lying down or the position assumed in lying down.

defibrillation (dee-**fib**-rih-**LAY**-shun): The use of electrical shock to restore the heart's normal rhythm; also known as cardioversion.

dehydration: A condition in which fluid loss exceeds fluid intake and disrupts the body's normal electrolyte balance.

delirium (dee-**LIR**-ee-um): A potentially reversible condition often associated with a high fever that comes on suddenly in which the patient is confused, disoriented, and unable to think clearly.

delirium tremens (dee-**LIR**-ee-um **TREE**-mens): A form of acute organic brain syndrome due to alcohol withdrawal that is characterized by sweating, tremor, restlessness, anxiety, mental confusion, and hallucinations.

delusion (dee-**LOO**-zhun): A false personal belief that is maintained despite obvious proof or evidence to the contrary.

dementia (dee-**MEN**-shee-ah): A slowly progressive decline in mental abilities including impaired memory, thinking, and judgment.

dental calculus (**KAL**-kyou-luhs): Hardened dental plaque on the teeth that irritates the surrounding tissues.

dental caries (**KAYR**-eez): An infectious disease that destroys the enamel and dentin of the tooth; also known as tooth decay or a cavity.

dental plaque (**PLACK**): A soft deposit consisting of bacteria and bacterial by-products that builds up on the teeth and is a major cause of dental caries and periodontal disease.

dentist: A specialist in diagnosing and treating diseases and disorders of teeth and tissues of the oral cavity.

dermabrasion (**der**-mah-**BRAY**-zhun): A form of abrasion involving the use of revolving wire brushes or sandpaper.

dermatitis (**der**-mah-**TYE**-tis): Inflammation of the upper layers of skin.

dermatitis, contact: A localized allergic response caused by contact with an irritant or allergen that causes redness, itching, and rash.

dermatologist (**der**-mah-**TOL**-oh-jist): A specialist in diagnosing and treating disorders of the skin.

dermatomycosis (**der**-mah-toh-my-**KOH**-sis): A fungal infection that causes white to light brown areas on the skin; also known as tinea versicolor.

dermatopathy (**der**-mah-**TOP**-ah-thee): Any disease of the skin.

dermatoplasty (**DER**-mah-toh-**plas**-tee): The replacement of damaged skin with tissue taken from a donor site on the patient's body; also known as a skin graft.

dermatosis (**der**-mah-**TOH**-sis): A general term used to denote any skin lesion or group of lesions or eruptions of any type that are *not* associated with inflammation.

detached retina: Condition in which the retina is pulled away from its normal position of being attached to the choroid in the back of the eye.

developmental disorder: An anomaly or malformation that is present at birth.

diabetes insipidus (**dye**-ah-**BEE**-teez in-**SIP**-ih-dus): A condition caused by insufficient production of antidiuretic hormone (ADH) or by the inability of the kidneys to respond to ADH that allows too much fluid to be excreted.

diabetes mellitus (**dye**-ah-**BEE**-teez mel-**EYE**-tus *or* **MEL**-ih-tus): A group of metabolic diseases characterized by hyperglycemia resulting from defects in insulin secretion, insulin action, or both.

diabetes mellitus, gestational: A form of diabetes that may occur during pregnancies and usually disappears after delivery.

diabetes mellitus, type 1: An insulin deficiency disorder; also known as insulin-dependent diabetes mellitus.

diabetes mellitus, type 2: An insulin resistance disorder; also known as non-insulin-dependent diabetes mellitus.

diabetic ketoacidosis (kee-toh-**ass-**ih-**DOH**-sis): An acute, life-threatening complication caused by a severe insulin deficiency.

diabetic nephropathy: Disease of the kidney caused by long-term diabetes mellitus.

dialysis (dye-AL-ih-sis): A procedure to remove waste products from the blood of patients whose kidneys no longer function.

diaphoresis (dye-ah-foh-**REE**-sis): Profuse sweating.

diarrhea (dye-ah-**REE**-ah): Abnormal frequency of loose or watery stools.

diffuse: Widespread.

digitalis (dij-ih-**TAL**-is): Medication administered to slow and strengthen the heart muscle contractions; also known as digoxin.

dilation (dye-LAY-shun): The expansion of an opening.

dilation and curettage: The dilation of the cervix and curettage of the uterus; also known as a D & C.

diopter (dye-AHP-tur): A unit of measurement of lens refractive power.

diphtheria (dif-THEE-ree-ah): An acute infectious disease of the throat and upper respiratory tract caused by the presence of diphtheria bacteria.

diplopia (dih-PLOH-pee-ah): The perception of two images of a single object; also known as double vision.

diskectomy (dis-KECK-toh-mee): Surgical removal of an intervertebral disk.

diuresis (dye-you-**REE**-sis): Increased excretion of urine.

diuretics (dye-you-**RET**-icks): Medications administered to increase urine secretion to rid the body of excess sodium and water.

diverticulectomy (dye-ver-**tick-**you-**LECK**-toh-mee): Surgical removal of a diverticulum.

diverticulitis (dye-ver-tick-you-**LYE**-tis): Inflammation of one or more diverticula.

diverticulum (dye-ver-**TICK**-you-lum): A pouch or sac occurring in the lining or wall of a tubular organ including the intestines.

dorsal recumbent position: Lying on the back with the knees bent.

Down syndrome: A genetic syndrome characterized by varying degrees of mental retardation and multiple physical abnormalities; also known as trisomy 21.

drug, adverse reaction: An undesirable drug response that accompanies the principal response for which the drug was taken.

drug, brand name: Medication sold under the name given by the manufacturer. A brand name is always spelled with a capital letter.

drug, generic: Medication named for its chemical structure and not protected by a brand name or trademark.

drug, interaction: A reaction that occurs when the effect of one drug is changed if it is administered at the same time as another drug.

drug, over-the-counter: A medication that may be dispensed without a written prescription.

drug, prescription: A medication that may be dispensed only with a prescription from an appropriately licensed professional.

dual x-ray absorptiometry (ab-**sorp-**shee-**OM**-eh-tree): Low-exposure radiographic measurement used to detect early signs of osteoporosis; also known as DXA.

Duchenne's muscular dystrophy (doo-**SHENZ**): A severe form of muscular dystrophy that appears between two and six years of age.

ductal carcinoma in situ: Breast cancer at its earliest stage before the cancer has broken through the wall of the duct.

duodenal ulcers (dew-oh-**DEE**-nal *or* dew-**ODD**-eh-nal **UL**-serz): Peptic ulcers occurring in the upper part of the small intestine.

dyschromia (dis-KROH-mee-ah): Any disorder of the pigmentation of the skin or hair.

dyscrasia (dis-KRAY-zee-ah): Any abnormal or pathologic condition of the blood.

dyskinesia (dis-kih-**NEE**-zee-ah): Distortion or impairment of voluntary movement as in a tic or spasm.

dyslexia (dis-LECK-see-ah): A learning disability characterized by reading achievement that falls substantially below that expected given the individual's chronological age, measured intelligence, and age-appropriate education.

dysmenorrhea (dis-men-oh-**REE**-ah): Abdominal pain caused by uterine cramps during a menstrual period.

dyspepsia (dis-PEP-see-ah): An impairment of digestion; also known as indigestion.

dysphagia (dis-FAY-jee-ah): Difficulty in swallowing.

dysphonia (dis-FOH-nee-ah): Any voice impairment including hoarseness, weakness, or loss of voice.

dysplasia (dis-PLAY-see-ah): Abnormal development or growth of cells.

dysplasia, cervical: The abnormal growth of cells of the cervix; also known as precancerous lesions.

dyspnea (DISP-nee-ah): Difficult or labored breathing; also known as shortness of breath.

dysrhythmia (dis-RITH-mee-ah): An irregularity or the loss of normal rhythm of the heartbeat; also known as cardiac arrhythmia.

dystaxia (dis-TACK-see-ah): Difficulty in controlling voluntary movement; also known as partial ataxia.

dystonia (dis-TOH-nee-ah): Condition of abnormal muscle tone.

dysuria (dis-YOU-ree-ah): Difficult or painful urination.

E

ecchymosis (**eck**-ih-**MOH**-sis): A purplish area caused by bleeding within the skin; also known as a bruise.

E. coli: An intestinal infection caused by the bacterium *Escherichia coli*.

echocardiography (**eck**-oh-**kar**-dee-**OG**-rah-fee): An ultrasonic diagnostic procedure used to evaluate the structures and motion of the heart.

echoencephalography (**eck**-oh-en-**sef**-ah-**LOG**-rah-fee): The use of ultrasound imaging to diagnose a shift in the midline structures of the brain.

eclampsia (eh-**KLAMP**-see-ah): A serious form of preeclampsia characterized by convulsions and sometimes coma.

ectopic pregnancy (eck-**TOP**-ick): A pregnancy in which the fertilized egg is implanted and begins to develop outside of the uterus; also known as an extrauterine pregnancy.

ectropion (eck-**TROH**-pee-on): The turning outward of the edge of the eyelid.

eczema (**ECK**-zeh-mah): An acute or chronic skin inflammation characterized by erythema, papules, vesicles, pustules, scales, crusts, scabs, and possibly itching.

edema (eh-**DEE**-mah): Excess fluid in body tissues, causing swelling.

effusion (eh-**FEW**-zhun): The escape of fluid from blood or lymphatic vessels into the tissues or a cavity.

effusion, pleural: Abnormal escape of fluid into the pleural cavity that prevents the lung from fully expanding.

electrocardiogram (ee-**leck**-troh-**KAR**-dee-oh-**gram**): A record of the electrical activity of the myocardium.

electroconvulsive therapy (ee-**leck**-troh-kon-**VUL**-siv): A controlled convulsion produced by the passage of an electric current through the brain to treat depression and mental disorders; also known as electroshock therapy.

electroencephalography (ee-**leck**-troh-en-**sef**-ah-**LOG**-rah-fee): The process of recording electrical brain-wave activity.

electromyography (ee-**leck**-troh-my-**OG**-rah-fee): Diagnostic test that records the strength of muscle contractions as the result of electrical stimulation.

electroneuromyography (ee-**leck**-troh-**new**-roh-my-**OG**-rah-fee): Recording neuromuscular activity by the electric stimulation of nerve trunk carrying fibers to and from the muscle; also known as nerve conduction studies.

electronic fetal monitor: A device used during labor to monitor the fetal heart rate and the maternal uterine contractions.

emaciated (ee-**MAY**-shee-ayt-ed): Abnormally thin.

embolism (**EM**-boh-lizm): Blockage of a vessel by an embolus.

embolus (**EM**-boh-lus): A foreign object, such as a blood clot, a quantity of air or gas, or a bit of tissue or tumor that is circulating in the blood.

embryo (**EM**-bree-oh): The developing child from implantation through the eighth week of pregnancy.

emesis (**EM**-eh-sis): The expelling of the contents of the stomach through the esophagus and out of the mouth; also known as vomiting.

emetic (eh-**MET**-ick): Medication administered to produce vomiting.

emmetropia (em-eh-**TROH**-pee-ah): The normal relationship between the refractive power of the eye and the shape of the eye that enables light rays to focus correctly on the retina.

empathy (**EM**-pah-thee): The ability to understand another person's mental and emotional state without becoming personally involved.

emphysema (**em**-fih-**SEE**-mah): The progressive loss of lung function due to a decrease in the total number of alveoli, the enlargement of the remaining alveoli, and then the progressive destruction of their walls.

empyema (**em**-pye-**EE**-mah): An accumulation of pus in the pleural cavity; also known as pyothorax.

encephalitis (**en**-sef-ah-**LYE**-tis): Inflammation of the brain.

encephalocele (en-**SEF**-ah-loh-**seel**): A congenital gap in the skull with herniation of brain substance; also known as a craniocele.

encephalography (en-**sef**-ah-**LOG**-rah-fee): A radiographic study demonstrating the intracranial fluid-containing spaces of the brain.

encephalomalacia (en-**sef**-ah-loh-mah-**LAY**-shee-ah): Abnormal softening of the brain.

encephalopathy (en-**sef**-ah-**LOP**-ah-thee): Any degenerative disease of the brain.

endarterectomy (**end**-ar-ter-**ECK**-toh-mee): Surgical removal of the lining of an artery that is clogged with plaque.

endemic (en-**DEM**-ick): Ongoing presence of a disease within a population, group, or area.

endocarditis (**en**-doh-kar-**DYE**-tis): Inflammation of the inner layer of the heart.

endocarditis, bacterial: Inflammation of the inner lining or valves of the heart caused by bacteria.

endocervicitis (**en**-doh-**ser**-vih-**SIGH**-tis): Inflammation of the mucous membrane lining of the cervix.

endocrinologist (**en**-doh-krih-**NOL**-oh-jist): A specialist in diagnosing and treating diseases and malfunctions of the glands of internal secretion.

endocrinology (**en**-doh-krih-**NOL**-oh-jee): Study of the endocrine glands and their secretions.

endocrinopathy (**en**-doh-krih-**NOP**-ah-thee): Any disease due to a disorder of the endocrine system.

endometriosis (**en**-doh-**mee**-tree-**OH**-sis): A condition in which endometrial tissue escapes the uterus and grows on other structures in the pelvic cavity.

endometritis (**en**-doh-mee-**TRY**-tis): Inflammation of the endometrium.

endoscopy (en-**DOS**-koh-pee): The visual examination of the interior of a body cavity with the use of an endoscope.

endotracheal intubation (**en**-doh-**TRAY**-kee-al **in**-too-**BAY**-shun): The passage of a tube through the nose or mouth into the trachea to establish an airway.

endovaginal ultrasound (**en**-doh-**VAJ**-ih-nal): An ultrasonic diagnostic test to determine the cause of abnormal vaginal bleeding.

enteritis (**en**-ter-**EYE**-tis): Inflammation of the small intestines.

entropion (en-**TROH**-pee-on): The turning inward of the edge of the eyelid.

enuresis (**en**-you-**REE**-sis): The involuntary discharge of urine.

enzyme-linked immunosorbent assay: A blood test to screen for the presence of HIV antibodies; also known as ELISA.

epicondylitis (**ep**-ih-**kon**-dih **LYE**-tis): Inflammation of the tissues surrounding the elbow.

epidemic (**ep**-ih-**DEM**-ick): Sudden and widespread outbreak of a disease within a population group or area.

epidemiologist (**ep**-ih-**dee**-mee-**OL**-oh-jist): A specialist in the study of outbreaks of disease within a population group.

epididymitis (**ep**-ih-did-ih-**MY**-tis): Inflammation of the epididymis.

epiglottitis (**ep**-ih-glot-**TYE**-tis): Inflammation of the epiglottis.

epilepsy (**EP**-ih-**lep**-see): A group of neurologic disorders characterized by recurrent episodes of seizures.

epilepsy, grand mal (**GRAN MAHL EP**-ih-**lep**-see): The more severe form of epilepsy that is characterized by generalized tonic-clonic seizures.

epilepsy, petit mal (pch **TEE MAHL EP**-ih-**lep**-see): The milder form of epilepsy in which there is a sudden, temporary loss of consciousness, lasting only a few seconds; also known as absence epilepsy.

epinephrine: A medication used as a vasoconstrictor to treat conditions such as heart dysrhythmias and asthma attacks.

episiorrhaphy (eh-**piz**-ee-**OR**-ah-fee): A sutured repair of an episiotomy.

episiotomy (eh-**piz**-ee-**OT**-oh-mee): A surgical incision of the perineum and vagina to facilitate delivery and prevent laceration of the tissues.

epispadias (**ep**-ih-**SPAY**-dee-as): In the male, a congenital abnormality in which the urethral opening is located on the upper surface of the penis. In the female with epispadias, the urethral opening is in the region of the clitoris.

epistaxis (**ep**-ih-**STACK**-sis): Bleeding from the nose; also known as a nosebleed.

epithelioma (**ep**-ih-thee-lee-**OH**-mah): A benign or malignant tumor originating in the epidermis that may occur on the skin or mucous membranes.

ergonomics (er-goh-**NOM**-icks): Study of human factors that affect the design and operation of tools and the work environment.

eructation (eh-ruk-**TAY**-shun): The act of belching or raising gas orally from the stomach.

erythema (**er**-ih-**THEE**-mah): Any redness of the skin such as a nervous blush, an inflammation, or a mild sunburn.

erythrocytosis (eh-**rith**-roh-sigh-**TOH**-sis): An abnormal increase in the number of circulating red blood cells.

esophagalgia (eh-**sof**-ah-**GAL**-jee-ah): Pain in the esophagus.

esophageal reflux (eh-**sof**-ah-**JEE**-al **REE**-flucks): The upward flow of stomach acid into the esophagus; also known as gastroesophageal reflux disease.

esophageal varices (eh-**sof**-ah-**JEE**-al **VAYR**-ih-seez): Enlarged and swollen veins at the lower end of the esophagus.

esophagogastrectomy (eh-**sof**-ah-goh-gas-**TRECK**-toh-mee): Surgical removal of all or part of the esophagus and stomach.

esophagoplasty (eh-**SOF**-ah-go-**plas**-tee): Surgical repair of the esophagus.

esotropia (**es**-oh-**TROH**-pee-ah): Strabismus characterized by an inward deviation of one eye in relation to the other; also known as cross-eyes.

etiology (**ee**-tee-**OL**-oh-jee): Study of the causes of diseases.

eupnea (youp-**NEE**-ah): Easy or normal breathing.

eustachitis (**you**-stay-**KYE**-tis): Inflammation of the eustachian tube.

Ewing's sarcoma (**YOU**-ingz sar-**KOH**-mah): Cancer usually occurring in the diaphyses of long bones in the arms and legs of children or adolescents.

excision (eck-**SIH**-zhun): The complete removal of a lesion or an organ.

exfoliative cytology (ecks-**FOH**-lee-**ay**-tiv sigh-**TOL**-oh-jee): A biopsy in which cells are scraped from the tissue and examined under a microscope.

exophthalmos (**eck**-sof-**THAL**-mos): Abnormal protrusion of the eyes.

exostosis (**eck**-sos-**TOH**-sis): Benign growth on the surface of a bone.

exotropia (**eck**-soh-**TROH**-pee-ah): Strabismus characterized by the outward deviation of one eye relative to the other; also known as wall-eye.

extracapsular cataract extraction: The removal of a cloudy lens that leaves the posterior lens capsule intact.

extracorporeal shock-wave lithotripsy (**LITH**-oh-**trip**-see): Destruction of a kidney stone with the use of ultrasonic waves traveling through water; also known as lithotripsy.

exudate (**ECKS**-you-dayt): Accumulated fluid in a cavity that has penetrated through vessel walls into the adjoining tissue.

F

fasciectomy (**fas**-ee-**ECK**-toh-mee): Surgical removal of fascia.

fasciitis (**fas**-ee-**EYE**-tis): Inflammation of a fascia.

fasciodesis (**fash**-ee-**ODD**-eh-sis): Binding fascia to a skeletal attachment.

fascioplasty (**FASH**-ee-oh-**plas**-tee): Surgical repair of a fascia.

fasciorrhaphy (**fash**-ee-**OR**-ah-fee): To suture torn fascia.

fasciotomy (**fash**-ee-**OT**-oh-mee): Surgical incision of fascia.

fasting blood sugar: A blood test used to screen for and to monitor treatment of diabetes mellitus.

fenestration (**fen**-es-**TRAY**-shun): A surgical procedure in which a new opening is made in the labyrinth of the inner ear to restore hearing.

fetus (**FEE**-tus): The developing child from the ninth week of pregnancy to the time of birth.

fibrillation (**fih**-brih-**LAY**-shun): Rapid, random, and ineffective contractions of the heart.

fibrillation, atrial: Condition in which the atria beat faster than the ventricles.

fibrillation, ventricular: The result of irregular contractions of the ventricles that is fatal unless reversed by electric defibrillation.

fibrocystic breast disease (**figh**-broh-**SIS**-tick): The presence of single or multiple cysts in the breasts.

fibroid: A benign tumor composed of muscle and fibrous tissue that occurs in the wall of the uterus; also known as a leiomyoma.

fibromyalgia syndrome (**figh**-broh-my-**AL**-jee-ah): A chronic disorder of unknown cause characterized by widespread aching pain, tender points, and fatigue.

fibrosis (figh-**BROH**-sis): The abnormal formation of fibrous tissue.

fissure: A groove or cracklike sore of the skin; normal folds in the contours of the brain.

fluorescein staining (**flew**-oh-**RES**-ee-in): A dye used to visualize a corneal abrasion.

fluoroscopy (**floo**-or-**OS**-koh-pee): An imaging technique used to visualize body parts in motion by projecting x-ray images on a luminous fluorescent screen.

flutter: A cardiac arrhythmia in which the atrial contractions are rapid but regular.

fructosamine test (fruck-**TOHS**-ah-meen): A blood test that measures average blood sugar levels over the previous three weeks.

functional: A disorder in which there are no detectable physical changes to explain the symptoms being experienced by the patient.

fungus (**FUNG**-gus): A simple parasitic plant; some fungi are pathogenic to humans.

furuncles (**FYOU**-rung-kuls): Large tender, swollen areas caused by staphylococcal infection around hair follicles; also known as boils.

G

galactocele (gah-**LACK**-toh-seel): A cystic enlargement of the mammary gland containing milk; also known as a galactoma.

galactoma (**gal**-ack-**TOH**-mah): See galactocele.

gallstone: A hard deposit that forms in the gallbladder and bile ducts; also known as biliary calculus.

gangrene (**GANG**-green): Tissue death usually associated with a loss of circulation.

gastralgia (gas-**TRAL**-jee-ah): Pain in the stomach.

gastrectomy (gas-**TRECK**-toh-mee): Surgical removal of all or a part of the stomach.

gastritis (gas-**TRY**-tis): Inflammation of the stomach.

gastroduodenostomy (**gas**-troh-**dew**-oh-deh-**NOS**-toh-mee): Removal of the pylorus of the stomach and the establishment of an anastomosis between the upper portion of the stomach and the duodenum.

gastrodynia (**gas**-troh-**DIN**-ee-ah): Pain in the stomach.

gastroenteritis (**gas**-troh-en-ter-**EYE**-tis): Inflammation of the stomach and small intestine.

gastroenterocolitis (**gas**-troh-**en**-ter-oh-koh-**LYE**-tis): Inflammation of the stomach, small intestine, and large intestine.

gastroenterologist (**gas**-troh-**en**-ter-**OL**-oh-jist): A specialist in diagnosing and treating diseases and disorders of the stomach and intestines.

gastroesophageal reflux disease: The upward flow of stomach acid into the esophagus; also known as esophageal reflux.

gastrointestinal endoscopy: Endoscopic examination of the interior of the esophagus, stomach, and duodenum.

gastropexy (**GAS**-troh-**peck**-see): Surgical fixation of the stomach to correct displacement.

gastrorrhagia (**gas**-troh-**RAY**-jee-ah): Bleeding from the stomach.

gastrorrhaphy (gas-**TROR**-ah-fee): To suture the stomach.

gastrorrhea (**gas**-troh-**REE**-ah): Excessive flow of gastric secretions.

gastrorrhexis (**gas**-troh-**RECK**-sis): Rupture of the stomach.

gastrosis (gas-**TROH**-sis): Any abnormal condition of the stomach.

gastrostomy (gas-**TROS**-toh-mee): Surgical creation of an artificial opening into the stomach.

gastrotomy (gas-**TROT**-oh-mee): A surgical incision into the stomach.

geneticist (jeh-**NET**-ih-sist): A specialist in the field of genetics.

genital herpes (**HER**-peez): A highly contagious sexually transmitted disease caused by the herpes simplex virus.

genital warts: A highly contagious sexually transmitted disease caused by the *human papillomavirus*.

gerontologist (**jer**-on-**TOL**-oh-jist): A specialist in diagnosing and treating diseases, disorders, and problems associated with aging.

gigantism (jigh-**GAN**-tiz-em *or* **JIGH**-en-tiz-em): Abnormal overgrowth of the body caused by excessive secretion of the growth hormone *before* puberty.

gingivectomy (**jin**-jih-**VECK**-toh-mee): Surgical removal of diseased gingival tissue.

gingivitis (**jin**-jih-**VYE**-tis): Inflammation of the gums that is the earliest stage of periodontal disease.

GI series, lower: A radiographic study of the lower portion of the digestive system using barium as a contrast medium; also known as a barium enema.

GI series, upper: A radiographic study of the upper portion of the digestive system using barium as a contrast medium; also known as a barium swallow.

glaucoma (glaw-**KOH**-mah): Increased intraocular pressure that damages the optic nerve and may cause the loss of peripheral vision and eventually blindness.

glomerulonephritis (gloh-**mer**-you-loh-neh-**FRY**-tis): Inflammation of the kidney involving primarily the glomeruli.

glucose tolerance test (**GLOO**-kohs): A blood test used to confirm diabetes mellitus and to aid in diagnosing hypoglycemia.

glycohemoglobin (**glye**-koh-**hee**-moh-**GLOH**-bin): The substance that forms when glucose in the blood attaches to the hemoglobin.

glycosuria (**glye**-koh-**SOO**-ree-ah): The presence of glucose in the urine that is commonly caused by diabetes.

goiter (**GOI**-ter): An abnormal enlargement of the thyroid gland that produces a swelling in the front part of the neck; also known as thyromegaly.

gonorrhea (**gon**-oh-**REE**-ah): A highly contagious sexually transmitted disease caused by the bacterium *Neisseria gonorrhoeae.*

granulation tissue: Tissue that forms during the healing of a wound to create what will become scar tissue.

granuloma (**gran**-you-**LOH**-mah): A general term used to describe small knot-like swellings of granulation tissue.

Graves' disease (**GRAYVZ** dih-**ZEEZ**): An autoimmune disorder characterized by hyperthyroidism, goiter, and exophthalmos.

Guillain-Barré syndrome (gee-**YAHN**-bah-**RAY**): A condition characterized by rapidly worsening muscle weakness that may lead to temporary paralysis.

gynecologist (**guy**-neh-**KOL**-oh-jist): A specialist in diagnosing and treating diseases and disorders of the female reproductive system.

gynecomastia (**guy**-neh-koh-**MAS**-tee-ah): The condition of excessive mammary development in the male.

H

halitosis (hal-ih-**TOH**-sis): An unpleasant breath odor that may be caused by dental diseases or respiratory or gastric disorders; also known as bad breath.

hallucination (hah-**loo**-sih-**NAY**-shun): A sense perception that has no basis in external stimulation.

hallux valgus (**HAL**-ucks **VAL**-guss): Abnormal enlargement of the joint at the base of the great toe; also known as a bunion.

hamstring injury: Strain or tear of the posterior femoral muscles.

Hashimoto's thyroiditis (hah-shee-**MOH**-tohz **thigh**-roi-**DYE**-tis): An autoimmune disorder in which the immune system mistakenly attacks thyroid tissue, setting up an inflammatory process that may progressively destroy the gland.

hearing loss, conductive: A hearing loss in which the outer or middle ear does not conduct sound vibrations to the inner ear normally.

hearing loss, noise-induced: Damage to sensitive hair-like cells of the inner ear caused by repeated exposure to very intense noise such as aircraft engines, noisy equipment, and loud music.

hearing loss, sensorineural: A hearing loss caused by problems affecting the inner ear; also known as nerve deafness.

hemangioma (hee-**man**-jee-**OH**-mah): A benign tumor made up of newly formed blood vessels.

hemangioma, strawberry: A dark reddish purple benign tumor made up of newly formed blood vessels that is usually present at birth; also known as a birthmark.

hematemesis (**hee**-mah-**TEM**-eh-sis *or* **hem**-ah-**TEM**-eh-sis): Vomiting blood.

hematocrit (hee-**MAT**-oh-krit): A laboratory test that measures the percentage by volume of packed red blood cells in a whole blood sample.

hematologist (**hee**-mah-**TOL**-oh-jist *or* **hem**-ah-**TOL**-oh-jist): A specialist in diagnosing and treating diseases and disorders of the blood and blood-forming tissues.

hematoma (**hee**-mah-**TOH**-mah): A collection of blood trapped within tissues.

hematoma, cranial: A collection of blood trapped in the tissues of the brain.

hematoma, subungual: A collection of blood trapped in the tissues under a nail.

hematopoietic (**hee**-mah-toh-poi-**ET**-ick *or* **hem**-ah-toh-poi-**ET**-ick): Pertaining to the formation of blood.

hematuria (**hee**-mah-**TOO**-ree-ah *or* **hem**-ah-**TOO**-ree-ah): The presence of blood in the urine.

hematuria, gross: The presence of blood in urine that can be detected without magnification.

hematuria, microscopic: The presence of blood in urine that can be seen only under a microscope.

hemianopia (**hem**-ee-ah-**NOH**-pee-ah): Blindness in one half of the visual field.

hemiparesis (**hem**-ee-pah-**REE**-sis): Slight paralysis of one side of the body.

hemiplegia (**hem**-ee-**PLEE**-jee-ah): Paralysis of one side of the body.

hemoccult (**HEE**-moh-kult): A laboratory test for hidden blood in the stools; also known as the fecal occult blood test.

hemochromatosis (hee-moh-kroh-mah-TOH-sis): A genetic disorder in which the intestines absorb too much iron and the excess accumulates in organs; also known as iron-overload disease.

hemodialysis (hee-moh-dye-AL-ih-sis): Removal of waste products by filtering the patient's blood.

hemoglobin A1c testing: A blood test that measures the average blood glucose level over the previous three to four months.

hemophilia (hee-moh-FILL-ee-ah): A group of hereditary bleeding disorders in which one of the factors needed to clot the blood is missing.

hemoptysis (hee-MOP-tih-sis): Spitting of blood or blood-stained sputum derived from the lungs or bronchial tubes as the result of a pulmonary or bronchial hemorrhage.

hemorrhage (HEM-or-idj): The loss of a large amount of blood in a short time.

hemorrhoidectomy (hem-oh-roid-ECK-toh-mee): Surgical removal of hemorrhoids.

hemorrhoids (HEM-oh-roids): Enlarged veins in or near the anus that may cause pain and bleeding; also known as piles.

hemostasis (hee-moh-STAY-sis): To control bleeding.

hemothorax (hee-moh-THOH-racks): An accumulation of blood in the pleural cavity.

hepatectomy (hep-ah-TECK-toh-mee): Surgical removal of all or part of the liver.

hepatitis (hep-ah-TYE-tis): Inflammation of the liver.

hepatoenteric (hep-ah-toh-en-TER-ick): Referring to the liver and intestines.

hepatomegaly (hep-ah-toh-MEG-ah-lee): Abnormal enlargement of the liver.

hepatorrhaphy (hep-ah-TOR-ah-fee): To suture the liver.

hepatorrhexis (hep-ah-toh-RECK-sis): Rupture of the liver.

hepatotomy (hep-ah-TOT-oh-mee): A surgical incision into the liver.

hereditary disorders: Diseases or conditions caused by a defective gene.

hernia (HER-nee-ah): Protrusion of a part or structure through the tissues normally containing it.

hernia, hiatal: Protrusion of part of the stomach through the esophageal sphincter in the diaphragm.

hernia, inguinal: Protrusion of a small loop of bowel through a weak place in the lower abdominal wall or groin.

herniated disk (HER-nee-ayt-ed): Rupture of the intervertebral disk resulting in pressure on spinal nerve roots; also known as a ruptured disk.

herniorrhaphy (her-nee-OR-ah-fee): To suture a defect in a muscular wall to repair a hernia.

herpes labialis (HER-peez lay-bee-AL-iss): Blisterlike sores caused by the herpes simplex virus that occur on the lips and adjacent tissue; also known as cold sores or fever blisters.

herpes zoster (HER-peez ZOS-ter): An acute viral infection characterized by painful skin eruptions that follow the underlying route of the inflamed nerve; also known as shingles.

hirsutism (HER-soot-izm): Abnormal hairiness; the appearance of male body or facial hair patterns in the female.

Hodgkin's lymphoma (HODJ-kinz): A form of lymphoma distinguished by the presence of Reed-Sternberg cells.

homocysteine (hoh-moh-SIS-teen): An amino acid normally found in the blood and used by the body to build and maintain tissues.

hordeolum (hor-DEE-oh-lum): An infection of one or more glands at the border of the eyelid; also known as a stye.

hormone replacement therapy: Administration during perimenopause and after menopause of artificially produced hormones to replace the estrogen and progesterone no longer produced.

human growth hormone therapy: A synthetic version of naturally occurring growth hormone that is administered to stimulate growth when the supply of growth hormone is insufficient for normal development.

human immunodeficiency virus: A bloodborne pathogen that invades and then progressively impairs or kills cells of the immune system; also known as HIV.

human papilloma virus (pap-ih-LOH-mah): A highly contagious sexually transmitted disease caused by the human papillomavirus; also known as genital warts.

Huntington's disease: A hereditary disorder with symptoms that first appear in midlife and cause the irreversible and progressive loss of muscle control and mental ability; also known as Huntington's chorea.

hydrocele (HIGH-droh-seel): A hernia filled with fluid in the testicles or the tubes leading from the testicles.

hydrocephalus (high-droh-SEF-ah-lus): An abnormally increased amount of cerebrospinal fluid within the brain.

hydronephrosis (high-droh-neh-FROH-sis): Dilation of the renal pelvis of one or both kidneys.

hydroureter (high-droh-you-REE-ter): Distention of the ureter with urine that cannot flow because the ureter is blocked.

hyperalbuminemia (high-per-al-byou-mih-NEE-mee-ah): Abnormally high level of albumin in the blood.

hypercalcemia (high-per-kal-SEE-mee-ah): A condition characterized by abnormally high concentrations of calcium circulating in the blood instead of being stored in the bones.

hypercrinism (high-per-KRY-nism): A condition caused by excessive secretion of any gland, especially an endocrine gland.

hyperemesis (high-per-EM-eh-sis): Excessive vomiting.

hyperesthesia (high-per-es-THEE-zee-ah): A condition of excessive sensitivity to stimuli.

hyperglycemia (high-per-glye-SEE-mee-ah): An abnormally high concentration of glucose in the blood.

hyperglycosuria (**high**-per-**glye**-koh-**SOO**-ree-ah): Presence of excess sugar in the urine.

hypergonadism (**high**-per-**GOH**-nad-izm): The condition of excessive secretion of hormones by the sex glands.

hyperhidrosis (**high**-per-high-**DROH**-sis): The condition of excessive sweating.

hyperinsulinism (**high**-per-**IN**-suh-lin-izm): A condition marked by excessive secretion of insulin that produces hypoglycemia.

hyperkinesia (**high**-per-kye-**NEE**-zee-ah): Abnormally increased motor function or activity; also known as hyperactivity.

hyperlipemia (**high**-per-lye-**PEE**-mee-ah). A general term for elevated plasma concentrations of cholesterol, triglycerides, and lipoproteins; also known as hyperlipidemia.

hyperlipidemia (**high**-per-**lip**-ih-**DEE**-mee-ah): See hyperlipemia.

hyperopia (**high**-per-**OH**-pee-ah): A defect in which light rays focus beyond the retina; also known as far-sightedness.

hyperparathyroidism (**high**-per-**par**-ah-**THIGH**-roid-izm): Overproduction of parathyroid hormone that causes hypercalcemia and may lead to weakened bones and the formation of kidney stones.

hyperpituitarism (**high**-per-pih-**TOO**-ih-tah-rizm): Pathology that results in excessive secretion by the anterior lobe of the pituitary gland.

hyperplasia (**high**-per-**PLAY**-zee-ah): An abnormal increase in the number of normal cells in normal arrangement in a tissue.

hyperpnea (**high**-perp-**NEE**-ah): An abnormal increase in the depth and rate of the respiratory movements.

hyperproteinuria (**high**-per-**proh**-tee-in-**YOU**-ree-ah): Presence of excess of protein in the urine.

hypertension: Consistent abnormally elevated blood pressure levels.

hyperthyroidism (**high**-per-**THIGH**-roid-izm): A condition of excessive thyroid hormones in the blood.

hypertonia (**high**-per-**TOH**-nee-ah): Condition of excessive tone of the skeletal muscles with increased resistance of muscle to passive stretching.

hyperventilation (**high**-per-**ven**-tih-**LAY**-shun): Abnormally rapid deep breathing, resulting in decreased levels of carbon dioxide at the cellular level.

hypnotic: Medication that depresses the central nervous system and usually produces sleep.

hypocalcemia (**high**-poh-kal-**SEE**-mee-ah): A condition characterized by abnormally low levels of calcium in the blood.

hypochondriasis (**high**-poh-kon-**DRY**-ah-sis): A preoccupation with fears of having, or the idea that one has, a serious disease based on misinterpretation of one or more bodily signs or symptoms.

hypocrinism (**high**-poh-**KRY**-nism): A condition caused by deficient secretion of any gland, especially an endocrine gland.

hypoglycemia (**high**-poh-glye-**SEE**-mee-ah): An abnormally low concentration of glucose in the blood.

hypogonadism (**high**-poh-**GOH**-nad-izm): The condition of deficient secretion of hormones by the sex glands.

hypohidrosis (**high**-poh-high-**DROH**-sis): Abnormal condition resulting in the diminished flow of perspiration.

hypokinesia (**high**-poh-kye-**NEE**-zee-ah): Abnormally decreased motor function or activity.

hypomenorrhea (**high**-poh-men-oh-**REE**-ah): A small amount of menstrual flow during a shortened regular menstrual period.

hypoparathyroidism (**high**-poh-**par**-ah-**THIGH**-roid-izm): A condition caused by an insufficient or absent secretion of the parathyroid glands.

hypoperfusion (**high**-poh-per-**FYOU**-zhun): A deficiency of blood passing through an organ or body part.

hypophysectomy (high-**pof**-ih-**SECK**-toh-mee): Removal of all or part of the pituitary gland by the use of radiation or surgery.

hypopituitarism (**high**-poh-pih-**TOO**-ih-tah-**rizm**): A condition of reduced secretion due to the partial or complete loss of the function of the anterior lobe of the pituitary gland.

hypoplasia (**high** poh **PLAY** zee ah): Incomplete development of an organ or tissue, but less severe in degree than aplasia.

hypopnea (**high**-poh-**NEE**-ah): Shallow or slow respiration.

hypospadias (**high**-poh-**SPAY**-dee-as): In the male, congenital abnormality in which the urethral opening is on the undersurface of the penis. In the female with hypospadias, the urethral opening is into the vagina.

hypotension (**high**-poh-**TEN**-shun): Lower than normal blood pressure.

hypothyroidism (**high**-poh-**THIGH**-roid-izm): A deficiency of thyroid secretion; also known as an underactive thyroid.

hypotonia (**high**-poh-**TOH**-nee-ah): Condition of diminished tone of the skeletal muscles with decreased resistance of muscle to passive stretching.

hypoxia (high-**POCK**-see-ah): Subnormal oxygen levels in the cells that is less severe than anoxia.

hysterectomy (**hiss**-teh-**RECK**-toh-mee): The surgical removal of the uterus that may or may not include the cervix.

hysterectomy, radical: Surgical removal of the uterus, tubes, ovaries, adjacent lymph nodes, and part of the vagina.

hysterectomy, total abdominal: A hysterectomy performed through an incision in the abdomen that includes the removal of the uterus, cervix, fallopian tubes, and ovaries.

hysterectomy, vaginal: A hysterectomy performed through the vagina.

hysterocele (**HISS**-ter-oh-seel): Hernia of the uterus, particularly during pregnancy.

hysteropexy (**HISS**-ter-oh-**peck**-see): Surgical fixation of a misplaced or abnormally movable uterus.

hysterorrhaphy (hiss-ter-**OR**-ah-fee): To suture the uterus.

hysterorrhexis (**hiss**-ter-oh-**RECK**-sis): Rupture of the uterus, particularly during pregnancy.

hysterosalpingography (hiss-ter-oh-**sal**-pin-**GOG**-rah-fee): A radiographic examination of the uterus and fallopian tubes after the injection of radiopaque material.

hysteroscopy (hiss-ter-**OSS**-koh-pee): The direct visual examination of the interior of the uterus using the magnification of a hysteroscope.

I

iatrogenic (eye-**at**-roh-**JEN**-ick): An unfavorable response to medical treatment for a different disorder.

icterus (**ICK**-ter-us): Yellow discoloration of the skin and other tissues caused by greater than normal amounts of bilirubin in the blood; also known as jaundice.

idiopathic (**id**-ee-oh-**PATH**-ick): Pertaining to an illness without known cause.

idiosyncratic reaction (**id**-ee-oh-sin-**KRAT**-ick): An unexpected reaction to a drug.

ileectomy (**ill**-ee-**ECK**-toh-mee): Surgical removal of the ileum.

ileitis (**ill**-ee-**EYE**-tis): Inflammation of the ileum.

ileostomy (**ill**-ee-**OS**-toh-mee): Surgical creation of an opening between the ileum, at the end of the small intestine, and the abdominal wall.

ileus (**ILL**-ee-us): A temporary stoppage of intestinal peristalsis.

immunodeficiency (**im**-you-noh-deh-**FISH**-en-see): A condition that occurs when one or more parts of the immune system are deficient or missing.

immunofluorescence (**im**-you-noh-**floo**-oh-**RES**-ens): A method of tagging antibodies with a fluorescent dye to detect or localize antigen-antibody combinations.

immunoglobulin (**im**-you-noh-**GLOB**-you-lin): A type of antibody produced naturally by the body; synthetic immunoglobulins are administered as a postexposure preventive measure against certain viruses such as rabies and some types of hepatitis.

immunologist (**im**-you-**NOL**-oh-jist): A specialist in the study, diagnosis, and treatment of disorders of the immune system.

immunology (**im**-you-**NOL**-oh-jee): Study of the immune system.

immunosuppressant (**im**-you-noh-soo-**PRES**-ant): Medication that prevents or reduces the body's normal reactions to invasion by disease or by foreign tissues.

immunosuppression (**im**-you-noh-sup-**PRESH**-un): Treatment used to interfere with the ability of the immune system to respond to antigen stimulation.

immunotherapy (ih-**myou**-noh-**THER**-ah-pee): Treatment of disease by either enhancing or repressing the immune response.

impacted cerumen: An accumulation of ear wax forming a solid mass adhering to the walls of the external auditory canal.

impetigo (im-peh-**TYE**-goh): A highly contagious bacterial skin infection characterized by isolated pustules that become crusted and rupture.

impingement syndrome (im-**PINJ**-ment): Inflammation of tendons caught in the narrow space between the bones within the shoulder joint.

impotence (**IM**-poh-tens): The inability of the male to achieve or maintain a penile erection; also known as erectile dysfunction.

incision and drainage: Cutting open a lesion such as an abscess and draining the contents.

incontinence (in-**KON**-tih-nents): The inability to control excretory functions.

incontinence, bowel: The inability to control the excretion of feces.

incontinence, urinary: The inability to control the voiding of urine.

infarct (**IN**-farkt): Localized area of necrosis (tissue death) caused by an interruption of the blood supply.

infectious (in-**FECK**-shus): Pertaining to an illness caused by a pathogenic organism.

infectious mononucleosis (**mon**-oh-**new**-klee-**OH**-sis): An infection caused by the Epstein-Barr virus (one of the herpes viruses) characterized by fever, a sore throat, and enlarged lymph nodes.

infertility: The inability of a couple to achieve pregnancy after one year of regular, unprotected intercourse or the inability of a woman to carry a pregnancy to a live birth.

infestation: The dwelling of a parasite on external surface tissue.

inflammation (in-flah-**MAY**-shun): A localized response to injury or destruction of tissues.

influenza (in-flew-**EN**-zah): An acute, highly contagious viral respiratory infection that is spread by respiratory droplets and occurs most commonly during the colder months.

injection, intradermal: An injection made into the middle layers of the skin.

injection, intramuscular: An injection made directly into muscle tissue.

injection, intravenous: An injection made directly into a vein.

injection, subcutaneous: An injection made into the fatty layer just below the skin.

insomnia: The prolonged or abnormal inability to sleep.

insulinemia (in-suh-lih-**NEE**-mee-ah): Abnormally high levels of insulin in the blood.

insulinoma (in-suh-lin-**OH**-mah): A benign tumor of the pancreas that causes hypoglycemia.

intermittent claudication (**klaw**-dih-**KAY**-shun): A complex of symptoms including cramplike pain of the leg muscles caused by poor circulation.

internist: A specialist in diagnosing and treating diseases and disorders of the internal organs.

interstitial cystitis (**in**-ter-**STISH**-al sis-**TYE**-tis): Inflammation within the wall of the bladder.

intestinal adhesions (ad-**HEE**-zhunz): Abnormally held together parts of the intestine where they normally should be separate.

intestinal obstruction: A complete stoppage or serious impairment of the passage of the intestinal contents.

intracapsular cataract extraction: The removal of a cloudy lens including the surrounding capsule.

intraocular lens: A plastic lens surgically implanted to replace the natural lens.

intravenous fluorescein angiography (**flew**-oh-**RES**-ee-in **an**-jee-**OG**-rah-fee): A diagnostic test in which a dye is injected into the arm and pictures are taken as the dye passes through the blood vessels in the retina.

intravenous pyelogram (**PYE**-eh-loh-**gram**): A radiographic examination of the kidneys and ureters using a contrast medium.

intravenous urography (you-**ROG**-rah-fee): A radiographic examination of the urinary tract with the use of a contrast medium.

intubation (**in**-too-**BAY**-shun): Insertion of a tube, usually for the passage of air or fluids.

intussusception (**in**-tus-sus-**SEP**-shun): Telescoping of one part of the intestine into the opening of an immediately adjacent part.

invasive ductal carcinoma: A form of breast cancer that starts in the milk duct, breaks through the wall of that duct, and invades fatty breast tissue; also known as infiltrating ductal carcinoma.

invasive lobular carcinoma: Breast cancer that starts in the milk glands, breaks through the wall of the gland, and invades the fatty tissue of the breast; also known as infiltrating lobular carcinoma.

iridalgia (**ir**-ih-**DAL**-jee-ah): Pain felt in the iris.

iridectomy (**ir**-ih-**DECK**-toh-mee): Surgical removal of a portion of the iris tissue.

iridopathy (**ir**-ih-**DOP**-ah-thee): Any disease of the iris.

iridotomy (**ir**-ih-**DOT**-oh-mee): Incision into the iris.

iritis (eye-**RYE**-tis): Inflammation of the iris.

irritable bowel syndrome: A disorder of the motility of the entire gastrointestinal tract characterized by abdominal pain, nausea, gas, constipation, and/or diarrhea; also known as spastic colon.

ischemia (iss-**KEE**-mee-ah): Deficiency in blood supply due to either the constriction or the obstruction of a blood vessel.

ischemic heart disease (iss-**KEE**-mick): A group of cardiac disabilities resulting from an insufficient supply of oxygenated blood to the heart.

J

jaundice (**JAWN**-dis): Yellow discoloration of the skin and other tissues caused by greater than normal amounts of bilirubin in the blood; also known as icterus.

K

Kaposi's sarcoma (**KAP**-oh-seez sar-**KOH**-mah): A form of sarcoma that is frequently associated with HIV and may affect the skin, mucous membranes, lymph nodes, and internal organs.

keloid (**KEE**-loid): An abnormally raised or thickened scar that is usually smooth and shiny.

keratitis (**ker**-ah-**TYE**-tis): Inflammation of the cornea of the eye.

keratoplasty (**KER**-ah-toh-**plas**-tee): The replacement of a scarred or diseased cornea with clear corneal tissue from a donor; also known as a corneal transplant.

keratosis (**kerr**-ah-**TOH**-sis): Any skin condition in which there are overgrowth and thickening of the skin.

ketonuria (**kee**-toh-**NEW**-ree-ah): The presence of ketones in the urine.

kidney transplant: The grafting of a donor kidney into the body to replace the recipient's failed kidneys; also known as a renal transplantation.

kleptomania (**klep**-toh-**MAY**-nee-ah): A personality disorder characterized by a recurrent failure to resist impulses to steal objects not for immediate use or their monetary value.

knee-chest position: Lying face down with the hips bent so the knees and chest rest on the table.

koilonychia (**koy**-loh-**NICK**-ee-ah): A malformation of the nails that is often indicative of iron-deficiency anemia in which the outer surface is scooped out; also known as spoon nail.

kyphosis (kye-**FOH**-sis): Abnormal increase in the outward curvature of the thoracic spine as viewed from the side; also known as humpback or dowager's hump.

L

labyrinthectomy (**lab**-ih-rin-**THECK**-toh-mee): Surgical removal of the labyrinth of the inner ear.

labyrinthitis (**lab**-ih-rin-**THIGH**-tis): Inflammation of the labyrinth resulting in vertigo.

labyrinthotomy (**lab**-ih-rin-**THOT**-oh-mee): A surgical incision into the labyrinth of the inner ear.

laceration (**lass**-er-**AY**-shun): A torn, ragged wound.

lacrimotomy (**lab**-ih-rin-**THOT**-oh-mee): Surgical incision into the lacrimal duct.

lactation (lack-**TAY**-shun): The process of forming and secreting milk from the breasts as nourishment for the infant.

laminectomy (**lam**-ih-**NECK**-toh-mee): Surgical removal of a lamina from a vertebra.

laparoscopic adrenalectomy (ah-**dree**-nal-**ECK**-toh-mee): A minimally invasive surgical procedure to remove one or both adrenal glands.

laparoscopic cholecystectomy (**koh**-lee-sis-**TECK**-toh-mee): Surgical removal of the gallbladder using a laparoscope and other instruments while working through very small openings in the abdominal wall.

laparoscopy (**lap**-ah-**ROS**-koh-pee): Visual examination of the interior of the abdomen with the use of a laparoscope.

laryngectomy (**lar**-in-**JECK**-toh-mee): Surgical removal of the larynx.

laryngitis (**lar**-in-**JIGH**-tis): Inflammation of the larynx.

laryngologist (**lar**-in-**GOL**-oh-jist): A specialist in the study of the larynx.

laryngoplasty (lah-**RING**-goh-**plas**-tee): Surgical repair of the larynx.

laryngoplegia (**lar**-ing-goh-**PLEE**-jee-ah): Paralysis of the larynx.

laryngorrhagia (**lar**-ing-goh-**RAY**-jee-ah): Bleeding from the larynx.

laryngoscopy (**lar**-ing-**GOS**-koh-pee): Visual examination of the larynx using a laryngoscope.

laryngospasm (lah-**RING**-goh-spazm): A sudden spasmodic closure of the larynx.

laser: The acronym for **l**ight **a**mplification by **s**timulated **e**mission of **r**adiation. Lasers are used to treat skin, eye, and many other conditions.

laser iridotomy (**ir**-ih-**DOT**-oh-mee): Laser treatment of closed-angle glaucoma.

laser trabeculoplasty (trah-**BECK**-you-loh-**plas**-tee): Laser treatment of open-angle glaucoma.

leiomyoma (**lye**-oh-my-**OH**-mah): A benign tumor composed of muscle and fibrous tissue that occurs in the wall of the uterus; also known as a fibroid.

lensectomy (len-**SECK**-toh-mee): The surgical removal of a cataract-clouded lens.

lesion (**LEE**-zhun): A pathologic change of the tissues due to disease or injury.

lethargy (**LETH**-ar-jee): A lowered level of consciousness marked by listlessness, drowsiness, and apathy.

leukemia (loo-**KEE**-mee-ah): A malignancy characterized by a progressive increase of abnormal leukocytes.

leukopenia (**loo**-koh-**PEE**-nee-ah): An abnormal decrease in the number of white blood cells.

leukorrhea (**loo**-koh-**REE**-ah): A profuse white mucus discharge from the uterus and vagina.

ligation (lye-**GAY**-shun): Binding or tying off of blood vessels or ducts.

lipectomy (lih-**PECK**-toh-mee): Surgical removal of fat beneath the skin.

lipedema (lip-eh-**DEE**-mah): An abnormal swelling due to the collection of fat and fluid under the skin, usually between the calf and ankle.

lipid tests: Laboratory tests to measure the amounts of cholesterol and triglycerides in a blood sample; also known as a lipid panel.

lipoma (lih-**POH**-mah): A benign fatty deposit under the skin, causing a bump.

liposuction (**LIP**-oh-**suck**-shun *or* **LYE**-poh-**suck**-shun): Surgical removal of fat beneath the skin with the aid of suction; also known as suction-assisted lipectomy.

lithotomy (lih-**THOT**-oh-mee): Surgical incision for the removal of a stone; an examination position.

lithotomy position (lih-**THOT**-oh-mee): Lying on the back with the feet and legs raised and supported in stirrups.

lithotripsy (**LITH**-oh-**trip**-see): Destruction of a kidney stone with the use of ultrasonic waves traveling through water; also known as extracorporeal shock-wave lithotripsy.

lobectomy (loh-**BECK**-toh-mee): Surgical removal of a lobe of the brain, liver, lung, or thyroid gland.

lochia (**LOH**-kee-ah): The vaginal discharge during the first week or two after childbirth.

lordosis (lor-**DOH**-sis): Abnormal increase in the forward curvature of the lower or lumbar spine; also known as swayback.

Lou Gehrig's disease: A degenerative disease of the motor neurons in which patients become progressively weaker until they are completely paralyzed; also known as amyotrophic lateral sclerosis.

lumbago (lum-**BAY**-goh): Pain of the lumbar region; also known as low back pain.

lumpectomy: Surgical removal of only the cancerous tissue and a margin of normal tissue.

lupus erythematosus (**LOO**-pus er-ih-**thee**-mah-**TOH**-sus): An autoimmune disorder characterized by a red, scaly rash on the face and upper trunk.

luxation (luck-**SAY**-shun): Dislocation or displacement of a bone from its joint.

lymphadenectomy (**lim**-fad-eh-**NECK**-toh-mee): Surgical removal of a lymph node.

lymphadenitis (lim-**fad**-eh-**NIGH**-tis): Inflammation of the lymph nodes; also known as swollen glands.

lymphadenopathy (lim-**fad**-eh-**NOP**-ah-thee): Any disease process usually involving enlargement of the lymph nodes.

lymphadenopathy, persistent generalized: The continued presence of enlarged lymph nodes that is often an indication of the presence of a malignancy or deficiency in immune system function.

lymphangiogram (lim-**FAN**-jee-oh-**gram**): A radiographic study of the lymphatic vessels and nodes with the use of a contrast medium to make these structures visible.

lymphangiography (lim-**fan**-jee-**OG**-rah-fee): A radiographic examination of the lymphatic vessels following the injection of a contrast medium.

lymphangioma (lim-**fan**-jee-**OH**-mah): A benign abnormal collection of lymphatic vessels forming a mass.

lymphangitis (**lim**-fan-**JIGH**-tis): Inflammation of the lymph vessel.

lymphedema (**lim**-feh-**DEE**-mah): An abnormal accumulation of lymphatic fluid that causes swelling usually in the arms or legs.

lymphoma (lim-**FOH**-mah): A general term applied to malignancies that develop in the lymphatic system.

M

macular degeneration (**MACK**-you-lar): A gradually progressive condition that results in the loss of central vision but not in total blindness.

macule (**MACK**-youl): A discolored, *flat* spot such as a freckle or flat mole that is *less than* 1 cm in diameter.

magnetic resonance imaging: The use of a combination of radio waves and a strong magnetic field to produce images of the structures of the body.

major depressive episode: A prolonged period during which there is either a depressed mood or the loss of interest or pleasure in nearly all activities.

malaria (mah-**LAY**-ree-ah): A disease caused by a parasite that lives within certain mosquitoes and is transferred to humans by the bite of the mosquito.

malignant: Harmful, tending to spread, becoming progressively worse, and life threatening.

malingering (mah-**LING**-ger-ing): The intentional creation of false or exaggerated physical or psychological symptoms, motivated by external incentives such as avoiding work.

malnutrition: Lack of proper food or nutrients in the body, due to either a shortage of food or the improper absorption or distribution of nutrients.

mammography (mam-**OG**-rah-fee): A radiographic study of the breasts. The resulting record is called a mammogram.

mammoplasty (**MAM**-oh-**plas**-tee): Surgical repair or restructuring of the breasts.

manic episode: A distinct period during which there is an abnormally, and persistently elevated, expansive and irritable mood.

mastitis (mas-**TYE**-tis): Inflammation of the breast usually associated with lactation but that may occur for other reasons.

mastodynia (**mas**-toh-**DIN**-ee-ah): Pain in the breast.

mastoidectomy (**mas**-toy-**DECK**-toh-mee): Surgical removal of mastoid cells.

mastoiditis (**mas**-toy-**DYE**-tis): Inflammation of any part of the mastoid process.

mastopexy (**MAS**-toh-**peck**-see): Surgery to affix sagging breasts in a more elevated position.

maxillofacial surgery (mack-**sill**-oh-**FAY**-shul): Specialized surgery of the face and jaws to correct deformities, treat diseases, and repair injuries.

measles: An acute, highly contagious viral disease transmitted by respiratory droplets that is characterized by Koplik's spots and a spreading skin rash.

meatotomy (**mee**-ah-**TOT**-oh-mee): An incision of the urinary meatus to enlarge the opening.

meconium (meh-**KOH**-nee-um): A greenish material that collects in the intestine of a fetus and forms the first stools of a newborn.

melanodermatitis (**mel**-ah-noh-**der**-mah-**TYE**-tis): Excess melanin present in an area of skin inflammation.

melanoma, malignant: Skin cancer derived from cells capable of forming melanin.

melanosis (**mel**-ah-**NOH**-sis): Any condition of unusual deposits of black pigment in different parts of the body.

melasma: A pigmentation disorder characterized by brownish spots on the face; also known as chloasma or the mask of pregnancy.

melena (meh-**LEE**-nah *or* **MEL**-eh-nah): The passage of black stools containing digested blood.

Ménière's syndrome (**men**-ee-**AYRZ** *or* men-**YEHRS**): A chronic disease of the inner ear characterized by three main symptoms: attacks of dizziness, a fluctuating hearing loss, and tinnitus.

meningitis (**men**-in-**JIGH**-tis): An inflammation of the meninges of the brain or spinal cord.

meningocele (meh-**NING**-goh-**seel**): The protrusion of the membranes of the brain or spinal cord through a defect in the skull or spinal column.

meningoencephalitis (meh-**ning**-goh-en-**sef**-ah-**LYE**-tis): Inflammation of the meninges and brain.

meningoencephalomyelitis (meh-**ning**-goh-en-**sef**-ah-loh-**my**-eh-**LYE**-tis): Inflammation of the meninges, brain, and spinal cord.

meningomalacia (meh-**ning**-goh-mah-**LAY**-shee-ah): Abnormal softening of the meninges.

menometrorrhagia (**men**-oh-**met**-roh-**RAY**-jee-ah): Excessive uterine bleeding occurring both during the menses and at irregular intervals.

menorrhagia (**men**-oh-**RAY**-jee-ah): An excessive amount of menstrual flow over a longer duration than a normal period.

mental retardation: Significantly below average general intellectual functioning that is accompanied by significant limitation in adaptive functioning.

metabolism (meh-**TAB**-oh-**lizm**): All of the processes involved in the body's use of nutrients; the rate at which the body uses energy and the speed at which body functions work.

metastasis (meh-**TAS**-tah-sis): The new cancer site that results from the spreading process.

metastasize (meh-**TAS**-tah-sighz): The process by which cancer spreads from one place to another.

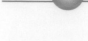

metrorrhea (**mee**-troh-**REE**-ah): An abnormal uterine discharge.

metrorrhexis (**mee**-troh-**RECK**-sis): Rupture of the uterus.

migraine headache (**MY**-grayn): A syndrome characterized by sudden, severe, sharp headache usually present on only one side.

miliaria (**mill**-ee-**AYR**-ee-ah): Trapped sweat that produces a skin rash and itching; also known as heat rash or prickly heat.

mitral stenosis (steh-**NOH**-sis): Abnormal narrowing of the opening of the mitral valve.

mitral valve prolapse: Abnormal protrusion of the mitral valve that results in the incomplete closure of the valve.

mittelschmerz (**MIT**-uhl-schmehrts): Pain between menstrual periods.

modified radical mastectomy: Surgical removal of the entire breast and lymph nodes under the arm.

Mohs' chemosurgery: A technique using a zinc chloride paste to remove recurrent tumors and scarlike basal cell carcinomas with a minimum of normal tissue loss but complete removal of the tumor.

monaural (mon-**AW**-rahl): Involving one ear.

monochromatism (**mon**-oh-**KROH**-mah-tizm): The lack of the ability to distinguish colors; also known as color blindness.

mucous (**MYOU**-kus): Specialized membranes that line the body cavities.

mucus (**MYOU**-kus): The substance secreted by the mucous membranes.

multiparous (mul-**TIP**-ah-rus): Referring to a woman who has given birth two or more times.

multiple sclerosis (skleh-**ROH**-sis): A progressive autoimmune disorder characterized by scattered patches of demyelination of nerve fibers of the brain and spinal cord.

mumps: An acute viral disease characterized by swelling of the parotid glands. (The parotid glands are salivary glands located on the face just in front of the ears.)

Munchausen syndrome (**MUHN**-chow-zen): A condition in which the "patient" repeatedly makes up clinically convincing simulations of disease for the purpose of gaining medical attention.

Munchausen syndrome by proxy: A form of child abuse in which the abusive parent will falsify an illness in a child by making up or creating symptoms and then seeking medical treatment.

muscle relaxant: Medication that acts on the central nervous system to relax muscle tone and relieve spasms.

muscular dystrophy (**DIS**-troh-fee): A group of inherited muscle disorders that cause muscle weakness without affecting the nervous system.

myalgia (my-**AL**-jee-ah): Muscle tenderness or pain.

myasthenia (**my**-as-**THEE**-nee-ah): Muscle weakness from any cause.

myasthenia gravis (**my**-as-**THEE**-nee-ah **GRAH**-vis): An autoimmune disease in which there is an abnormality in the neuromuscular function causing episodes of muscle weakness.

mycoplasma pneumonia (**my**-koh-**PLAZ**-mah new-**MOH**-nee-ah): A milder but longer-lasting form of the pneumonia caused by the fungus *Mycoplasma pneumoniae;* also known as walking pneumonia.

mycosis (my-**KOH**-sis): Any disease caused by a fungus.

mydriatic drops (**mid**-ree-**AT**-ick): Medication placed in the eye to produce temporary paralysis that forces the pupils to remain wide open even in the presence of bright light.

myectomy (my-**ECK**-toh-mee): Surgical removal of a portion of a muscle.

myelitis (**my**-eh-**LYE**-tis): Inflammation of the spinal cord; also inflammation of bone marrow.

myelography (**my**-eh-**LOG**-rah-fee): A radiographic study of the spinal cord after the injection of a contrast medium.

myeloma (**my**-eh-**LOH**-mah): A malignant tumor composed of cells derived from hemopoietic tissues of the bone marrow.

myelopathy (**my**-eh-**LOP**-ah-thee): Any pathologic condition of the spinal cord.

myelosis (**my**-eh-**LOH**-sis): A tumor of the spinal cord; also an abnormal proliferation of bone marrow tissue.

myocardial infarction (**my**-oh-**KAR**-dee-al in-**FARK**-shun): Occlusion of a coronary artery resulting in an infarct of the affected myocardium; also known as a heart attack.

myocarditis (**my**-oh-kar-**DYE**-tis): Inflammation of the myocardium.

myocele (**MY**-oh-seel): Protrusion of a muscle through its ruptured sheath or fascia.

myoclonus (**my**-oh-**KLOH**-nus *or* my-**OCK**-loh-nus): Spasm or twitching of a muscle or group of muscles.

myofascial damage (**my**-oh-**FASH**-ee-ahl): Tenderness and swelling of the muscles and their surrounding tissues that is caused by overworking the muscles.

myolysis (my-**OL**-ih-sis): Degeneration of muscle tissue.

myoma (my-**OH**-mah): A benign neoplasm made up of muscle tissue.

myomalacia (**my**-oh-mah-**LAY**-shee-ah): Abnormal softening of muscle tissue.

myonecrosis (**my**-oh-neh-**KROH**-sis): Death of individual muscle fibers.

myoparesis (**my**-oh-**PAR**-eh-sis): Weakness or slight paralysis of a muscle.

myopathy (my-**OP**-ah-thee): Any pathologic change or disease of muscle tissue.

myopia (my-**OH**-pee-ah): A defect in which light rays focus in front of the retina; also known as nearsightedness.

myoplasty (**MY**-oh-**plas**-tee): Surgical repair of a muscle.

myorrhaphy (my-**OR**-ah-fee): To suture a muscle wound.

myorrhexis (**my**-oh-**RECK**-sis): Rupture of a muscle.

myosarcoma (**my**-oh-sahr-**KOH**-mah): A malignant tumor derived from muscle tissue.

myosclerosis (**my**-oh-skleh-**ROH**-sis): Abnormal hardening of muscle tissue.

myositis (**my**-oh-**SIGH**-tis): Inflammation of skeletal muscle tissue.

myotomy (my-**OT**-oh-mee): Surgical incision into, or division of, a muscle.

myotonia (**my**-oh-**TOH**-nee-ah): Delayed relaxation of a muscle after a strong contraction.

myringectomy (**mir**-in-**JECK**-toh-mee): Surgical removal of all or part of the tympanic membrane; also known as a tympanectomy.

myringitis (**mir**-in-**JIGH**-tis): Inflammation of the tympanic membrane.

myringotomy (**mir**-in-**GOT**-oh-mee): A surgical incision of the eardrum to create an opening for the placement of tympanostomy tubes.

myxedema (**mick**-seh-**DEE**-mah): A severe form of hypothyroidism in adults.

N

narcissistic personality disorder (**nahr**-sih-**SIS**-tick): A pattern of an exaggerated need for admiration and complete lack of empathy.

narcolepsy (**NAR**-koh-**lep**-see): A syndrome characterized by recurrent uncontrollable seizures of drowsiness and sleep.

nasogastric intubation (**nay**-zoh-**GAS**-trick **in**-too-**BAY**-shun): Placement of a tube through the nose and into the stomach.

natal (**NAY**-tal): Pertaining to birth.

nausea (**NAW**-see-ah): The sensation that leads to the urge to vomit.

neonate (**NEE**-oh-nayt): An infant during the first four weeks after birth.

neonatologist (**nee**-oh-nay-**TOL**-oh-jist): A specialist in diagnosing and treating disorders of the newborn.

neonatology (**nee**-oh-nay-**TOL**-oh-jee): Study of disorders of the newborn.

neoplasm (**NEE**-oh-plazm): A new and abnormal tissue formation that may be benign or malignant; also known as a tumor.

nephrectasis (neh-**FRECK**-tah-sis): Distention of a kidney.

nephrectomy (neh-**FRECK**-toh-mee): Surgical removal of a kidney.

nephritis (neh-**FRY**-tis): Inflammation of the kidney.

nephrolith (**NEF**-roh-lith): Presence of stones in the kidney; also known as renal calculus or a kidney stone.

nephrolithiasis (**nef**-roh-lih-**THIGH**-ah-sis): A disorder characterized by the presence of stones in the kidney.

nephrolithotomy (**nef**-roh-lih-**THOT**-oh-mee): Surgical removal of a kidney stone through an incision in the kidney.

nephrologist (neh-**FROL**-oh-jist): A specialist in diagnosing and treating diseases and disorders of the kidneys.

nephrolysis (neh-**FROL**-ih-sis): Freeing of a kidney from adhesions.

nephromalacia (**nef**-roh-mah-**LAY**-shee-ah): Abnormal softening of the kidney.

nephropathy (neh-**FROP**-ah-thee): Disease of the kidney.

nephropexy (**NEF**-roh-**peck**-see): Surgical fixation of a floating kidney.

nephroptosis (**nef**-rop-**TOH**-sis): The downward displacement of the kidney; also known as a floating kidney.

nephropyosis (**nef**-roh-pye-**OH**-sis): Formation or discharge of pus from the kidney.

nephrosclerosis (**nef**-roh-skleh-**ROH**-sis): Abnormal hardening of the kidney.

nephrosis (neh-**FROH**-sis): Any abnormal condition of the kidney.

nephrostomy (neh-**FROS**-toh-mee): Surgical establishment of an opening between the pelvis of the kidney through its cortex to the exterior of the body.

nephrotic syndrome (neh-**FROT**-ick): A group of kidney diseases characterized by edema, hyperproteinuria, hypoproteinemia, and hyperlipidemia.

nephrotomy (neh-**FROT**-oh-mee): Surgical incision into the kidney.

neuralgia (new-**RAL**-jee-ah): Pain in a nerve or nerves.

neurectomy (new-**RECK**-toh-mee): The surgical removal of a nerve.

neuritis (new-**RYE**-tis): Inflammation of a nerve or nerves.

neuroblastoma (**new**-roh-blas-**TOH**-mah): A sarcoma of nervous system origin.

neurologist (new-**ROL**-oh-jist): A specialist in diagnosing and treating disorders of the central nervous system.

neuroma (new-**ROH**-mah): A benign tumor made up of nerve tissue.

neuromalacia (**new**-roh-mah-**LAY**-shee-ah): Abnormal softening of a nerve or nerves.

neuroplasty (**NEW**-roh-**plas**-tee): Surgical repair of a nerve or nerves.

neurorrhaphy (new-**ROR**-ah-fee): To suture the ends of a severed nerve.

neurosurgeon: A physician who specializes in surgery of the nervous system.

neurotomy (new-**ROT**-oh-mee): A surgical incision or the dissection of a nerve.

nevi (**NEE**-vye): Small dark skin growths that develop from melanocytes in the skin; also known as moles.

nevi, dysplastic: Atypical moles that may develop into skin cancer.

nitroglycerin: A vasodilator used to relieve the pain of angina.

nocturia (nock-**TOO**-ree-ah): Excessive urination during the night.

nocturnal enuresis: The involuntary discharge of urine during sleep; also known as bedwetting.

nocturnal myoclonus (nock-**TER**-nal **my**-oh-**KLOH**-nus *or* my-**OCK**-loh-nus): Jerking of the limbs that may occur normally as a person is falling asleep.

nodule (**NOD**-youl): A small *solid* bump that may be felt within the skin or may be raised as if it had formed below the surface of the skin and pushed upward.

non-Hodgkin's lymphomas: The term used to describe all lymphomas *other than* Hodgkin's lymphoma.

nonsteroidal anti-inflammatory drugs: Medication to control pain and to reduce inflammation and swelling: also known as NSAIDs.

nosocomial (**nos**-oh-**KOH**-mee-al): Pertaining to a hospital-acquired infection that was not present on admission but appears 72 hours or more after hospitalization.

nuclear medicine: A diagnostic technique that focuses on physiologic processes to determine how well body organs or systems are functioning; also known as radionuclide imaging.

nuclear scan: The use of radionucleide tracers to gather information about the structure and function of organs or systems that cannot be seen on conventional x-rays; also known as a scintigram.

nulligravida (**null**-ih-**GRAV**-ih-dah): Pertaining to a woman who has never been pregnant.

nullipara (nuh-**LIP**-ah-rah): Pertaining to a woman who has never borne a viable child.

nyctalopia (**nick**-tah-**LOH**-pee-ah): A condition in which the individual has difficulty seeing at night; also known as night blindness.

nystagmus (nis-**TAG**-mus): Involuntary, constant, rhythmic movement of the eyeball.

O

obesity (oh-**BEE**-sih-tee): An excessive accumulation of fat in the body.

obsessions: Persistent ideas, thoughts, or images that cause the individual anxiety or distress.

obsessive-compulsive disorder: A pattern of specific behaviors such as repeated hand washing that are caused by obsessions and compulsions.

obstetrician (**ob**-steh-**TRISH**-un): A specialist in providing medical care to women during pregnancy, childbirth, and immediately thereafter.

occlusion (ah-**KLOO**-zhun): Blockage in a canal, vessel, or passageway in the body; coming together.

oligomenorrhea (ol-ih-goh-**men**-oh-**REE**-ah): Markedly reduced menstrual flow and abnormally infrequent menstruation.

oligospermia (ol-ih-goh-**SPER**-mee-ah): An abnormally low number of sperm in the ejaculate; also known as a low sperm count.

oliguria (ol-ih-**GOO**-ree-ah): Scanty urination.

oncologist (ong-**KOL**-oh-jist): A specialist in diagnosing and treating malignant disorders such as tumors and cancer.

oncology (ong-**KOL**-oh-jee): The study of the prevention, causes, and treatment of tumors and cancer.

onychectomy (on-ih-**KECK**-toh-mee): Surgical removal of a fingernail or toenail.

onychia (oh-**NICK**-ee-ah): Inflammation of the matrix of the nail; also known as onychitis.

onychitis (on-ih-**KYE**-tis): See onychia.

onychocryptosis (on-ih-koh-krip-**TOH**-sis): Ingrown toenail.

onychoma (on-ih-**KOH**-mah): A tumor arising from the nail bed.

onychomalacia (on-ih-koh-mah-**LAY**-shee-ah): Abnormal softening of the nails.

onychomycosis (on-ih-koh-my-**KOH**-sis): Any fungal infection of the nail.

onychophagia (on-ih-koh-**FAY**-jee-ah): Nail biting or eating.

oophorectomy (**oh**-ahf-oh-**RECK**-toh-mee): Surgical removal of one or both ovaries; also known as an ovariectomy.

oophoritis (**oh**-ahf-oh-**RYE**-tis): Inflammation of an ovary.

oophoropexy (oh-**AHF**-oh-roh-**peck**-see): Surgical fixation of a displaced ovary.

oophoroplasty (oh-**AHF**-oh-roh-**plas**-tee): Surgical repair of an ovary.

ophthalmologist (ahf-thal-**MOL**-oh-jist): A specialist in diagnosing and treating diseases and disorders of the eye.

ophthalmology (ahf-thal-**MOL**-oh-jee): Study of the eye.

ophthalmoscope (ahf-**THAL**-moh-skope): An instrument used to examine the interior of the eye.

optometrist (op-**TOM**-eh-trist): A specialist in measuring the accuracy of vision to determine if corrective lenses or eyeglasses are needed.

oral rehydration therapy: Treatment in which a solution of electrolytes is administered orally to counteract dehydration that may accompany severe diarrhea.

orbitotomy (or-bih-**TOT**-oh-mee): A surgical incision into the orbit for biopsy, abscess drainage, and removal of a tumor mass or foreign object.

orchidectomy (**or**-kih-**DECK**-toh-mee): Surgical removal of one or both testicles; also known as an orchiectomy or testectomy.

orchiectomy (**or**-kee-**ECK**-toh-mee): See orchidectomy.

orchitis (or-**KYE**-tis): Inflammation of one or both testicles; also known as testitis.

organic (or-**GAN**-ick): Pertaining to a disorder in which there are pathologic physical changes that explain the symptoms being experienced by the patient.

orthodontist (**or**-thoh-**DON**-tist): A dental specialist in the prevention or correction of abnormalities in the positioning of the teeth and related facial structures.

orthopedic surgeon: A specialist in diagnosing and treating diseases and disorders involving the bones, joints, and muscles; also known as an orthopedist.

orthopedist (**or**-thoh-**PEE**-dist): See orthopedic surgeon.

ostealgia (**oss**-tee-**AL**-jee-ah): Pain linked to an abnormal condition within a bone.

ostectomy (oss-**TECK**-toh-mee): Surgical removal of bone.

osteitis (**oss**-tee-**EYE**-tis): Inflammation of bone.

osteitis deformans (**oss**-tee-**EYE**-tis dee-**FOR**-manz): A disease of unknown cause characterized by extensive bone destruction followed by abnormal bone repair; also known as Paget's disease.

osteoarthritis (**oss**-tee-oh-ar-**THRIGH**-tis): Form of arthritis commonly associated with aging; also known as wear-and-tear arthritis.

osteoarthropathy (**oss**-tee-oh-ar-**THROP**-ah-thee): Any disease involving the bones and joints.

osteochondroma (**oss**-tee-oh-kon-**DROH**-mah): Benign bone tumors that occur as growths on the surface of a bone that protrude as hard lumps covered with a cap of cartilage.

osteoclasis (**oss**-tee-**OCK**-lah-sis): Surgical fracture of a bone to correct a deformity.

osteomalacia (**oss**-tee-oh-mah-**LAY**-shee-ah): Abnormal softening of bones due to disease.

osteomyelitis (**oss**-tee-oh-**my**-eh-**LYE**-tis): Inflammation of the bone and bone marrow.

osteonecrosis (**oss**-tee-oh-neh-**KROH**-sis): Death of bone tissue caused by an insufficient blood supply, infection, malignancy, or trauma.

osteopathic physician (**oss**-tee-oh-**PATH**-ick): A specialist in treating health problems by manipulation (changing the positions of the bones); may also use traditional forms of medical treatment.

osteoplasty (**OSS**-tee-oh-**plas**-tee): Surgical repair of bones.

osteoporosis (**oss**-tee-oh-poh-**ROH**-sis): Loss of bone density and an increase in bone porosity frequently associated with aging.

osteorrhaphy (**oss**-tee-**OR**-ah-fee): Suturing or wiring together of bones.

osteosarcoma (**oss**-tee-oh-sar-**KOH**-mah): A malignant tumor usually involving the upper shaft of long bones, the pelvis, or the knee.

osteosclerosis (**oss**-tee-oh-skleh-**ROH**-sis): Abnormal hardening of bone.

osteotomy (**oss**-tee-**OT**-oh-mee): Surgical incision or sectioning of a bone.

ostomy (**OSS**-toh-mee): Surgical procedure to create an artificial opening between an organ and the body surface.

otalgia (oh-**TAL**-gee-ah): Pain in the ear.

otitis (oh-**TYE**-tis): Inflammation of the ear.

otitis externa: Inflammation of the outer ear.

otitis media, acute (oh-**TYE**-tis **MEE**-dee-ah): Inflammation of the middle ear usually associated with an upper respiratory infection that is most commonly seen in young children.

otitis media, purulent (**PYOU**-roo-lent): A buildup of pus within the middle ear.

otitis media, serous: A fluid buildup in the middle ear that may follow acute otitis media or be caused by obstruction of the eustachian tube.

otolaryngologist (**oh**-toh-**lar**-in-**GOL**-oh-jist): A specialist in diagnosing and treating diseases and disorders of the ears, nose, and throat; also known as an otorhinolaryngologist.

otomycosis (**oh**-toh-my-**KOH**-sis): A fungal infection of the external auditory canal.

otoplasty (**OH**-toh-**plas**-tee): Surgical repair of the pinna of the outer ear.

otopyorrhea (**oh**-toh-**pye**-oh-**REE**-ah): The flow of pus from the ear.

otorhinolaryngologist (**oh**-toh-**rye**-noh-**lar**-in-**GOL**-oh-jist): See otolaryngologist.

otorhinolaryngology (**oh**-toh-**rye**-noh-**lar**-in-**GOL**-oh-jee): Study of the ears, nose, and throat.

otorrhagia (**oh**-toh-**RAY**-jee-ah): Bleeding from the ear.

otosclerosis (**oh**-toh-skleh-**ROH**-sis): Ankylosis of the bones of the middle ear resulting in a conductive hearing loss.

otoscope (**OH**-toh-skope): An instrument used to visually examine the external ear canal and tympanic membrane.

ovariectomy (**oh**-vay-ree-**ECK**-toh-me): Surgical removal of one or both ovaries; also known as an oophorectomy.

ovariorrhexis (**oh**-vay-ree-oh-**RECK**-sis): Rupture of an ovary.

 P

pacemaker: An electronic device to regulate the heartbeat to treat bradycardia or atrial fibrillation.

Paget's disease (**PAJ**-its): Disease of unknown cause characterized by extensive bone destruction followed by abnormal bone repair; also known as osteitis deformans.

palatoplasty (**PAL**-ah-toh-**plas**-tee): Surgical repair of a cleft palate.

palliative (**PAL**-ee-**ay**-tiv *or* **PAL**-ee-ah-tiv): A substance that eases the pain or severity of a disease but does not cure it.

palpation (pal-**PAY**-shun): An examination technique in which the examiner's hands are used to feel the texture, size, consistency, and location of certain body parts.

palpitation (**pal**-pih-**TAY**-shun): A pounding or racing heart.

pancreatalgia (**pan**-kree-ah-**TAL**-jee-ah): Pain in the pancreas.

pancreatectomy (**pan**-kree-ah-**TECK**-toh-mee): Surgical removal of the pancreas.

pancreatitis (**pan**-kree-ah-**TYE**-tis): Inflammation of the pancreas.

pancreatotomy (**pan**-kree-ah-**TOT**-oh-mee): Surgical incision into the pancreas.

pandemic (pan-**DEM**-ick): A disease outbreak occurring over a large geographic area, possibly worldwide.

panic attack: A mental state that includes intense feelings of apprehension, fearfulness, terror, and impending doom plus physical symptoms that include shortness of breath and heart palpitations.

Papanicolaou test (**pap**-ah-**nick**-oh-**LAY**-ooh): An exfoliative test for the detection and diagnosis of conditions of the cervix and surrounding tissues: also known as a Pap smear.

papilledema (**pap**-ill-eh-**DEE**-mah): Swelling and inflammation of the optic nerve at the point of entrance through the optic disk; also known as choked disk.

papilloma (**pap**-ih-**LOH**-mah): A benign epithelial tumor that projects from the surrounding surface.

papule (**PAP**-youl): A small, solid, raised skin lesion that is *less than* 0.5 cm in diameter; also known as a pimple.

paralysis (pah-**RAL**-ih-sis): Loss of sensation and voluntary muscle movements through disease or injury to the muscle's nerve supply.

paraplegia (**par**-ah-**PLEE**-jee-ah): Paralysis of both legs and the lower part of the body.

parasite (**PAR**-ah-sight): A plant or animal that lives on or within another living organism at the expense of that organism.

paraspadias (**par**-ah-**SPAY**-dee-as): A congenital male abnormality in which the urethral opening is on one side of the penis.

parathyroidectomy (**par**-ah-**thigh**-roi-**DECK**-toh-mee): Surgical removal of one or more of the parathyroid glands.

paresthesia (**par**-es-**THEE**-zee-ah): An abnormal sensation, such as burning, tingling, or numbness, for no apparent reason.

Parkinson's disease: A chronic slowly progressive, degenerative, central nervous system disorder character-ized by fine muscle tremors, a masklike facial expression, and a shuffling gait.

paronychia (**par**-oh-**NICK**-ee-ah): An acute or chronic infection of the skin fold at the margin of a nail.

paroxysm (**PAR**-ock-sizm): A sudden convulsion, seizure, or spasm.

paroxysmal (**par**-ock-**SIZ**-mal): Sudden or spasmlike.

paroxysmal tachycardia: A fast heartbeat of sudden onset.

parturition (**par**-tyou-**RISH**-un): The act of giving birth to an offspring; also known as labor and childbirth.

pathogen (**PATH**-oh-jen): A microorganism that causes a disease.

pathologist (pah-**THOL**-oh-jist): A specialist in the laboratory analysis of tissue samples to confirm or establish a diagnosis.

pathology (pah-**THOL**-oh-jee): A condition caused by disease; the study of structural and functional changes caused by disease.

pattern baldness, female: A condition in which the hair thins in the front and on the sides and sometimes on the crown.

pattern baldness, male: A condition in which the hairline recedes from the front to the back until only a horseshoe-shaped area of hair remains in the back and on the temples.

patulous eustachian tube (**PAT**-you-lus): Distention of the eustachian tube.

pediatrician (**pee**-dee-ah-**TRISH**-un): A specialist in diagnosing, treating, and preventing disorders and diseases of children.

pediculosis (pee-**dick**-you-**LOH**-sis): An infestation with lice.

pediculosis capitis: An infestation with head lice.

pediculosis corporis: An infestation with body lice.

pediculosis pubis: An infestation with lice in the pubic hair and pubic region.

pelvic inflammatory disease: Any inflammation of the female reproductive organs not associated with surgery or pregnancy; also known as PID.

pelvimetry (pel-**VIM**-eh-tree): The measurement of the dimensions of the pelvis to determine its capacity to allow passage of the fetus through the birth canal.

peptic ulcer: A lesion of the mucous membranes of the digestive system caused by the bacterium *Helicobacter pylori*.

percussion (per-**KUSH**-un): A diagnostic procedure to determine the density of a body area by the sound produced by tapping the surface with the finger or instrument.

percutaneous (per-kyou-**TAY**-nee-us): A procedure performed through the skin.

percutaneous transluminal coronary angioplasty (**AN**-jee-oh-**plas**-tee): A procedure in which a small balloon on the end of a catheter is used to open a partially blocked coronary artery; also known as balloon angioplasty.

perfusion (per-**FYOU**-zuhn): The flow of blood through the vessels of an organ.

pericardiectomy (pehr-ih-**kar**-dee-**ECK**-toh-mee): Surgical removal of a portion of the tissue surrounding the heart.

pericardiocentesis (**pehr**-ih-**kar**-dee-oh-sen-**TEE**-sis): Drawing of fluid from the pericardial sac.

pericardiorrhaphy (**pehr**-ih-**kar**-dee-**OR**-ah-fee): To suture the tissue surrounding the heart.

pericarditis (**pehr**-ih-kar-**DYE**-tis): Inflammation of the pericardium.

perinatal (**pehr**-ih-**NAY**-tal): Time and events just before, during, and just after birth.

periodontal disease: Inflammation of the tissues that surround and support the teeth; also known as periodontitis.

periodontist (**pehr**-ee-oh-**DON**-tist): A dental specialist in the prevention and treatment of disorders of the tissues surrounding the teeth.

periodontitis (**pehr**-ee-oh-don-**TYE**-tis): Inflammation of the tissues that surround and support the teeth; also known as periodontal disease.

periosteotomy (**peer**-ee-**oss**-tee-**OT**-oh-mee): Surgical incision through the periosteum.

periostitis (**pehr**-ee-oss-**TYE**-tis): Inflammation of the periosteum.

peripheral neuritis (new-**RYE**-tis): A painful condition of the nerves of the hands and feet due to peripheral nerve damage; also known as peripheral neuropathy.

peripheral neuropathy (new-**ROP**-ah-thee): See peripheral neuritis.

peritoneal dialysis (**pehr**-ih-toh-**NEE**-al dye-**AL**-ih-sis): Removal of waste products through fluid exchange in the peritoneal cavity.

personality disorder: An enduring pattern of inner experience and behavior that deviates markedly from the expectations of the individual's culture.

pertussis (per-**TUS**-is): A contagious bacterial infection of the upper respiratory tract that is characterized by a paroxysmal cough; also known as whooping cough.

petechiae (pee-**TEE**-kee-ee): Small pinpoint hemorrhages; smaller versions of bruises.

phacoemulsification (**fay**-koh-ee-**mul**-sih-fih-**KAY**-shun or **fack**-koh-ee-**mul**-sih-fih-**KAY**-shun): The use of ultrasonic vibration to shatter and break up a cataract, making it easier to remove.

pharmacist: A specialist who is licensed in formulating and dispensing medications.

pharmacology: The study of the nature, uses, and effects of drugs for medical purposes.

pharyngitis (**far**-in-**JIGH**-tis): Inflammation of the pharynx; also known as a sore throat.

pharyngolaryngitis (fah-**ring**-goh-**lar**-in-**JIGH**-tis): Inflammation of both the pharynx and the larynx.

pharyngoplasty (fah-**RING**-goh-**plas**-tee): Surgical repair of the pharynx.

pharyngorrhagia (**far**-ing-goh-**RAY**-jee-ah): Bleeding from the pharynx.

pharyngorrhea (**far**-ing-goh-**REE**-ah): An abnormal discharge from the pharynx.

pharyngostomy (**far**-ing-**GOSS**-toh-mee): Surgical creation of an artificial opening into the pharynx.

pharyngotomy (**far**-ing-**GOT**-oh-mee): A surgical incision of the pharynx.

phenobarbital (**fee**-noh-**BAR**-bih-tal): A barbiturate used as a sedative and as an anticonvulsant.

phenylketonuria (**fen**-il-**kee**-toh-**NEW**-ree-ah): A genetic disorder in which an essential digestive enzyme is missing.

pheochromocytoma (fee-oh-**kroh**-moh-sigh-**TOH**-mah): A benign tumor of the adrenal medulla that causes the gland to produce excess epinephrine.

phimosis (figh-**MOH**-sis): A narrowing of the opening of the foreskin so it cannot be retracted to expose the glans penis.

phlebitis (fleh-**BYE**-tis): Inflammation of a vein or veins.

phlebography (fleh-**BOG**-rah-fee): A radiograph study of the veins with the use of a contrast medium.

phleborrhexis (**fleb**-oh-**RECK**-sis): Rupture of a vein.

phlebostenosis (**fleb**-oh-steh-**NOH**-sis): Abnormal narrowing of the lumen of a vein.

phlebotomist (fleh-**BOT**-oh-mist): An individual trained and skilled in phlebotomy.

phlebotomy (fleh-**BOT**-oh-mee): The puncture of a vein for the purpose of drawing blood; also known as venipuncture.

phlegm (**FLEM**): Thick mucus secreted by the tissues lining the respiratory passages.

phobia (**FOH**-bee-ah): A persistent irrational fear of a specific thing or situation. This fear is strong enough to cause avoidance of that thing or situation.

photorefractive keratectomy (**ker**-ah-**TECK**-toh-mee): Laser treatment to correct refraction disorders by reshaping of the top layer of the cornea.

pica (**PYE**-kah): An eating disorder in which there is persistent eating of nonnutritional substances such as clay.

pinealectomy (**pin**-ee-al-**ECK**-toh-mee): Surgical removal of the pineal gland.

pinealoma (**pin**-ee-ah-**LOH**-mah): Tumor of the pineal gland.

pinealopathy (**pin**-ee-ah-**LOP**-ah-thee): Any disorder of the pineal gland.

pituitarism (pih-**TOO**-ih-tar-izm): Any disorder of pituitary function.

placebo (plah-**SEE**-boh): A substance containing no active ingredients that is given for its suggestive effects.

placenta previa (plah-**SEN**-tah **PREE**-vee-ah): Abnormal implantation of the placenta in the lower portion of the uterus.

plaque (**PLACK**): A solid raised area of skin that is different from the area around it and *greater than* 0.5 cm in diameter.

plasmapheresis (**plaz**-mah-feh-**REE**-sis): A procedure in which the plasma is removed from donated blood and the red blood cells are returned to the donor.

platelet count: A laboratory test that measures the number of platelets in a specified amount of blood.

pleuralgia (ploor-**AL**-jee-ah): Pain in the pleura or in the side.

pleurectomy (ploor-**ECK**-toh-mee): Surgical removal of part of the pleura.

pleurisy (**PLOOR**-ih-see): Inflammation of the visceral and parietal pleura in the thoracic cavity.

pneumoconiosis (**new**-moh-**koh**-nee-**OH**-sis): An abnormal condition caused by dust in the lungs that usually develops after years of environmental or occupational contact.

pneumocystis carinii pneumonia (**new**-moh-**SIS**-tis kah-**RYE**-nee-eye new-**MOH**-nee-ah): A form of pneumonia caused by an infection with the fungus *Pneumocystis carinii*.

pneumonectomy (**new**-moh-**NECK**-toh-mee): Surgical removal of all or part of a lung.

pneumonia (new-**MOH**-nee-ah): Inflammation of the lungs in which the air sacs fill with pus and other liquid.

pneumonitis (**new**-moh-**NIGH**-tis): Inflammation of the lungs.

pneumorrhagia (**new**-moh-**RAY**-jee-ah): Bleeding from the lungs.

pneumothorax (**new**-moh-**THOR**-racks): An accumulation of air or gas in the pleural space causing the lung to collapse.

podiatrist (poh-**DYE**-ah-trist): A specialist in diagnosing, treating, and correcting disorders of the feet.

poliomyelitis (**poh**-lee-oh-**my**-eh-**LYE**-tis): A viral infection of the gray matter of the spinal cord that may result in paralysis.

polyarteritis (**pol**-ee-**ar**-teh-**RYE**-tis): Inflammation involving several arteries.

polyarthritis (**pol**-ee-ar-**THRIGH**-tis): Inflammation of more than one joint.

polycystic ovary syndrome: Enlargement of the ovaries caused by the presence of many cysts.

polydipsia (**pol**-ee-**DIP**-see-ah): Excessive thirst.

polymenorrhea (**pol**-ee-**men**-oh-**REE**-ah): Abnormally frequent menstruation.

polymyalgia (**pol**-ee-my-**AL**-jee-ah): Pain in several muscle groups.

polymyositis (**pol**-ee-**my**-oh-**SIGH**-tis): A chronic, progressive disease affecting the skeletal muscles that is characterized by muscle weakness and atrophy.

polyneuritis (**pol**-ee-new-**RYE**-tis): Inflammation affecting many nerves.

polyp (**POL**-ip): A general term describing a mushroom-like growth from the surface of a mucous membrane.

polyuria (pol-ee-**YOU**-ree-ah): Excessive urination.

port-wine stain: A large reddish purple discoloration of the face or neck that is present at birth and will not resolve without treatment; also known as a birthmark.

positioning: In radiography, the body placement and the part of the body closest to the film.

positron emission tomography: The combination of tomography with radionuclide tracers to produce enhanced images of selected body organs or areas; also known as PET.

postnatal (pohst-**NAY**-tal): Time and events after birth.

postpolio syndrome: Recurrence later in life of some polio symptoms in individuals who have had poliomyelitis and have recovered from it.

posttraumatic stress disorder: The development of symptoms such as sleep disorders and anxiety after a psychologically traumatic event such as witnessing a shooting, surviving a natural disaster, or being held as a hostage.

potentiation (poh-**ten**-shee-**AY**-shun): An interaction occuring when the effect of one drug is increased by another drug; also known as synergism.

preeclampsia (**pree**-ee-**KLAMP**-see-ah): A complication of pregnancy characterized by hypertension, edema, and proteinuria; also known as toxemia of pregnancy.

premenstrual syndrome: Symptoms occurring within the two-week period before menstruation; also known as PMS.

prenatal (pre-**NAY**-tal): The time and events before birth.

presbycusis (**pres**-beh-**KOO**-sis): A progressive hearing loss occurring in old age.

presbyopia (**pres**-bee-**OH**-pee-ah): Changes in the eyes that occur with aging.

prescription: An order for medication, therapy, or a therapeutic device given by an authorized person to a person properly authorized to dispense or perform the order.

primigravida (**prye**-mih-**GRAV**-ih-dah): Pertaining to a woman during her first pregnancy.

primipara (prye-**MIP**-ah-rah): Pertaining to a woman who has borne one child.

proctalgia (prock-**TAL**-jee-ah): Pain in and around the anus and rectum.

proctectomy (prock-**TECK**-toh-mee): Surgical removal of the rectum.

proctologist (prock-**TOL**-oh-jist): A specialist in disorders of the colon, rectum, and anus.

proctopexy (**PROCK**-toh-**peck**-see): Surgical fixation of the rectum to an adjacent tissue or organ.

proctoplasty (**PROCK**-toh-**plas**-tee): Surgical repair of the rectum.

proctoscopy: Visual examination of the rectum and anus.

profile: Laboratory tests frequently performed as a group on automated multichannel laboratory testing equipment.

projection: In radiography, the path that the x-ray beam follows through the body from entrance to exit.

prolactinoma (proh-**lack**-tih-**NOH**-mah): A benign tumor of the pituitary gland that causes it to produce too much prolactin; also known as a prolactin-producing adenoma.

prolapse (proh-**LAPS**): Downward placement.

prolapse of uterus: Falling or sinking down of the uterus until it protrudes through the vaginal opening.

prone: Lying on the belly with the *face down*.

prostatectomy (**pros**-tah-**TECK**-toh-mee): Surgical removal of all or part of the prostate gland.

prostatectomy, radical: Surgical removal of the entire prostate gland, the seminal vesicles, and some surrounding tissue.

prostatectomy, transurethral: Removal of all or part of the prostate through the urethra; also known as transurethral resection of the prostate.

prostate-specific antigen: A blood test to screen for prostate cancer; also known as PSA.

prostatitis (**pros**-tah-**TYE**-tis): Inflammation of the prostate gland.

prostatomegaly (**pros**-tah-toh-**MEG**-ah-lee): Abnormal enlargement of the prostate gland that may be benign or malignant.

prostatorrhea (**pros**-tah-toh-**REE**-ah): An abnormal flow of prostatic fluid discharged through the urethra.

prostrate (**PROS**-trayt): To collapse or to be overcome with exhaustion.

proteinuria (**proh**-tee-in-**YOU**-ree-ah): An abnormally high level of serum protein in the urine.

prothrombin time (proh-**THROM**-bin): A laboratory test to diagnose conditions associated with abnormal bleeding and to monitor anticoagulant therapy.

pruritus (proo-**RYE**-tus): Itching.

pruritus vulvae (proo-**RYE**-tus **VUL**-vee): A condition of severe itching of the external female genitalia.

pseudophakia (**soo**-doh-**FAY**-kee-ah): An eye in which the natural lens is replaced with an intraocular lens.

psoriasis (soh-**RYE**-uh-sis): A chronic autoimmune disorder of the skin characterized by red papules covered with silvery scales that occur predominantly on the elbows, knees, scalp, back, and buttocks.

psychiatrist (sigh-**KYE**-ah-trist): A physician who specializes in diagnosing and treating chemical dependencies, emotional problems, and mental illness.

psychologist (sigh-**KOL**-oh-jist): A specialist, other than a physician, in evaluating and treating emotional problems.

psychotic disorder (sigh-**KOT**-ick): The derangement of personality, loss of contact with reality, and deterioration of normal social functioning.

psychotropic drugs (**sigh**-koh-**TROP**-pick): Drugs that are capable of affecting the mind, emotions, and behavior.

puerperium (**pyou**-er-**PEE**-ree-um): The period of three to six weeks after childbirth until the uterus returns to its normal size.

pulmonary edema (eh-**DEE**-mah): An accumulation of fluid in lung tissues.

pulmonary fibrosis: The formation of scar tissue that replaces the pulmonary alveolar walls.

pulmonary function tests: A group of tests that measure the capacity of the lungs to hold air, their ability to move air in and out, and their ability to exchange oxygen and carbon dioxide.

pulmonologist (**pull**-mah-**NOL**-oh-jist): A specialist in diagnosing and treating diseases and disorders of the lungs and associated tissues.

puncture wound: A deep hole made by a sharp object such as a nail.

purpura (**PUR**-pew-rah): A condition characterized by hemorrhage into the skin that causes spontaneous bruising.

purulent (**PYOU**-roo-lent): Producing or containing pus.

pustule (**PUS**-tyoul): A small, circumscribed elevation of the skin containing pus.

putrefaction (**pyou**-treh-**FACK**-shun): Decay that produces foul-smelling odors.

pyelitis (**pye**-eh-**LYE**-tis): Inflammation of the renal pelvis.

pyelonephritis (**pye**-eh-loh-neh-**FRY**-tis): Inflammation of the renal pelvis and of the kidney.

pyeloplasty (**PYE**-eh-loh-**plas**-tee): Surgical repair of the renal pelvis.

pyelotomy (**pye**-eh-**LOT**-oh-mee): A surgical incision into the renal pelvis.

pyemia (pye-**EE**-mee-ah): Presence of pus-forming organisms in the blood.

pyoderma (**pye**-oh-**DER**-mah): Any pus-forming skin disease.

pyometritis (**pye**-oh-meh-**TRY**-tis): A pus-containing inflammation of the uterus.

pyosalpinx (**pye**-oh-**SAL**-pinks): An accumulation of pus in the fallopian tube.

pyothorax (**pye**-oh-**THOH**-racks): An accumulation of pus in the pleural cavity; also known as empyema.

pyromania (**pye**-roh-**MAY**-nee-ah): A personality disorder characterized by a recurrent failure to resist impulses to set fires.

pyrosis (pye-**ROH**-sis): Regurgitation of stomach acid upward into the esophagus; also known as heartburn.

pyuria (pye-**YOU**-ree-ah): The presence of pus in the urine.

quadriplegia (**kwad**-rih-**PLEE**-jee-ah): Paralysis of all four extremities.

R

rabies (**RAY**-beez): An acute viral infection that may be transmitted to humans by the blood, tissue, or saliva of an infected animal.

radial keratotomy (**ker**-ah-**TOT**-oh-mee): Surgery used to correct myopia by making partial incisions in the cornea causing it to flatten.

radiation therapy: Cancer treatment with the use of x-radiation.

radiculitis (rah-**dick**-you-**LYE**-tis): Inflammation of the root of a spinal nerve; also known as a pinched nerve.

radioassay: A laboratory technique in which a radioactively labeled substance is mixed with a blood specimen; also known as radioimmunoassay.

radiographs, bitewing: Intraoral radiographs that show the crowns of teeth in both arches.

radiographs, periapical: Intraoral radiographs that show the entire tooth and some surrounding tissue.

radiography: The use of x-rays to expose a film that shows the body in profile.

radiography, extraoral: In dentistry, radiographic projections in which the film is placed outside of the mouth.

radiography, intraoral: In dentistry, radiographic projections in which the film is placed within the mouth.

radioimmunoassay (**ray**-dee-oh-**im**-you-noh-**ASS**-ay): A laboratory technique in which a radioactively labeled substance is mixed with a blood specimen; also known as radioassay.

radiologist (**ray**-dee-**OL**-oh-jist): A specialist in diagnosing and treating diseases and disorders with x-rays and other forms of radiant energy.

radiology (**ray**-dee-**OL**-oh-jee): The use of radiant energy and radioactive substances in medicine for diagnosis and treatment.

radionuclide imaging (**ray**-dee-oh-**NEW**-klyd): A diagnostic technique that focuses on physiologic processes to determine how well body organs or systems are functioning; also known as nuclear medicine.

rale (**RAHL**): An abnormal rattle or crackle-like respiratory sound heard while breathing in.

Raynaud's phenomenon (ray-**NOHZ**): Intermittent attacks of pallor (paleness), cyanosis (blue color), and redness of the fingers and toes.

recumbent (ree-**KUM**-bent): Any position in which the patient is lying down.

red blood cell count: A laboratory test to determine the number of erythrocytes in the blood.

reflux (**REE**-flucks): A backward or return flow.

refraction: An examination procedure to determine the ability of the lens of the eye to bend light rays so they focus on the retina.

refractive disorder: A condition in which the lens and cornea do not bend light so that it focuses properly on the retina.

regimen (**REJ**-ih-men): Directions or rules.

regurgitation (ree-**gur**-jih-**TAY**-shun): The return of swallowed food into the mouth.

renal colic (**REE**-nal **KOLL**-ick): Acute pain in the kidney area caused by blockage during the passage of a kidney stone.

renal failure: Inability of the kidney or kidneys to perform their functions; also known as kidney failure.

renal failure, acute: Sudden onset of renal failure that is characterized by uremia.

renal failure, chronic: A progressive disease that may be caused by a variety of conditions.

restenosis: The condition in which an artery that has been opened by angioplasty becomes blocked again.

retinal tear: A hole that develops in the retina when the retina is pulled away from its normal position.

retinitis (ret-ih-**NIGH**-tis): Inflammation of the retina.

retinoblastoma (**ret**-ih-noh-blas-**TOH**-mah): A malignant tumor of childhood arising from cells of the retina of the eye.

retinopathy (**ret**-ih-**NOP**-ah-thee): Any disease of the retina.

retinopathy, diabetic: A complication of diabetes causing damage to the retina of the eye.

retinopexy (**RET**-ih-noh-**peck**-see): Laser treatment to reattach a detached retina.

retroflexion (**ret**-roh-**FLECK**-shun): Abnormal tipping, with the body of the uterus bent forming an angle with the cervix.

retroversion (**ret**-roh-**VER**-zhun): Abnormal tipping of the entire uterus backward, with the cervix pointing forward.

rheumatologist (roo-mah-**TOL**-oh-jist): A specialist in the diagnosis and treatment of rheumatic diseases characterized by inflammation in the connective tissues.

rhinitis (rye-**NIGH**-tis): Inflammation of the nose.

rhinophyma (**rye**-noh-**FIGH**-muh): Hyperplasia of the nose; also known as bulbous nose.

rhinoplasty (**RYE**-noh-**plas**-tee): Plastic surgery to change the shape or size of the nose.

rhinorrhea (**rye**-noh-**REE**-ah): An excessive flow of mucus from the nose; also known as a runny nose.

rhonchus (**RONG**-kus): An added sound with a musical pitch occurring during inspiration or expiration that results from a partially obstructed airway; also known as wheezing.

rhytidectomy (**rit**-ih-**DECK**-toh-mee): Surgical removal of excess skin to eliminate wrinkles; also known as a facelift.

rickets (**RICK**-ets): Bone disorder caused by calcium and vitamin D deficiencies in early childhood.

rickettsia (rih-**KET**-see-ah): Small bacterium that lives in lice, fleas, ticks, and mites.

rosacea (roh-**ZAY**-shee-ah): A chronic condition of unknown cause that produces redness, tiny pimples, and broken blood vessels.

rotator cuff tendinitis (ten-dih-**NIGH**-tis): Inflammation of the tendons of the rotator cuff.

rubella (roo-**BELL**-ah): A viral infection characterized by fever and a diffuse, fine, red rash; also known as German measles or three-day measles.

S

salmonella (**sal**-moh-**NEL**-ah): An intestinal bacterial infection caused by nontyphoidal *Salmonella*.

salpingectomy (**sal**-pin-**JECK**-toh-mee): Surgical removal of a fallopian tube or tubes.

salpingitis (**sal**-pin-**JIGH**-tis): Inflammation of a fallopian tube; inflammation of the eustachian tube.

sarcoma (sar-**KOH**-mah): A malignant tumor arising from connective tissue.

scabies (**SKAY**-beez): A skin infection caused by an infestation with the itch mite.

scale: A flaking or dry patch made up of excess dead epidermal cells.

schizophrenia (**skit**-soh-**FREE**-nee-ah): A psychotic disorder characterized by delusions, hallucinations, disorganized speech that is often incoherent, and disruptive or catatonic behavior.

sciatica (sigh-**AT**-ih-kah): Inflammation of the sciatic nerve that results in pain along the course of the nerve through the thigh and leg.

scintigram (**SIN**-tih-gram): The use of radionucleide tracers to gather information about the structure and function of organs or systems that cannot be seen on conventional x-rays; also known as a nuclear scan.

scleritis (skleh-**RYE**-tis): Inflammation of the sclera of the eye.

scleroderma (**sklehr**-oh-**DER**-mah *or* **skleer**-oh-**DER**-mah): An autoimmune disorder that causes abnormal tissue thickening usually starting on the hands, feet, or face.

sclerotherapy (**sklehr**-oh-**THER**-ah-pee): Injection of a sclerosing solution to treat spider veins.

scoliosis (**skoh**-lee-**OH**-sis): Abnormal lateral curvature of the spine.

scotoma (skoh-**TOH**-mah): Abnormal area of absent or depressed vision surrounded by an area of normal vision.

scratch test: A diagnostic test to identify commonly troublesome allergens such as tree pollen and ragweed.

sebaceous cyst (seh-**BAY**-shus): A cyst of a sebaceous gland, containing yellow, fatty material.

seborrhea (**seb**-oh-**REE**-ah): Any of several common skin conditions in which there is an overproduction of sebum.

seborrheic dermatitis (**seb**-oh-**REE**-ick **der**-mah-**TYE**-tis): An inflammation of the upper layers of the skin, caused by seborrhea.

seborrheic keratosis (**seb**-oh-**REE**-ick **kerr**-ah-**TOH**-sis): A benign flesh-colored, brown, or black skin tumor.

sedative: Medication that depresses the central nervous system and produces calm and diminished responsiveness without producing sleep.

sedimentation rate: A laboratory test based on the rate at which the red blood cells separate from plasma and settle to the bottom of the container; also known as erythrocyte sedimentation rate.

seizure (**SEE**-zhur): A sudden, violent, involuntary contraction of a group of muscles caused by a disturbance in brain function; also known as a convulsion.

seizure, generalized tonic-clonic: A loss of consciousness and tonic convulsions followed by clonic convulsions; also known as a generalized seizure. See also convulsion, tonic and convulsion, clonic.

seizure, localized: A state that begins with specific motor, sensory, or psychomotor phenomena without loss of consciousness; also known as a partial seizure.

septicemia (**sep**-tih-**SEE**-mee-ah): The presence of pathogenic microorganisms or their toxins in the blood; also known as blood poisoning.

septoplasty (**SEP**-toh-**plas**-tee): Surgical reconstruction of the nasal septum.

serum bilirubin test: A laboratory test to measure how well red blood cells are being broken down by the liver.

serum enzyme tests: Laboratory tests to measure the blood enzymes.

sexually transmitted diseases: Diseases transmitted through sexual intercourse or other genital contact; also known as venereal diseases.

shin splint: Pain caused by the muscle's tearing away from the tibia.

sigmoidectomy (**sig**-moi-**DECK**-toh-mee): Surgical removal of all or part of the sigmoid colon.

sigmoiditis (**sig**-moi-**DYE**-tis): Inflammation of the sigmoid colon.

sigmoidoscopy (**sig**-moi-**DOS**-koh-pee): Visual examination of the interior of the entire rectum, sigmoid colon, and possibly a portion of the descending colon.

silicosis (**sill**-ih-**KOH**-sis): A form of pneumoconiosis caused by silica dust or glass in the lungs; also known as grinder's disease.

Sims' position: Lying on the left side with the right knee and thigh drawn up with the left arm placed along the back.

single photon emission computed tomography: A nuclear imaging technique in which pictures are taken by one to three gamma cameras after a radionuclide tracer has been injected into the blood.

singultus (sing-**GUL**-tus): Myoclonus of the diaphragm that causes the characteristic hiccup sound with each spasm; also known as hiccups.

sinusitis (**sigh**-nuh-**SIGH**-tis): Inflammation of the sinuses.

sinusotomy (**sigh**-nuhs-**OT**-oh-mee): A surgical incision into a sinus.

skin tags: Small flesh-colored or light brown growths that hang from the body by fine stalks.

sleep apnea syndromes: A group of potentially deadly disorders in which breathing repeatedly stops during sleep for periods long enough to cause a measurable decrease in blood oxygen levels.

smoker's respiratory syndrome: A group of symptoms seen in smokers that include a cough, wheezing, vocal hoarseness, pharyngitis, difficult breathing, and susceptibility to respiratory infections.

somatoform (soh-**MAT**-oh-**form**): The presence of physical symptoms that suggest general medical conditions but are not explained by the patient's actual medical condition.

somnambulism (som-**NAM**-byou-lizm): The condition of walking without awakening; also known as sleepwalking.

somnolence (**SOM**-noh-lens): A condition of unnatural sleepiness or semiconsciousness approaching coma.

spasm: A sudden, violent, involuntary contraction of a muscle or a group of muscles; also known as a cramp.

spasmodic torticollis (spaz-**MOD**-ick **tor**-tih-**KOL**-is): A stiff neck due to spasmodic contractions of the neck muscles that pull the head toward the affected side; also known as wryneck.

speculum (**SPECK**-you-lum): An instrument used to enlarge the opening of any canal or cavity to make it possible to inspect its interior.

sperm analysis: A diagnostic test of freshly ejaculated sperm to determine the count, shape, size, and motility.

sphincterotomy (**sfink**-ter-**OT**-oh-mee): An incision into or division of a sphincter muscle.

sphygmomanometer (**sfig**-moh-mah-**NOM**-eh-ter): An instrument used to measure blood pressure.

spina bifida (**SPY**-nah **BIF**-ih-dah): A congenital defect in which the spinal canal fails to close around the spinal cord.

spirochetes (**SPY**-roh-keets): Spiral-shaped bacteria that have flexible walls and are capable of movement.

spirometry (spy-**ROM**-eh-tree): A testing method to record the volume of air inhaled or exhaled and the length of time each breath takes.

splenectomy (splee-**NECK**-toh-mee): Surgical removal of the spleen.

splenitis (splee-**NIGH**-tis): Inflammation of the spleen.

splenomegaly (**splee**-noh-**MEG**-ah-lee): Abnormal enlargement of the spleen.

splenorrhagia (**splee**-noh-**RAY**-jee-ah): Bleeding from the spleen.

splenorrhaphy (splee-**NOR**-ah-fee): To suture the spleen.

spondylitis (**spon**-dih-**LYE**-tis): Inflammation of the vertebrae.

spondylolisthesis (**spon**-dih-loh-liss-**THEE**-sis): Forward movement of the body of one of the lower lumbar vertebra on the vertebra below it or on the sacrum.

spondylosis (**spon**-dih-**LOH**-sis): Any degenerative condition of the vertebrae.

sprain: Injury to a joint such as an ankle, knee, or wrist involving stretched or torn ligaments.

sputum (**SPYOU**-tum): Phlegm that is ejected through the mouth.

staging: The process of classifying tumors with respect to how far the disease has progressed.

stapedectomy (**stay**-peh-**DECK**-toh-mee): Surgical removal of the stapes, which is a bone of the middle ear.

staphylococci (**staf**-ih-loh-**KOCK**-sigh): Bacteria that form irregular groups or clusters.

statins: Medications administered to reduce low-density lipoprotein (LDL) cholesterol or other lipids in the blood; also known as cholesterol-lowering drugs.

steroids (**STEHR**-oidz): Naturally occurring hormones that help control metabolism, inflammation, immune functions, salt and water balance, development of sexual characteristics, and the ability to withstand illness and injury; artificially produced hormones used as medications to duplicate the action of naturally occurring steroids.

steroids, anabolic: Artificially produced hormones that are chemically related to the male sex hormone testosterone and have been used illegally by athletes to increase strength and muscle mass.

stethoscope (**STETH**-oh-skope): An instrument used to listen to sounds within the body and during the measurement of blood pressure.

: A fetus that died before or during delivery.

stoma (**STOH**-mah): An opening on a body surface that can occur naturally or may be created surgically.

strabismus (strah-**BIZ**-mus): A disorder in which the eyes cannot be directed in a parallel manner toward the same object.

strain: Injury to the body of the muscle or attachment of the tendon.

streptococci (**strep**-toh-**KOCK**-sigh): Bacteria that form a chain.

stricture: An abnormal band of tissue narrowing a body passage.

stridor (**STRYE**-dor): An abnormal, high-pitched, harsh or crowing sound heard during inspiration that results from a partial blockage of the pharynx, larynx, and trachea.

stroke: Damage to the brain that occurs when the blood flow to the brain is disrupted because a blood vessel supplying it is either blocked or has ruptured.

stroke, hemorrhagic (**hem**-oh-**RAJ**-ick): Damage to brain tissue caused by the rupture or leaking of a blood vessel within the brain; also known as a bleed.

stroke, ischemic: Damage to the brain caused by narrowing or blockage of the carotid artery and the resulting decreased flow of blood to the brain; also known as a cerebrovascular accident.

stupor (**STOO**-per): A state of impaired consciousness marked by a lack of responsiveness to environmental stimuli.

subluxation (**sub**-luck-**SAY**-shun): Partial displacement of a bone from its joint.

sudden infant death syndrome: The unexplainable death of an apparently healthy infant that typically occurs while the infant is sleeping; also known as SIDS or crib death.

supine (**SUE**-pine): Lying on the back with the *face up;* also known as the horizontal recumbent position.

suppuration (**sup**-you-**RAY**-shun): Formation or discharge of pus.

suturing (**SOO**-chur-ing): Closing a wound or incision by stitching or a similar means.

syncope (**SIN**-koh-pee): The brief loss of consciousness caused by brief lack of oxygen in the brain; also known as fainting.

synechia (sigh-**NECK**-ee-ah): An adhesion that binds the iris to any adjacent structure.

synergism (**SIN**-er-jizm): An interaction that occurs when the effect of one drug is increased by another drug; also known as potentiation.

synovectomy (sin-oh-**VECK**-toh-mee): Surgical removal of a synovial membrane from a joint.

synovitis (sin-oh-**VYE** tiss): Inflammation of the synovial membrane that results in swelling and pain.

syphilis (**SIF**-ih-lis): A highly contagious sexually transmitted disease caused by the spirochete *Treponema pallidum.*

T

tachycardia (**tack**-ee-**KAR**-dee-ah): An abnormally fast heartbeat.

tachypnea (**tack**-ihp-**NEE**-ah): An abnormally rapid rate of respiration usually of more than 20 breaths per minute.

talipes (**TAL**-ih-peez): Congenital deformity in which the foot may be turned outward or inward; also known as a clubfoot.

tardive dyskinesia (**TAHR**-div **dis**-kih-**NEE**-zee-ah): Late appearance of dyskinesia as a side effect of long-term treatment with certain antipsychotic drugs.

tarsectomy (tahr-**SECK**-toh-mee): Surgical removal of a segment of the tarsal plate of the upper or lower eyelid.

tarsorrhaphy (tahr-**SOR**-ah-fee): Partially or completely suturing together of the upper and lower eyelids to provide protection to the eye when the lids are paralyzed and unable to close normally.

Tay-Sachs disease: A hereditary disease marked by progressive physical degeneration, mental retardation, and early death.

teletherapy (**tel**-eh-**THER**-ah-pee): Radiation therapy administered at a distance from the body.

temporomandibular disorders (**tem**-poh-roh-man-**DIB**-you-lar): A group of complex symptoms related to the malfunctioning of the temporomandibular joint; also known as myofascial pain dysfunction.

tenalgia (ten-**AL**-jee-ah): Pain in a tendon; also known as tenodynia.

tendinitis (**ten**-dih-**NIGH**-tis): Inflammation of the tendons caused by excessive or unusual use of the joint; is also known as tendonitis.

tendonitis (**ten**-doh-**NIGH**-itis): See tendinitis.

tendoplasty: Surgical repair of a tendon; also known as tenoplasty.

tendotomy: Surgical division of a tendon for relief of a deformity; also known as tenotomy.

tenectomy (teh-**NECK**-toh-mee): Surgical removal of a lesion from a tendon or tendon sheath.

tenodesis (ten-**ODD**-eh-sis): To suture the end of a tendon to bone.

tenodynia (**ten**-oh-**DIN**-ee-ah): Pain in a tendon; also known as tenalgia.

tenolysis (ten-**OL**-ih-sis): To free a tendon from adhesions.

tenonectomy (**ten**-oh-**NECK**-toh-mee): Surgical removal of part of a tendon for the purpose of shortening it.

tenoplasty (**TEN**-oh-**plas**-tee): Surgical repair of a tendon; also known as tendoplasty.

tenorrhaphy (ten-**OR**-ah-fee): Suturing of a divided tendon.

tenotomy (teh-**NOT**-oh-mee): Surgical division of a tendon for relief of a deformity; also known as tendotomy.

testectomy: Surgical removal of one or both testicles; also known as an orchidectomy.

testicular self-examination: An important self-help step in early detection of testicular cancer.

testitis (tes-**TYE** tis): Inflammation of one or both testicles; also known as orchitis.

tetanus (**TET**-ah-nus): An acute and potentially fatal bacterial infection of the central nervous system caused by the tetanus bacillus.

tetany (**TET**-ah-nee): An abnormal condition characterized by periodic painful muscle spasms and tremors.

thalamotomy (**thal**-ah-**MOT**-oh-mee): A surgical incision into the thalamus to quiet the tremors of Parkinson's disease, to treat some psychotic disorders, or to stop intractable pain.

thalassemia (**thal**-ah-**SEE**-mee-ah): A group of genetic disorders characterized by short-lived red blood cells that lack the normal ability to produce hemoglobin; also known as Cooley's anemia.

thoracentesis (**thoh**-rah-sen-**TEE**-sis): Puncture of the chest wall with a needle to obtain fluid from the pleural cavity for diagnostic purposes, to drain pleural effusions, or to reexpand a collapsed lung.

thoracostomy (**thoh**-rah-**KOS**-toh-mee): Surgical creation of an opening into the chest.

thoracotomy (**thoh**-rah-**KOT**-toh-mee): A surgical incision into the wall of the chest.

thrombocytopenia (**throm**-boh-**sigh**-toh-**PEE**-nee-ah): An abnormal decrease in the number of platelets; also known as thrombopenia.

thrombolytic (**throm**-boh-**LIT**-ick): Medication administered to slow blood clotting and to prevent new clots from forming; also known as an anticoagulant.

thrombopenia: An abnormal decrease in the number of platelets; also known as thrombocytopenia.

thrombosis (throm-**BOH**-sis): An abnormal condition in which a thrombus develops within a blood vessel.

thrombotic occlusion (throm-**BOT**-ick ah-**KLOO**-zhun): Blocking of an artery by a clot.

thrombus (**THROM**-bus): A blood clot attached to the interior wall of a vein or artery.

thymectomy (thigh-**MECK**-toh-mee): Surgical removal of the thymus gland.

thymitis (thigh-**MY**-tis): Inflammation of the thymus gland.

thymoma (thigh-**MOH**-mah): A benign tumor originating in the thymus.

thymopathy (thigh-**MOP**-ah-thee): Any disease of the thymus gland.

thyroidectomy, chemical: The administration of radioactive iodine to suppress the function of the thyroid; also known as radioactive iodine therapy.

thyroiditis (thigh-roi-**DYE**-tis): Inflammation of the thyroid gland.

thyroidotomy (thigh-roi-**DOT**-oh-mee): Surgical incision into the thyroid gland.

thyroid-stimulating hormone assay: A laboratory test that measures circulating blood levels of thyroid-stimulating hormone.

thyromegaly (**thigh**-roh-**MEG**-ah-lee): An abnormal enlargement of the thyroid gland that produces a swelling in the front part of the neck; also known as goiter.

thyrotoxicosis (**thy**-roh-**tock**-sih-**KOH**-sis): A life-threatening condition resulting from the presence of excessive quantities of the thyroid hormones; also known as thyroid storm.

tic douloureux (**TICK** doo-loo-**ROO**): Inflammation of the trigeminal nerve characterized by sudden, intense, sharp pain on one side of the face; also known as trigeminal neuralgia.

tinea (**TIN**-ee-ah): A fungal skin disease affecting different areas of the body; also known as ringworm.

tinea capitis: A fungal infection found on the scalps of children.

tinea cruris: A fungal infection of the genital area; also known as jock itch.

tinea pedis: A fungal infection found between the toes and on the feet; also known as athlete's foot.

tinnitus (tih-**NIGH**-tus): A ringing, buzzing, or roaring sound in the ears.

tissue plasminogen activator (**TISH**-you plaz-**MIN**-oh-jen **ACK**-tih-**vay**-tor): A clot-dissolving enzyme used for the immediate treatment of heart attack victims.

tonometry (toh-**NOM**-eh-tree): A test that measures intraocular pressure (IOP).

tonsillectomy (ton-sih-**LECK**-toh-mee): Surgical removal of the tonsils.

tonsillitis (ton-sih-**LYE**-tis): Inflammation of the tonsils.

total hemoglobin: A laboratory test that measures the amount of hemoglobin found in whole blood.

toxemia of pregnancy: A complication of pregnancy characterized by hypertension, edema, and proteinuria; also known as preeclampsia.

tracheitis (tray-kee-**EYE**-tis): Inflammation of the trachea.

tracheobronchoscopy (tray-kee-oh-brong-**KOS**-koh-pee): Inspection of both the trachea and bronchi through a bronchoscope.

tracheoplasty (**TRAY**-kee-oh-**plas**-tee): Surgical repair of the trachea.

tracheorrhagia (tray-kee-oh-**RAY**-jee-ah): Bleeding from the trachea.

tracheorrhaphy (tray-kee-**OR**-ah-fee): Suturing of the trachea.

tracheostenosis (tray-kee-oh-steh-**NOH**-sis): Abnormal narrowing of the lumen of the trachea.

tracheostomy (tray-kee-**OS**-toh-mee): Creating an opening into the trachea and inserting a tube to facilitate the passage of air or the removal of secretions.

tracheotomy (tray-kee-**OT**-oh-mee): An emergency procedure in which an incision is made into the trachea to gain access to the airway below a blockage.

tranquilizers: Medications administered to suppress anxiety and relax muscles; also known as antianxiety drugs.

transcutaneous electronic nerve stimulation: A method of pain control by the application of electronic impulses to the nerve endings through the skin.

transesophageal echocardiography (**trans**-eh-**sof**-ah-**JEE**-al **eck**-oh-**kar**-dee-**OG**-rah-fee): An ultrasonic procedure that images the heart from inside the esophagus.

transient ischemic attack (iss-**KEE**-mick): The temporary interruption in the blood supply to the brain that may be a warning of an impending stroke.

transurethral resection of the prostate: Surgical removal of all or part of the prostate gland through the urethra; also known as a prostatectomy.

trauma (**TRAW**-mah): Wound or injury.

Trendelenburg position: Lying on the back with the knees bent and the legs elevated slightly higher than the head.

triage (tree-**AHZH**): Medical screening of patients to determine their relative priority of need and the proper place of treatment.

trichomonas (**trick**-oh-**MOH**-nas): A vaginal inflammation caused by the protozoan parasite *Trichomonas vagnalis*.

tricuspid stenosis: Abnormal narrowing of the opening of the tricuspid valve.

trigeminal neuralgia: Inflammation of the trigeminal nerve that is characterized by sudden, intense, sharp pain on one side of the face; also known as tic douloureux.

triglycerides (try-**GLIS**-er-eyeds): Combinations of fatty acids attached to glycerol that are also found normally in the blood in limited quantities.

tubal ligation: A surgical procedure performed for the purpose of female sterilization.

tuberculin skin testing: A screening test to detect tuberculosis.

tuberculosis (too-**ber**-kew-**LOH**-sis): An infectious disease caused by *Mycobacterium tuberculosis* that usually attacks the lungs.

twins, fraternal: Two embryos resulting from the fertilization of separate ova by separate sperm cells.

twins, identical: Two embryos resulting from the fertilization of a single egg cell by a single sperm that has separated into two separate parts.

tympanectomy (**tim**-pah-**NECK**-toh-me): Surgical removal of all or part of the tympanic membrane; also known as a myringectomy.

tympanocentesis (**tim**-pah-noh-sen-**TEE**-sis): Surgical puncture of the tympanic membrane to remove fluid from the middle ear.

tympanometry (**tim**-pah-**NOM**-eh-tree): An indirect measurement of acoustical energy absorbed or reflected by the middle ear.

tympanoplasty (**tim**-pah-noh-**PLAS**-tee): Surgical correction of a damaged middle ear.

tympanostomy tubes (**tim**-pan-**OSS**-toh-mee): Tiny ventilating tubes placed through the eardrum to provide ongoing drainage for fluids and to relieve pressure that can build up after ear infections.

typhoid fever: An intestinal infection caused by *Salmonella typhi*; also known as enteric fever.

U

ulcer (**UL**-ser): An open sore or erosion of the skin or mucous membrane resulting in tissue loss and usually with inflammation.

ulcer, decubitus: An ulcerated area caused by prolonged pressure that cuts off circulation to a body part; also known as a pressure ulcer or bedsore.

ultrasonography (**ul**-trah-son-**OG**-rah-fee): The imaging of deep body structures by recording the echoes of pulses of sound waves above the range of human hearing; also known as diagnostic ultrasound.

uremia (you-**REE**-mee-ah): A toxic condition caused by excessive amounts of urea and other waste products in the bloodstream; also known as uremic poisoning.

ureterectasis (you-**ree**-ter-**ECK**-tah-sis): Distention of a ureter.

ureterectomy (**you**-ree-ter-**ECK**-toh-mee): Surgical removal of a ureter.

ureterolith (you-**REE**-ter-oh-**lith**): Presence of stones in a ureter.

ureterolysis (you-**ree**-ter-**OL**-ih-sis): Procedure to separate adhesions around a ureter.

ureteroplasty (you-**REE**-ter-oh-**plas**-tee): Surgical repair of a ureter.

ureterorrhagia (you-**ree**-ter-oh-**RAY**-jee-ah): Bleeding from the ureter.

ureterorrhaphy (**you**-ree-ter-**OR**-ah-fee): To suture a ureter.

ureterostenosis (you-**ree**-ter-oh-steh-**NOH**-sis): A stricture of the ureter.

urethralgia (**you**-ree-**THRAL**-jee-ah): Pain in the urethra.

urethritis (**you**-reh-**THRIGH**-tis): Inflammation of the urethra.

urethrocele (you-**REE**-throh-seel): Hernia in the urethral wall.

urethropexy (you-**REE**-throh-**peck**-see): Surgical fixation of the urethra usually for the correction of urinary stress incontinence.

urethroplasty (you-**REE**-throh-**plas**-tee): Surgical repair of the urethra.

urethrorrhagia (you-**ree**-throh-**RAY**-jee-ah): Bleeding from the urethra.

urethrorrhea (you-**ree**-throh-**REE**-ah): An abnormal discharge from the urethra.

urethrostenosis (you-**ree**-throh-steh-**NOH**-sis): A stricture of the urethra.

urethrostomy (**you**-reh-**THROS**-toh-mee): Surgical creation of a permanent opening between the urethra and the skin.

urethrotomy (**you**-reh-**THROT**-oh-mee): A surgical incision into the urethra for relief of a stricture.

urinalysis (**you**-rih-**NAL**-ih-sis): Laboratory examination of the physical and chemical properties of urine to determine the presence of abnormal elements.

urography, excretory: A radiographic examination that traces the action of the kidney as it processes and excretes dye injected into the bloodstream.

urography, retrograde: A radiographic examination of the urinary system taken after dye has been placed in the urethra through a sterile catheter and caused to flow upward through the urinary tract.

urologist (you-**ROL**-oh-jist): A specialist in diagnosing and treating diseases and disorders of the urinary system of females and the genitourinary system of males.

urology (you-**ROL**-oh-jee): The study of the urinary system.

urticaria (**ur**-tih-**KAR**-ree-ah): A skin condition characterized by localized areas of swelling accompanied by itching that is associated with an allergic reaction; also known as hives.

uveitis (**you**-vee-**EYE**-tis): Inflammation anywhere in the uveal tract.

V

vaginal candidiasis (**kan**-dih-**DYE**-ah-sis): A vaginal yeast infection caused by *Candida albicans*.

vaginitis (**vaj**-ih-**NIGH**-tis): Inflammation of the lining of the vagina; also known as colpitis.

vaginocele (**VAJ**-ih-noh-**seel**): Hernia protruding into the vagina; prolapse or falling down of the vagina.

vaginodynia (vaj-ih-noh-**DIN**-ee-ah): Pain in the vagina.

vaginoplasty (vah-**JIGH**-noh-**plas**-tee): Surgical repair of the vagina.

vaginosis, bacterial: A sexually transmitted bacterial infection of the vagina.

valvoplasty (**VAL**-voh-**plas**-tee): Surgical repair or replacement of a heart valve; also known as valvuloplasty.

valvulitis (val-view-**LYE**-tis): Inflammation of a heart valve.

valvuloplasty (**VAL**-view-loh-**plas**-tee). Surgical repair or replacement of a heart valve; also known as valvoplasty.

varicocele (**VAR**-ih-koh-**seel**): A varicose vein of the testicles that may cause male infertility.

varicocelectomy (**var**-ih-koh-sih-**LECK**-toh-mee): Surgical removal of a portion of an enlarged vein to relieve a varicocele.

varicose veins (**VAR**-ih-kohs **VAYNS**): Abnormally swollen veins.

vasculitis (vas-kyou-**LYE**-tis): Inflammation of a blood or lymph vessel; also known as angiitis and vasculitis.

vasectomy (vah-**SECK**-toh-mee): A male sterilization procedure in which a portion of the vas deferens is surgically removed.

vasoconstrictor (vas-oh-kon-**STRICK**-tor): Medication that constricts (narrows) the blood vessels.

vasodilator (vas-oh-dye-**LAYT**-or): Medication that dilates (expands) the blood vessels.

vasovasostomy (**vas**-oh-vah-**ZOS**-toh-mee *or* **vay**-zoh-vay-**ZOS**-toh-mee): A procedure to restore fertility to a vasectomized male.

venereal diseases (veh-**NEER**-ee-ahl): Diseases transmitted through sexual intercourse or other genital contact; also known as sexually transmitted diseases.

venipuncture (**VEN**-ih-**punk**-tyour): The puncture of a vein for the purpose of drawing blood; also known as phlebotomy.

verrucae (veh-**ROO**-see): Skin lesions caused by the human papilloma virus; also known as warts.

vertigo (**VER**-tih-goh): A sense of whirling, dizziness, and the loss of balance.

vesicle (**VES**-ih-kul): A circumscribed elevation of skin containing fluid that is *less than* 0.5 cm in diameter; also known as a blister.

vesicovaginal fissure (**ves**-ih-koh-**VAG**-ih-nahl): An abnormal opening between the bladder and vagina.

viral (**VYE**-ral): Pertaining to a virus.

virile (**VIR**-ill): Possessing masculine traits.

viruses (**VYE**-rus-ez): Very small infectious agents that live only by invading cells.

visual acuity: The ability to distinguish object details and shape at a distance.

visual acuity measurement (ah-**KYOU**-ih-tee): An evaluation of the eye's ability to distinguish object details and shape.

visual field test: A diagnostic test to determine losses in peripheral vision.

vitiligo (**vit**-ih-**LYE**-goh): A condition in which a loss of melanocytes results in whitish areas of skin bordered by normally pigmented areas.

volvulus (**VOL**-view-lus): Twisting of the intestine on itself that causes an obstruction.

vulvitis (vul-**VYE**-tis): Inflammation of the vulva.

vulvodynia (vul-voh-**DIN**-ee-ah): A nonspecific syndrome of unknown cause characterized by chronic burning, pain during sexual intercourse, itching, or stinging irritation of the vulva.

vulvovaginitis (**vul**-voh-**vaj**-ih-**NIGH**-tis): Inflammation of the vulva and the vagina.

W

Western blot test: A blood test to confirm the diagnosis of HIV positive.

wheal (**WHEEL**): A smooth, *slightly elevated,* swollen area that is redder or paler than the surrounding skin that is usually accompanied by itching.

white blood cell differential: A laboratory test to determine what percentage of the total white blood cell count is composed of each of the five types of leukocytes.

white blood count: A laboratory test to determine the number of leukocytes in the blood.

X

xeroderma (zee-roh-**DER**-mah): Excessively dry skin.

xerophthalmia (**zeer**-ahf-**THAL**-mee-ah): Drying of eye surfaces characterized by the loss of luster of the conjunctiva and cornea.

Index

Page numbers in boldface refer to tables.

Set-Up Instructions

1. Double-click My Computer.
2. Double-click the Control Panel icon.
3. Double-click Add/Remove Programs.
4. Click the Install button and follow the on-screen prompts from there.

System Requirements

- Operating System: Microsoft® Windows® 95 or better
- Pentium processor or faster
- Memory: 24 MB or more
- Hard disk space: 10 MB or more
- CD-ROM drive: 2x or faster

License Agreement for Delmar Learning, a division of Thomson Learning, Educational Software/Data

You, the customer, and Delmar Learning, a division of Thomson Learning, Inc., incur certain benefits, rights, and obligations to each other when you open this package and use the software/data it contains. BE SURE YOU READ THE LICENSE AGREEMENT CAREFULLY, SINCE BY USING THE SOFTWARE/DATA YOU INDICATE YOU HAVE READ, UNDERSTOOD, AND ACCEPTED THE TERMS OF THIS AGREEMENT.

Your rights:

1. You enjoy a non-exclusive license to use the software/data on a single microcomputer in consideration for payment of the required license fee, (which may be included in the purchase price of an accompanying print component), or receipt of this software/data, and your acceptance of the terms and conditions of this agreement.
2. You acknowledge that you do not own the aforesaid software/data. You also acknowledge that the software/data is furnished "as is," and contains copyrighted and/or proprietary and confidential information of Delmar Learning, a division of Thomson Learning, Inc., or its licensors.

There are limitations on your rights:

1. You may not copy or print the software/data for any reason whatsoever, except to install it on a hard drive on a single microcomputer and to make one archival copy, unless copying or printing is expressly permitted in writing or statements recorded on the diskette(s).
2. You may not revise, translate, convert, disassemble or otherwise reverse engineer the software/data except that you may add to or rearrange any data recorded on the media as part of the normal use of the software/data.
3. You may not sell, license, lease, rent, loan, or otherwise distribute or network the software/data except that you may give the software/data to a student or and instructor for use at school or, temporarily at home.

Should you fail to abide by the Copyright Law of the United States as it applies to this software/data your license to use it will become invalid. You agree to erase or otherwise destroy the software/data immediately after receiving note of Delmar Learning, a division of Thomson Learning, Inc., termination of this agreement for violation of its provisions.

Delmar Learning, a division of Thomson Learning, Inc., gives you a LIMITED WARRANTY covering the enclosed software/data. The LIMITED WARRANTY follows this License.

This license is the entire agreement between you and Delmar Learning, a division of Thomson Learning, Inc. interpreted and enforced under New York law.

This warranty does not extend to the software or information recorded on the media. The software and information are provided "AS IS." Any statements made about the utility of the software or information are not to be considered as express or implied warranties. Delmar Learning, a division of Thomson Learning, Inc., will not be liable for incidental or consequential damages of any kind incurred by you, the consumer, or any other user.

Some states do not allow the exclusion or limitation of incidental or consequential damages, or limitations on the duration of implied warranties, so the above limitation or exclusion may not apply to you. This warranty gives you specific legal rights, and you may also have other rights which vary from state to state. Address all correspondence to Delmar Learning, 5 Maxwell Drive, Clifton Park, NY 12065-2919. Attention: Technology Department.

LIMITED WARRANTY

Delmar Learning, a division of Thomson Learning, Inc. warrants to the original licensee/purchaser of this copy of microcomputer software/data and the media on which it is recorded that the media will be free from defects in material and workmanship for ninety (90) days from the date of original purchase. All implied warranties are limited in duration to this ninety (90) day period. THEREAFTER, ANY IMPLIED WARRANTIES, INCLUDING IMPLIED WARRANTIES OF MERCHANTABILITY AND FITNESS FOR A PARTICULAR PURPOSE, ARE EXCLUDED. THIS WARRANTY IS IN LIEU OF ALL OTHER WARRANTIES, WHETHER ORAL OR WRITTEN, EXPRESS OR IMPLIED.

If you believe the media is defective please return it during the ninety day period to the address shown below. Defective media will be replaced without charge provided that it has not been subjected to misuse or damage.

This warranty does not extend to the software or information recorded on the media. The software and information are provided "AS IS." Any statements made about the utility of the software or information are not to be considered as express or implied warranties.

Limitation of liability: Our liability to you for any losses shall be limited to direct damages, and shall not exceed the amount you paid for the software. In no event will we be liable to you for any indirect, special, incidental, or consequential damages (including loss of profits) even if we have been advised of the possibility of such damages.

Some states do not allow the exclusion or limitation of incidental or consequential damages, or limitations on the duration of implied warranties, so the above limitation or exclusion may not apply to you. This warranty gives you specific legal rights, and you may also have other rights which vary from state to state. Address all correspondence to: Delmar Learning, 5 Maxwell Drive, Clifton Park, NY 12065-2919. Attention: Technology Department.